OTONEUROSURGERY AND LATERAL SKULL BASE SURGERY

OTONEUROSURGERY AND LATERAL SKULL BASE SURGERY

Fabrizio Salvinelli, M.D.

Assistant Clinical Professor of Otolaryngology
Catholic University of Sacred Heart
University of Rome Medical School, Italy

Antonio De la Cruz, M.D.

Clinical Professor of Otolaryngology, University of Southern California
St. Vincent Medical Center LAC/USC Medical Center
USC University Hospital, Los Angeles, California

Foreword by
William F. House

W.B. SAUNDERS COMPANY
A Division of Harcourt Brace & Company
PHILADELPHIA • LONDON • TORONTO • MONTREAL • SYDNEY • TOKYO

W.B. SAUNDERS COMPANY
A Division of Harcourt Brace & Company

The Curtis Center
Indipendence Square West
Philadelphia, PA 19106

Library of Congress Cataloging-in-Publication Data

Otoneurosurgery and lateral skull base surgery/Salvinelli, De la Cruz

p. cm.

Includes bibliographical references and index.

ISBN 0-7216-7051-2

1. otoneurosurgery. 2. skull base surgery. 3. otolaryngology.

Otoneurosurgery and Lateral Skull Base Surgery ISBN 0-7216-7051-2

Printed in Italy

Last digit is the print number: 9 8 7 6 5 4 3 2 1

To my wife Alessandra and our children Emanuele and Beatrice. The greatest sacrifice that went into the making of this book was the time I was away from them. To Emanuele and Beatrice, in the hope that they learn to follow their dreams and make them real, in the joy that only true commitment can give.

FABRIZIO SALVINELLI

Dedication

This book is dedicated to Maurizio Maurizi, Head of the ENT Department of the Catholic University of Sacred Heart, that so many contributions has made to the field of Otolaryngology. With him, I have been able to live, to learn, to grow.

It was he who inspired my trip to the House Ear Institute in 1990, 1991, and it was his encouragement that gave me the opportunity to dedicate myself completely to Skull Base Surgery and finish in Italy the book begun in the United States.

The joy I feel today, upon the completion of this 6-year project, is overwhelming. I know that my former teacher Maurizio Maurizi shares my delight and my satisfaction. All the sacrifices made have been worthwhile, since perseverance and faith are as important in making a dream a reality as is the ability to dream itself.

This book is dedicated to Maurizio Maurizi, who has done for me the greatest thing that one man can do for another: he has given life to my dreams.

FABRIZIO SALVINELLI

Dedication

It is a special pleasure to dedicate this book to Dr. William House, my teacher, my associate and my friend. I had the good fortune of not only being trained by him, but to participate with him in the struggles for the introduction of this new field of neurotology and skull base surgery. Bill introduced the operating microscope to neurotology and opened brand new surgical fields in the early 1960s and 1970s that allowed the mortality rate for acoustic tumors to drop from 40% to less then 0.5% today.
Two basic approaches allowed for the removal of lesions with hearing preservation and without greater cranial nerve deficit or cerebellar injury: the extended middle fossa approach and the translabyrinthine-transcochlear approach, not only for lesions of the clivus, but intradural lesions which cross the midline. About the time when the transcochlear approach was being published, Bill's creative genius turned to perfecting a clinically usable cochlear implant. His association with Dr. William Hitselberger led to the development of the auditory brainstem implant in 1979 for patients who do not have auditory nerves, creating the first direct stimulation of the brain to replace a sensory organ. As a teacher Bill is single-handedly responsible for the training of a whole generation of colleagues. He most unselfishly educated, trained, and shared every technique and device that he ever developed with other professionals, without compensation. Today, Bill continues to work in cochlear implants, guided by one of his mottoes: "What is better for the patient is, in the long run, better for the surgeon", in his quest to fulfill his mission in life: that every deaf child in the world will be able to afford a cochlear implant.
There is much to be admired in such an unselfish teacher and creative genius. This book is dedicated to William F. House, M.D., the father of Otoneurosurgery and Lateral Skull Base Surgery.

ANTONIO DE LA CRUZ

I would like to express the admiration and gratitude I feel towards William F. House. I have had the honor of learning from him the basis of Otoneurosurgery and Skull Base Surgery, on which this book was built. Someday, I will tell my children: I Knew him: he was one of my teachers.
Thank you, Dr. House. My experience with you inspired me to grow both as a physician and as a person.

FABRIZIO SALVINELLI

Preface

Neurotology and lateral skull base surgery have achieved a considerable measure of maturity in the last 20 years due to the cooperation of otorhinolaryngologists, neurosurgeons, facial plastic surgeons, reconstructive surgeons, endoscopists and through the monumental advances in imaging. This has been accomplished in large part through the efforts of increasingly ingenious, creative, energetic physicians who have decided to blur specialty boundaries and work as part of a team supported by post-residency fellowships in this field. Cooperation with radiologists and interventional radiologists has relieved patients from excessive morbidity, mortality and excessive blood loss. It has led the surgeon to resect masses with a minimum of cranial nerve deficit and infection.

Our goal was to produce a volume that reflected the current state of our knowledge and the prospectives in such a rapidly-evolving field. To make it useful for surgical practice, it is equipped with hand-drawn and computer-generated designs, and more than 300 anatomical and intraoperative dissections, all laid out in a progressive sequence, illustrating the surgical phases explained in the text.

We hope in this way to encourage many surgeons to become more involved in this most exciting field of cranial base surgery. We realize that a book such as this is only the initial part of the learning process which must be continued by the improvement of knowledge of skull base anatomy by repeated anatomical dissections and training with individuals who are experienced in the field of cranial base surgery.

We wish to thank the hundreds of authors and medical artists whose publications are cited in this book and our medical artist, Silvano di Meo.

Saunders and Verduci, respectively the International and Italian publishers, believed in our book and have made every effort to ensure its top quality; sincere thanks to them both.

A final thought to our families, for their lifelong love and support.

FABRIZIO SALVINELLI
ANTONIO DE LA CRUZ

Foreword

I am pleased to be asked to write a foreword for this very comprehensive book on the ever emerging and expanding field of Otoneurosurgery and Lateral Skull Base Surgery. The authors, whom I know and admire, asked that I write a personal history of my career in Otology and in Otoneurosurgery. It does not seem possible to me that is now a 40 years saga.

In July 1956 I finished a 3 year residency at LA County Hospital and started practice with my brother Howard. June and I had been married for 10 years and Karen and David were in grammar school. It was the start of a great adventure that has lasted until this very day. It has taken us all over the world an given us many dear friends from countries everywhere.

Through Howard's influence I had decided to limit my practice to the fledgling field of Otology. I could not have had a better teacher to give me hands on training in the art and practice of medicine, and to show me what was then state of the art and practice of Otology. Howard was very busy doing Fenestration surgery and it kept Jim Sheehy, Fred Linthicum and I busy working up his patients and taking care of them after surgery. He was very willing to turn over his chronic ear and dizzy patients to Fred, Jim and I and would encourage these patients to let us do their surgery.

I can remember taking 4 or 5 hours to do a radical mastoid with the headlight and loops, the 2 hands on the drill, and the squirt and suck techniques that was the way that mastoid surgery was done. But times were changing. The Zeiss microscope had just been introduced from Germany and soon Howard had several of them including one at the L.A. County morgue. Stapes mobilization was started by Rosen, and soon the mobilizing the stapes through an otoscope was replaced by the John Shea Stapedectomy using the microscope. I became a microscope aficionado and spent many evenings with June at the morgue developing instrumentation to allow the suction irrigator to be used in one hand and the drill in the other. My dental background that taught me to use a mirror in one hand and a drill in the other helped me here. Within a couple of years I was doing 2 or 3 mastoids a week. Howard encouraged me but I remember many of Howard's students and visitors being aghast at such reckless technique. Several told we they could not understand why a young man with a good eyesight should need a microscope just to drill out the mastoid.

Fortunately, I did not have a residency staff to take care of my patients, so I worked them up, treated or operated them and took care of their cavities post op. Tympanoplasty with middle ear skin grafting was coming into vogue. I remember an older colleague telling me that he had decided, "Timpanoplasty" was the new name for a 3 stage radical mastoid. I must say I felt obliged to agree with him. Gradually, over the years, the concept of meticulous removal of all diseased middle ear and mastoid tissue, the facial recess approach with the intact canal wall, aeration of the middle ear and mastoid and reconstruction of the ossicular chain developed. I remember presenting some of these concepts at a meeting of the American Otologic and in the discussion an older colleague asking, "What's wrong with the tried and true radical mastoid". The audience cheered. Seeing the sheer volume of otosclerosis patients that came to Howard, and had been treated by him over the years convinced me that progressive sensorineural hearing loss was a part of otosclerosis. Howard had developed a temporal bone banks program that has now become a national effort. Fred Linthicum in his early work with these willed temporal bones, also became convinced that otosclerosis could cause sensorineural hearing loss and showed me temporal bones with extensive otosclerosis around the cochlea. At the time this concept was strongly opposed by Hal Sckuknecht. I became curious about how otosclerosis could cause progressive sensorineural hearing loss. A review of the literature on otosclerosis that had been collected by the American Otologic Society into a two volume book provided some interesting leads. I was fascinated by several studies that showed otosclerotic lesions over the lateral end of the internal auditory canal that the authors ascribed to progressive sensorineural hearing loss due to cochlear nerve compression. The thought came to me that if only we could drill out these lesions somewhat like we drill out oval window otosclerotic lesions maybe we could reverse the hearing loss. The trick would be to get to the lateral end of the internal auditory canal without injuring the cochlea or the facial nerve. I began a series of dissections in the morgue that ultimately led me to using the superior petrosal and facial nerve with continuous irrigation and diamond stones to guide me to the internal auditory canal. This has become known as the middle fossa approach. With a neurosurgeon colleague, Dr. Kurze, I first tried this on a totally deaf patient that I knew had otosclerosis from the studies done over the previous years in our office. I remember the date, because June was helping me in the OR on her birthday August 1, 1958. Unfortunately the patient did not regain any hearing, but in the later years was to become one of my first 10 cochlea implant patients.

In 1959 at an otosclerosis symposium in Detroit that was sponsored by Hal Schuknecht, I presented 3 patients who had middle fossa decompression of the internal auditory canal. None of them regained any hearing. I did indicate, however, that the approach could have other uses in terms of facial nerve problems or vestibular nerve section. I showed a slide of the incision with the patients head upside down. I was crushed when during the discussion a doctor stated that it was the first time he had seen a patient operated upside-down. The audience laughed. Another discussant said he thought this was "Ruthless human vivisection". This criticism affected my willingness to report my early work on cochlear implants that was just beginning and had resulted in two failures, but convinced me that cochlear implants had great promise. I simply did not want to be looked at like a crazy human vivisectionest. Fortunately, Howard backed me up and encouraged me to continue my efforts.

During my residency I came under the influence of Gilbert Roy Owens, a wonderful otolaryngologist who invited me on a regular basis to his office to learn about sinus and mastoid Xray techniques. He even had a special mastoid view called the Owen view that showed the petrous apex in a special way. He was a strong advocate of Xraying all unilateral sensorineural hearing losses. He showed me Xray studies of cases with blown out internal auditory canals that were later operated for acoustic neuroma. I remember one of my teachers, Victor Goodhill, being an advocate of early diagnosis of acoustic neuromas. In my first year of practice I diagnosed, in a young fireman, an acoustic neuroma based on the Xrays and unilateral hearing loss. I sent him to a neurosurgical colleague who told me he agreed with my diagnosis, but he did not feel the patient would be willing to trade a little hearing loss and tinnitus for a facial paralysis and a significant chance of mortality. A year later, the patient developed papilledema and was operated. I witnessed the very blood operation with the patient in a seated position. He never regained consciousness. The surgeon remark was "Of course you realize he had a very big tumor". It occurred to me that the only solution to early treatment of acoustic neuromas was to save the facial nerve. In the ensuing years my first acoustic tumor approaches, that were done as a team with neurosurgeons, were in the sitting position through the middle fossa. It soon became apparent that it would be better to use a more otologic approach through the mastoid with the patient lying on the table, the translabyrinthine approach. A most unfortunate turf war developed with hearings before the executive committee of St. Vincent's hospital, in which the neurosurgical staff was insisting that all acoustics admitted to the hospital would be evaluated by them and they would decide the approach to be used. By then I was working very harmoniously with Bill Hitselberger and through Howard's intervention we were allowed to continue our acoustic neuroma work. One neurosurgeon who was chairman of Neurosurgery at USC resigned from St. Vincent's staff over the dispute.

I was fortunate to have the L.A. County library near by and I remember deciding to peruse the literature on Mèniére's. I came across an interesting article by Georges Portmann published in 1925 about comparing Mèniére's to glaucoma and therefore draining the endolymphatic sac to release the endolymphatic pressure. This prompted a series of dissections to surgically locate the endolymphatic sac and see if it could be opened. Over the next few years I developed endolymphatic sac surgery as a method of controlling the vertigo by correcting the endolymphatic fluid pressure and at the same time conserving the hearing. This surgical management of Mèniére's was considerably different then the trans oval window destructive procedures of Day and Cauthorne or the vestibular nerve section of Dandy. In the discussion of this work when I first presented it at a medical meeting a prominent Otologist stated he had never seen a Mèniére's patient who needed surgery. I had seen a patient treated by this doctor, and the patient stated he had been told that nothing could be done for the dizzy spells, he would simply have to learn to live with them. I was surprised that the Otologist did not realize that once a patient is told that nothing could be done they are not likely to return with a request for more treatment. To assume that their lack of return was because they were cured seemed illogical to me. Today my emphasis is on the alleviation of sensorineural hearing loss through the cochlea implant. This has been an interesting saga of how clinical observations can lead to a different approach than would seem logical from trying to apply the theories of how the cochlea works.

To understand the management of any Otologic problem you must continue long term observation of the patients and do your best to try to help them. This commitment to clinical observation constantly pressures you to face the limitation of the present management of a particular clinical entity and think the problem through. You will be amazed at how this approach leads you to new solutions to difficult cases. Realize, there will be criticism, but overcome this by keeping your eye on what you are trying to achieve. I only hope that the pressure of cost cutting medicine does not eliminate this time consuming, hands on doctor patient relationship and the commitment constantly improve what can be done for our patients.

I am very disturbed by the ruthless cost cutting and emphasis on mass production medicine that we are seeing today.

I urge you as young doctors to realize how gratifying it can be, to above all else, work with your patient's problems and come up with better ways of solving their needs. I can tell you from personal experience that your patient's gratitude is very rewarding. The constant challenge to find new solutions to seemingly impossible problems will keep you from the burn out of monotony and make you proud to be a healer.

William Fitgerald House

Contents

1

Temporal bone anatomy

The House Ear Institute is like Mecca for Muslims; if you don't go at least once during your lifetime, you don't enter Paradise.

SALVINELLI F.

The temporal bone is composed of a squamous part, a petrous part, a tympanic part, and the styloid bone (Fig. 1-1).

THE SQUAMOUS BONE

The squamous bone is composed of a superior and an inferior part.
The superior (or vertical) part of the squamous temporal bone includes the zygomatic process.
The inferior part is divided into an anterior and a posterior part. The anterior (or horizontal) part is separated from the vertical portion by the zygomatic process. The zygomatic process forms the glenoid cavity, the condyles, part of the infratemporal fossa and the roof of the external auditory canal. The posterior part is also the retromeatal part of the squama, which makes up the posterior wall of the external auditory canal. The spine of Henle is found at the beginning of the osseous part of the EAC in a posterior-superior position.
The superior part joins the petrous portion at the petrosquamous suture to make up the mastoid region.
The tympanic bone makes up the anterior and inferior portions of the external auditory canal. It is also the bone structure which accommodates the tympanic cavity.

THE FOUR FACES OF THE PETROSAL PYRAMID

The four faces of the petrosal pyramid are as follows: external, inferior, posterior, and anterior.

THE EXTERNAL FACE

The external face of the petrosal pyramid is composed of the mastoid, the external auditory canal porus and the root of the zygomatic bone. The squama of the temporal bone is found above. From top to bottom, the following structures are observed:
The zygomatic root: Its superior margin begins at the temporal line and continues on to the temporo-parietal suture.
The temporal line is the lower boundary of temporalis muscle insertion and approximately marks the location of the meninges in the middle cranial fossa.
The external auditory canal: Its posterior-superior boundary is delineated by the spine of Henle. Posterior-inferior to it is the tympano-mastoid suture. Behind the spine of Henle there is a cribriform area transversed by numerous vessels. This is called the retromeatal cribriform area.

THE INFERIOR FACE

The inferior face of the petrosal pyramid is composed of part of the skull base. The inferior part of the tympanic bone and the tympano-mastoid suture can be observed.
The stylo-mastoid foramen is here; the facial nerve emerges from it and enters in the parotid gland; the stylo-mastoid artery lies in the same canal. The styloid process is close to the stylo-mastoid foramen and is related laterally to the parotid gland.
The jugular fossa accommodates the jugular bulb.
The pyramidal depression is located medial to the jugular fossa. The cochlear duct opens into its superior wall, and connects the subarachnoid spaces with the endolymph of the scala tympani.
The carotic foramen is the place where the carotid becomes endocranial.
The digastric root is found posteriorly-laterally.

THE ANTERIOR FACE

The anterior face of the petrosal pyramid is a triangle with a medial vertex. Posteriorly it unites with the greater wing of the sphenoid bone. Its lateral base unites with the temporal squama.
The following features are observed:
The arcuate eminence is a bony ridge approximately twice as far from the vertex as from the base. Inside this structure is the superior semicir-

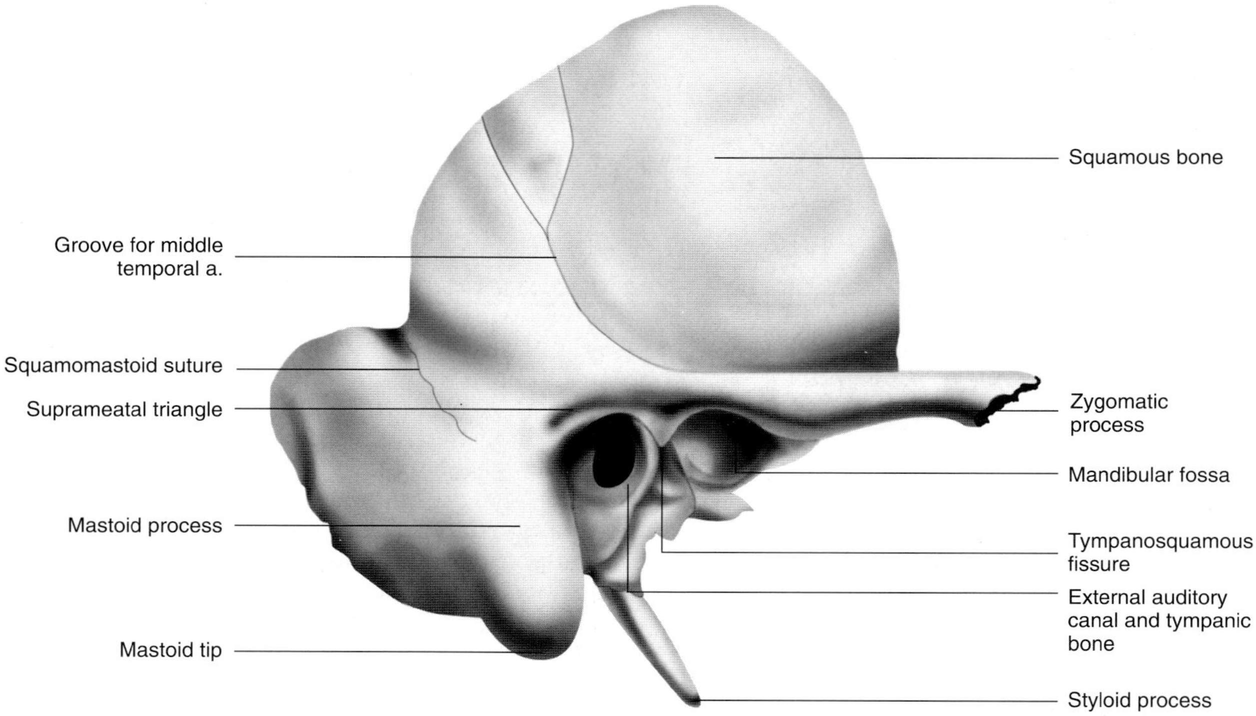

Fig. 1-1. The right temporal bone.

cular canal, an important landmark in the middle cranial fossa approach. A thin plate of bone is found above:- this is the tegmen tympani-.

Princeteau's tuberculum is a bony ridge located almost at the petrous apex. Beyond it is the gasserian ganglion.

The falloppian hiatus is a small aperture, approx. 1 mm in diameter. It is anterior and medial to Princeteau's tuberculum, and opens into the canal where the greater superficial petrosal nerve is found.

Between the arcuate eminence and the greater superficial petrosal nerve is the internal auditory canal. Its porus is found on the posterior face. Above the porus on the margin of the petrous bone, a bony protruberance can be observed: this is the eminentia suprauditiva.

THE POSTERIOR FACE

The posterior face is triangular with an external base, where the lateral sinus is found (Fig. 1-2).

Below is the posterior foramen lacerum where the jugular bulb is located (Figs. 1-3, 1-4). Superior to the foramen lacerum, the groove of the inferior petrosal sinus can be observed.

The porus of the internal auditory canal is found above the foramen lacerum and has an approximate diameter of 8 mm wide and 4 mm high. Here pass the vestibulo-cochlear nerve and the facial nerves. Supralaterally to the porus is the subarcuate fossa. Its fundus accommodates the petromastoid canal, which connects the antrum to the posterior labyrinth. The subarcuate artery runs through the posterior labyrinth to vascularize these structures.

The endolymphatic depression is the orifice which connects the vestibular canal with the endolymphatic sac. It is found halfway between the porus of the

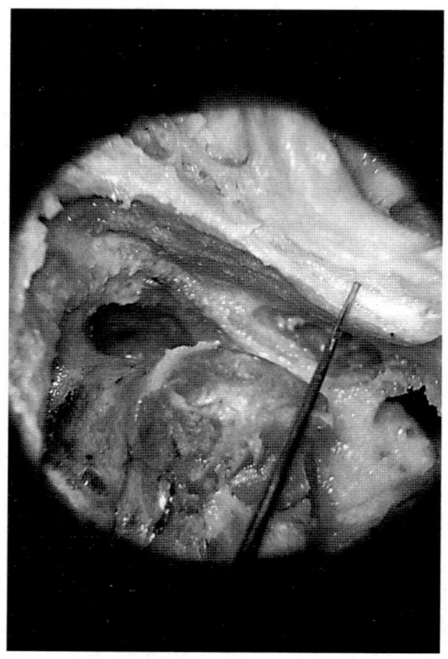

Fig. 1-2. Left ear. A high sigmoid sinus (injured), just under the mastoid cortical bone.

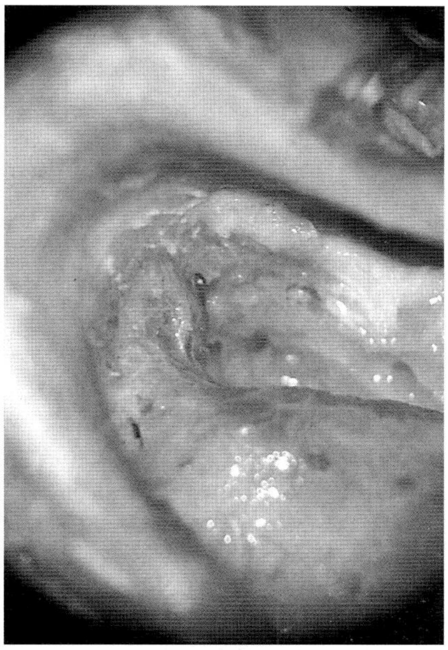

Fig. 1-3. Left ear. Normal position of the jugular bulb.

internal auditory canal and the posterior foramen lacerum, and is lateral to these structures.

THE PETROSAL CAVITIES
The temporal bone contains the cavities of the external, middle and inner ear (Fig. 1-5).

THE EXTERNAL EAR

The external ear is composed of the auricle and the external auditory canal (Fig. 1-6).

AURICLE
The function of this structure is to collect air vibrations and bring them inside in the form of soundwaves. These waves pass through the external auditory meatus to the eardrum. The average vertical diameter of the auricle is 55-65 mm, while its transversal diameter is approx. 25-35 mm. It originates in the lateral part of the cranium, and proceeds slightly anteriorly to form a cephalo-auricular angle. This is generally 20-30°, but can be up to 90° in lop-ears. It is composed of several peaks and valleys, described below:
Helix. This is the curved perimeter of the auricle, which goes from the anterior concha to the posterior lobe. In this anterior-posterior curve, it forms an oft-noted protruberance: Darwin's tuberculum.
Antihelix. This makes up most of the auricle's surface. The antihelix's insertion is located in the auricle, and together they form the scaphoid fossa. Below, one of its ridges defines the triangular fossa.
Auricular concha. The auricular concha is found in the center of the antihelix, touching the external auditory meatus. The anterior insertion of the helix is also the upper boundary of the cymba conchae, located above the suprameatal triangle. The latter is, in turn, superior to the mastoid antrum.
Tragus. The tragus is the anterior margin of the concha and partially masks the external auditory meatus.
Antitragus. The antitragus is found on the inferior-posterior edge of the concha, opposite the tragus. The intertragal scissure separates the tragus and the antitragus.
Lobe. The lobe is composed exclusively of fibrous and adipose tissue. It has a soft consistency.
The auricle is made up of skin, cartilage, and ligaments. The skin is thin and adherent to the cartilage. It is rich in fine hairs and sebaceous glands, particularly in the concha. It is continuous with the skin of the external auditory canal.

EXTERNAL AUDITORY CANAL
This is an oval canal which connects the concha externally to the tympanic membrane internally. At its widest point, its diameter can be from 8.13 to 9.08 mm, while its diameter at the narrowest point ranges from 4.60 to 6.54 mm. Its posterior wall is approx. 25 mm long, while the anterior wall is slightly longer (approx. 35 mm) due to the oblique position of the tympanic membrane.
The external auditory canal penetrates medially into the temporal bone and follows an S-shaped path. The external and medial parts have an ante-

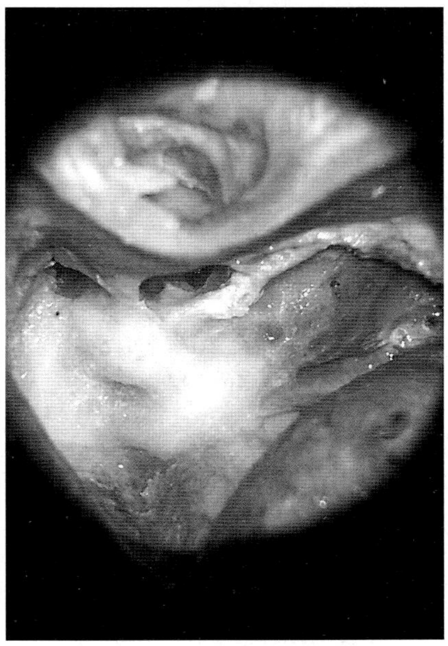

Fig. 1-4. Right ear. High jugular bulb. The jugular bulb is in contact with the posterior semicircular canal. In the translabyrinthine approach, the jugular bulb must be decompressed to obtain a sufficient exposure of the IAC.

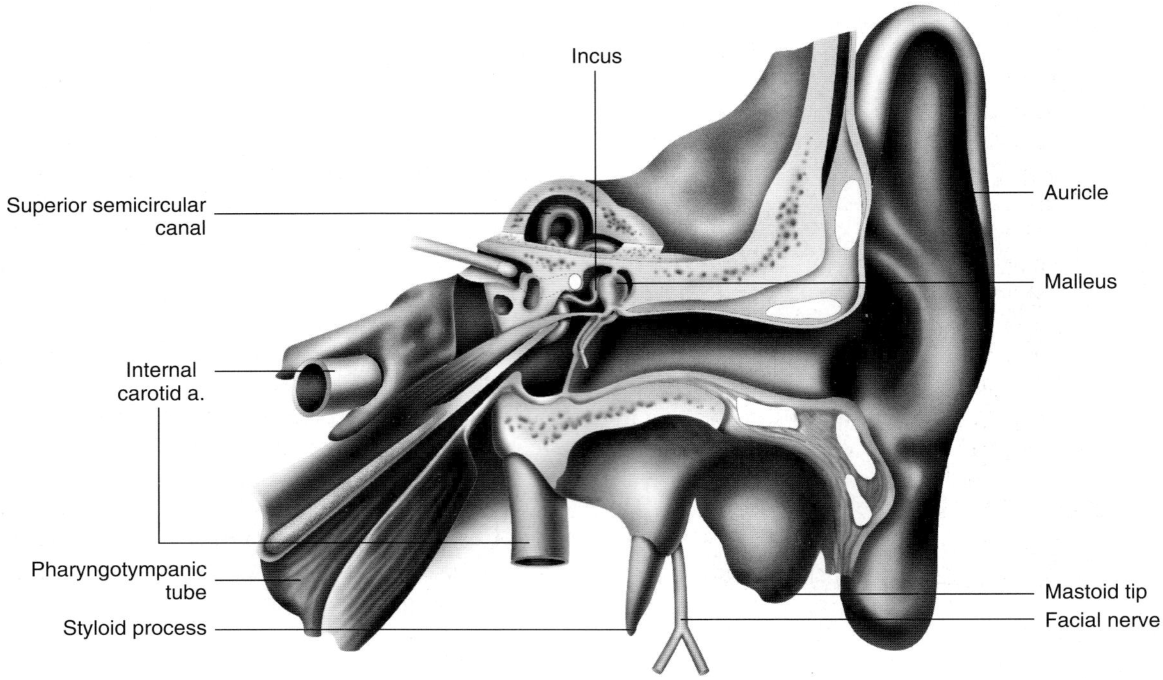

Fig. 1-5. The external, middle and inner ear.

rior-superior path, while the internal portion goes in a posterior-superior direction. The lateral third of the canal is cartilaginous, whereas the medial two-thirds are bony. Two concavities may be observed: a posterior and an anterior one. The posterior concavity (formed by the tragus) can be modified by stretching the auricle back. The anterior concavity is in the osseous part.

The cartilaginous part continues the cartilage of the auricle. It is smaller at its fundus.

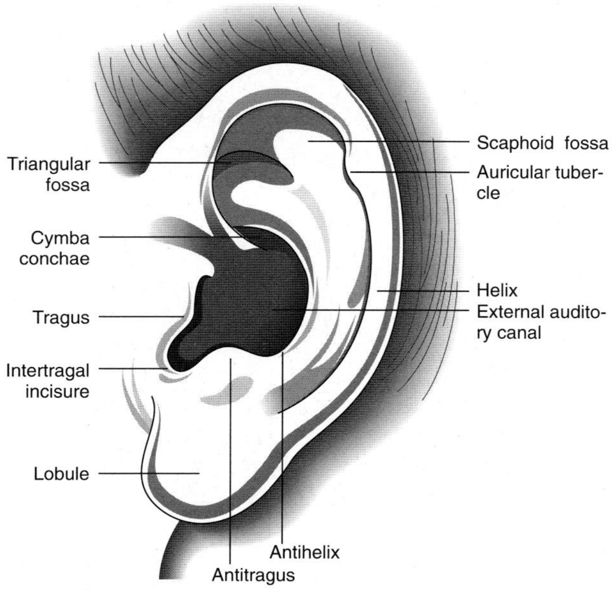

Fig. 1-6. The auricle.

The narrower (bony) part has an isthmus at approx. 5 mm from the insertion of the tympanic membrane into the posterior wall. Most of the osseous part of the external auditory canal (EAC) is formed by tympanic bone, except for the posterior-superior part which is formed by squamous bone. The EAC has four walls, as follows:

The posterior (or mastoid) wall is formed by a 4-5 mm layer of compact bony tissue. This separates the external canal from the mastoid cells. It communicates with the facial nerve canal, where the third section of the facial nerve is found, and accommodates the intraosseous part of the chorda tympani.

The anterior (or mandibular) wall is continuous to the mandibular condyle, which forms an endocanalar convexity.

The superior (or cranial) wall is near the middle cranial fossa.

The inferior (parotid) wall is near the parotid gland and its niche. In its cartilaginous part it is transversed by two furrows (Santorini's grooves), sealed by fibrous tissue.

The skin of the auricle continues into the external auditory canal and covers the tympanic membrane. It is thin and stretches over the underlying cartilaginous structures, making even the slightest inflammation very painful. The ceruminous glands are found in the subcutaneous cartilaginous part. These glands open either onto the epithelial surface or into the orifice of a hair follicle, along with the sebaceous glands. They secrete

cerumen (earwax), which protects against insects and small foreign bodies.
The arterial vascularization of the EAC is provided by the posterior auricular branch of the external carotid, the deep auricular branch of the maxillary artery, and the auricular branches of the superficial temporal artery. Reflux venous blood goes to the external jugular vein, the maxillary veins and to the pterygoid plexus.
The EAC is innervated by branches of the cervical plexus: The auriculo-temporal nerve separates from the mandibular branch of the trigeminal nerve and innervates the anterior and superior walls of the meatus. The auricular branch of the vagus nerve innervates the posterior and inferior parts.

TYMPANIC MEMBRANE

The tympanic membrane (TM) makes up the lateral wall of the tympanic cavity. The membrane forms an obtuse angle with the posterior wall of the EAC (posterior tympano-meatal angle). It then proceeds forward and medially to form an acute angle (40-50°) with the anterior wall (anterior tympano-meatal angle).
It has an elliptical shape, with a maximum diameter of 8-10 mm back to front. Its smallest diameter is vertical: 7-9 mm. It is approx. 0.07 mm thick. The membrane is composed of three layers: The external (cutaneous) layer, the intermediate (fibrous) layer, and the internal (mucosal) layer (Fig. 1-7).
The external layer is formed by stratified squamous epithelium, continuing the skin of the EAC. Its thickness is 50-60 μ.
The fibrous layer has the most important function. Fibers radiate from the manubrium of the malleus to attach to the fibrous annulus, and give the membrane its cone shape.

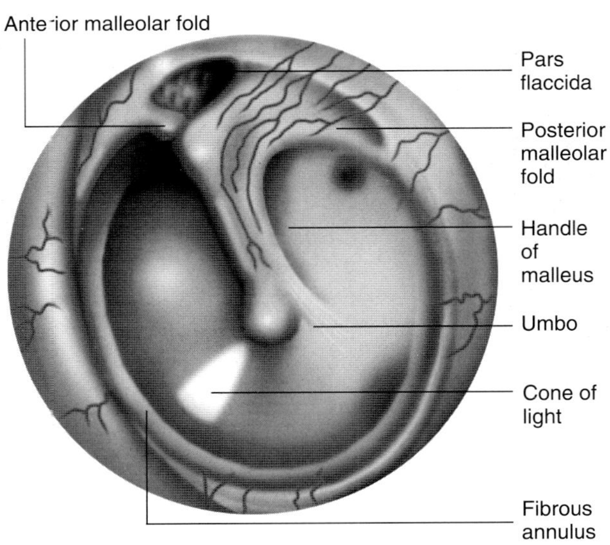

Fig. 1-7. Otoscopy of the left tympanic membrane.

Medially, the circular fibers (more numerous around the circumference, less numerous around the center) form loops which wind around the manubrium of the malleus.
Medially, parabolic fibers connect the short process of the malleus to the fibro-cartilaginous ring.
Transverse and semilunar fibers are spread through the inferior part.
The mucosal layer, 20-40 μ thick, is a continuation of the mucosa of the tympanic cavity. It is composed of cuboidal or squamous epithelium.

VASCULARIZATION

From the deep auricular branch of the maxillary artery, some branches separate and penetrate the cutaneous layer.
From the stylomastoid branch of the posterior auricular artery and the tympanic branch of the maxillary artery, some vessels separate to enter the mucosal layer.
The veins of the medial part drain partially into the tubaric venous plexus, and partially into the veins of the dura mater and the transverse sinus.

INNERVATION

The auriculotemporal branch of the mandibular nerve, the tympanic branch of the glossopharyngeal nerve, and the auricular branch of the vagus nerve, all innervate the tympanic membrane.
The circumference of the TM is thickened and forms the fibrous annulus which inserts into a bone furrow (sulcus tympanicus). The bone furrow is not found superiorly; nor is the fibrous annulus. The malleolar folds (anterior and posterior) connect the superior margins of the osseous ring to the lateral process of the malleus. The triangular part of the membrane, with its base on the malleolar folds and its vertex on the superior EAC wall, is called the pars flaccida. It is made up of skin and mucosa, and is flaccid due to its lack of muscular tissue.
The pars tensa has a lateral surface which forms a concavity with the vertex called the umbo. The latter has an internal depression due to its proximity to the manubrium of the malleus.
Two lines, one drawn along the manubrium of the malleus, and another transversing the umbo and parallel to the malleolar folds, divide the membrane into four sectors: the anterior-superior, the anterior-inferior, the posterior-superior, and the posterior-inferior quadrants.
During otoscopy a "shiny triangle" is seen in the anterior-inferior quadrant, due to light reflection during otoscopy.
Here the manubrium of the malleus, the fibrous annulus, and the anterior and posterior malleolar folds can be observed until they join the short process of the malleus.

THE MIDDLE EAR

The middle ear is composed of the tympanic cavity, the mastoid, and the eustachian (pharyngotympanic or auditory) tube (Fig. 1-8).

THE TYMPANIC CAVITY

The tympanic cavity is shaped roughly like a biconcave lens. Internally it has a longitudinal and anterior-posterior diameter of approx. 1.5 cm and transverse diameters of 6 mm above and approx. 4 mm below. Its central diameter, below the umbo, is approx. 2 mm.
Six walls can be distinguished: the lateral, medial, anterior, posterior, superior, and inferior walls.

Lateral wall

The eardrum makes up most of the lateral wall. Other structures involved are the tympanic bone ring (into which the membrane inserts), the squamous part of the temporal bone forming the lateral wall of the epitympanic recess, and the epitympanic recess: the hypotympanum.
In the superior part of the bone ring, three fissures can be distinguished: the petrotympanic fissure and the anterior and posterior canaliculi for the chorda tympani.
The petrotympanic fissure opens superiorly near the pars flaccida. It is approx. 2 mm in length and contains the anterior process and the anterior ligament of the malleus. It is transversed by the anterior tympanic branch of the maxillary artery on its way to the tympanic cavity.
The posterior canaliculus is located at the junction between the lateral and the posterior walls. It almost touches the posterior fibrous annulus of the tympanic membrane at the same level as the lateral process of the malleus.
The anterior canaliculus is found in the petrotympanic fissure, in a medial position.
The chorda tympani separates from the facial nerve approx. 6 mm from the stylomastoid foramen, and passes through a bony canal to form an acute angle with nerve V. It then enters the posterior canaliculus along with a branch of the stylomastoid artery, and passes through the tympanic cavity just medial to the tympanic membrane. It then enters into the petrotympanic fissure and proceeds toward the oral cavity (see chapter 6).

Medial wall

Also called the labyrinthine wall, this is the lateral face of the bony labyrinth. In it the following structures can be seen: the promontory, the oval window (fenestra vestibuli), the round window

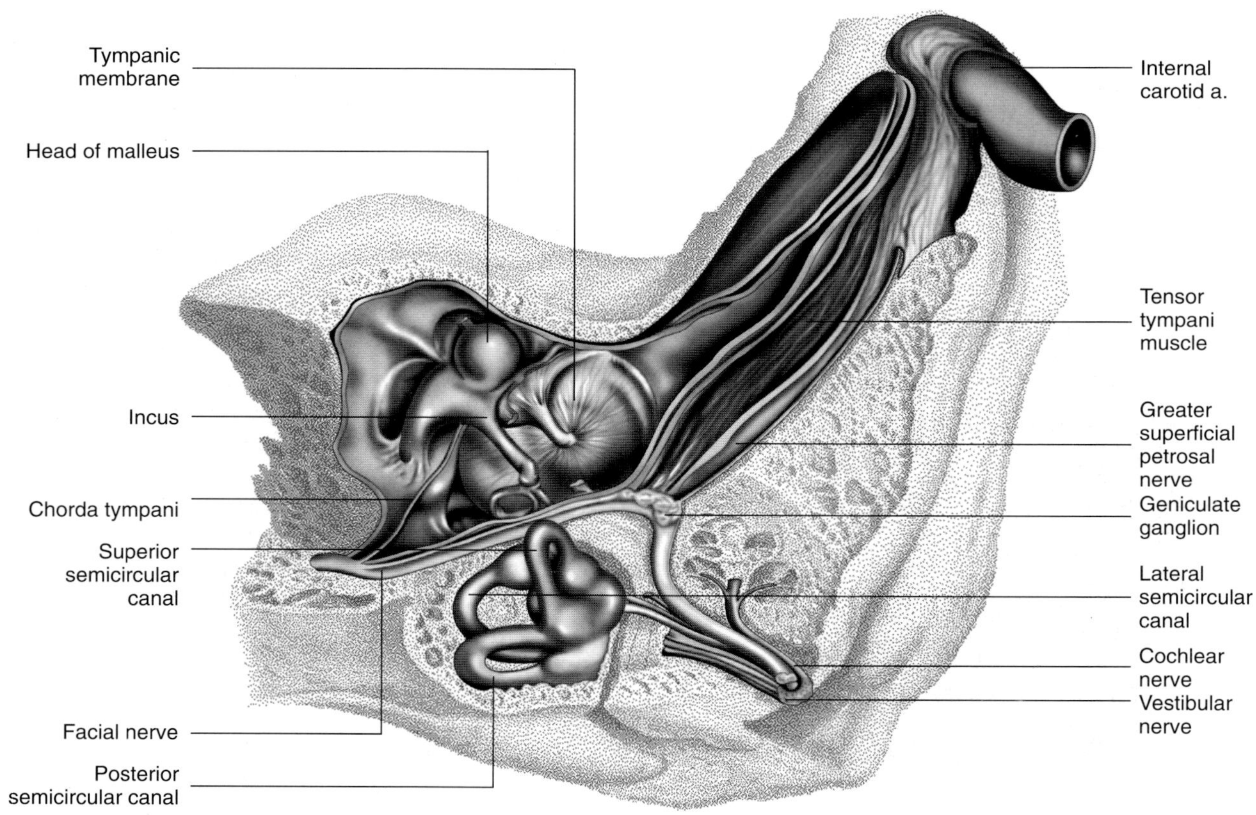

Fig. 1-8. The middle and inner ear. Internal aspect. (Adapted from Sobotta's anatomy).

(fenestra cochlea), the canal of the tensor tympani muscle, and the second segment of the facial nerve.

The oval window is shaped like a kidney bean. It touches the vestibule of the bony labyrinth of the inner ear. Its longitudinal diameter is approx. 3-3.7 mm while its transversal diameter is approx. 1.2-2 mm. It is parallel to the tympanic membrane, and accommodates the footplate of the stapes and the surrounding annular ligament.

The promontory is a round osseous relief formed by the basal turn of the cochlea. It is delineated superiorly by the oval window, and below by the niche of the round window. On its surface many grooves can be observed. These serve for the branches of Jacobson's nerve, itself a branch of the glossopharyngeal nerve.

The niche of the round window is oval in shape and inclined obliquely. Its average length is 2.25 mm and its width is approx. 1mm. The fundus of the niche is hidden anteriorly by the promontory. The niche is closed by the secondary tympanic membrane, which closes the tympanic ramp of the basal turn of the cochlea. This membrane forms a convexity lateral to the junction of its posterior third with its two anterior thirds. It is composed of an external layer originating in the mucosa of the tympanic cavity; an intermediate (fibrous) layer; and an internal layer, derived from the membrane surrounding the cochlea.

The prominence of the second segment of the facial nerve goes from the posterior margin of the lateral semicircular canal to the geniculate ganglion. It follows the superior margin of the oval window and often protrudes into it. Its superior ridge and that of the promontory below form a niche of the oval window.

Superior to the facial canal is harder and whiter compact bone: the lateral semicircular canal.

The pyramidal eminence and the inferior margin of the oval window are connected by an osseous bridge called the ponticulus. A similar osseous bridge goes from the posterior margin of the niche of the oval window to the styloid eminence (subiculum). The sinus tympani (infrapyramidal depression) is found between the two osseous margins. Its size varies. Above the ponticulus is the posterior tympanic sinus. In some cases the ponticulus is completely absent, and a single cavity is observed. The latter is composed of the sinus tympani and the posterior tympanic sinus.

Behind the pyramidal eminence, between it and the descending tract of the facial nerve, is the facial sinus.

The tensor tympani canal runs inferior to the tegmen. Posteriorly it touches the facial nerve canal. Near the facial nerve it curves externally to form the cochleariform process, where the tensor tendon detaches from the tympanum. The canal runs anteriorly to reach the carotic canal.

Superior wall

The superior wall is formed by the tegmen tympani, which separates the tympanic cavity from the middle cranial fossa. At times the bony wall is so thin that it shows dehiscences of the dura. The tegmen tympani goes from the petrous part to the temporal squama. Posteriorly, the junction of the superior and lateral walls forms the petrosquamous suture. In adults, veins from the tympanic cavity transverse this suture to reach the superior petrosal sinus. Posteriorly-superiorly, the tegmen tympani forms the roof of the attic, delineated in part by the medial and the lateral walls (the internal part of the temporal squama). The attic accommodates the body of the incus and the head and body of the malleus. The facial nerve runs below to the geniculate ganglion, and the aditus ad antrum is found posteriorly.

Inferior wall

Also called the jugular wall, the inferior wall is included in the petrous bone. It separates the jugular bulb from the tympanic cavity. The osseous part may be thick or thin, high or low, depending on the jugular bulb's position, which may in some cases protrude directly into the tympanic cavity. Here the junction of the medial (tympanic) wall and the lateral (petrous) wall may give rise to an hypotympanic sinus. If the suture is on the same level as the sulcus tympanicus, the sinus is absent. The sinus's size increases with the more posterior relationship of the suture to the sulcus tympanicus.

Posterior wall

Inferiorly, the wall is composed of irregular but continuous bone. In it we find the styloid complex, derived from the second branchial arch. It is composed of the chordal eminence (the exiting point of the chorda tympani), the pyramidal eminence (stapes tendon exit), and the styloid eminence. The relationship between these three prominences and other structures delineates the sinus tympani, the posterior tympanic sinus, the facial sinus (see medial wall...).

An aperture is observed above: this is the aditus ad antrum. Inferiorly it approaches the lateral semicircular canal, which connects the antrum with the epitympanic cavity.

The mastoid antrum is the largest cavity of all the mastoid cells. Anteriorly it touches the aditus ad antrum, medially it touches the lateral and posterior canals, and laterally it approaches the temporal squama, which is the surgical wall. The latter is approx. 12-15 mm thick (see suprameatal triangle...). Posteriorly and inferiorly it is surrounded by mastoid cells. Superiorly it is separated from the middle cranial fossa by a bony plate of variable thickness and the tegmen antri cells.

THE MASTOID

The dimensions of a newborn's antrum are similar to those of an adult. The mastoid cells, like other sinus cavities, grow later. Mastoid development becomes significant around 2 years of age, when the cells spread into the mastoid. At four years of age the cells are well-formed, but most of their development takes place in puberty. Thus the lateral wall of the antrum is rather undeveloped and both the facial nerve and the stylomastoid foramen are much more superficial than in the adult.

The adult mastoid may be seen in the following forms: pneumatized (many cells), sclerotic (composed of compact bone), and mixed (combination of the two previous types).

The mastoid cell system may be defined as follows:

Mastoid antrum.

Periantral cells. These cells surround the antrum and occupy the anterior-superior part of the mastoid bone.

Tegmen area cells. These cells are located in the superior part of the mastoid bone, near the tegmen.

Sino-dural angle cells. These cells occupy the angle delineated by the bone which covers the middle cranial fossa superiorly and the sigmoid sinus inferiorly.

Intersinuso-facial cells. These cells are found between the lateral sinus and the facial nerve.

Retrosinusal cells. These cells are located in the mastoid bone between the sigmoid sinus and the posterior cranial fossa dura.

Mastoid tip cells. These cells reach the digastric crest.

Zygomatic root cells. These are usually few in number or completely absent.

THE EUSTACHIAN TUBE

The eustachian tube connects the tympanic cavity with the rhinopharynx. Its direction is oblique, and it forms a 30-40° angle with the horizontal plane. The pharyngeal orifice lies approx. 15 mm below the tympanic orifice. It forms a 45° angle with the sagittal plane. This is composed of a posterolateral osseous part (protympanum) and an anteromedial cartilaginous part.

The tube is approx. 36 mm long. The osseous part (1/3 of the whole) is approx. 12 mm in length, while the cartilaginous part is approx. 24 mm long (Fig. 1-9).

Osseous part

The transition between the tympanic cavity and the bony entrance to the tube (protympanum) is

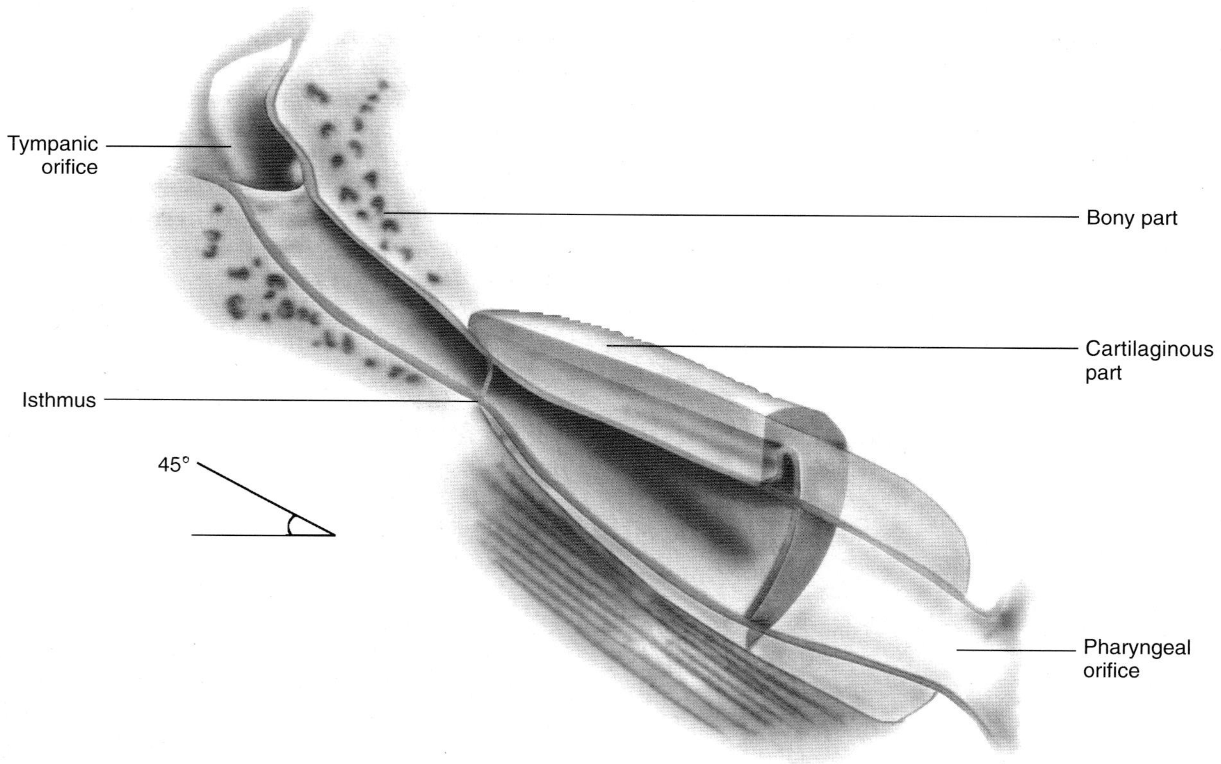

Fig. 1-9. The eustachian tube.

indistinct. The ostium tubaricus, located in the anterior wall, is approx. 4.5 mm high and 3.3 mm wide. The lumen of the osseous canal is approx. 2 mm wide and narrows slightly at the isthmus, i.e. at the junction of the cartilaginous part of the tube.
The lateral wall of the protympanum is a thin plate of tympanic bone. Under the medial wall, which is thin and often crossed by carotic-tympanic vessels, lies the internal carotid artery, which may be dehiscent.
The osseous portion terminates in the angle formed by the squamous and petrous osseous parts.
Fibrocartilaginous part
This portion attaches to the medial extremity of the osseous part and opens into the lateral wall of the rhinopharynx. It lies in a groove called the sulcus tubaricus, between the petrous part and the greater sphenoid wing, and is suspended from the skull base by the superior tubaric ligament. The pharyngeal orifice is approx. 10 mm high and 5 mm wide.
Eustachian tube musculature
Though the opening and closing mechanisms of the eustachian tube are unclear even today, we do know the role of some muscles: the tensor and the levator veli palatini, the superior pharyngeal constrictor, the salpingopharyngeal muscle, and the tensor tympani.
The *tensor veli palatini* muscle runs anterior to the tube. It arches the palate and opens the tube.
The *tensor tympani* opens the tubaric lumen.
These two extrapharyngeal muscles are innervated by the mandibular branch of nerve V and dilate the lateral segment of the tubaric lumen.
The *levator veli palatini* elevates the tube and the palate during swallowing.
The *superior pharyngeal constrictor* also lifts the tube during swallowing.
The *salpingopharyngeal* muscle opens the tube.
The intrapharyngeal muscles, innervated by IX-X-XI, open the pharygeal ostium and dilate the medial segment of the tubaric lumen.

Anterior and lateral to the tube are the vascular-nervous structures: the medial meningeal artery, the chorda tympani, the mandibular nerve, and the otic ganglion of the glossopharyngeal nerve. Posteriorly the tube is in contact to the petrous part of the temporal bone.
The eustachian tube's mucosa is histologically analogous to that of the rhinopharynx and the tympanic cavity: ciliated cylindric epithelium with calyciform cells.
Branches of the ascending pharyngeal artery (a branch of the external carotid) supply blood to the tube, together with the middle meningeal artery and the pterygoid canal artery (branches of the maxillary artery). The veins drain into the pterygoid venous plexus.
The eustachian tube is innervated by Bock's pharyngeal nerve exiting the palatine sinus, and by branches of nerve IX, derived from the pharyngeal plexus and the tympanic nerve.
Lymph drains into the retropharyngeal and parotid lymphnodes.

THE OSSICULAR CHAIN

The ossicular chain is composed of three ossicles: the malleus, the incus, and the stapes (Figs. 1-10, 1-11).

Malleus
The malleus, approx. 8-9 mm in length, is composed of the head, the body, and the manubrium. The first two are contained in the epitympanum, while the latter is attached to the tympanic membrane. The oval-shaped head has an articulated face for the incus. This consists of two parts, forming a straight angle: a larger (superior) part, and an inferior part.
The neck is below the head. At its transition extremity with the manubrium, it has a lateral process and an anterior process. The lateral process (or short process) is attached to the superior part of the tympanic membrane, pointing out. The malleolar folds are attached to it. The anterior (or long) process, enters the petro-tympanic fissure which is connected to it by ligaments.
The manubrium is connected to the tympanic membrane on its lateral surface. It proceeds obliquely, medially, and posteriorly. Medially, near the neck, is an osseous ridge where the tendon of the tensor tympani muscle attaches.
Ligaments connect the ossicles to the walls of the tympanic cavity. The malleus contains the lateral, superior, and anterior ligaments.

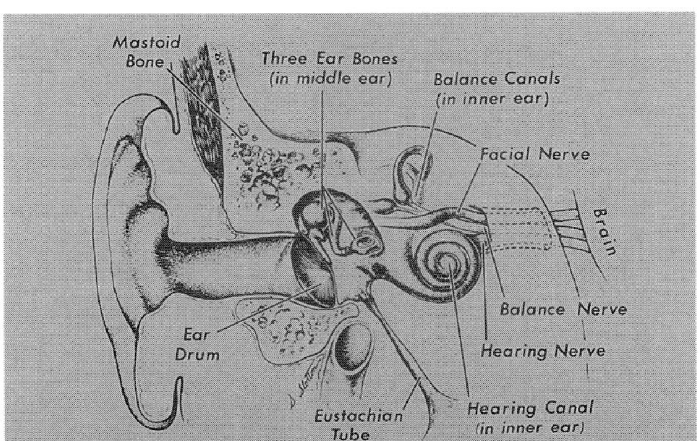

Fig. 1-10. Hearing mechanism.

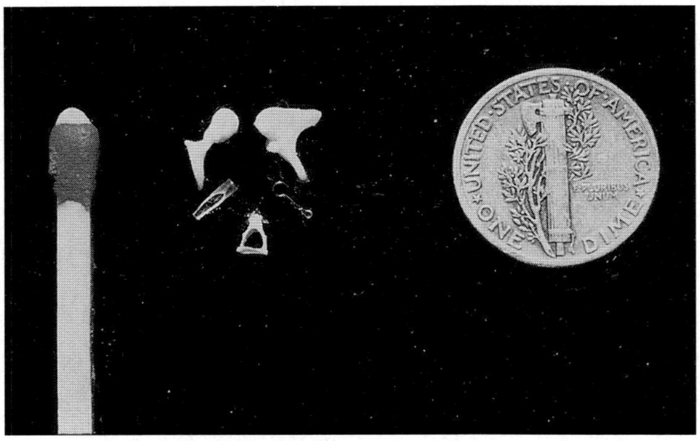

Fig. 1-11. The ossicles.

The lateral ligaments connect the head of the malleus to the posterior region of the tympanic groove.
The superior ligament connects the head of the malleus to the epitympanum.
The anterior ligament connects the anterior wall of the tympanic cavity, near the petrotympanic fissure, to the neck of the malleus.

Incus
The incus has a roughly triangular shape. The body, short process, and long process can be distinguished here. On the body, the anterior face has an articulated saddle-shaped face for the malleus.
The short process goes in the same direction as the posterior osseous wall of the EAC and its extremity indicates a triangular space between the facial nerve and the chorda tympani: this is the posterior tympanotomy.
The long process proceeds downward, then takes a medial and curved direction and forms the lenticular process. It has an articulated cartilaginous surface for the head of the stapes.
The posterior ligament connects the fossa incudis to the end of the short process of the incus.
The superior ligament, which is very thin, connects the body of the incus with the epitympanum.

Stapes
The stapes has a head, neck, two arches (anterior and posterior), and a footplate.
The head faces laterally. Its surface is basically flat, and covered with cartilage, upon which the lenticular process articulates. The posterior portion of the neck is the site of stapedial muscle insertion. From the neck, two arches detach and attach to the footplate. The first arch is anterior, smaller and straighter; and the second is posterior. There is an oval-shaped osseous surface, inserted into the oval window (fenestra vestibuli). A ring-shaped ligament is connected to its margins.

The muscles of the tympanic cavity are the tensor tympani muscle and the stapedial muscle.
The tensor tympani originates in the cartilaginous part of the auditory canal and the greater wing of the sphenoid bone. It runs in an osseous semicanal (tensor tympani semicanal), turns laterally and emits the tensor tympani tendon at the exit of a bony prominence of the cochleariform process. This tendon attaches to the medial surface of the malleus, near the neck.
This muscle originates at the Ist branchial arch, and is innervated by a branch of the mandibular nerve of the trigeminal nerve. When it contracts, the malleus moves downward, taking the tympanic membrane with it. This increases the depth of the cone formed by it. The membrane stretches and the stapes enters the oval window. This last effect is contrasted by the simultaneous action of the stapedial muscle.
The stapedial muscle detaches medially from the third part of the facial nerve and emerges from the apex of an osseous pyramid called the pyramidal eminence. It attaches posteriorly to the neck of the stapes. The stapedial muscle originates at the IInd branchial arch, is innervated by the facial nerve, and its contraction reduces the stapes' penetration into the round window (Figs. 1-12, 1-13, 1-14).

THE INNER EAR

The inner ear is composed of two parts: an osseous part, called the bony labyrinth, located in the medial third of the petrous part; and a membranous part, inside the bony labyrinth, called the membranous labyrinth.

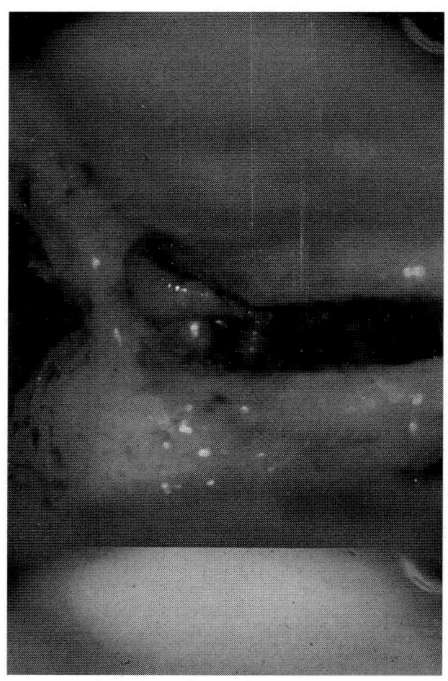

Fig. 1-12. Right ear. The incus and the incudo-stapedial joint as seen through the facial recess.

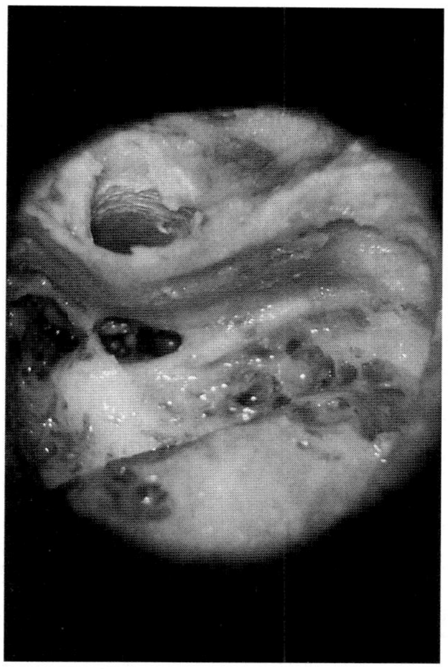

Fig. 1-13. Right ear. The mastoid (third) part of the facial nerve and the facial recess.

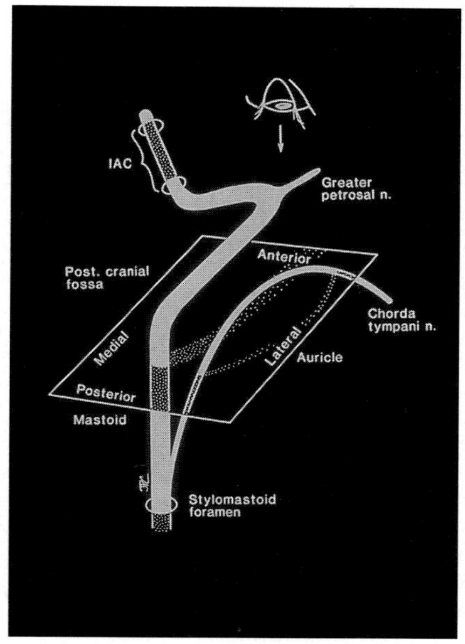

Fig. 1-14. Diagram of facial nerve anatomy.

BONY LABYRINTH

The bony labyrinth is composed of harder and more compact bone than the petrous bone. It consists of the semicircular canals posteriorly, the vestibule in the middle, and the cochlea anteriorly (Figs. 1-15, 1-16).

THE VESTIBULE

The vestibule is an oval cavity with a vertical diameter of approx. 6 mm, an anterior-posterior diameter of approx. 6 mm, and a depth of approx. 3 mm. It is made up of a lateral, a medial, an anterior, a posterior, a superior and an inferior wall.

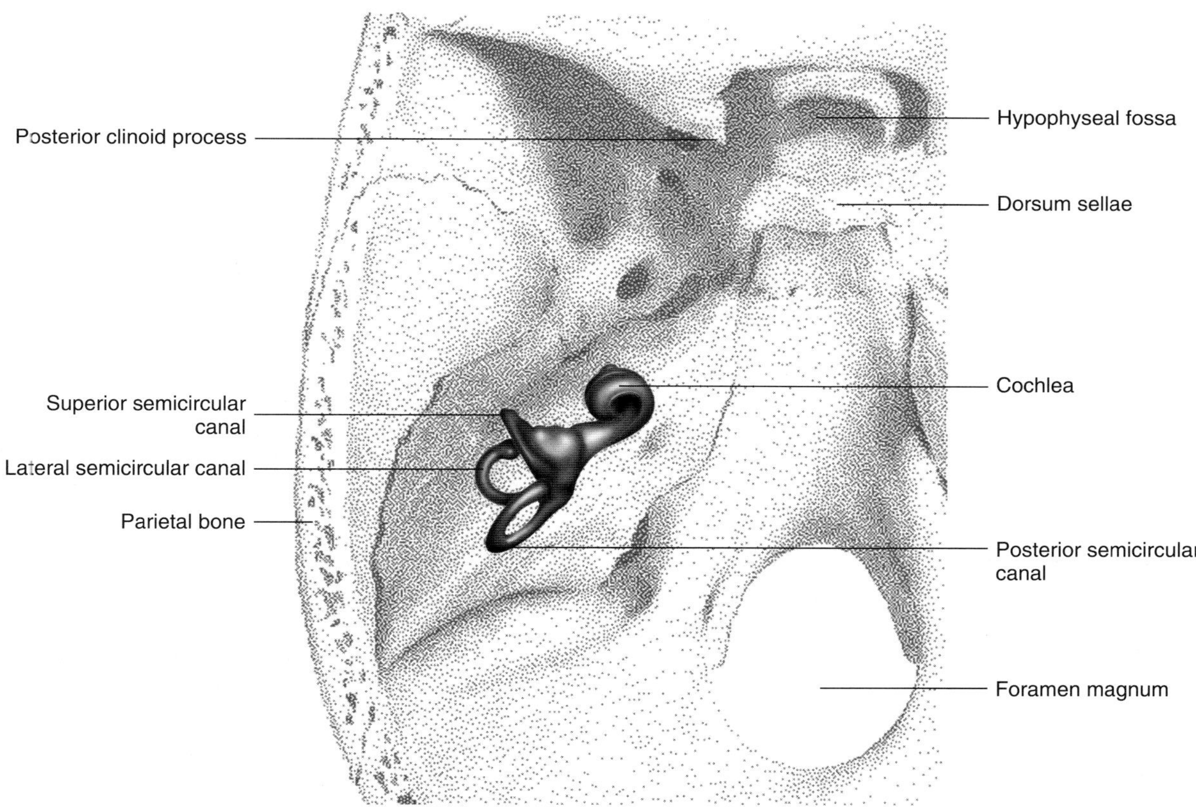

Fig. 1-15. The left bony labyrinth in the temporal bone.

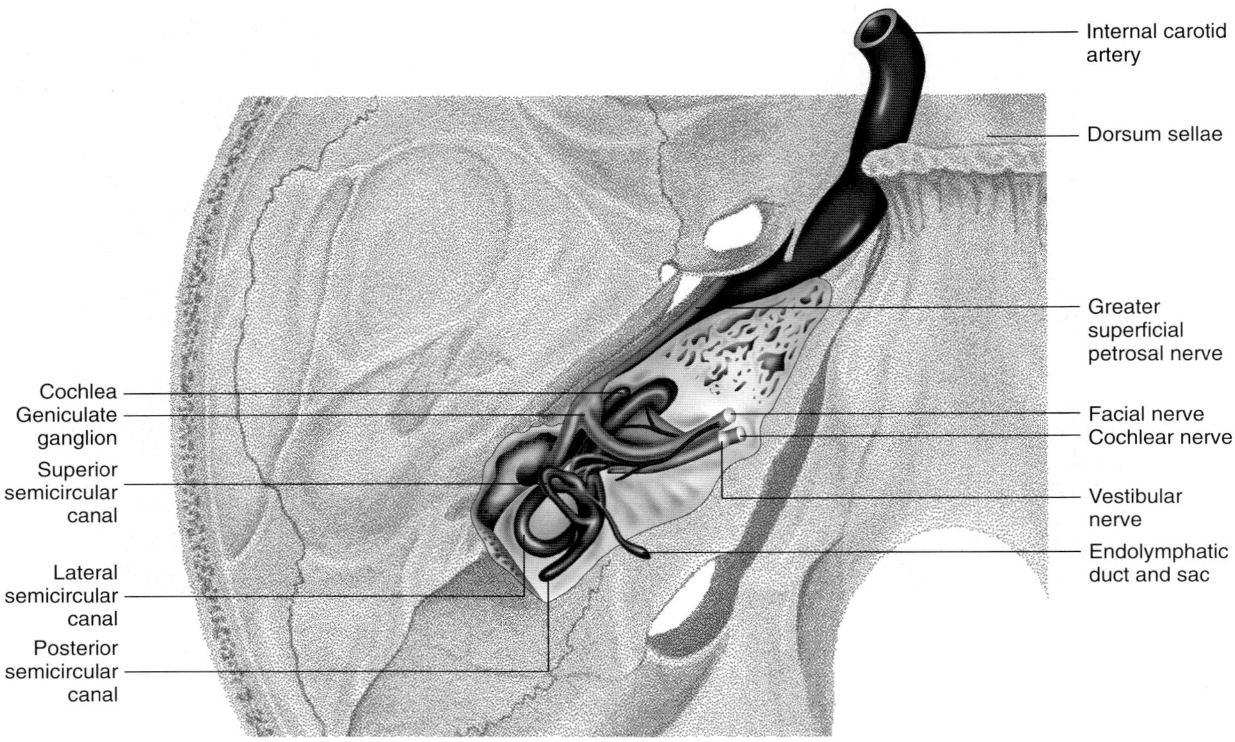

Fig. 1-16. The left bony labyrinth: position in the skull base. (Adapted from Sobotta's anatomy).

LATERAL WALL

The oval window is found in an anterior-inferior position. It is approx. 1.5 mm thick, and opens into the tympanic cavity. The ampullar orifice of the lateral semicircular canal is found in an anterior-superior position, with the non-ampullar orifice in a posterior-superior position.

MEDIAL WALL

The medial wall separates the vestibule from the internal auditory canal (Fig. 1-17).

The spherical (saccular) recess is found in an anterior position. It contains the saccule. Its central part has numerous small perforations (macula cribrosa media), through which filaments of the vestibulo-cochlear nerve reach the saccule. This area, just under the oval window, is the origin of the inferior vestibular nerve, at the bottom of the middle meatus.

Above and behind the spherical recess, there is an osseous ridge called the vestibular crest or the transverse crest. At its anterior end there is a triangular bony prominence, the vestibular pyramid. The transverse crest divides the spherical recess from the elliptical recess, which is in a posterior-superior position. Both the pyramid and the continuous part of the elliptical recess represent the emergence of the inferior vestibular nerve, at the fundus of the auditory canal. The falciform crest, which proceeds medially, divides the superior and the inferior vestibular nerves in the fundus of the internal auditory canal.

The elliptical (utricular) recess and the vestibular pyramid have a cribriform area. This area is full of perforations and is called the macula cribrosa superior. The nervous terminations from the utricle and from the ampullae of the superior and lat-

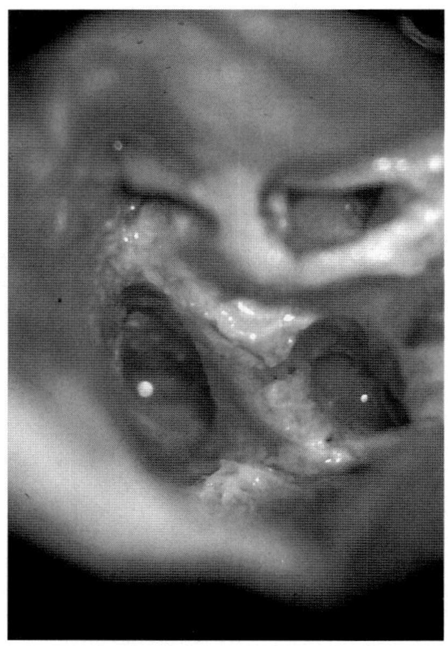

Fig. 1-17. Right ear. The facial recess, the facial nerve (mastoid part), the exposed internal auditory canal.

eral semicircular canals reach the superior vestibular nerve by passing through these perforations (across the pyramid and through the elliptical recess, respectively).
The orifice of the vestibular aqueduct opens below the elliptical recess. It reaches the posterior petrosal region (mastoid) and contains an endolymphatic evagination of the membranous labyrinth and the endolymphatic duct, along with small veins.

The endolymphatic duct
The endolymphatic duct goes from the vestibule to the endolymphatic sac. It is contained in the vestibular aqueduct. It communicates in the vestibule with the saccule and the utricle through the utricular and saccular ducts.

The endolymphatic sac
The endolymphatic sac is found in a small niche, called the foveate impression, and is located on the posterior surface of the petrous pyramid. Most of the sac is extraosseous, held between two sheets of dura mater. Its internal surface is smooth, regular, and flat. Part of it is intraosseous, inside the vestibular aqueduct, with a similar histological aspect. An intermediate wrinkled (rugose) part is found, with an irregular internal surface covered by epithelial folds.

SUPERIOR WALL

The ampullar orifice of the superior semicircular canal is found at the anterior extremity, the orifice of the crus communis of the canals superior and posterior to the extreme posterior extremity.

INFERIOR WALL

The inferior wall connects the medial wall to the lateral wall of the vestibule. Anteriorly is the aperture of the scala vestibuli, while the ampullar orifice of the posterior semicircular canal is located posteriorly.

ANTERIOR WALL

The anterior wall goes from the margins of the round window below to the superior ampullar crest above.

POSTERIOR WALL

The posterior wall is found between the orifice of the crus communis and the ampullar orifice of the posterior semicircular canal.

SEMICIRCULAR CANALS

The three semicircular canals make up 60-65% of a circle, hence their name. They are perpendicular to one another and have an average diameter of 0.8 mm. Each canal has an ampullated end with a diameter of approx. 1.6 mm, dilated to contain the ampulla of the membranous labyrinth. There are two orifices of the non-ampullated end, since the arm of the posterior canal and that of the superior canal join to open together into the vestibule (crus communis) (Figs. 1-18, 1-19).

LATERAL SEMICIRCULAR CANAL

The lateral semicircular canal has a horizontal path. Shorter than the other canals (12-15 mm in length), it is nonetheless wider. It opens into the lateral wall of the vestibule, with the ampullated arm projecting anteriorly-superiorly and the non-ampullated arm projecting posteriorly-superiorly.

SUPERIOR SEMICIRCULAR CANAL

This canal is 15-18 mm long and has a vertical path. The ampullated end of the canal opens onto the medial wall of the vestibule. The opposite extreme fuses with the non-ampullated end of the posterior canal and together they open at the posterior end of the superior vestibular wall.

POSTERIOR SEMICIRCULAR CANAL

The longest of the canals (16-20 mm), the posterior semicircular canal has a vertical course.
Its ampullated end opens posteriorly onto the inferior wall of the vestibule, in the area of the macula cribrosa inferioris. This macula cribrosa has minute perforations, which are threaded with nervous filaments forming the singular nerve. This exits the fundus of the internal auditory canal from the singular foramen. The posterior extremity contributes to the formation of the crus communis.

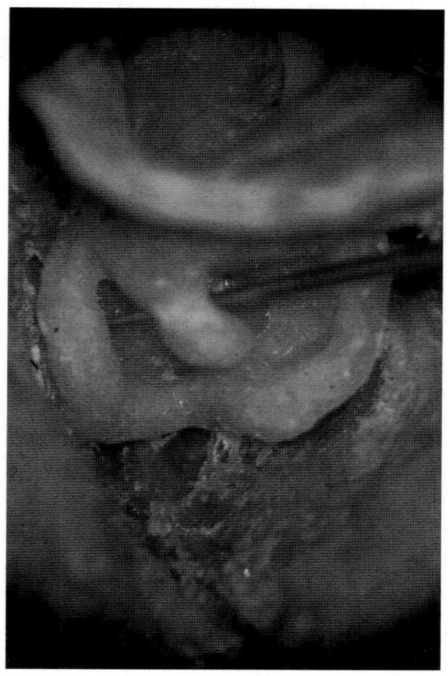

Fig. 1-18. Right ear. The semicircular canals.

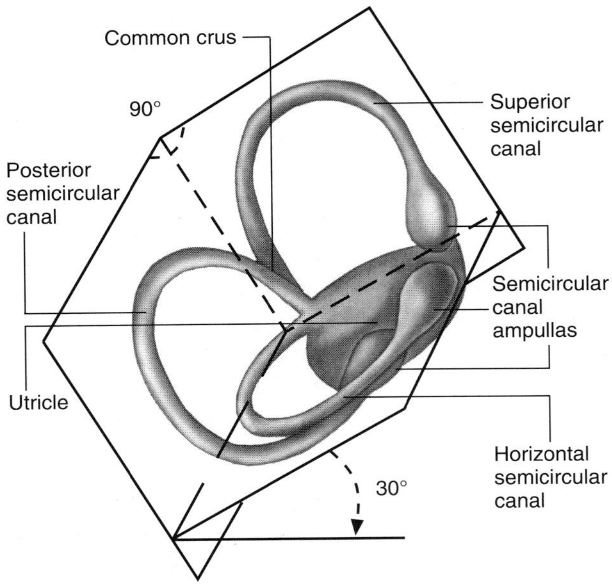

Fig. 1-19. Spatial disposition of the semicircular canals.

THE COCHLEA

This spiral-shaped structure rests on the medial wall of the vestibule. It is approx. 10 mm wide and 5 mm high (Fig. 1-20).

The cochlea is cone-shaped, with a 30 mm-long osseous canal that turns on itself two and a half times, with the basal turn, the intermediate turn, the apical turn, and finally the helicotrema. The basal turn protrudes into the tympanic cavity forming the promontory. The diameter of the cochlear canal is approx. 4 mm at the basal turn, and decreases progressively until narrowing to 1 mm at the apex. The first turn is more medial and for the first 4 mm it is below the level of the vestibule. The last turn is more lateral. The osseous canal turns around an osseous axis: the modiolus.

A thin osseous lamina exits the modiolus. This is called the osseous spiral lamina, which follows the cochlear canal and partially divides it into two parts. This division is completed by the cochlear canal, which goes from the free margin of the osseous spiral lamina to the external wall of the cochlea.

The modiolus has an enlarged base, consisting of the tractus spiralis foraminosum.

This cribriform area, located at the fundus of the internal auditory canal, allows the terminal branches of the cochlear nerve to pass through its foramina. A canaliculus enters the cochlea from each foramen, conducting axons from the cochlear nerve to the ganglion of Corti. The central foramen continues into a canal that enters the modiolus and ends at its apex. Osseous canals enter the cochlea from other foramina and enter the spiral canal, which follows the margin of the osseous spiral lamina, distal to the attachment to the modiolus. The spiral canal also terminates at the apex of the cochlea.

At the entrance of the osseous canal of the cochlea, three apertures can be observed: the fenestra vestibuli (oval window), the fenestra cochleae (round window), and the orifice of the cochlear canaliculus.

The fenestra vestibuli accommodates the footplate of the stapes in the tympanic cavity. The fenestra cochleae is closed in the tympanic cavity by the secondary tympanic membrane. The cochlear canaliculus connects the scala tympani to the inferior surface of the petrous ridge. Thus it connects the perilymph of the scala tympani with the subarachnoid space. The cochlear canaliculus also contains a vein which flows into the inferior petrosal sinus.

Bipolar cells in the spiral canal are found. Their bodies make up the ganglion of Corti, also called the spiral ganglion (see chapter 6, vestibulocochlear nerve) (Figs. 1-21, 1-22).

THE MEMBRANOUS LABYRINTH

The membranous labyrinth is contained in the bony labyrinth. It is composed of the utricle, saccule, semicircular ducts, and the cochlear duct. The semicircular ducts, comprised in the semicircular canals, open into the utricle. The latter communicates with the saccule by means of the utriculosaccular duct, which flows into the endolymphatic sac. The saccule, in turn, is connected to the endolymphatic sac by means of the endolymphatic duct. The utriculosaccular duct connects the endolymphatic sac with the cochlear duct (Fig. 1-23).

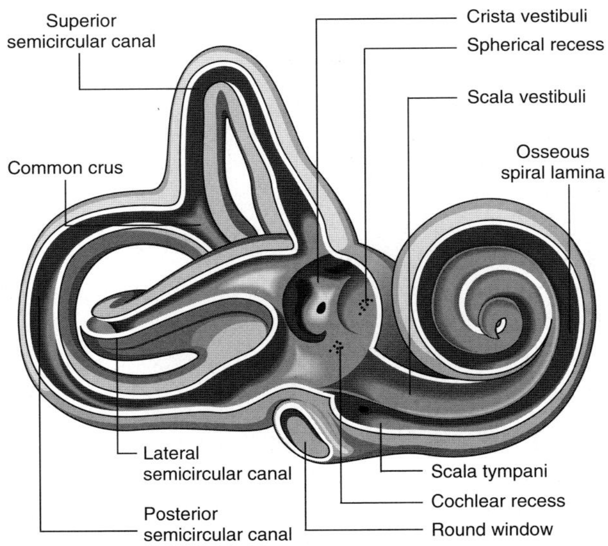

Fig. 1-20. The right osseous labyrinth, interior aspect. (Adapted from Gray's anatomy).

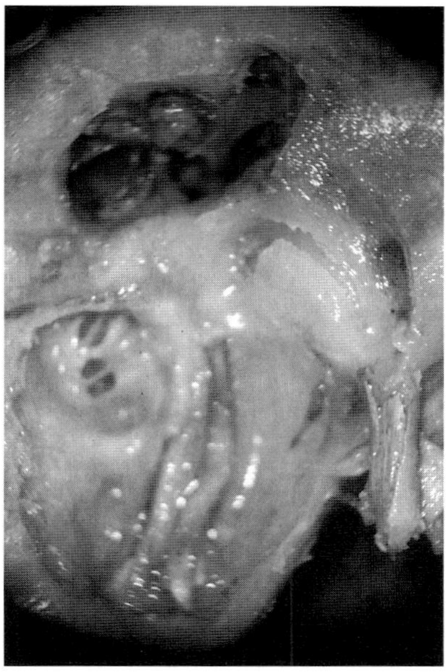

Fig. 1-21. Right ear. Middle fossa approach. For anatomical purposes the cochlea and the epitympanum have been opened and the superior semicircular canal has been fenestrated.

The perilymphatic space is found between the bony and membranous labyrinths. It is filled with perilymph, similar in composition to cerebrospinal fluid. The perilymph contained in the semicircular canals communicates with the perilymph of the vestibule, which fills the scala vestibuli to its apex, the helicotrema. Here it communicates with the scala tympani. The scala tympani communicates in turn with the subarachnoid space through the cochlear canaliculus.

UTRICLE

The utricle is found in the vestibule, superiorly and posteriorly. It touches the elliptical recess. The non-ampullated arms of the semicircular canals and the ampulla of the posterior canal open into the medial wall of the utricle. The ampullae of the superior and lateral canals open into its lateral wall.
In its point of contact with the elliptical recess, an organ is found called the macula of the utricle. This is where the superior vestibular nerve fibers begin.

The macula of the utricle

The macula of the utricle is composed of hair cells and supporting cells. The hair cells are the sensory cells. Their free surface has 40-100 microvilli and there is a kinocilium at one end. The stereocilia, shorter than the kinocilium, decrease progressively from those near the kinocilium (100 microns approx.) to those farthest away (1 micron) (Fig. 1-24).
A central strip (striola) has no hair cells.
The sensory cells are always electrically active. The inclination of the cilia toward the kinocilium provokes a depolarization and thus an increased discharge frequency, whereas an inclination in the opposite direction provokes hyperpolarization and thus inhibition.
The cilia are immersed in a gelatinous layer, called the otolithic membrane. On its apex, calcium carbonate stones are found, called otocones and otoliths. (If they say you have rocks in your head, they're right! H. House).

SACCULE

The saccule rests in the spherical recess of the vestibule.
The ductus reuniens (in communication with the scala vestibuli) detaches from its inferior wall.
The endolymphatic duct exits from the posterior-superior area.
The macula of the saccule is on the anterior wall.
The structure of the macula of the saccule is similar to that of the utricle.

PHYSIOLOGY

The maculae of the utricle and saccule are stimulated by the force of gravity (weight of the otolithic membrane) and by straightforward accelerations.
The flexed extension of the head modifies the pressure and the traction exerted by the otolithic membrane on the stereocilial bundles of the sensory cells of the maculae. This influences flexor and extensor muscle tone.
Lateral head movements modify the pressure and the stretching exerted by the otolytic membrane

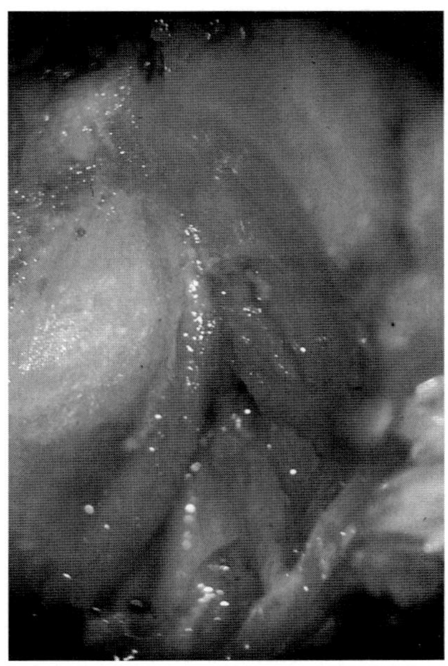

Fig. 1-22. Right ear. Middle fossa approach. Cochlea is outlined, IAC dura is opened, VII-VIII CNs can be seen.

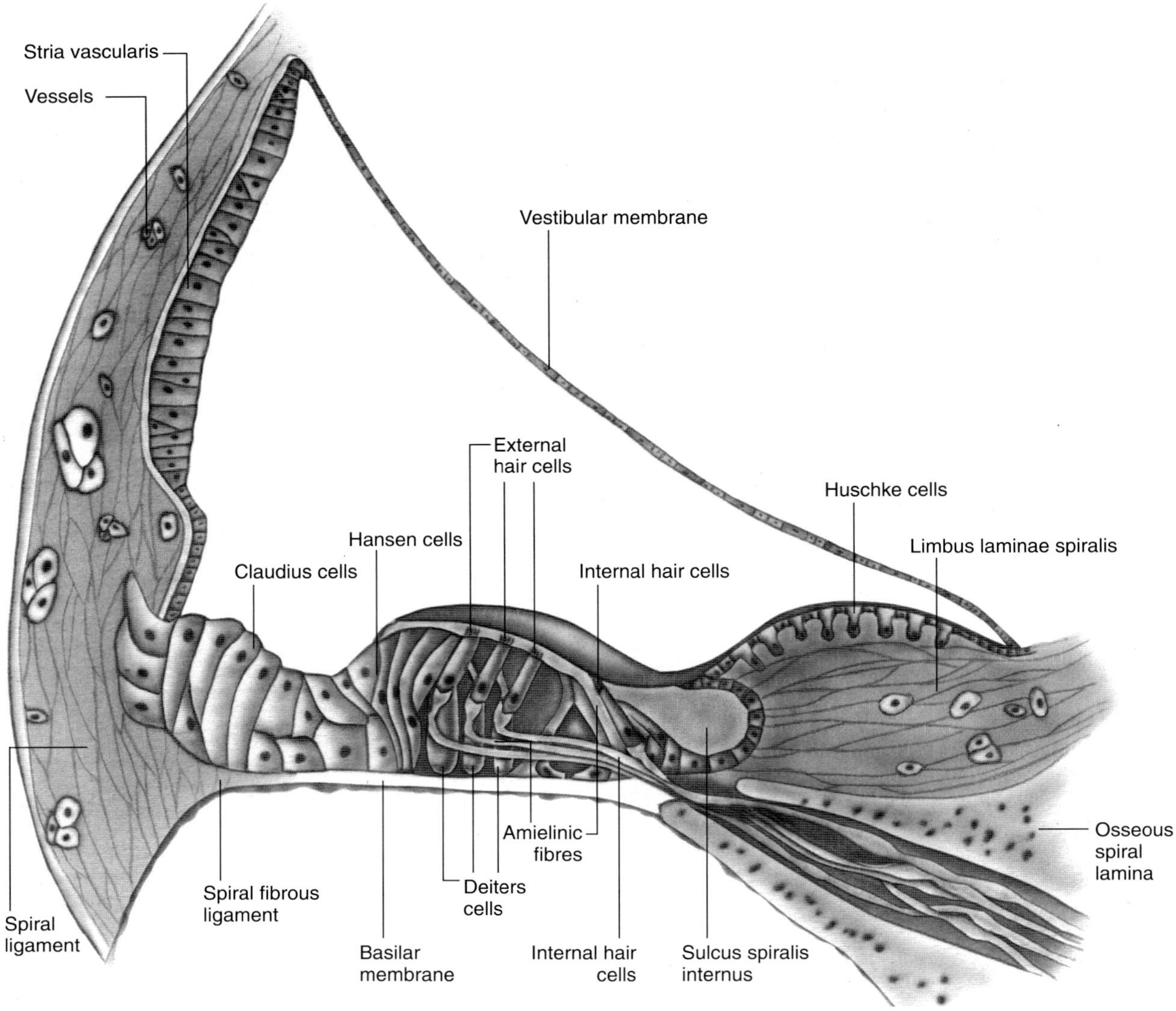

Fig. 1-23. The cochlear duct and related structures.

on the cilia of the macula of the saccule. This influences the abductor and adductive muscles tone.

The ampullae of the semicircular canals contain the ampullary crests, which have structures similar to the maculae of utricule and saccule. The crests are elevated by the osseous plane and have hair cells and supporting cells. The cilia are longer than those of the maculae. The disposition of the cilia and the kinocilium is the same as that of the macular cells.

At the center of the crest the cilia have a vertical path, whereas peripherically they have an oblique path. The cellular surface is surrounded by a gelatinous substance, called the cupula due to its shape.

In each canal ampulla there are hair cells, similar to those of the maculas of utricule and saccule (Fig. 1-25). The movement of endolymph, caused by angular movements of the head, deflect the cupola of each crista and bend the stereocilial-kinocilial bundles. The stimulus pass to the primary sensory neurons of the vestibular nerve. The body of the primary sensory neurons forms the vestibular ganglion (chapter 6).

The ampullary receptors of the semicircular canals are connected to the superior and medial vestibular nuclei and then, along the medial longitudinal bundle, with motor neurons of the III, IV, VI nerves nuclei, directed to the extrinsic ocular muscles: (superior, inferior, medial and lateral recti muscles and superior and inferior obliqui muscles). This is the tri-neuronal basis for the vestibulo-oculomotor reflex.

VASCULARIZATION OF THE LABYRINTH

The labyrinthine artery is a branch of the basilar artery, or, more frequently, of the anterior-inferi-

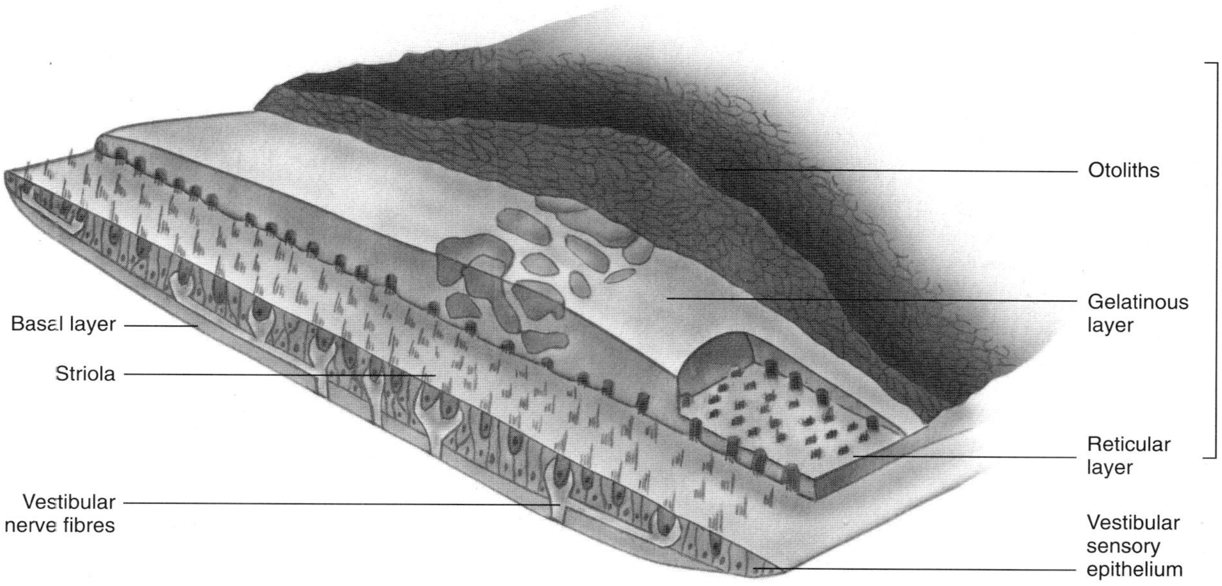

Fig. 1-24. Morphological organization of the macula of the utricle.

or cerebellar artery (AICA). It proceeds from the cerebellopontine angle to the internal auditory canal at the porus. It then runs from the facial nerve to the vestibulocochlear nerve, reaches the fundus of the internal auditory canal, and divides into a cochlear branch and a vestibular branch. The vestibular branch subdivides to supply the saccule, the utricle, and the semicircular canals.

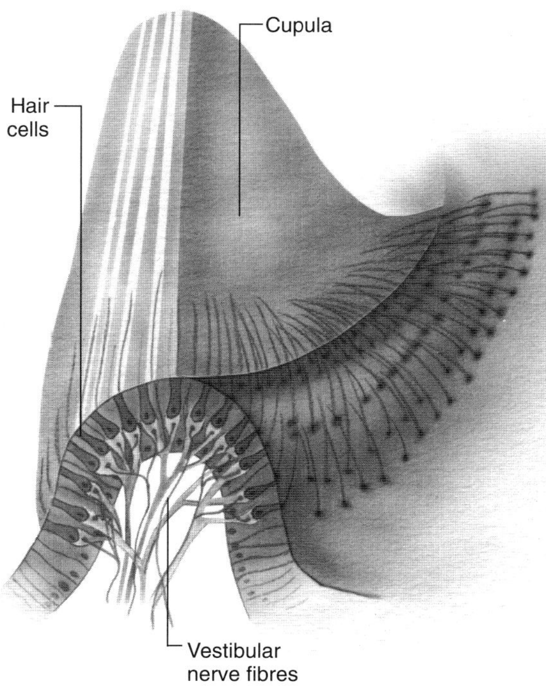

Fig. 1-25. The ampullary crest of a semicircular canal.

The cochlear branch subdivides into small branches which transverse the canals of the tractus spiralis foraminosum and spread, in the form of minute capillaries, to the spiral lamina and the basilar membrane.

The veins carrying reflux blood from the cochlea, the semicircular canals, and the vestibule accompany the arterial vessels. At the base of the modiolus they flow into the labyrinthine vein, which enters either the superior petrosal sinus or the transverse sinus.

A small vein goes from the basal turn of the cochlea to the internal jugular vein through the cochlear canaliculus.

REFERENCES

Allam AF: Pneumatisation of the temporal bone. Annals Otol Rhinol Laryngol 78: 49-64, 1969.

Anson BJ, Donaldson JA: Surgical anatomy of the temporal bone. Third edition. WB Saunders Company. Publisher. Philadelphia, 1981.

Bagger-Sjoback D, Friberg U, Rask Andersen H: The human endolymphatic sac. Arch Otolaryng Head Neck Surg 112: 398-409, 1986.

Cannoni M, Pech A, Pellet W, Zanaret M, Triglia JM: Les procidences veineuses et meningees au cours des voies trans-labyrinthiques elargies. Ann Oto Laryng (Paris) 103: 303-308, 1986.

Cawthorne T: Bell's palsies. Ann Otol (St Louis) 72: 774-779, 1963.

Charachon R, Accoyer B: Note technique sur le reperage du conduit auditif interne. Acta Otolaryng. Belgica 30/1: 76-83, 1976.

Chouard CH: Wrisberg intermediary nerve. In facial nerve surgery. Edit U Fisch-Kugler Med Pub Amstelveen. Aesculapius Pub; Comp Birmingham (Alab): 24-39, 1977.

Coates AE: A note on the superior petrosal sinus and its relation to the sensory root of the trigeminal nerve. J Anat 68: 428-430, 1934.

Das AC, Hasan M: The occipital sinus. J Neuro Surg 33: 307-311, 1970.

Di Chiro G, Fisher RL, Nelson KB: The jugular foramen. J Neurosurg 21:447-60, 1964.

Di Chiro G, Fisher RL, Nelson KB: The jugular foramen. J Neurosurg 21: 447-460, 1964.

Domb GH, Chole RA: Anatomical studies of the posterior petrous apex with regard to hearing preservation in acoustic neuroma removal. Laryngoscope 90: 1769-1776, 1980.

Domb GH, Chole RA: Anatomical studies of the posterior petrous apex with regard to hearing preservation in acoustic neuroma removal. Laryngoscope 90:1769-76, 1980.

Domb GH, Chole RA: Anatomical studies of the posterior petrous apex with regard to hearing preservation in acoustic neuroma removal. Laryngoscope 90: 1769-1776, 1980.

Donaldson A, Duckert LG, Lambert PM, Rubel EW: Anson and Donaldson surgical anatomy of the temporal bone. New York: Raven Press, 1992.

Droissart A: Les anomalies vasculaires a incidence otologique. J Head Neck Pathol 1: 39-44, 1982.

Duvernoy HM: Human Brainstem Vessels, Springer-Verlag (New York) Edit 188pp. 1977.

Duvernoy HM: The superficial veins of the human brain. Springer-Verlag (New York) Edit 11 Opp, 1975.

Eyries CH, Chouard CH: Les origines reelles du nerf facial. Ann Otolaryng 87/6: 321-326, 1970.

Fisch U: Infratemporal fossa approach to tumors of the temporal bone and base of the skull. J Laryng Otol 92: 949-967, 1978.

Fisch U: L'anatomie chirurgicale du systeme arteriel du conduit auditif interne chez l'homme. Rev Laryngol (Bordeaux) 89/11,12: 659-671, 1968.

Graham MD: The jugular bulb: Its anatomic and clinical considerations in contemporary otology. Laryngoscope 87/1: 105-125, 1977.

Guerkink NA: Surgical anatomy of the temporal bone posterior to the internal auditory canal: an operative approach. Laryngoscope 87:975 -86, 1977.

Guerkink NA: Surgical anatomy of the temporal bone posterior to the internal auditory canal: an operative approach. Laryngoscope 87: 975-986, 1977.

Guerrier Y, Guerrier B: Anatomie topographique et chirurgicale du rocher. Acta oto-rhino-Laryngol. Belgica 30/1: 22-50, 1976.

Guerrier Y: Surgical anatomy, particularly vascular supply of the facial nerve. In facial nerve surgery. Edit U Fisch. Kugler Med Pub (Amstelveen). Aesculapius Pub Comp Birmingham Alab: 13-23, 1977.

Guild SR: A hitherto unrecognised structure, the glomus jugularis in man. Anat Rec 79: Suppl 2-28, 1941.

Hall GM, Pulec JL, Rhoton AL: Geniculate ganglion anatomy for the otologist. Arch Otolaryng 90: 568-571, 1969.

Harris FS, Rhoton AL: Anatomy of the cavernous sinus. A microsurgical study. J Neurosurg 45: 169-180, 1976.

House WF, Hitselberger WE: The transcochlear approach to the skull base. Arch Otolaryngol 102: 334-342, 1976.

House WF, Luetje CM: Acoustic tumors. Univ Park press (Baltimore) Vol I Diagnosis 289pp. Vol II management 280pp, 1979.

House WF: Monograph II: Acoustic neuroma. Arch Otolaryngol 88/6: 575-715, 1968.

House WF: Surgical exposure of the internal auditory canal and its contents, through the middle cranial fossa. Laryngoscope 71: 1363-1385, 1961.

House WF: Monograph of trans-temporal removal of acoustic neuromas. Arch Oto-Laryngol 80: 587-756, 1964.

Kapur TR, Bangash W: Tegmental and petro-mastoid defects in the temporal bone. J Laryngol Otol 100: 1129-1132, 1986.

Kartush JM, Telian SA, Graham MD, Kemink JL: Anatomic basis for labyrinthine preservation during posterior fossa acoustic tumor surgery. Laryngoscope 96: 1024-1028, 1986.

Korner O: Uber die fossa jugularis und die Knochenlucken im Boden der Paukenhohle. Arch Ohr Nas U Keblkheilk 30: 236-239, 1890.

Legent F, Perlemuter L, Vandenbrouck C: Cahiers d'Anatomie ORL. Masson Edit 1-125, 1979.

Mercier Ph, Fardoun R, Cadou B, Le Patezour A, Guy G: Etude microchirurgicale du nerf facial intra-cranien. In diagnostic et traitement des neurinomes de l'acoustique. Lazorthes Y, Clanet M, Fraysse B Edit. Fournie Imp Toulouse: 61-70, 1983.

Moret J: La vascularisation de l'appareil auditif. Normal-variantes-tumeurs glomiques. J Neuroradiol (Paris) 9: 213-260, 1982.

Nadol JB: Causes of failure of mastoidectomy for chronic otitis media. Laryngoscope 95:410-413, 1985.

Nager GT, Nager M: The arteries of the human middle ear with particular regard to the blood supply of the auditory ossicles. Ann Otol Rhinol Laryngol 62/4: 923-949, 1953.

Naguib M, Aristegui M, Saleh E, Cokkeser Y, Landolfi M, Sanna M: Surgical anatomy of the petrous apex as it relates to the enlarged middle cranial fossa approaches. Otolaryngol Head Neck Surg, 111:488-493, 1994.

Ogura Y, Clemis JD: A study of the gross anatomy of the human vestibular aqueduct. Ann Otol Rhinol Laryngol 80/6: 813 825, 1971.

Pait TG, Zeal A, Harns FS, Paullus WS, Rhoton AL: Microdissection anatomy and dissection of the temporal bone. Sur Neurol 8: 363-391, 1977.

Palva T, Palva A: Size of the human mastoid air cell system. Acta Oto-Laryng 62: 237-251, 1966.

Parisier SC: The middle cranial fossa approach to the internal auditory canal. An anatomical study stressing critical distances between surgical landmarks. Laryngoscope 84: 1-20, 1974.

Paullus WC, Pait TG, Rhoton AL: Microsurgical exposure of the petrous portion of the carotid artery. J Neurosurg 47: 713-726, 1977.

Pertuiset B: Les neurinomes de l'acoustique. Neuro-Chir (Paris) 16: Supp 1, 1-147, 1970.

Pialoux P: Contribution a l'anatomie stereotaxique du conduit auditif interne. Ann Oto-Laryng Paris 90/7-8: 409-422, 1973.

Pool JL, Pava AA, Greenfield EC: Acoustic nerve tumors. Early diagnosis and treatment. Second edition. Ch Thomas. Pub Spingfield III, 1-161,1970.

Portmann M: Quelques observations sur la systematisation des nerfs transpetreux. Revue Laryngol 76: 281-298, 1955.

Proctor B: Surgical anatomy of the posterior tympanum. Ann Otol Rhinol Laryngol 78: 1026-1241, 1969.

Proctor B: Surgical anatomy of the posterior tympanum. Ann Otol-Rhinol-Laryngol 78: 1026-1040, 1969.

Rask-Andersen M, Stahle J, Wilbrand H: Human cochlear aqueduct and its accessory canal. Ann-Otol-Rhinol-Laryngol 86/5: part 2: 2-16, 1977.

Rhoton AL, Buza R: Microsurgical anatomy of the jugular foramen. J neurosurg 42 541-550, 1975.

Rhoton AL, Pulec JL, Hall GM, Boyd A: Absence of bone over the geniculate ganglion. J Neurosurg 28:48-53, 1968.

Rhoton AL, Pulec JL, Hall GM, Boyd AS: Absence of bone over the geniculate ganglion. J Neurosurg 28/1: 48-53, 1968.

Rhoton AL: Microsurgery of the internal auditory meatus. Surg Neurol 2: 311-318, 1974.

Roland PS, Meyerhoff WL, Wright CG, Mickey B: Anatomic considerations in the posterior approach to the internal auditory canal. Ann Otol Rhinol Laryngol 97:621-625, 1988.

Rougerie J, Guyot JF: Essai de conservation du nerf facial dans l'ablation des neurinomes de l'angle ponto-cerebelleux. Neuro-Chir (Paris) 10/1: 13-21, 1964.

Sanna M, Shea C, Gamoletti R, Russo A: Surgery of the "only hearing ear" with chronic ear disease. J Laryngol Otol 106:n-n, 1992.

Sanna M: Anatomy of the posterior mesotympanum. In: Zini C, Sheehy JL, Sanna M, eds. Microsurgery of cholesteatoma of the middle ear. Milan: Ghedini, 1980:69-73.

Santini JJ: Atlas d'osteologie du crane. Masson Edit Paris 1-129, 1980.

Savie D, Djerie D: Morphological variations and relations of the epitympanum. Rev Laryngol 107/1: 61-64, 1986.

Schuknecht HF, Gylya JA: Anatomy of the temporal bone with surgical implications. Philadelphia: Lea and Febiger, 1986.

Shapiro R: Compartimentation of the jugular foramen. J Neurosurg 36/3: 340-343, 1972.

Shea DA, Chole RA, Paparella MM: The endolymphatic sac: anatomical considerations. Laryngoscope 89: 88-93, 1979.

Shrontz C, Dujouny M, Ausman Jl, Diaz FG, Pearce JE, Berman SK, Hirsch E, Mirchandani HG: Surgical anatomy of the arteries of the posterior fossa. J Neurosurg 65/4: 540-544, 1986.

Sterkers JM: Technique simplifee de decouverte du conduit auditif interne par voi temporale. Ann Otol Laryngol (Paris) 90:232-235, 1973.

Sunderland S: Some anatomical and pathophysiological data relevant to facial nerve surgery and repair. In facial nerve surgery. U Fisch Edit Kugler Med Pub Amstelveen. Aesculapius Pub Comp Birmingham (alab): 47-61, 1977.

Vernick DM: Labyrinthectomy. In: Nadol JB, Schuknecht HF eds. Surgery of the ear and temporal bone. New York: Raven Press, 275 -280, 1993.

Waltner JG: Anatomic variations of the lateral and sigmoid sinuses. Arch Otol 39: 307, 1944.

Weinberg J, Sade J: Posterior wall atrophy. Am J Otol 3:315-317, 1982.

Wigand ME, Rettinger G, Haid T, Berg M: Die Ausraumung von Oktavus Neurinomen des Kleinhirnbruckenwinkels mit transtemporalem Zugang uber die mittlere Schadelgrube. HNO 33: 11-16, 1985.

Wigand ME, Trillsch K: Surgical anatomy of the sinus epitympani. Ann Otol Rhinol Laryngol 82:378-384, 1973.

Winkler G: Le nerf facial. Morphologie, topographie, structure et systematisation fonctionnelle. CR Ass Anat 125b: 11-50, 1965.

Woodhall B: Anatomy of the cranial blood sinuses with particular reference to the lateral. Laryngoscope 49: 966-1009, 1939.

Woodhall B: Variations of the cranial venous sinuses in the region of the torcular Herophili. Arch Surg 33: 297-314, 1936.

Yasargil MG, Kasdaglis K, Jain KK, Weber HP: Anatomical observations of the sub-arachnoid cisterns of the brain during surgery. J Neurosurg 44/3: 298-302, 1976.

Yasargil MG, Smith RD, Gasser JC: Microsurgical approach to acoustic neurinomas. Adv Tech Standards Neurosurg 4: 93-129, 1977.

2

Anatomy of the skull base

Surgery of the skull base moves from a known point towards an unknown point, proceeding from the certain to the uncertain. If you lose your way, you have to turn back and begin again from the known point.

The external surface of the skull base extends from the incisor teeth anteriorly to the nuchal line of the occipital bone posteriorly.
In an overhead view, the skull base divides into three parts, going downward: the anterior, middle, and posterior cranial fossa (Figs. 2-1, 2-2, 2-3).

Anterior cranial fossa

The frontal, ethmoidal, and sphenoidal bones contribute to form the floor of the anterior cranial fossa, which is primarily composed of a convex and rugose surface of the frontal bone. On its anterior edge, in a vertical position, the posterior walls of the frontal sinuses are found. The roof with the ethmoid sinuses is found medially, and more medial still is the cribriform plate of the ethmoid. This is dimpled and bordered laterally by the medial wall of the sphenoid sinus and transversed medially by the crista galli. Olfactory fibers pass through the foramina of the cribriform plate, as do the anterior and posterior ethmoidal arteries and nerves.
Posterior to the cribriform plate is the sphenoid plane, which proceeds to the tuberculum sellae. The sphenoid plane continues laterally with the lesser wing of the sphenoid bone, which represents the posterior boundary of the anterior fossa. The frontal, ethmoidal, and sphenoid sinuses thus relate to the floor of the anterior cranial fossa.

THE INFERIOR SKULL BASE

The anterior (palatine) region is composed of the palatine processes of the maxillary bone and the horizontal part of the palatine bones. In the hard palate, on the midline (anteriorly), the fossa incisiva is found where the incisive canal opens. The major and minor fori palatini are found posteriorly-laterally, where the pterygopalatine and palatine canals open.

DURA MATER

On the cribriform plate of the ethmoid, the dura of the anterior cranial fossa is thin and difficult to dissect, whereas it is thicker on the sphenoid plane and behind the lesser wing of the sphenoid bone.

VESSELS OF DURA AND FLOOR OF ANTERIOR CRANIAL FOSSA.

The ethmoidal arteries. Their branches cross the cribriform plate to reach the walls of the medial and lateral nasal fossae.
The frontal branch of the middle meningeal artery, which often reaches the orbit across the meningo-orbitary foramen.
The internal carotid artery.

REFERENCES

(see references of anatomy of middle cranial fossa).

Middle cranial fossa

The osseous floor of the skull base of the middle fossa is made up of the greater wing of the sphenoid bone, the parietal bone, the temporal bone (squamous part) and the anterior surface of the petrous part. The petrous component is the posterior boundary, whereas the anterior limit is the lesser wing of the sphenoid bone and its lateral prominence, the alaris crest. The body of the sphenoid is medial. It is bounded by the sella turgica above and the cavernous sinus and its contents below.
The floor of the middle cranial fossa is supplied mainly by branches of the middle meningeal artery.

HYPOPHYSEAL FOSSA AND CAVERNOUS SINUS

The hypophyseal fossa is found at the center of the skull base, on the superior face of the sphenoid body. The sphenoid body is found between

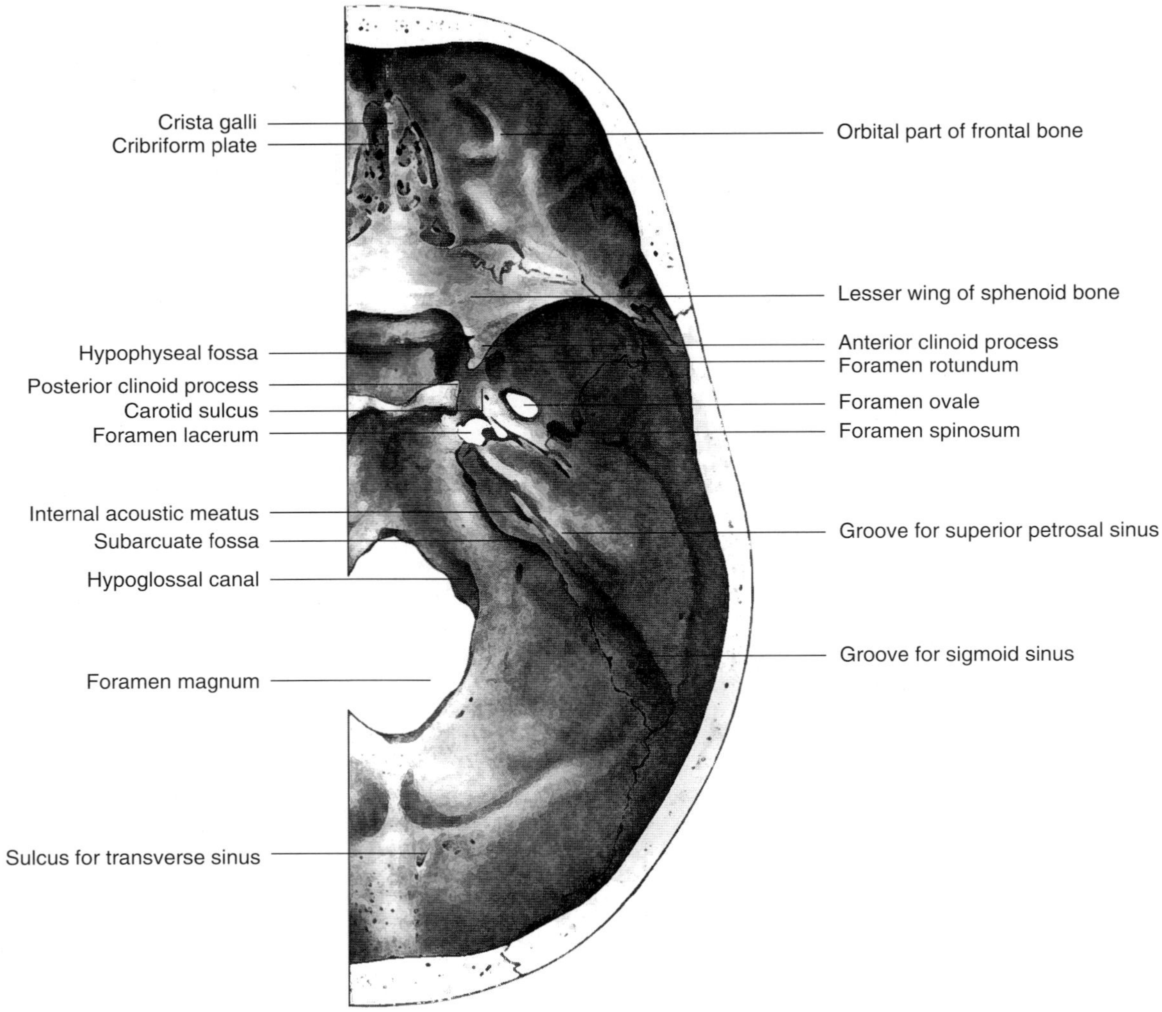

Fig. 2-1. The base of the skull: Internal aspect.

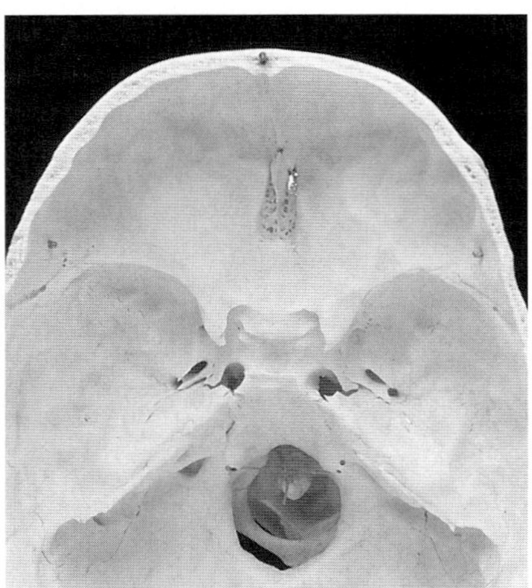

Fig. 2-2. The skull base.

the basilar part of the occipital bone posteriorly and the ethmoid anteriorly.

The sphenoid body makes up the posterior part of the vault of the nasal cavities and the medial orbital wall.

The inner part of the sphenoid body is occupied by two cavities: the sphenoid sinuses (see chapter 5).

The superior face of the body is concave and is called the sella turgica. In the bottom of the sella the hypophyseal fossa accommodates the hypophysis. Posterior to the sella is a bony structure, the dorsum of the sella. Its superior free margins terminate laterally in two ridges called the posterior clinoid processes. The sella slopes laterally to the floor of the middle cranial fossa. Lateral to the sella turgica the sphenoid has a groove for the internal carotid artery, which turns anteriorly from the foramen lacerum.

Hypophyseal cisterns

The arachnoid transverses the diaphragmatic foramen (see chapter 3) to reach the anterior

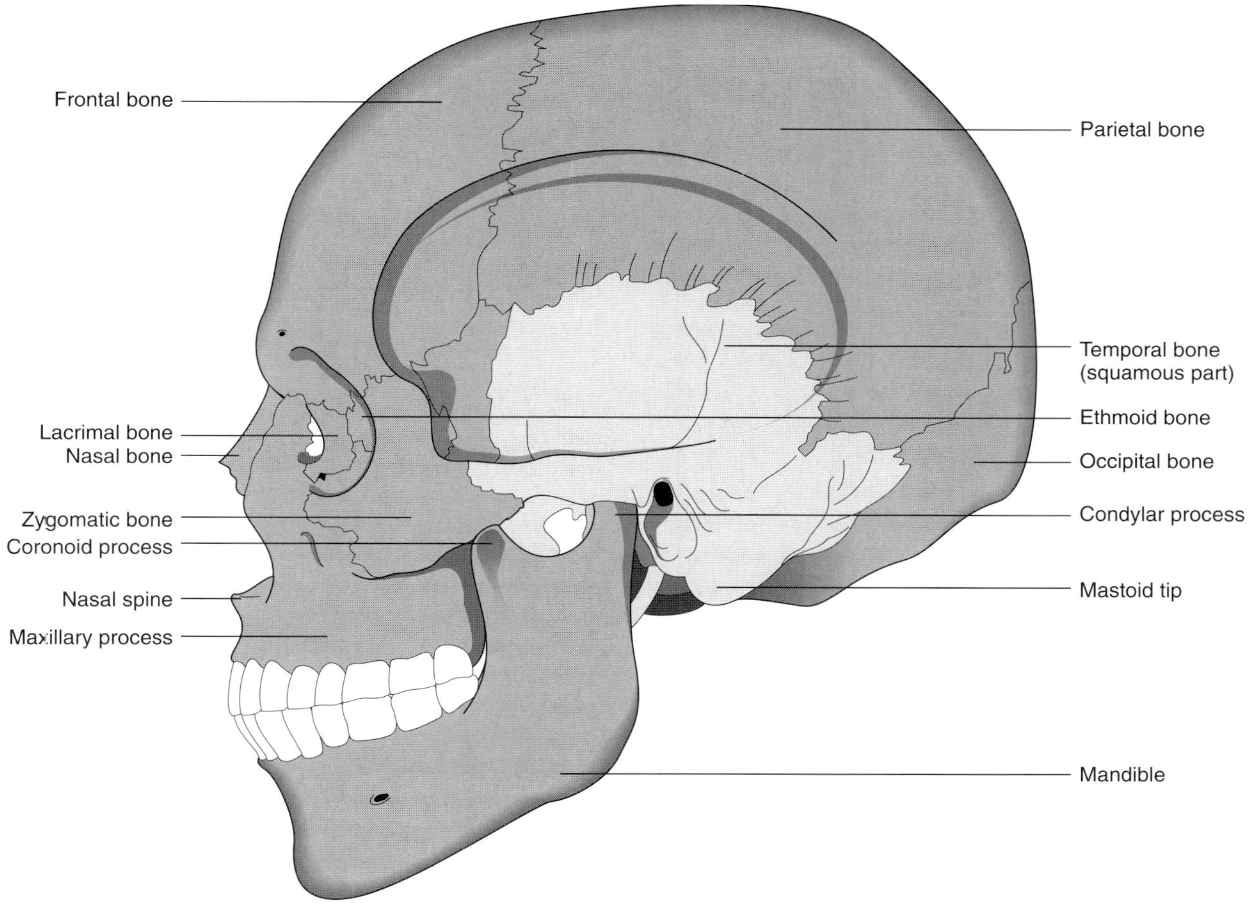

Fig. 2-3. The skull. Lateral aspect.

lobe of the hypophysis. In adults, this space is full of liquid and is called the hypophyseal cistern.

Hypophyseal arteries

There may be from one to four hypophyseal arteries, but generally there are two. They exit the ICA, which transverses the diaphragm of the sella in its subarachnoid tract. The arteries lie posteriorly and inferiorly, near the infundibulum. They emit branches under the optic chiasma and the optic nerve. They run anteriorly and laterally to the hypophyseal peduncle, around which an arterial circle is formed where the true superior hypophyseal arteries originate.

Carotico-cavernous arteries

When the ICA transverses the cavernous sinus, it emits two collateral branches, or trunks. The posterior carotico-cavernous trunk (or meningeal-hypophyseal trunk) has a retrograde direction. It emits the inferior hypophyseal artery whose branches supply the hypophysis, the dura of the clivus and part of the tentorium. It emits the capsular arteries, which at times detach directly from the ICA to supply the hypophysis, the hypophyseal fossa floor, and the mucosa of the sphenoid sinus.

The inferolateral trunk originates in the inferior part of the intracavernous carotid artery and supplies the dura and the cranial nerves in this area.

HYPOPHYSEAL VEINS

Reflux blood from the hypophysis is drained into the cavernous sinus.

CAVERNOUS SINUS

The lateral wall of the cavernous sinus is formed by the dura of the middle cranial fossa, in contact with the brain. Just underneath are the oculomotor, trochlear, ophthalmic, abducens, and maxillary nerves (see chapter 6).

Superior orbitary fissure

Located between the greater and lesser wings of the sphenoid bone, this groove connects the orbit with the middle cranial fossa. It is transversed by nerves III, IV, V1, VI, the superior ophthalmic vein, and the meningeal arteries.

It connects the middle fossa with the inferior orbitary fissure and the pterygopalatine fossa.

MIDDLE CRANIAL FOSSA FORAMINA

Foramen rotundum

This foramen is inferior to the superior orbitary fissure. With a diameter of approx. 4 mm, it is transversed by the maxillary nerve (V2) which enters the pterygopalatine fossa.
SPINOSUM OVALE ROTUNDUM LACERUM. Acronym to remember the name of the foramens: S-O-R-ry, LACER-ated.
Meningeal Artery, Mandibular nerve, Maxillary nerve, Internal Carotid artery. Acronym to remember the contents of the foramen: MA-M-Ma x ICe. (I call Mamma for ice). The foramen spinosum transmits the middle meningeal artery, the foramen ovale transmits the mandibular nerve, the foramen rotundum trasmits the maxillary nerve, the foramen lacerum trasmits the internal carotid artery (Fig. 2-1).

Foramen ovale

Posterior to the foramen rotundum, this foramen connects the floor of the middle cranial fossa with the infratemporal fossa. It is transversed by the mandibular nerve of the trigeminal (V3) and by a venous plexus. This venous plexus connects the cavernous sinus and the middle meningeal vein (generally) in the endocranium with the venous pterygoid plexus extracranially.
The foramen ovale is the anterior dissecting boundary in the enlarged middle fossa approach. A line drawn from the foramen spinosum to the foramen ovale is parallel and lateral to the course of the internal carotid artery.

Foramen spinosum

The foramen spinosum is posterior and lateral to the foramen ovale. It is transversed by the middle meningeal artery, which continues from the middle fossa to the infratemporal fossa. The middle meningeal veins, shaped like sinuses, course with the artery.

Foramen lacerum

The foramen lacerum is located between the foramen ovale anteriorly and the anterior-inferior part of the carotic canal posteriorly. It is bordered by the petrous apex, the sphenoid body and the occipital base. It is a possible connection between the rhinopharynx and the middle fossa, closed in nature by a fibrocartilaginous layer. The tongue of the sphenoid projects into the foramen and divides it into a lateral and a medial part. Upon exiting the carotic canal, the internal carotid with its accompanying sympathetic and venous plexuses goes through the middle tract to penetrate the cranial cavity.

Carotid canal

A large, circular foramen is posterior-lateral to the foramen lacerum and opens into the carotid canal. The internal carotid artery ascends in this canal, bends anteriorly-medially and then superiorly-medially and becomes endocranial.

Trigeminal path

Near the petrous apex and on the anterior surface of the petrous bone, there is a groove which accommodates the semilunar ganglion.
The superior surface of the petrous apex makes up the posterior and medial parts of the middle fossa floor.
The petrosquamous suture divides the petrous and squamous parts of the temporal bone. When dissecting the dura in the middle fossa approach, the petrosquamous suture often represents an area of adherence.

The greater superficial petrous nerve (GSPN)

This nerve comes from the geniculate ganglion after having crossed the geniculate foramen (or facial hiatus). It runs in a sulcus, medial to the petrosquamous suture, and passes below the trigeminal ganglion to reach the foramen lacerum. It transverses the lateral wall of the foramen lacerum to reach the pterygoid canal. Here it receives the deep petrous nerve and forms the nerve of the pterygoid canal. This canal lies in the base of the middle pterygoid lamina of the sphenoid. The nerve reaches the pterygopalatine ganglion, suspended from V2 in the pterygopalatine fossa. The GSPN is usually accompanied by the petrous artery, a branch of the middle meningeal artery, which supplies the geniculate ganglion and the labyrinthine and tympanic segments of VII.
The small petrous nerve lies inferior and anterior to the GSPN. Wrapped in dura, it proceeds to the otic ganglion. It is usually accompanied by the superior tympanic artery, a branch of the middle meningeal artery, which supplies the tympanic cavity and the tensor tympani muscle.
The arcuate eminence is found posterior to the facial hiatus in the surgical position. It accommodates the prominence of the superior semicircular canal, which has a variable and thus unpredictable location. The bisector of the angle between the GSPN and the blue line of the superior semicircular canal (SSC) indicates the IAC's path. According to Fisch, if drawing a 60° angle with the SSC blue line as the posterior side and its center on the ampulla, a meatal plane is defined, below which lies the IAC. The danger of injuring the anterior cochlea is avoided, by keeping in this plane.
Lateral to the arcuate eminence is the tegmen tympani, which is usually very thin. When opening the tegmen tympani we can identify the head of the malleus, the body of the incus, the tympanic segment of the facial nerve and the superior and lateral semicircular canals.

Along the crest of the petrous apex lies the superior petrosal sinus.
The floor of the middle cranial fossa receives blood mostly from the middle meningeal artery.

SURGICAL ANATOMICAL NOTES ON THE PETROUS APEX

The petrous apex is medial to the bony labyrinth and the ICA. The tip of the apex is attached to the posterior clinoid process by means of the petroclinoid ligament. It is located near the foramen lacerum. Its posterior boundary is the posterior cranial fossa, while its superior limit is made up of the middle cranial fossa, the middle meningeal artery, and the gasserian ganglion. Its inferior border is delineated by the jugular bulb and the inferior petrosal sinus.
The dura covering the posterior wall of the petrosal apex, anterior to the IAC, is not transversed by any structure. Within the petrosal apex and anterior to the IAC are the cochlea and the internal carotid artery.

THE TENTORIUM

The tentorium is attached to the petrous margin and the anterior and posterior clinoid processes. It divides the middle and posterior cranial fossae. Posteriorly it is attached to the transverse sinus, while anteriorly-laterally it touches the petrous ridge. Posterior to the brainstem, it terminates in a free edge. The space between this free edge and the brainstem is called the tentorial notch.
When the tentorium is incised as in the transpetrous middle fossa approach and the modified transcochlear approach (type C), access is notably enlarged. Some structures in particular must not be injured, however:
The trochlear nerve runs infratentorially and parallel to the free edge. It proceeds then through the tentorium to become supratentorial.
Labbé's vein (or inferior anastomotic vein) runs infratentorially connecting the middle cerebral vein to the transverse sinus or the lateral sinus and is extremely fragile. It collects the flow of veins draining the posterior temporal lobe and the inferior parietal lobe, then enters the transverse sinus above the junction of the superior petrosal sinus and sigmoid sinus. Here its walls are very thin. Injury to this vein may cause seizures and aphasia on the dominant side. In rare instances uncal herniation may occur, causing edema and death.
The superior cerebellar artery (SCA) and the petrosal vein, or vein of Dandy, runs infratentorially.
The posterior cerebral artery courses supratentorially.
The oculomotor nerve runs at the level of the tentorial notch.

REFERENCES

(Anatomy of anterior and middle cranial fossa)

Ciric I: On the origin and nature of the pituitary gland capsule. J Neurosurg 46:596-600, 1977.

Corner EM: On the temporal fossa. J Anat Physiol 30:377-385, 1896.

Dietemann JL, Lang J, Francke JP, Bonneville JF, Clarisse J, Wackenheim A: Anatomy and radiology of the sellar spine. Neuroradiology 21:5-7, 1981.

Goldenberg R: Surgeon's view of the skull base from the lateral approach. Laryngoscope 94(suppl 36):1-21, 1984.

Guild SR: A hitherto unrecognized structure, the glomus jugularis, in man. Anat Rec 79:29, 1941.

Hagen PT, Scholz DG, Edwards W: Incidence and size of patent foramen during the first decades of life: an autopsy study of 965 normal heads. Mayo Clin Proc 59: 17-50, 1984.

Hardy J: Transsphenoidal microsurgery of the normal and pathological pituitary. Clin Neurosurg 16: 185-217, 1969.

Hitselberger WE, Horn K, Hankinson H, Brackmann DE, House WF: The middle fossa transpetrous approach for petroclival meningioma. Skull Base Surg 3:130-5, 1993.

Honee GLJM: The anatomy of the lateral pterygoid muscle. Acta Morphol Neerl Scand 10:331-340, 1972.

House WF: Middle cranial fossa approach to the petrous pyramid: report of 50 cases. Arch Otolaryngol 78:460-468, 1963.

House WF: Surgical exposure of the internal auditory canal and its contents through the middle cranial fossa. Laryngoscope 71:1363-1935, 1961.

Jung A: Resection de l'articulation uncovertebrale et ouverture de trou de conjugaison par voie anterieure dans le traitment de la nevralgie cervico-brachiale. Technique operatoire. Mem Acad Chir 89:361-367, 1963.

Juniper RP: The superior pterygoid muscle. Br J Oral Surg 19:121-128, 1981.

Kanzaki J, Ogawa K, Tsuchihashi N, Inoue Y, Yamamoto M, Ikeda S: Postoperative complications in acoustic neuroma surgery by the extended middle cranial fossa approach. Acta Otolaryngol Suppl Stockh 487:75-79, 1991.

Kanzaki J, Shiobara R, Toya S: Classification of the extended middle cranial fossa approach. Acta Otolaryngol Suppl Stockh 487: 6-16, 1991.

Kartush JM, Telian SA, Graham MD, Kemink JL: Anatomic basis for labyirinthine preservation during posterior fossa acoustic tumor surgery. Laryngoscope 96:1024-1028, 1986.

Kinney SE, Hughes GB, Little JR: Retrolabyrinthine transtentorial approach to lesions of the anterior cerebellopontine angle. Am J Otol 13:426-30, 1992.

Koornneef L: New insights in the human orbital connective tissue. Arch Ophthalmol 95: 1269-1273, 1977.

Koval J, Molcan M, Bowdler AD, Sterkers JM: Retrosigmoid transmeatal approach: an anatomic study of an approach used for preservation of hearing in acoustic neuroma surgery and vestibular neurectomy. Skull Base Surg 3:16-21, 1993.

Krizan Z: Uber die fraglichen Korrelationen und uber die Entwicklung einiger Typen der A. Maxillaris. Acta Anat 42:71-87, 1960.

Krmpotic-Nemanic J, Draf W, Helms J: Surgical anatomy of the head and neck. Berlin: Springer, 1985.

Kveton JF, Cooper MH: Microsurgical anatomy of the jugular foramen region. Am J Otol 9:109-112, 1988.

Lang J, Heilek E: Anatomische-klinische befunde zur a. pharyngeal ascendens. Anat Anz 156: 177-207, 1984.

Lang J, Kageyama I: Clinical anatomy of the ophthalmic artery and cavernous sinus. In: Samii M, ed. Surgery of the sellar region, vol 2. Springer 145- 148, 1991.

Lang J, Maier R, Schafhauser O: On the postnatal magnification of the foramina rotundum, ovale and spinosum and their topographical changes. Anat Anz 156:351-387, 1984.

Lang J, Tisch-Rottensteiner KF: Uber form und formvarianten der sella turcica. Verh Anat Ges 71: 1279- 1282, 1977.

Lang J: Clinical anatomy of the head. Neurocranium-orbit-craniocervical regions. New York: Springer, 1983.
Lang J: Clinical anatomy of the posterior cranial fossa and its foramina. New York: Thieme, 1991.
Lang J: Structure and postnatal organization of heretofore uninvestigated and infrequent ossifications of the sella turcica region. 99:121-139, 1977.
Lang J: Topographical anatomy of the skull base and adjacent tissues. In: Scheunemann H, Schurmann K, Helms J, eds. Tumors of the skull base. Berlin: de Gruyter, 3-28, 1986.
Lindblom K: A roentgenographic study of the vascular channels of the skull. Acta Radiol 30: 146, 1936.
Maroon JC, Kennerdell JS: Lateral microsurgical approach to intraorbital tumors. J. Neurosurg 44:556-561, 1976.
Ogawa K, Inoue Y, Yamamoto M, Ikeda S, Kanzaki J: Surgical anatomy for the extended middle cranial fossa approach. Acta Otolaryngol Suppl Stockh 487: 41-47, 1991.
Oliviera E, Rhoton AL, Peace D: Microsurgical anatomy of the foramen magnum. Surg Neurol 24:293-352, 1985.
Parisier SC: The middle cranial fossa approach to the internal auditory canal: an anatomic study stressing critical distances between surgical landmarks. Laryngoscope 87(suppl):1-19, 1977.
Paullus WS, Pait TG, Rhoton AL: Microsurgical exposure of the petrous portion of the carotid artery. J Neurosurg 47:713-26, 1977.
Pearson BW, MacKenzie RG, Goodman WS: The anatomical basis of the transantral ligation of the maxillary artery in severe epistaxis. Laryngoscope 79: 969-984, 1969.
Pickrell KL: Reconstructive plastic surgery of the face. In: Walton JH ed. Clinical symposia, vol 20. Canada: Ciba, 1968.
Sekhar LN, Estonillo R: Transtemporal approach to the skull base: an anatomical study. Neurosurgery 19: 799-808, 1986.
Simoes S: Relacoes anatomicas do seio emisario do forame ovale suas implicacoes clinico-chirurgicas. Arq Neuropsiquiatr 31: 1-9, 1973.
Sondheimer FK: Basal foramina and canals. In: Newton TH, Pott DG, eds. Radiology of the skull and brain. The skull. St Louis: CV Mosby, 287-347, 1971.
Whitaker SR, Sprinkle PM, Chou SM: Nasal glioma. Arch Otolaryngol 107:550-554, 1981.

Posterior cranial fossa

The posterior cranial fossa is the largest of the three cranial fossae. It is bounded by the parietal bone, the temporal bone, the occipital bone, and the sphenoid bone.

Anterior Medial Limit

Near the midline, anteriorly, the dorsum sellae of the sphenoid separates the posterior and middle fossae.

Posterior Medial Limit

Inferior and posteriorly, near the midline, the clivus and the basal occipital bone are found.

Anterior Lateral Limit

The superior margin of the petrous part of the temporal bone, up to the apex and the anterior clinoid process, is the point where the cerebellar tentorium attaches to the cerebellum. This represents the anterior and lateral boundaries.

Posterior Lateral Limit

The posterior limit consists of the transverse sinus which runs in the occipital and parietal bones.

MAIN STRUCTURES OF THE POSTERIOR FOSSA FLOOR

Foramen magnum

The foramen magnum is surrounded by occipital bone. The apical ligament of the dens is anterior and lateral to the foramen magnum, while posteriorly the medulla oblongata is contained.

Petro-occipital fissure

The petro-occipital fissure separates the occipital bone from the petrous part of the temporal bone, where the inferior petrous sinus is found.

Jugular foramen

Located at the posterior extremity of the petro-occipital fissure, this foramen is transversed posteriorly by the sigmoid sinus, which continues with the internal jugular vein and anteriorly with nerves IX, X, and XI, from back to front.

The superior part of the foramen is transversed by a septum (see chapter 6, glossopharyngeal nerve). The deepest part of the septum is transversed by the cochlear canaliculus, which contains perilymph.

Hypoglossal canal

The hypoglossal canal is medial to the jugular foramen, between the jugular tubercle above and the occipital condyle below. It is transversed by the hypoglossal nerve and by a meningeal branch of the ascending pharyngeal artery.

Stylomastoid foramen

It is posterior to the root of the styloid process; the facial nerve exit the mastoid through this foramen, together with the stylomastoid artery, and enters in the parotid gland.

Internal auditory canal

The internal auditory canal lies superior to the anterior part of the jugular foramen by approx. 1 cm, in the posterior wall of the petrosal pyramid.

Sigmoid sulcus

The mastoid part of the petrous ridge makes up the lateral wall of the temporal bone. The sigmoid sulcus is found here, and contains the sigmoid sinus.

Internal occipital crest

The internal occipital crest is found medially, behind the foramen magnum. It terminates posteriorly in a ridge, called the internal occipital protuberance. There are furrows on both sides, accommodating the transverse sinus. The crest delineates the cerebellar fossae at its two sides.

Internal auditory canal

The four nerves of the internal auditory canal, visible from the lateral-most fundus, are the following: the superior vestibular nerve, the inferior vestibular nerve, the cochlear nerve, and the facial nerve.

The meatal fundus is divided by an osseous crest, called the falciform or transverse crest. It has a superior and an inferior part.

The superior vestibular nerve is found posteriorly-superiorly in its superior part, while the facial

nerve is found anteriorly-superiorly. An osseous crest, called the vertical crest or Bill's bar, separates the superior vestibular nerve from the facial nerve.
In the inferior part there are the inferior vestibular nerve, the posterior-inferior nerve (singular nerve), and the cochlear nerve in anterior-superior position.
The vestibular nerve then unites in one single trunk below the transverse crest, and runs with and superior to the cochlear nerve to the pons (vestibulo-cochlear nerve) (Fig. 2-4).

Clivus anatomy

The clivus slopes in an anterior-posterior direction. It is formed by the dorsal surface of the dorsum sellae and the endocranial face of the basilar part of the occipital bone.
The sella turgica is bounded anteriorly by an osseous crest with a ridge in the center, the tubercle of the sella. Facing it is a transverse sulcus, the sulcus of the optic chiasma. Here lies the chiasma of the optic nerves. The sulcus extends on both sides to the optic canal. The optic nerve and the ophthalmic artery enter the orbitary cavity via this canal that pass through the inferior orbital fissure. On the superior face of the sphenoid body, anterior to the sulcus of the chiasma, there are two depressions. These are the olfactory grooves, where the olfactory tracts are located.

For surgical purposes, the clivus may be divided into three regions: superior, middle, and inferior (Fig. 2-5).

SUPERIOR CLIVUS
The superior clivus includes the dorsum of the sella and the posterior clinoid processes. It is superior to the exits of the trigeminal and abducens nerves.
Anterior limit: sella turgica and sphenoid bone.
Posterior limit: basilar artery, midbrain.
Lateral limit: intracavernous segment of the carotid arteries and cavernous sinuses.

MIDCLIVUS
The midclivus goes from the emergence of the trigeminal nerve to that of the mixed nerves.
Anterior limit: rhinopharynx.
Posterior limit: basilar artery, vertebrobasilar junction, pons.

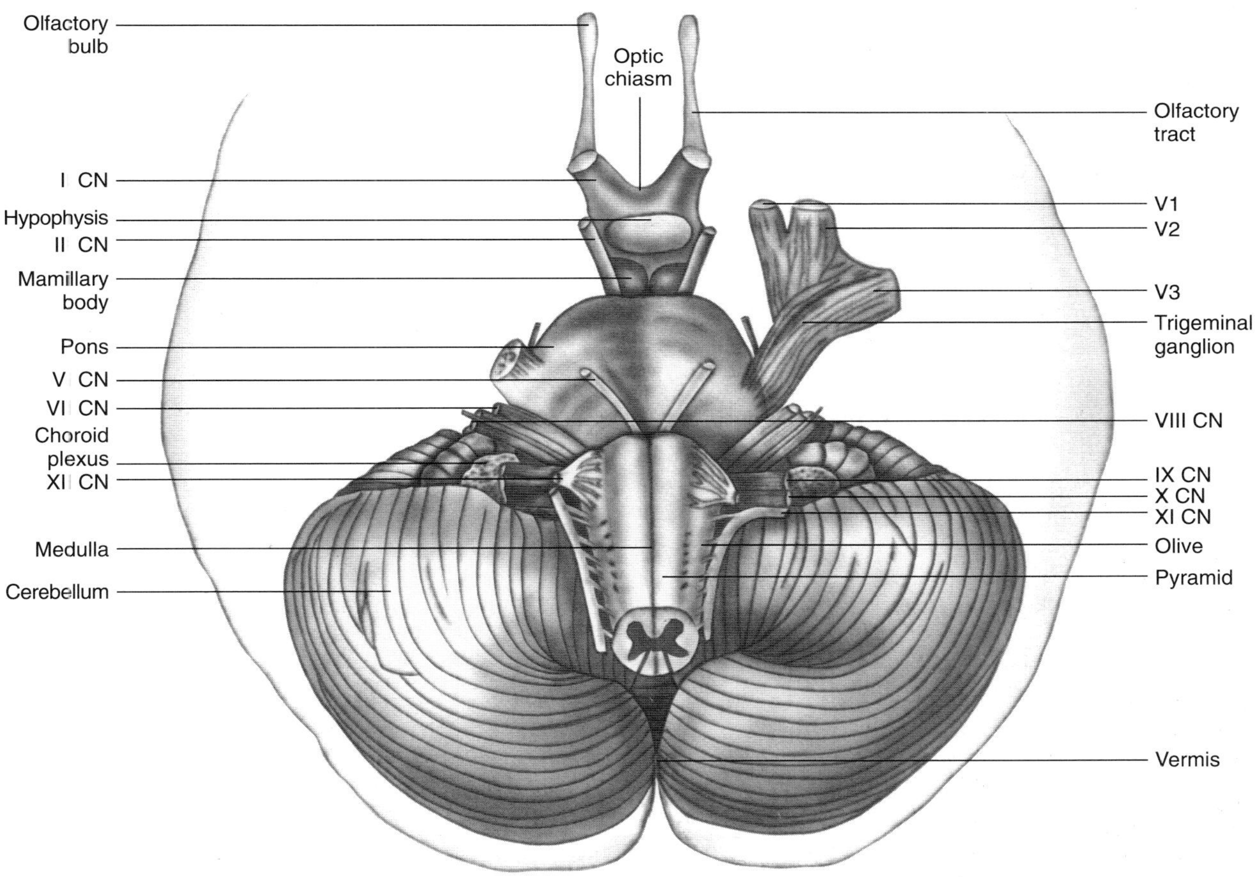

Fig. 2-4. A basal view of the cranial nerves and related structures.

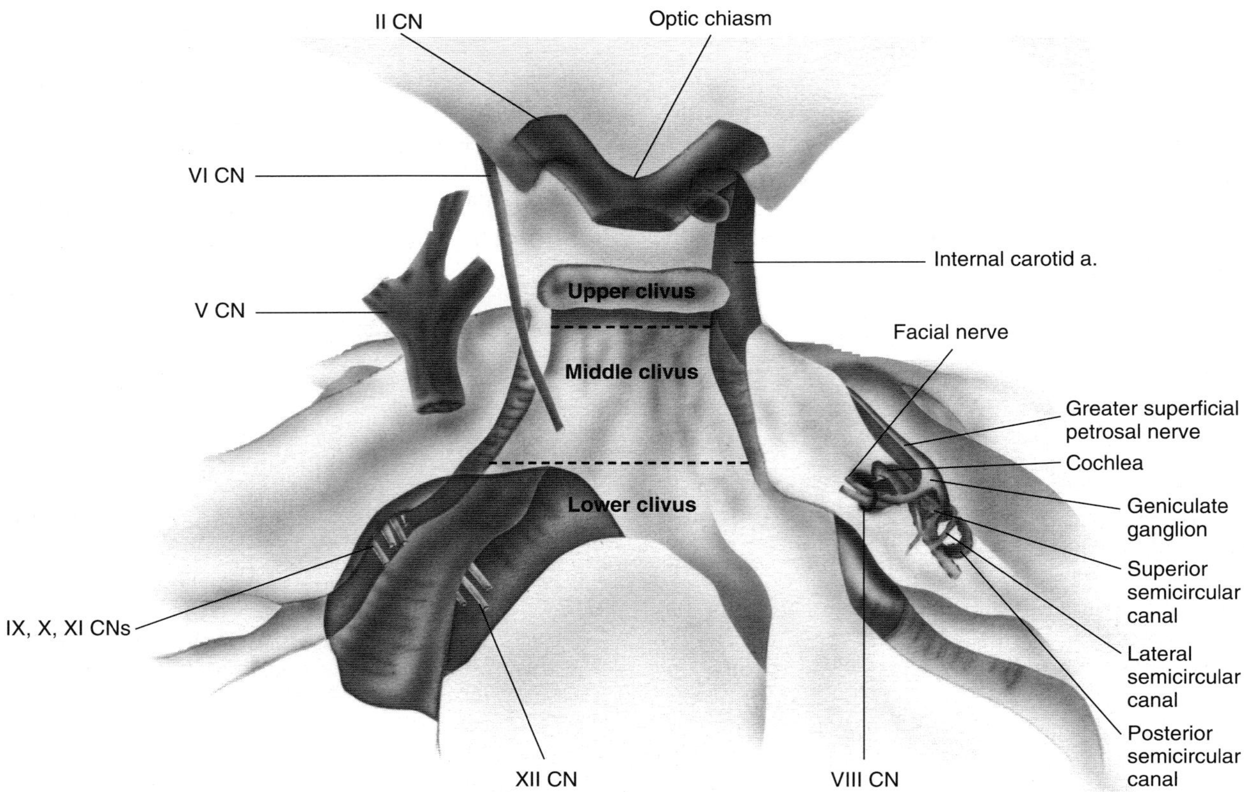

Fig. 2-5. Clivus and related structures.

Lateral limit: Posterior surface of the petrous bone, from the apex to the exits of nerves VII and VIII and the superior petrosal sinuses.

INFERIOR CLIVUS

The inferior clivus goes from the internal auditory meatus to the foramen magnum, the hypoglossal canals and the occipital condyles.
Anterior limit: rhinopharynx.
Posterior limit: vertebral arteries, bulb with its superior junctions, pontine and inferior bulb, spinal bulb.
Lateral limit: lateral sinus and jugular bulb, hypoglossal nerve.

REFERENCES

Arnold G, Lang J: Masse des Schadels, Korrelation von Leitungsbahnen und Beispiele ihrer praktischen Bedeutung. Acta Anat 73:98-108, 1969.

Camins MB, Oppenheim JS: Anatomy and surgical techniques in the suboccipital transmeatal approach to acoustic neuromas. Clin Neurosurg 38: 567-588, 1992.

Gabrielsen TO, Bookstein JJ: Jugular venography by catheter approach from the arm. Radiology 91:378-379, 1968.

Glasscock ME, Woods CI, Jackson CG, et al: Management of bilateral acoustic tumors. Laryngoscope 99:475, 1989.

Hardy DG, Rhoton AL Jr: Microsurgical relationship of the superior cerebellar artery and the trigeminal nerve. J Neurosurg 49: 669-678, 1978.

Howieson J, Norrell H: Angiographic findings in congenital infantile hydrocephalus. Acta Radiol Diagn (Stockh) 9:322-326, 1969.

Hyrtl J: Der Sinus ophthalmo-petrosus. Wien Med Wochenschr 19:291-292, 1862.

Jackler RK, Pitts LH: Selection of surgical approach to acoustic neuroma. Otolaryngol Clin North Am 25: 361-387, 1992.

Jannetta PJ: Arterial compression of the trigeminal nerve at the pons on patients with trigeminal neuralgia. J Neurosurg 26: 159-162, 1967.

Kemink JL, LaRouere MJ, Kileny RP, et al: Hearing preservation following suboccipital removal of acoustic neuromas. Laryngoscope 100:597, 1990.

Kimmel DL: Innervation of spinal dura mater and dura mater of the posterior cranial fossa. Neurology 11: 800-809, 1961.

Lack H: The endocranial equivalents of the Frankfurt plane and the exocranial position of the internal auditory meatus. J Anat 65:96-97, 1930/31.

Lang J Jr, Samii A: Retrosigmoidal approach to the posterior cranial fossa. An anatomical study. Acta Neurochir (Wien) 111:147-153, 1991.

Lang J, Reiter U: Uber die intrazisternale lange der hirnnerven VII-XII. Neurochirurgia (Stuttg);28: 153- 157, 1985.

Lang J, Schaffrath H, Fischer G: Weiters befunde zu den rami diencephalici. Neurochirurgia (Stuttg);30: 103-107, 1987.

Lang J: Clinical anatomy of the posterior cranial fossa and its foramina. New York: Thieme, 1991.

Lang J: Clinical anatomy of the head. ln: Wilson RR, Winstanley DP trans. Neurocranium-orbit-craniocervical regions. Berlin: Springer, 1983.

Lang J: Kollmannsberger A. Beitrag zur Anatomie der Kleinhirnarterien. Gegenbaurs Morphol Jahrb 102: 170-179, 1961.

Mangham CA, Skalabrin TA: Indications for hearing preservation in acoustic tumor surgery. Presented at the Annual

Meeting of the American Neurotology Society, Kona, Hawaii, May 4, 1991.
Mazzoni A: Internal auditory canal arterial relations at the porus acusticus. Ann Otol Rhinol Laryngol 78:797-814, 1969.
Mazzoni A: The subarcuate artery in man. Laryngoscope 80:69-79, 1970.
Mizuno N, Akimoto C, Mochizuki K, Matsuschima R: Experimental studies of efferent fibers in the hypoglossal nerve in the cat: a scanning electron microscopic observation in the lingual mucosa following transsection of the nerve, and a degeneration study with silver impregnation methods. Arch Histol Jpn 35: 99-113, 1973.
Rhoton AL, Kobayashi S, Hollinshead HW: Nervus intermedius. J Neurosurg 29:609-618, 1968.
Rhoton AL: Microsurgical anatomy of the brainstem surface facing an acoustic neuroma. Surg Neurol 25: 326-339, 1986.
Rhoton AL: The suboccipital approach to removal of acoustic neuromas. Otolaryngol Head Neck Surg 1: 313-333, 1979.
Ring A, Waddington M: Intraluminal diameters of the intracranial arteries. Vasc Surg 1/3:137-151, 1967.
Saleh E, Naguib M, Aristegui M, Cokkeser Y, Russo A, Sanna M: Surgical anatomy of the jugular foramen area. In: Mazzoni A, Sanna M, eds. Skull base surgery Update, 1. Amsterdam: Kugler, 1995 pp. 3-8.
Saleh E, Naguib M, Aristegui M, Cokkeser Y, Sanna M: The lower skull base: anatomical study with surgical implications. Ann Otol Rhinol Laryngol 104:57-61, 1995.
Saleh E, Taibah A, Achilli V, Aristegui M, Mazzoni A, Sanna M: Posterior fossa meningioma: surgical strategy. Skull Base Surg 4:209-219, 1994.
Silverstein H, Morrell H, Smouha E, Jones R: Combined retrolab-retrosigmoid vestibular neurectomy. An evolution in approach. Am J Otol 10: 166-169, 1989.
Silverstein H, Norrell H, Rosenberg S: An evolution of approach in vestibular neurectomy. Otolaryngol Head Neck Surg 102: 374-381, 1990.
Silverstein H, Norrell H, Rosenberg S: The resurrection of vestibular neurectomy: A 10-year experience with 115 cases. J Neurosurg 72: 533-539,1990.
Silverstein H, Norrell H, Smouha E, Jones R: Combined retrolab-retrosigmoid vestibular neurectomy: An evolution in approach. Am J Otol 10: 166-169, 1989.
Silverstein H, Rosenberg S: Vestibular neurectomy via the posterior fossa. In Silverstein H, Rosenberg S (eds): Surgical techniques of the temporal bone and skull base. Philadelphia, Lea & Febiger, 1992, pp 175-194.
Silverstein H, Wanamaker H, Flanzer J, Rosenberg S: Vestibular neurectomy in the USA 1990. Am J Otol 13: 23-30, 1992.
Silverstein H: Transmeatal labyrinthectomy with and without cochleovestibular neurectomy. Laryngoscope 86: 1777-1791, 1976.
Stopford JSB: The arteries of the pons and medulla oblongata. J Anat Physiol 50:131-164, 1916.
Sunderland S: Arterial relations of the internal auditory meatus. Brain 1945;68:23-27.
Sunderland S: Neurovascular relations and anomalies at the base of the brain. J Neurol Neurosurg Psychiatry 11 :243-257, 1948.
Takahashi M: Atlas of vertebral angiography. Berlin: Urban & Schwarzenberg/Tokyo: Igaku Shoin Ltd, 1974.
Tarlov IM: Structure of the nerve root. I. Nature of the junction between the central and peripheral nervous system. Arch Neurol Psychiatry 37:555-583, 1937.
Tarlov IM: Structure of the nerve root. II. Differentiation of sensory from motor roots; observations on identification of function in roots of mixed cranial nerves. Arch Neurol Psychiatry; 37:1338-1355, 1937.

The inferior skull base

The anterior part of the inferior skull base is formed by the bony palate. Between the posterior margin of the hard palate and the anterior limit of the occipital orifice there are the choanae. These are the posterior apertures of the nasal cavities, separated by the posterior margin of the vomer.
Behind the third molar tooth, the medial and lateral pterygoid plates of the pterygoid process border the pterygoid fossa. The lateral surface of the lateral pterygoid plate is the medial limit of the infratemporal fossa.

Infratemporal fossa

The lateral part of the middle fossa floor, or the greater wing of the sphenoid bone, forms the roof of the infratemporal fossa, comprised between the orbitary fissure anteriorly, the lateral pterygoid lamina laterally, and the temporo-mandibular articulation posteriorly.
The inferior orbitary fissure connects the infratemporal fossa with the orbitary cavity. The medial part of this fissure continues in another fissure, found between the maxillary tuberosity and the pterygoid process, called the sphenomaxillary fissure, which leads to the pterygopalatine fossa.
In the infratemporal fossa vessels and nerves are contained: the maxillary artery, the mandibular nerve (V3) with its posterior branch (auricolotemporal nerve), the chorda tympani nerve, the deep temporal nerves, the masseter nerve, the buccal nerve, the lingual nerve and the inferior alveolar nerves. These explains symptoms of infratemporal fossa tumors: deafness, anesthesia of the mandibular nerve distribution, external auditory canal pain.

Pterygopalatine fossa

This structure is bounded anteriorly by the maxillary tuberosity, medially by the perpendicular lamina of the palatine bone, and posteriorly by the pterygoid process.
The pterygopalatine ganglion is contained in this fossa, suspended from the maxillary branch of V. Some veins and one-third of the internal maxillary artery run here. The foramen rotundum opens posteriorly into the fossa.
Behind and lateral to the pterygopalatine fossa is the squamous part of the temporal bone. Behind the squama is the tympanic part of the temporal bone and the tegmen tympani.
Posterior and lateral is the mandibular fossa, where the mandibular condyle is articulated. Behind the mandibular fossa there is the tympanic part of the petrous ridge, connected to the squamous part by the tympano-squamous suture.

The styloid process is an osseous cylinder anterior and medial to the stylomastoid foramen and the tip of the mastoid.
The mastoid is located posteriorly.

Inferior skull base foramina
See middle fossa anatomy.

MUSCLES OF THE INFERIOR SKULL BASE

Lateral pterygoid muscle
This muscle transverses the infratemporal fossa to reach the mandibular cranium. It is made up of two parts. The smaller (posterior) part originates in the infratemporal crest and the infratemporal surface of the greater wing of the sphenoid. The inferior part originates in the lateral lamina of the pterygoid process. These two fasciae join running lateral and posterior to reach the pterygoid depression of the mandibular condyle and the capsule of the mandibular articulation.
The muscle contraction from both sides causes the mandible to slide forward, with the head of the mandible rotating on the articulated disk.
Temporalis muscle
The temporalis muscle occupies the temporal fossa and descends into the infratemporal fossa. All the fibers converge in a tendon attached to the edge and to the medial face of the coronal process of the mandible.
It is covered by the temporal fascia in the temporal fossa, and adheres to the osseous part.
It moves in synergy with the masseter and internal pterygoid muscles, elevating the mandible. It has the most effective action of all these muscles.
Masseter muscle
The superficial layer originates in the anterior two-thirds of the inferior margin of the zygomatic arch, and goes toward the lateral face of the mandibular angle. The deep layer is covered by the superficial layer.
The parotid gland is near the posterior margin of the muscle. The parotid-masseteric fascia covers the surface of the parotid gland and the masseter muscle.
Medial pterygoid muscle
The medial pterygoid muscle originates in the pterygoid fossa and the pyramidal process of the palatine bone. Some fasciae come from the maxillary tuberosity.
Levator veli palatini muscle
This muscle originates anterior to the external aperture of the carotid canal, the inferior face of the temporal pyramid, and the lateral lamina of the tubaric cartilage. It attaches to the lower part of the palatine aponeurosis. It elevates the soft palate and constricts the pharyngeal orifice of the auditory tube.
Tensor veli palatini muscle
This muscle originates in the greater wing of the sphenoid bone, the pterygoid process, and the cartilage of the auditory canal. It proceeds to the posterior margin of the horizontal part of the palatine bone.
It is the tensor of the soft palate and dilatator of the tubaric orifice.
Uvula muscle
This muscle originates near the posterior nasal spine and terminates thinning at the apex of the uvula.

NERVES OF THE INFERIOR SKULL BASE

The sympathetic trunk is immersed in the prevertebral cervical fascia.
The superior cervical ganglion of the sympathetic trunk, located between the first and third cervical vertebrae, is supplied by branches of the ascending pharyngeal artery.
The ventral branches of the cervical nerves transverse the deep cervical fascia. Branches of the superior cervical ganglion and the first (C1) and second (C2) cervical nerves go to the hypoglossal nerve in front of the atlas.
At the jugular foramen, the IX-X-XI-XII cranial nerves run between the internal carotid artery and the internal jugular vein.
The pathways of nerves V, VII, VIII, IX, X, XI, XII have anatomical relationships with the inferior skull base (see chapter 6).

VEINS OF THE INFERIOR SKULL BASE

The internal jugular vein courses in the parapharyngeal space. The bulb is lateral to the margin of the jugular foramen, and extends upward from there. When the bulb is very high, it may reach the ampulla of the lateral canal, in contact with the IAC (if lateral). If medial, it may touch the hypotympanum. A high jugular bulb may reduce the surgical field in the translabyrinthine approach (see Fig. 1-4).

REFERENCES

Farrior JB: Infra-temporal approach to skull base for glomus tumors: anatomic considerations. Ann Otol Rhinol Laryngol 93: 616-622, 1984.
Hakuba A, Hashi K, Fujotani K, Ikuno H, Nakamura T, Inoue Y: Jugular foramen neurinomas. Surg Neurol 11: 83 - 94, 1984.
Schwaber MK, Netterville JL, Maciunas R: Microsurgical anatomy of the lower skull base: a morphometric analysis. Am J Otol 11:401-405, 1990.
Wackym PA, Blackwell KE: Abnormalities of the craniovertebral junction. In: Jackler RK, Brackmann DE, eds. Neuro-Otology. Baltimore: Mosby, 1993:1203-31.

3

Anatomy of cisterns, meninges, venous sinuses and arteries

THE CISTERNS

Wherever the brain and the cranial bone are not in close contact with each other, the arachnoid is separated from the pia mater by a space that forms the subarachnoid cisterns.
The cisterns connect the subarachnoid spaces. The cephalorachidian fluid contained in the spaces between the gyri flows to these great anfractuosities of the brain.

Cistern of the chiasma

This cistern is found between the chiasma and the rostrum of the corpus callosum. Anteriorly it receives the cistern of the corpus callosum.

Interpeduncular cistern

This cistern is located between the chiasma and the superior limit of the pons and communicates with the cistern with the middle and lateral faces of the pons. Bilaterally it touches the cistern of the great cerebral vein.

Cistern of the great cerebral vein

This cistern is found between the cerebellum and the splenium of the corpus callosum. It is transversed by the great cerebral vein.

Cerebellomedullary cistern

This is the largest cistern, also called the cisterna magna. It occupies the cerebellomedullary scissure and is located between the inferior side of the cerebellum and the dorsal face of the bulb. It communicates with the IVth ventricle through the medial foramen (of Magendie) and the lateral foramen (of Luschka).

Pontine cistern

This cistern is located on the anterior face of the pons. It is continuous behind with the cerebellomedullary cistern, anteriorly with the interpeduncolary cistern and below with the spinal subarachnoid space. The basilar artery and the venous vessels of the basilar plexus run through it.

Cerebellopontine cistern

This cistern is lateral to the middle cistern of the pons and reaches the surface of the cerebellum. It continues from here with the subarachnoid spaces around the bulb and the subarachnoid space of the brainstem. The trigeminal, facial and acoustic nerves run through this cistern.

Sylvian cistern

The sylvian cistern is located in the scissure of Sylvius. The sylvian artery runs inside.

ENCEPHALIC MENINGES

The cranial dura mater adheres to the periosteum covering the internal surface of the cranial cavity. The venous sinuses are located in the dura mater. The internal surface of the dura mater faces the arachnoid.
The venous sinuses are contained within the thickness of the dura mater.
Septums leave the internal surface of the dura. These are called tentoria or tents if they are horizontal, and falx if they are vertical.

Falx cerebri

This is a septum of dura mater extended sagittally on the midline of the cranium, from the frontal bone to the occipital bone. Its superior (convex) margin adheres to the cranial vault and terminates posterior to the level of the internal occipital protruberance. The inferior margin is concave, and the anterior extremity reaches the crista galli process of the ethmoid, while the posterior extremity adheres to the tentorium of the cerebellum for its entire length. The lateral faces, in the intrahemispheric fissure, are in contact with the medial faces of the two hemispheres. The superior longitudinal sinus runs within the falx cerebri. The free and delicate inferior margin approaches the corpus callosum and duplicates to accommodate the inferior longitudinal sinus. The straight sinus is inside the base.

Falx cerebelli
This is a median septum which goes from the internal occipital protruberance to the posterior margin of the occipital foramen. The anterior margin goes toward the vermis superior and the hilum of the cerebellum. The posterior margin, attached to the internal occipital crest, contains the occipital venous sinus.

Cerebellar tentorium
This separates the occipital lobes (superior) from the cerebellar hemispheres below. It has a semilunar shape, concave in the front.
The falx cerebri attaches to its superior face medially. Its inferior face faces the vermis and the cerebellar hemispheres.
The anterior margin is concave, and lies on the apex of the petrous ridge. It attaches to the anterior clinoid process and the oculomotor nerve passes in the groove between them. The posterior margin adheres to the internal occipital protruberance, the transverses sulcus of the occipital bone and the superior margin of the petrous ridge. In a duplication it accommodates the transverse sinus anteriorly and the superior petrosal sinus posteriorly.
Near the petrous apex the lower layer of the tentorium forms a recess, the Meckel's cave, containing the roots and ganglion of the trigeminal nerve.

Diaphragm of the sella
This is a transverse septum which proceeds from the sulcus of the optic chiasma to the anterior and posterior clinoid processes, and to the dorsum of the sella turgica. On the dorsum of the sella the dura mater divides into two laminae. The deep lamina covers the hypophyseal fossa, and its sides are contiguous to the wall of the cavernous sinus. The superficial lamina makes up the diaphragm of the sella. The aperture at its center is called the diaphragmatic foramen. The hypophyseal peduncle passes through here. It is transversed by the intercavernous sinus, which connects the cavernous sinuses from both sides.

Olfactory tent
There is a dural septum in the olfactory fossa called the olfactory bulb tent. It lies over the cribriform plate of the ethmoid and covers the corresponding olfactory bulb.

VENOUS SINUSES OF THE DURA

These are venous canals running in the dura mater. They carry blood to the cerebral veins. The venous flow comes about by means of the internal jugular vein, and partially by the emissary veins (Figs. 3-1, 3-2, 3-3).

Superior sagittal sinus
This sinus lies in the fixed margin of the encephalic falx, from the blind foramen of the frontal bone to the confluent of the sinuses at the internal occipital protruberance. It originates in the veins of the foramen caecum, and receives the superior cerebral veins, the diploic veins, and the meningeal veins. It emits the parietal emissary vein.

Inferior sagittal sinus
This sinus begins as a cul-de-sac and runs in the free edge of the encephalic falx, where it reaches the anterior edge of the rectus sinus. It receives veins from the falx and corpus callosum.

Straight sinus
This sinus receives the inferior sagittal sinus anteriorly, and runs along the line of junction of the encephalic falx with the cerebellar tentorium. It then opens posteriorly into the transverse sinus or in the confluent of the sinuses. Other affluents are the great cerebral vein of Galenus and the veins of the tentorium.

Occipital sinus
This sinus originates in the transverse sinus, and runs in the fixed margin of the falx cerebelli; it is occasionally paired. Here it divides into two branches, each of which encircles the great occipital foramen and terminates at the inferior edge of the homolateral transverse sinus. The occipital sinus receives dural, diploic, and cerebellar veins.

Transverse sinuses.
They originate at the internal occipital protuberance, the left continuous with the straight sinus, the right, which is the larger, with the superior sagittal sinus. Each runs in the transverse sulcus of the occipital and parietal bones and turns down as a sigmoid sinus. The transverse sinus receives inferior cerebral veins and cerebellar veins. Where the transverse sinuses continue as sigmoid sinuses, receive the superior petrosal sinus. They emit the occipital emissary vein.

Sigmoid sinuses
The sigmoid sinus runs in the sigmoid sulcus of the temporal bone, and emits the mastoid emissary vein posteriorly. It then reaches the jugular

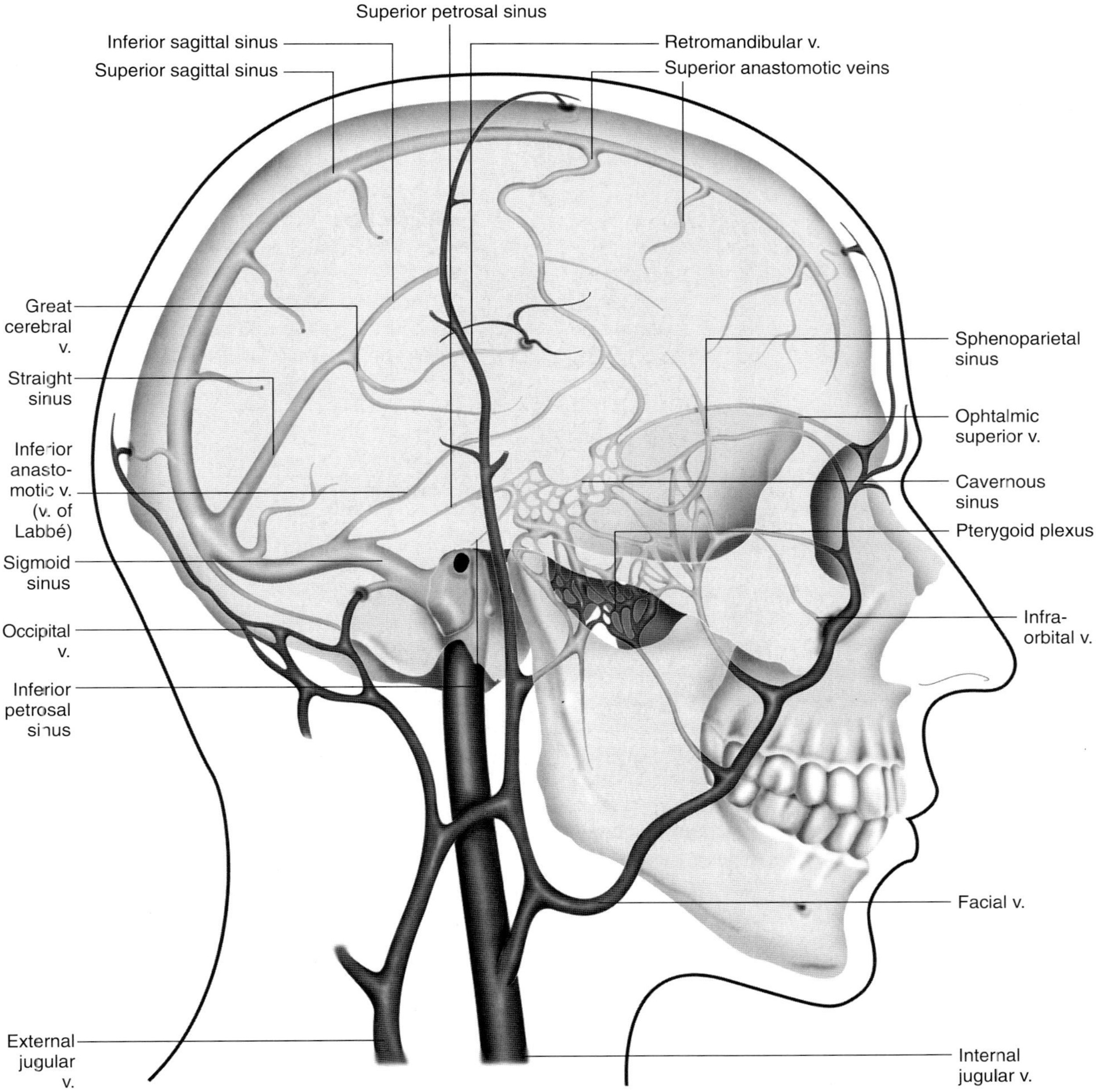

Fig. 3-1. Venous relationship in the head. Adapted from Ferner-Kautzky.

foramen and continues with the jugular bulb and the internal jugular vein.

ANATOMY OF THE ARTERIES

EXTERNAL CAROTID ARTERY

The external carotid artery originates from the common carotid, which divides at the level of the superior margin of the thyroid cartilage.

It ascends vertically to the mandibular angle, where it proceeds outward, then encounters the internal carotid and proceeds laterally to it.

It straightens, then curves with a lateral and posterior convexity until it divides into its terminal branches, the superficial temporal artery and the internal maxillary artery.

This artery also supplies collateral branches. From bottom to top, these are: the superior thyroid, lingual, occipital, pharyngeal-meningeal, external maxillary, posterior auricular, and parotid arteries.

Superficial temporal artery

The superficial temporal artery is the branch dividing the lateral and superficial external carotid (ECA). It originates in the ECA approx. 4 cm

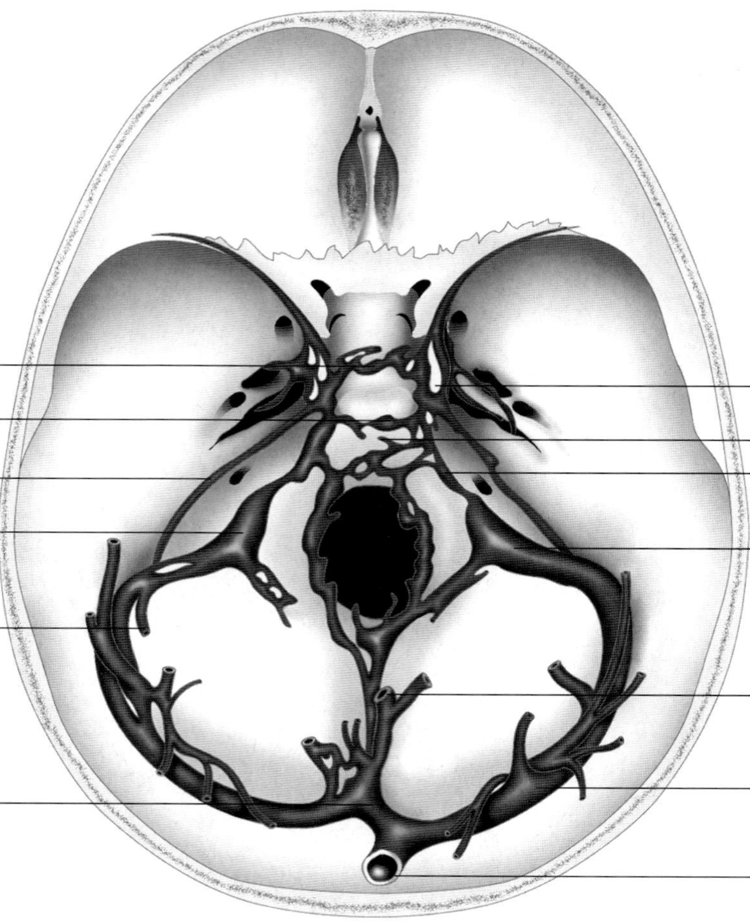

Fig. 3-2. Skull base: venous sinuses.

from the mandibular angle. It courses upward, parallel to the ECA, and passes before the tragus on the posterior root of the zygomatic process. It terminates by branching into the soft tissues of the temporalis region (Fig. 3-4).

Internal maxillary artery

The internal maxillary artery originates 4 cm above the mandibular angle. It transverses the infratemporal fossa and the pterygopalatine fossa where it terminates, at the fundus. It then continues with the sphenopalatine artery.

First (or retromandibular) part. The artery courses behind the mandible and sends branches to the tympanic membrane and the following arteries: deep auricular, anterior tympanic, middle meningeal and branches of the tympanic membrane arteries.

Second (or pterygoid) part. The pterygoid part courses on the lateral or medial face of the external pterygoid muscle. It encounters the lingual nerve and then, with the buccal nerve, passes between the two extremities of the external pterygoid muscle.

Third (pterygopalatine) part. The third part passes through the sphenopalatine fissure and courses in the pterygopalatine fossa to the sphenopalatine foramen, where it ends. Its collateral branches are the deep anterior temporal, the posterior-superior alveolar, the infraorbital, the greater palatine, and the sphenopalatine arteries.

INTERNAL CAROTID ARTERY

The internal carotid artery (ICA) originates at the bifurcation of the common carotid. It may be divided into four tracts: the cervical, petrous, cavernous, and cerebral tracts.

Cervical tract

The cervical tract ascends in the neck. The transverse processes of the first three cervical vertebrae are posterior. Anterior and lateral is the external carotid artery. It is medial to the parotid gland, the sternocleidomastoid muscle, and the digastric and styloid muscles.

The vagus nerve and the internal jugular vein run laterally.

The ICA rests on the posterior wall of the pharynx medially, with the interposition of fat, con-

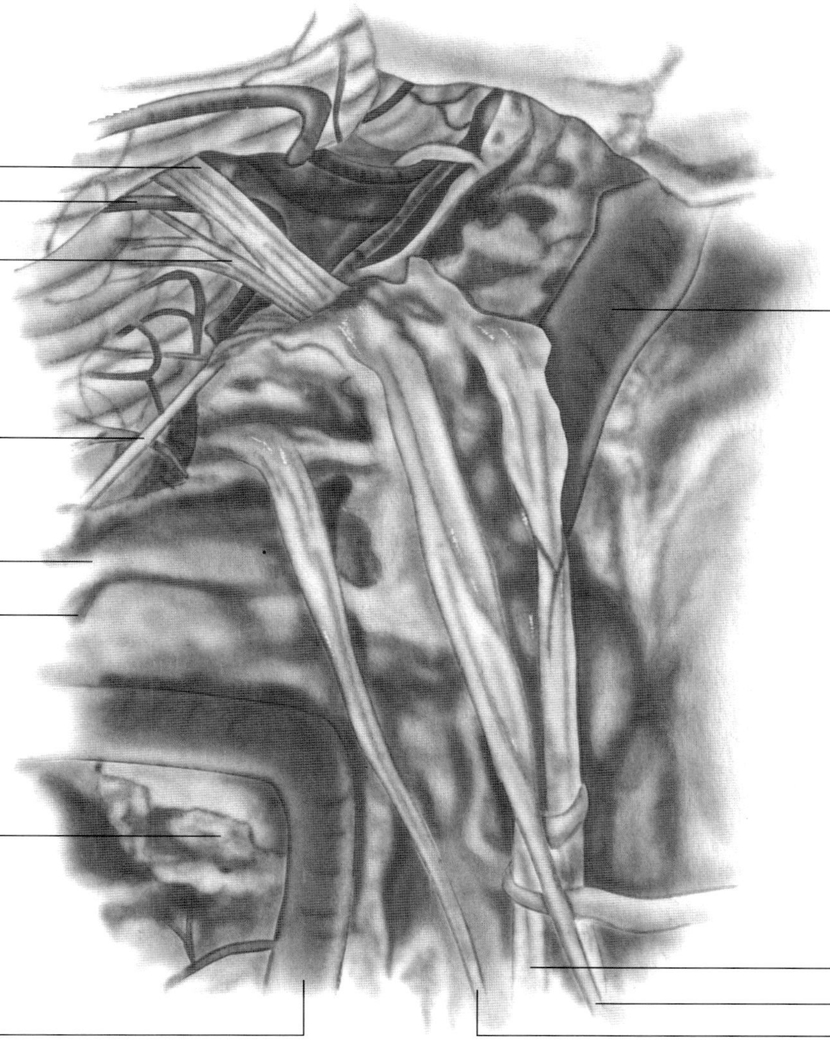

Fig. 3-3. Lateral view of opened jugular foramen and neuro-vascular relationship. Adapted from Koos.

nective tissue, the superior laryngeal nerve, and the ascending pharyngeal artery and vein.

Upon reaching the skull base, it enters the carotid canal. Posteriorly, it leaves the internal jugular vein. Between the two vessels, the following cranial nerves are found (from front to back): IX, X, and XI. Nerve XII and the superior root of the cervical loop run under the digastric muscle, superior to the artery.

Petrous tract

The petrosal carotid artery enters the inferior orifice of the carotid canal in this canal, ascending vertically briefly. Laterally, the basal turn of the cochlea is contiguous, and separated from the artery by 1-2 mm of bone. The artery then curves anteriorly-medially and becomes horizontal. Inside the canal, it is surrounded by the carotid plexus of the sympathetic nerve and by several veins. These veins (the internal carotid venous plexus) communicate with the cavernous sinus above. The eustachian tube runs above. Near the petrous apex, this artery is contiguous to the middle meningeal artery and the semilunar ganglion, which rests on the superior wall of the canal.

The artery exits at the level of the petrous apex and takes a vertical course towards the posterior clinoid process. It then enters the cavernous sinus beside the lateral wall of the sphenoid sinus. Here it runs medial to the oculomotor nerve, the abducens nerve, and the trochlear and ophthalmic branches of the trigeminal nerve.

It ascends medial to the anterior clinoid process, crosses the dura, courses on the roof of the sphenoid, and becomes the cerebral tract.

Cerebral tract

The artery takes a retrograde path, and passes between the optic (II) and oculomotor (III) nerves. It then reaches the anterior perforated substance and divides into the anterior and middle cerebral arteries.

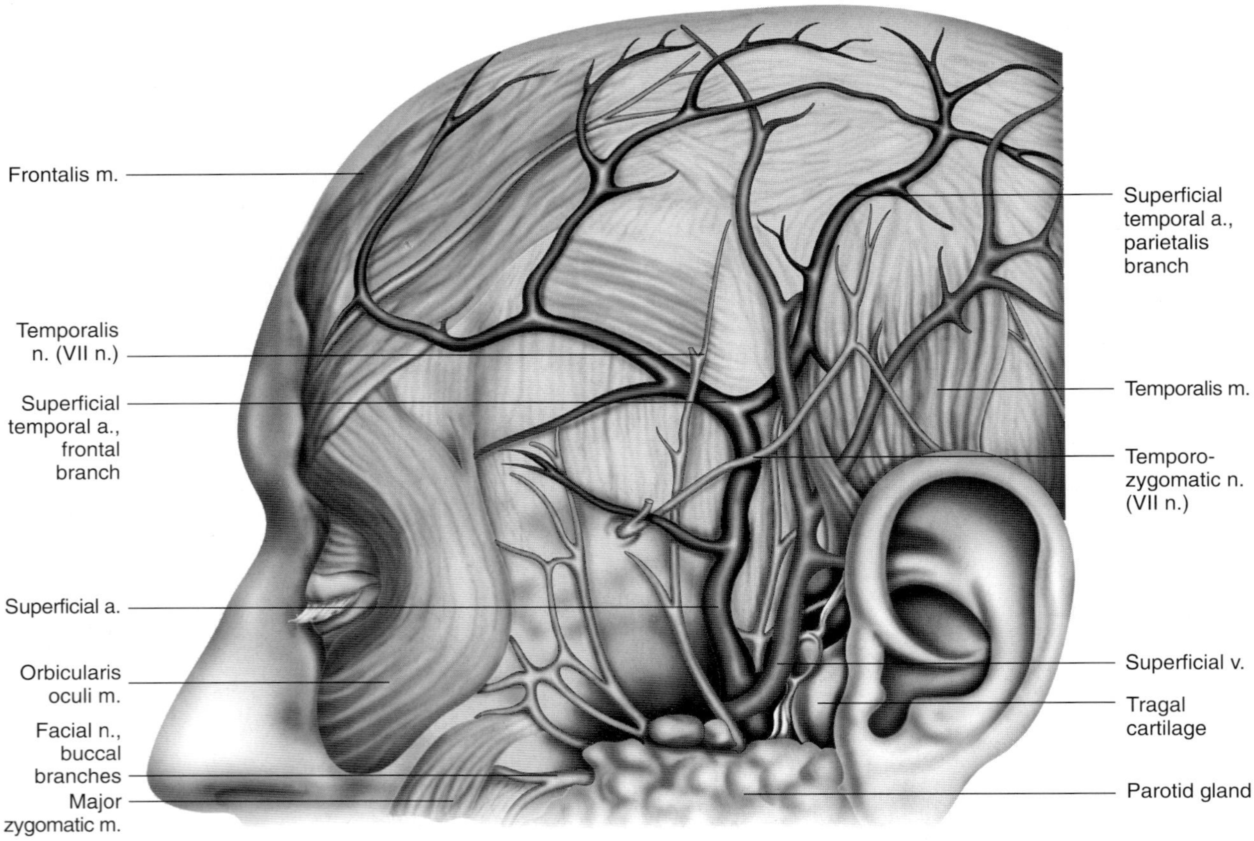

Fig. 3-4. Vascularization of the left temporal region. (Adapted from Sobotta's anatomy).

BRANCHES OF THE INTERNAL CAROTID ARTERY

Cervical tract: No branches.

Petrous tract:

- *Carotico-tympanic branch*: This branch transverses the carotid canal and enters the tympanic cavity. Here it anastomoses with the stylomastoid artery and the tympanic branch of the maxillary artery. It may be ectatic in tympanojugular glomi.
- *Pterygoid (vidian) branch*: This branch enters the pterygoid canal with the pterygoid nerve. It anastomoses with a branch of the sphenopalatine artery.

Cavernous tract

- *Cavernous branches*: These branches carry blood to the walls of the inferior petrosal sinus, the cavernous sinus, and the trigeminal ganglion.
- *Superior hypophyseal artery*: This artery supplies blood to the optic chiasma and the anterior lobe of the hypophysis, which it then anastomoses with the contralateral artery.
- *Meningeal branch*: The meningeal branch supplies blood to the dura mater and the bone of the anterior cranial fossa.

Cerebral tract

- *Ophthalmic artery*: The ophthalmic artery originates in the internal carotid artery at its exit from the cavernous sinus. It crosses the optic canal inferiorly and the optic nerve laterally, and enters the orbit lateral to the optic nerve and medial to the oculomotor and trochlear nerves. It then passes above the optic nerve and divides into two branches, the supratrochlear and the branch of the nasal dorsum. Branches of the ophthalmic artery are the following: central artery of the retina, lacrimal artery, long and short posterior ciliary arteries, long and short anterior ciliary arteries, muscular arteries, lateral palpebral arteries, posterior and anterior ethmoid arteries, the meningeal branch, the medial palpebral arteries, the supratrochlear artery, the artery of the nasal dorsum.
- *Anterior cerebral artery*: This is a terminal branch. It begins medial to the bifurcation of the internal carotid artery, supraclinoid. Posteriorly it is connected to another cerebral artery anterior to the communicating anterior artery. It courses in the longitudinal cerebral fissure, surrounds the genu of the corpus callosum and anastomoses with the posterior cerebral artery. It supplies the anterior surface of the brainstem, with branches called: central, cortical, orbital, frontal, and parietal.
- *Middle cerebral artery*: This is a terminal branch. It begins at the supraclinoid carotic

branch, beside the optic chiasma. It passes anterior to the anterior perforated substance and enters the lateral sylvian fissure where it divides into collateral branches: central, parietal, cortical, and temporal. The lateral and medial lenticulostriated arteries depart from the superior surface of the artery. It supplies the lateral surface of the cerebral hemisphere.

- *Posterior communicating artery*: This artery runs in a retrograde course from the middle cerebral artery to the posterior cerebral artery (a branch of the basilar artery). Its secondary branches supply the optic tract, the optic chiasma, the medial surface of the thalamus, and the walls of the third ventricle.
- *Choroid artery*: This artery originates near the internal carotid and takes a retrograde pathway to the inferior horn of the lateral ventricle, terminating in the choroid plexus. Its branches supply the geniculate body, the globus pallidus, the radiations and the optic tract, the fimbria, and the hippocampus.

VERTEBRAL ARTERY

Prevertebral tract

The prevertebral tract exits the subclavian artery and courses between the long muscles of the neck and the anterior scalene muscles. It enters the transverse foramen of the VIth cervical vertebra.
Posteriorly it relates to the cervicothoracic ganglion and the ventral branches of the cervical nerves VII and VIII.
Anteriorly it relates to the common carotid, the vertebral, and inferior thyroid arteries, and to the left it relates to the thoracic duct.

Transverse tract

The transverse tract courses in the intervertebral foramen to C3, and to the intravertebral space between C3 and C2. It is accompanied by a branch of the cervicothoracic sympathetic plexus and by veins which flow into the vertebral vein below.

Third tract

The third tract goes from the transverse foramen of C2 to the dura of the posterior fossa. It crosses the transverse foramen of the atlas, skirts the body of the atlas posteriorly, and perforates the posterior atlantooccipital membrane and the dura mater. It then penetrates the endocranium, passing between the posterior arch of the atlas and the occipital bone.

Fourth tract

The fourth tract courses lateral to the medulla oblongata and then unites with the contralateral artery, on its ventral face. At the level of the bulbopontine sulcus, the two vessels unite to form the basilar artery (Fig. 3-5).

COLLATERAL BRANCHES OF THE VERTEBRAL ARTERY

Cervical branches

- *Spinal branches*: These cross the intervertebral orificium.
- *Muscular branches*: These supply the prevertebral muscles.

Endocranial branches

- *Meningeal branches*: These are for the dura mater of the posterior fossa.
- *Posterior spinal artery*: This artery descends along the lateral margin of the brainstem in two branches, one anterior and the other posterior to the roots of the cranial nerves.
- *Anterior spinal artery*: This artery descends on the anterior surface of the medulla. It unites with the contralateral artery at the level of the bulbar olive, forming a single trunk. This trunk occupies the anterior median fissure of the brainstem.
- *Posterior inferior cerebellar artery*: This artery originates at the level of the bulbar olive. It ascends on the lateral surface of the bulb, passing between the roots of nerves XII and IX. It encounters the inferior cerebellar peduncle at the inferior margin of the pons, where it divides into a lateral and a medial branch. The lateral branch supplies the inferior face of the cerebellar hemisphere and its lateral margin. The medial branch primarily supplies the cerebellar vermis and runs between it and the cerebellar hemisphere.

BASILAR ARTERY

The basilar artery is formed by the union of the two vertebral arteries (Fig. 3-6). It goes from the bulbopontine sulcus to the superior margin of the pons. It courses on the ventral surface of the pons, in the basilar sulcus and terminates by dividing into the two posterior cerebral arteries (Fig. 3-7).
Its collateral branches are as follows:

- *Pontine branches*, for the pons.

Internal auditory (labyrinthine) artery: This artery penetrates the internal auditory canal and supplies the membranous labyrinth with its three branches: the cochlear, cochleovestibular, and vestibular arteries.

- *Anteriorinferior cerebellar artery* (see chapter 28).
- *Superior cerebellar artery* (see chapters 28; 38).
- *Posterior cerebral artery*: Frequently double, each of these arteries courses laterally, parallel to the superior cerebellar artery, and receives the communicating posterior artery. It skirts the cerebral peduncle, courses between the occipital and temporal lobes, and terminates near the cuneus, becoming a calcarine artery. Collateral branches are: cortical branches for the temporal

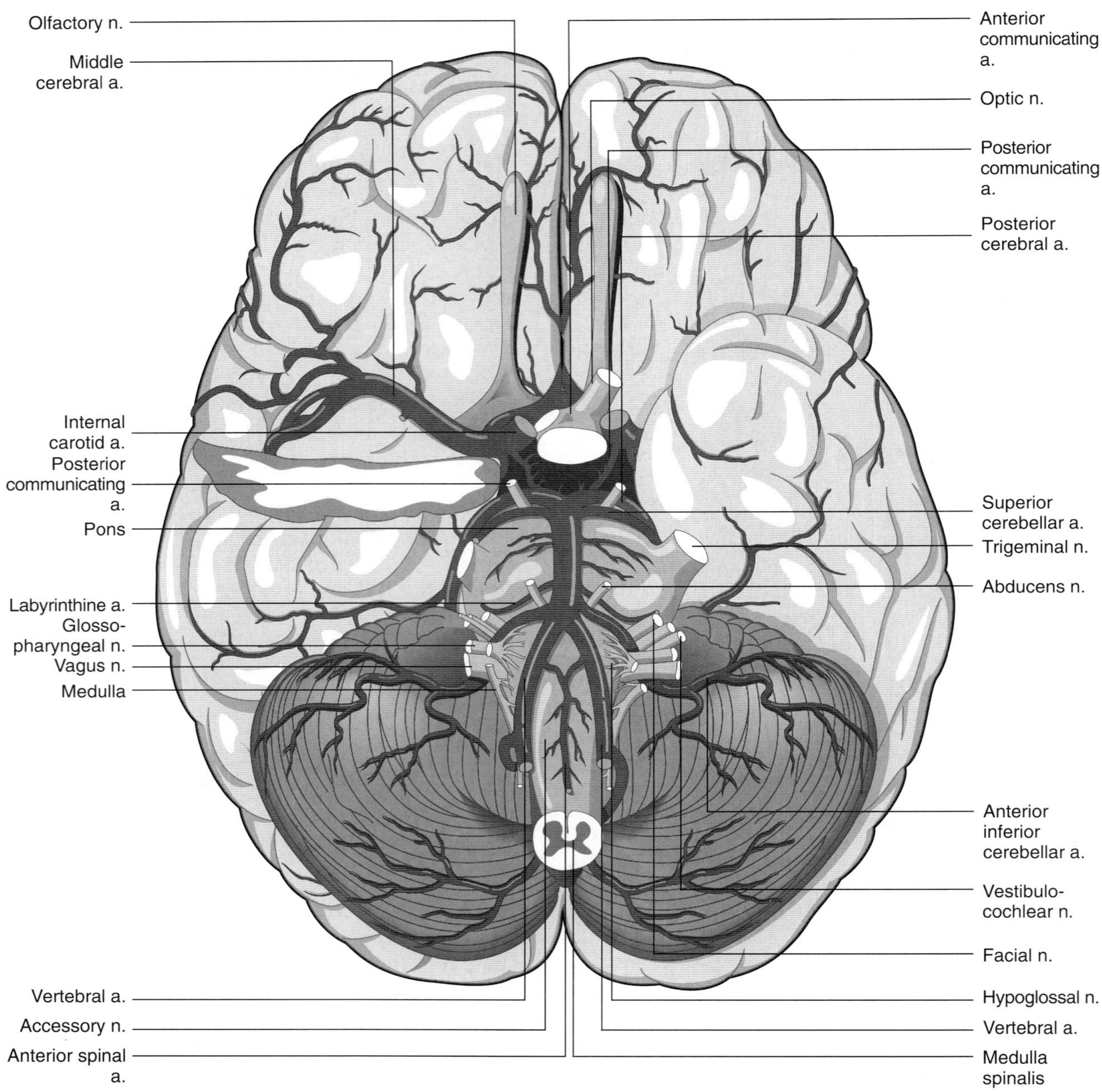

Fig. 3-5. Neurovascular relationship on the brain. Basal view.

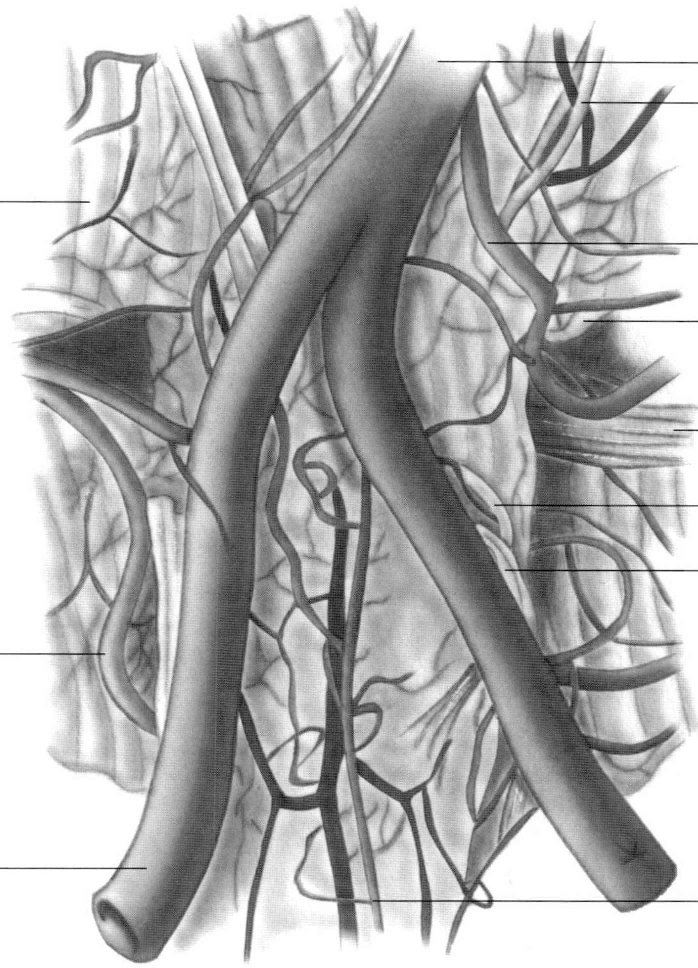

Fig. 3-6. The vertebrobasilar junction. Basal view.

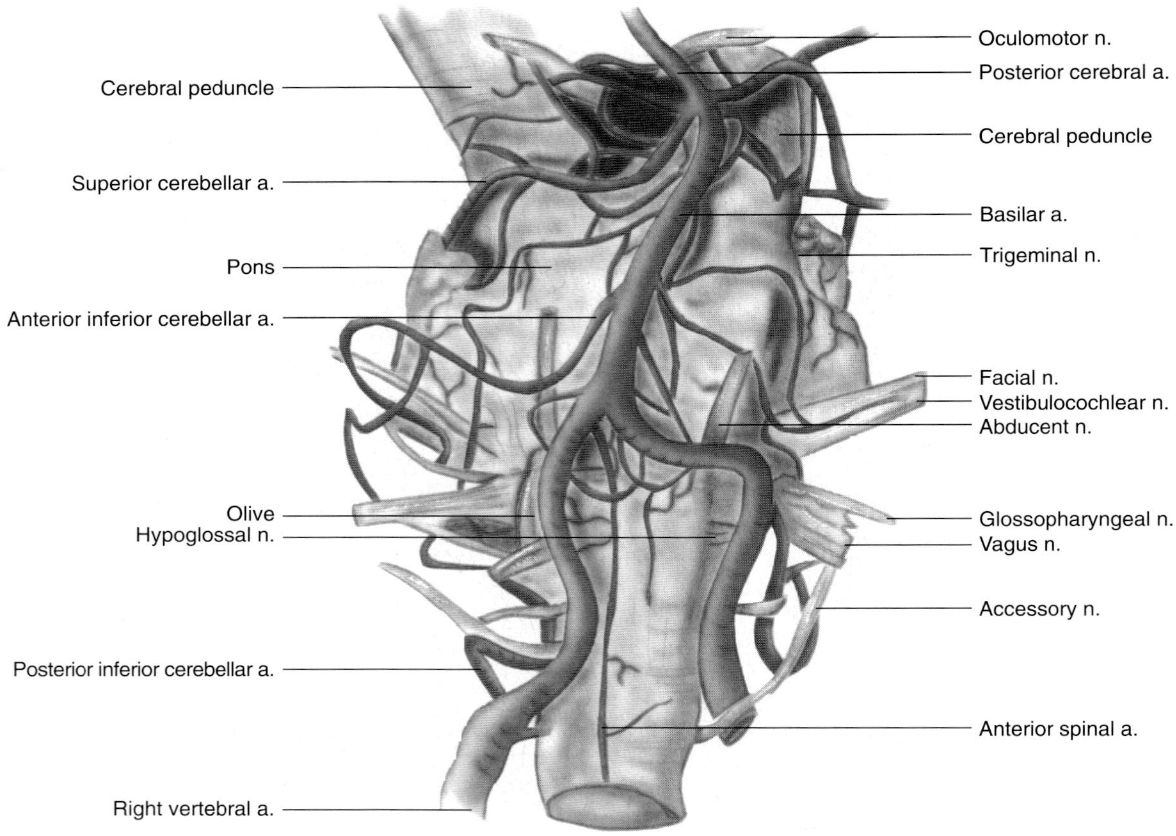

Fig. 3-7. Vertebral arteries and basilar artery. Basal view.

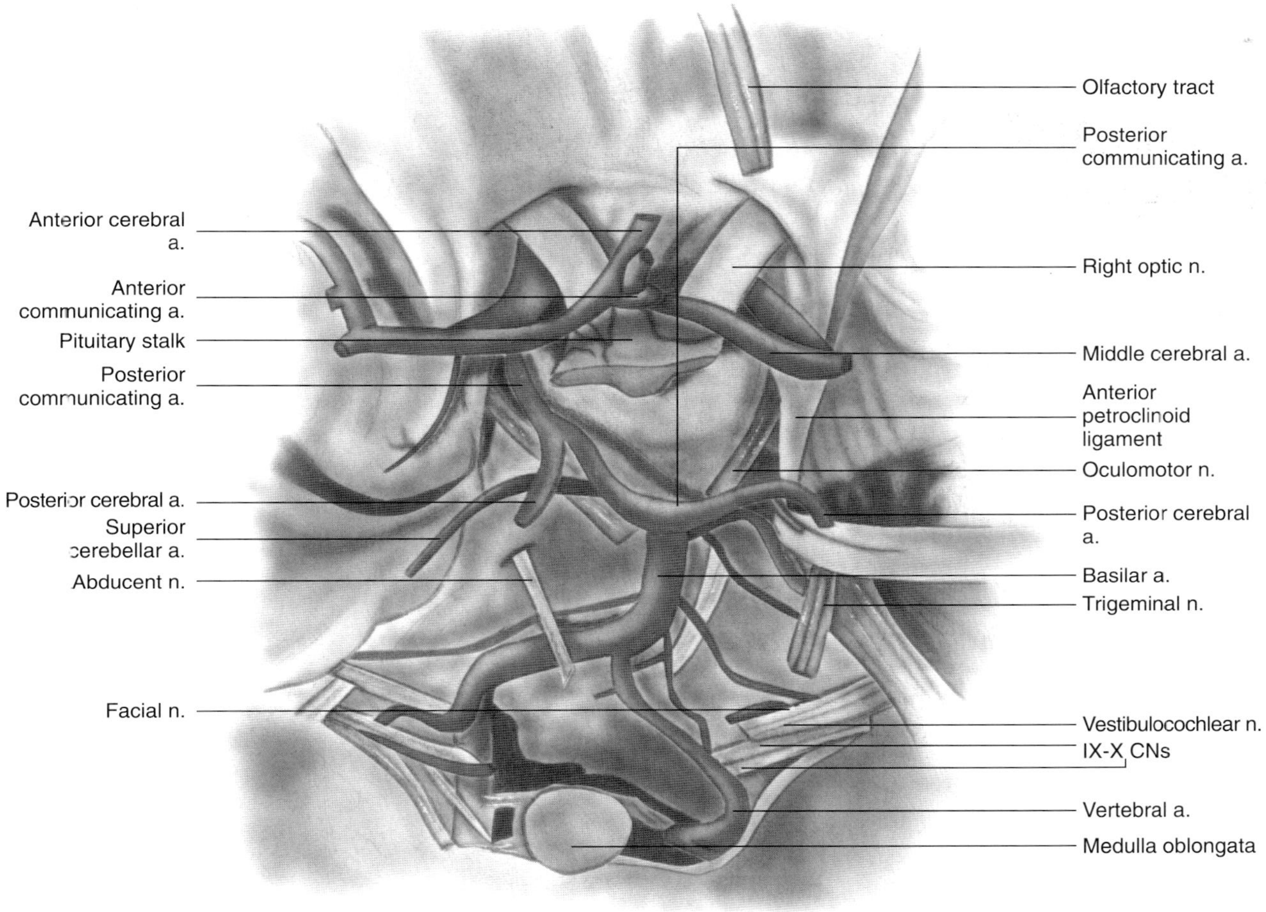

Fig. 3-8. Skull base view from above. The circle of Willis.

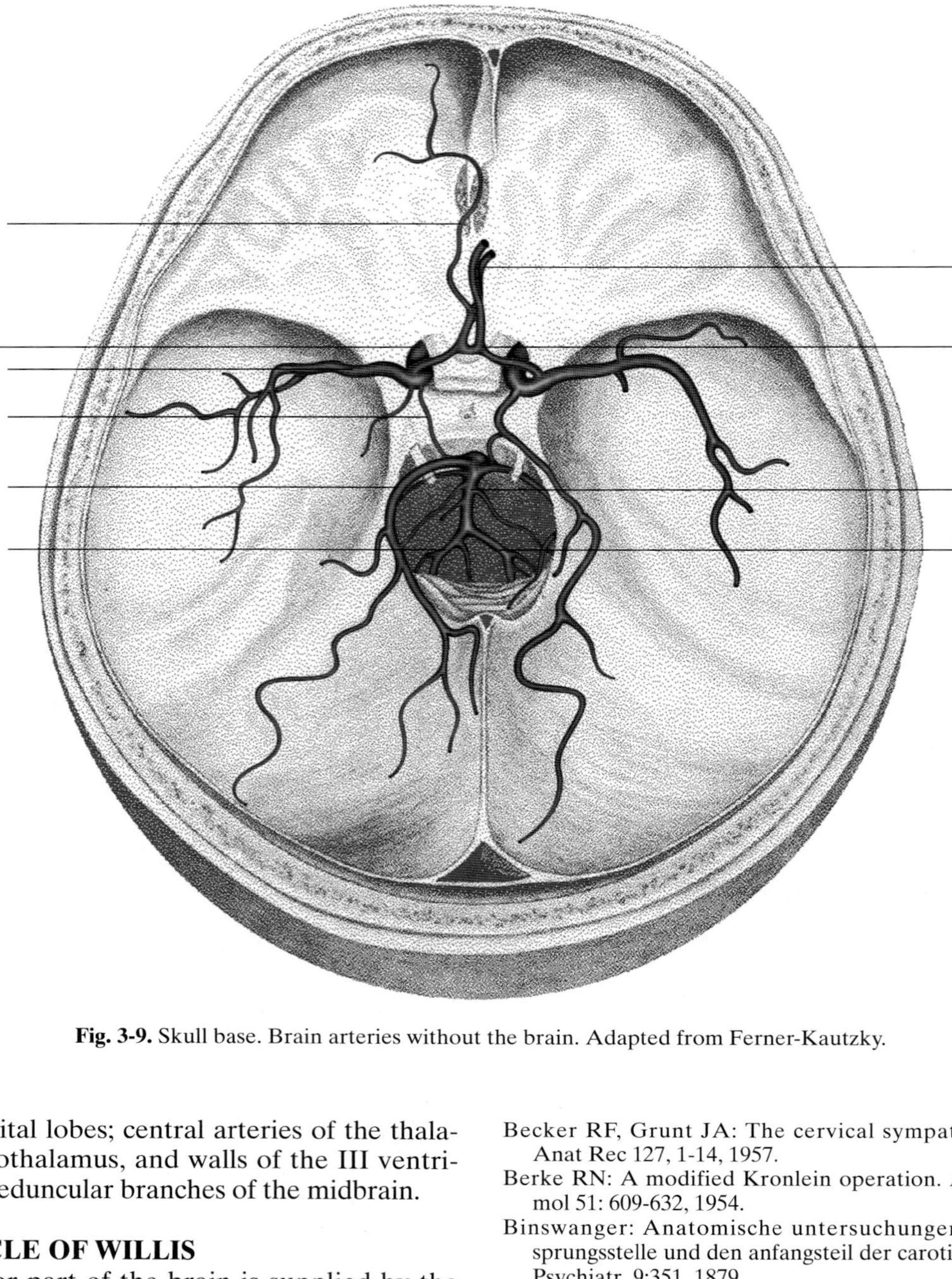

Fig. 3-9. Skull base. Brain arteries without the brain. Adapted from Ferner-Kautzky.

and occipital lobes; central arteries of the thalamus, hypothalamus, and walls of the III ventricle; and peduncular branches of the midbrain.

THE CIRCLE OF WILLIS

The anterior part of the brain is supplied by the internal carotid artery, the posterior part by the vertebro-basilar system. At the skull base, these two systems anastomose in a circle called the Circle of Willis (Fig. 3-8).

The anterior cerebral arteries run anteriorly to their anterior communicating artery.

Laterally, the communicating posterior arteries run from the internal carotids to the posterior cerebral arteries. Posteriorly, the posterior cerebral arteries flow into the basilar artery (Fig. 3-9).

REFERENCES

Argenson C, Francke JP, Sylla S, Dintimille H, Papasian S, di Manno V: The vertebral arteries (segments V, and V2). Anat Clin 2:29-41, 1980.

Becker RF, Grunt JA: The cervical sympathetic ganglia. Anat Rec 127, 1-14, 1957.

Berke RN: A modified Kronlein operation. Arch Ophthalmol 51: 609-632, 1954.

Binswanger: Anatomische untersuchungen uber die ursprungsstelle und den anfangsteil der carotis interna. Arch Psychiatr 9:351, 1879.

Cannoni M, Pech A, Pellet W, Zanaret M, Triglia JM: Les procidences veineuses et meningees au cours des voies trans-labyrinthiques elargies. Ann Oto Laryng (Paris) 103: 303-308, 1986.

Chandler SB, Derezinski CF: The variations of the middle meningeal artery within the middle cranial fossa. Anat Rec 62:309-319, 1935.

Coates AE: A note on the superior petrosal sinus and its relation to the sensory root of the trigeminal nerve. J Anat 68: 428-430, 1934.

Crawford E, de Baker M, Fields W: Roetgenographic diagnosis and surgical treatment of the basilar artery insufficiency. JAMA 168:509-514, 1958.

Das AC, Hasan M: The occipital sinus. J Neuro Surg 33: 307-311, 1970.

Di Chiro G, Fisher RL, Nelson KB: The jugular foramen. J Neurosurg 21: 447-460, 1964.

Droissart A: Les anomalies vasculaires a incidence otologique. J Head Neck Pathol 1: 39-44, 1982.

Duvernoy HM: Human Brainstem Vessels, Springer-Verlag (New York) Edit 188pp. 1977.
Duvernoy HM: The superficial veins of the human brain. Springer-Verlag (New York) Edit 11 Opp, 1975.
Elkin DC, Harns MH: Arteriovenous aneurysm of the vertebral vessels. Report of 10 cases. Ann Surg 124: 934-951, 1946.
Fisher AG: Case of complete absence of both internal carotid arteries with a preliminary note on development of stapedial artery. J Anat Physiol 48:37-46, 1914.
Hardin C, Wilimason W, Steegmann A: Vertebral artery insufficiency produced by cervical osteoarthritic spurs. Neurolog 10: 855-858, 1960.
Harris FS, Rhoton AL: Anatomy of the cavernous sinus. A microsurgical study. J Neurosurg 45: 169-180, 1976.
Hayreh SS, Dass R: The ophthalmic artery. I. Origin and intracranial and intra-canalicular course. Br J Ophthalmol 46:65-98, 1962.
Hayreh SS, Dass R: The ophthalmic artery. II. Intraorbital course. Br J Ophthalmol 46, 165-185, 1962.
Henle J: Handbuch der Nervenlehre des Menschen. Braunschweig: Vieweg & Sohn, 1871.
Kartush JM, Telian SA, Graham MD, Kemink JL: Anatomic basis for labyrinthine preservation during posterior fossa acoustic tumor surgery. Laryngoscope 96: 1024-1028, 1986.
Knott JF: On the cerebral sinuses and their variations. J Anat Physiol 16:27-42, 1881.
Korner O: Uber die fossa jugularis und die knochenlucken im boden der paukenhohle. Arch Ohr Nas U Keblkheilk 30: 236-239, 1890.
Lang J, Koth R, Reiss G: Uber die Bildung, die Zuflusse und den Verlauf der V. basalis und der V. cerebri interna. Anat Anz 150:385-423, 1981.
Lang J, Kessler B: About the suboccipital part of the vertebral artery and the neighbouring bone-joint and nerve relationships. Skull Base Surg 1:64-71, 1991.
Lang J: Eintritt und verlauf der hirnnerven (III, IV, VI) "im sinus cavernosus. Z Anat Entwicklungsgesch 145:87-99, 1974.
Lang J: Uber die vascularisation der periorbita. Gegenbaurs Morphol Jahrb 121:174-191, 1975.
Lang J: Zur vascularisation der dura mater cerebri. II. Vascularisierte durazotten am eingang in den canalis opticus. Z anat Entwicklungsgesch 141: 223-236, 1973.
Legent F, Perlemuter L, Vandenbrouck C: Cahiers d'anatomie ORL. Masson Edit 1-125, 1979.
Leonetti JP, Smith PG, Linthicum FH: The petrous carotid artery: anatomic relationships in skull base surgery. Otolaryngol Head Neck Surg 102:3-12, 1990.
Lindblom K: A roentgenographic study of the vascular channels of the skull. Acta Radiol 30: 146, 1936.
Mercier Ph, Fardoun R, Cadou B, Le Patezour A, Guy G: Etude microchirurgicale du nerf facial intra-cranien. In diagnostic et traitement des neurinomes de l'acoustique. Lazorthes Y, Clanet M, Fraysse B Edit. Fournie Imp Toulouse: 61-70, 1983.
Moret J: La vascularisation de l'appareil auditif. Normal-variantes-tumeurs glomiques. J Neuroradiol (Paris) 9: 213-260, 1982.
Nager GT, Nager M: The arteries of the human middle ear with particular regard to the blood supply of the auditory ossicles. Ann Otol Rhinol Laryngol 62/4: 923-949, 1953.
Ogura Y, Clemis JD: A study of the gross anatomy of the human vestibular aqueduct. Ann Otol Rhinol Laryngol 80/6: 813 825, 1971.
Overton SB, Ritter FN: A high placed jugular bulb in the middle ear: a clinical and temporal bone study. Laryngoscope 83: 1986-1991, 1973.
Perese DM: Superficial veins of the brain from a surgical point of view. J Neurosurg 17:402-412, 1960.
Platzer W: Zur Anatomie der "Sellabrucke und ihrer Beziehung zur A. carotis interna. ROFO 87:613-616, 1957.
Saleh E, Miguel M, Taibah A, Mazzoni A, Sanna M: Management of the high jugular bulb in the translabyrinthine approach. Otolaryngol Head Neck Surg 110:397-99, 1994.
Shapiro R: Compartimentation of the jugular foramen. J Neurosurg 36/3: 340-343, 1972.
Wackym PA, Blackwell KE: Abnormalities of the craniovertebral junction. In:Jackler RK, Brackmann DE, eds. Neuro-Otology. Baltimore: Mosby, 1993:1203-31.
Woodhall B: Anatomy of the cranial blood sinuses with particular reference to the lateral. Laryngoscope 49: 966-1009, 1939.
Woodhall B: Variations of the cranial venous sinuses in the region of the torcular Herophili. Arch Surg 33: 297-314, 1936.
Yasargil MG, Kasdaglis K, Jain KK, Weber HP: Anatomical observations of the sub-arachnoid cisterns of the brain during surgery. J Neurosurg 44/3: 298-302, 1976.

4

Anatomy of the cerebello-pontine angle

The pons and the medulla oblongata are comprised in the posterior cranial fossa, where they rest on the clivus. The cerebellar hemispheres are posterior, resting on the inferior cerebellar fissures. The cerebellum, the pons and the medulla oblongata form an angle: this is the *cerebellopontine angle*.
Nerves V to XII are contained in this space (Fig. 4-1).

The following is seen in the surgical perspective of a translabyrinthine or retrosigmoid approach:
The cerebellopontine angle is bordered superiorly by the superior part of the cerebellopontine fissure, and inferiorly by the inferior part of the cerebellopontine fissure. The inferior part of the latter contacts the medulla oblongata and becomes cerebello-medullary. These fissures are shaped like a triangle, with the inside of the triangle being the middle cerebral peduncle. The base of the triangle is the basilar artery, which runs along the pons.
The following nerves are found between the two arms of the cerebellopontine fissure: V, VI, VII, VIII, and IX. V is the only nerve anterior to the superior arm of the fissure, while the others are anterior to the inferior arm. VII and VIII are near to the vertex of this triangle.
VII emerges from the posterior extremity of the ponto-medullary sulcus. This groove, which divides the surface of the pons from the bulb, ends just posterior to the emergence of VII. It is in contact with the floccule, the choroid plexus, the foramen of Luschka, and the lateral recess of the fourth ventricle.
The vestibulo-cochlear nerve emerges 1-2 mm lateral to the VII, from the same sulcus. The two nerves near each other as they leave the trunk behind.
The foramen of Luschka is not readily visible with a translabyrinthine or retrosigmoid approach, but the choroid plexus, lateral to it, is easily observed. The latter is in contact with the emergence of the trunk of nerves IX and X. The cerebellar floccule is superior to the choroid plexus and the encephalic emergence of nerve VIII.

In the translabyrinthine approach view:
The pons is the structure just medial. It is white in color. The lateral prominence is the pyramidal eminence, in which the pyramidal fibers are located. When compressed, these provoke pyramidal symptoms.
IV emerges from the pons in a cranial position with respect to the surgical field, while V is more caudal and medial. The tentorium is superior.
The medulla oblongata follows the pons inferiorly. It is grayish in color, very vascularized, and covered with arachnoid.
VI exits medially to the bulb, near the midline.
Nerve VIII exits from the lateral extremity of the pontomedullary sulcus. Nerve VII exits approx. 2 mm caudally and approx. 3-4 mm medially to nerve VIII. An imaginary line along the entrance point of the roots of the mixed nerves proceeds 3 mm superiorly to nerve VII. The presence of nerve VIII, lateral to VII, is heralded by the cerebellar floccule.
IX, X, XI are visible caudally to the field, but their entrance into the bulb is masked by the cerebellum.
The pathway of the nerves is as follows:

- IV: medial to lateral direction.
- V: medial to lateral direction.
- VI: caudal to cranial direction, along the basilar artery.
- VII and VIII: medial to lateral, with a slight inferior-superior inclination.
- IX, X, XI: posterior to anterior.

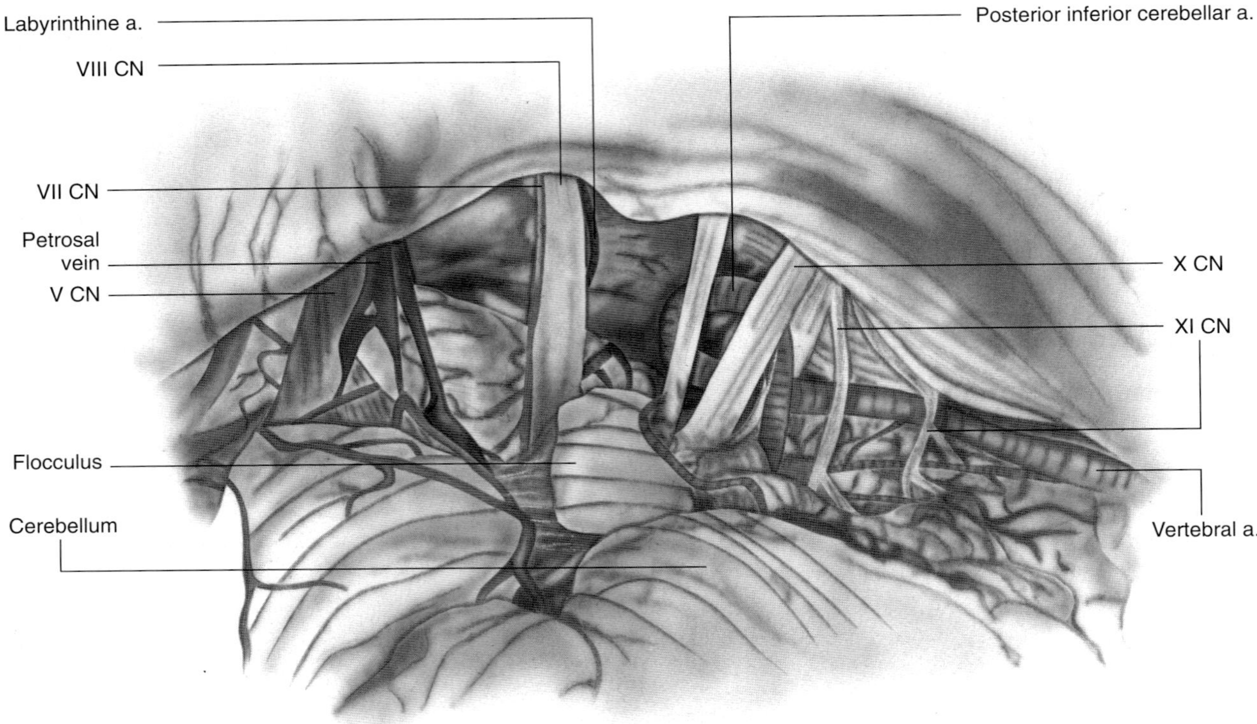

Fig. 4-1. View of the cerebello-pontine angle with a retrosigmoid approach.

ARTERIAL RELATIONSHIPS

The length of the basilar artery is approx. 3 cm.
The anterior-inferior cerebellar artery (AICA) almost always originates in the inferior or medial third of the basilar artery; only very rarely does it originate in the superior third (2% of cases). It runs near the pontomedullary sulcus, and is thus in contact with nerves VI, VII, and VIII. It surrounds the floccule, supplies the cerebellopontine fissure, sends branches to the choroid plexus, and terminates on the cerebellar surface in contact with the temporal bone (petrous part). Near VII and VIII the AICA forms a loop, which may be found in the internal auditory canal. It may be in the porus acusticus or near the porus. Collateral branches go from this loop to the acoustic meatus (labyrinthine artery and subarcuate artery).
The superior cerebellar artery (SCA) originates in the superior third of the basilar artery, near its divarication. It runs between nerve III and IV superiorly and V inferiorly. It then divides in two branches in the interpeduncular fossa, or proximally to it, and primarily supplies the cerebellum, as well as the pons and the pineal body. Tumors in the CPA usually dislocate the SCA superiorly.
The posterior-inferior cerebellar artery (PICA) originates in the proximal third of the intracisternal part of the vertebral artery, at the level of C1-C2. In rare instances, it may originate medially or distally. It runs on the medulla, first anteriorly and then laterally, and finally posteriorly. The artery sends branches to the choroid plexus of the fourth ventricle, the cerebellar tonsils, the medial and lateral surfaces of the medulla. Tumors in CPA usually dislocate the PICA inferiorly.

VENOUS RELATIONSHIPS

The petrosal vein (of Dandy) has varying points of origin. It may originate posterior to the entrance of the sensory root of the trigeminal nerve into the pons (48% of the time), at the anterolateral margin of the floccule (25%), dorsal to the sensory root of the trigeminal nerve (18%), or at the level of the horizontal fissure of the cerebellum (9%) (Lang). It receives veins from the superior and middle cerebellar peduncles, from the inferior surface of the cerebellum, from the bulb, the pons, the floccule, and from lateral veins of the IVth ventricle and the lateral mesencephalic vein.
They are:
Vein of the cerebello-medullary fissure.
Vein of the cerebellopontine fissure.
Vein of the ponto-medullary sulcus.
Lateral medullary vein.
Vein of the middle cerebellar peduncle.

These veins flow into the petrosal vein at the level of the entrance of the greater root of V into the pons. The petrosal vein opens into the superior petrosal sinus, draining the trunk of the brain and the cerebellar hemisphere. The superior petrosal sinus runs in the free margin of the petrous crest.

REFERENCES

Amjad AH, Scheer AA, Rosenthal J: Human internal auditory canal. Arch Otolaryng 89: 709-714, 1969.

Atkinson WJ: The anterior inferior cerebellar artery. J Neurol Neurosurg Psychiatry 12: 137- 151, 1949.

Atkinson WJ: Anterior inferior cerebellar artery: its variation, pontine distribution and significance in surgery of the cerebello-pontine angle tumors. J Neurol Neurosurg Psychiatry 12: 137-151, 1949.

Bebin J: Pathophysiology of acoustic tumors. In acoustic tumors - Volume I Diagnosis. Edit House WF, Lutje CH. University Park Press. Baltimore Chap 5: 45-83, 1979.

Brackmann DE: Middle cranial fossa approach. In acoustic tumors. Volume II Management. Edit House WF, Luetje CH University Park Press. Baltimore: 15-41, 1979.

Bucy PC: Surgical treatment of acoustic tumors. J Neurosurg 8: 547-555, 1951.

Dutillo MV, Malkasian D, Rand DW: A critical comparison of neurosurgical and otolaryngological approaches to acoustic neuromas. J Neurosurg 48: 1-12, 1978.

Friedman WA, Bova FJ: The University of Florida Radiosurgery System. Surg Neurol 32:334-342, 1989.

Friedman WA, Kaplan BJ, Gravenstein D, Rhoton AL Jr: Intraoperative brain-stem auditory evoked potentials during posterior fossa microvascular decompression. J Neurosurg 62: 552-557, 1985.

Fujii K, Lenkey C, Rhoton AL Jr: Microsurgical anatomy of the choroidal arteries: fourth ventricle and cerebellopontine angles. J Neurosurg 52:504-524, 1980;

Hardy DG, Peace DA, Rhoton AL Jr: Microsurgical anatomy of the superior cerebellar artery. Neurosurgery 6: 10-28, 1980.

House WF, Hitselberger WE: The transcochlear approach to the skull base. Arch Otolaryngol 102: 334-342, 1976.

House WF, Luetje CM: Acoustic tumors. Univ Park press (Baltimore) Vol I Diagnosis 289pp. Vol II management 280pp, 1979.

House WF: Monograph II. Acoustic neuroma. Arch Otolaryngol 88/6: 575-715, 1968.

House WF: Surgical exposure of the internal auditory canal and its contents, through the middle cranial fossa. Laryngoscope 71: 1363-1385, 1961.

House WF: Monograph II. Acoustic neuroma. Arch Otolaryngol 88: 575-715, 1968.

House WF: Monograph of trans-temporal removal of acoustic neuromas. Arch Oto-Laryngol 80: 587-756, 1964.

House WF: Surgical exposure of the internal auditory canal and its contents through the middle cranial fossa. Laryngoscope 71: 1363-1385, 1961.

Kartush JM, Telian SA, Graham MD, Kemink JL: Anatomic basis for labyrinthine preservation during posterior fossa acoustic tumor surgery. Laryngoscope 96: 1024-1028, 1986.

Koos W, Perneczky A: Pathomorphologie et pathophysiologie des neurinomes de l'acoustique. In: diagnostic et traitement des neurinomes de l'acoustique. Edit Lazorthes Y, Clanet M, Fraysse B, Foumie impr: 37-59, 1983.

Linskey ME, Lunsford LD, Flickinger JC: Radiosurgery for acoustic neuromas, neurinomas: early experience. Neurosurgery 26:736-745, 1990.

Lister JR, Rhoton AL Jr, Matsushima T, Peace DA: Microsurgical anatomy of the posterior inferior cerebellar artery. Neurosurgery 10:170-199, 1982.

Marquet JM: Contribution a l'angiologie du conduit auditif interne. Inn Progresos en Radiologia ORL, M Trujillo. Editorial Marban. Hilarion Eslava, 55 Madrid 15: 374-379, 1973.

Martin RG, Grant JL, Peace D, Theiss C, Rhoton AL: Microsurgical relationships of the anterior cerebellar artery and the facial vestibulo-cochlear nerve complex. Neurosurgery 6: 483-507, 1980.

Matsushima T, Rhoton AL Jr, de Oliveira E, Peace D: Microsurgical anatomy of the veins of the posterior fossa. J Neurosurg 59:63-105, 1983.

Matsushima T, Rhoton AL Jr, Lenkey C: Microsurgery of the fourth ventricle: part 1. Microsurgical anatomy. Neurosurgery 11:621-667, 1982.

Matsushima T, Rhoton AL, De Oliveira E, Peace D: Microsurgical anatomy of the veins of the posterior fossa. J Neurosurg 59: 63-105, 1983.

Mazzoni A: The subarcuate artery in man. Laryngoscope 80:69-79, 1970.

Mazzoni A: Internal auditory canal arterial relations at the porus acusticus. Ann Otol Rhinol Laryngol 78:797-814, 1969.

Ojemann RG, Levine RA, Montgomery WM, McGaffigan P: Use of intraoperative auditory evoked potentials to preserve hearing in unilateral acoustic neuroma removal. J Neurosurg 61: 938-948, 1984.

Pait TG, Zeal A, Harris FS, Paullus WS, Rhoton AL Jr: Microsurgical anatomy of dissection of the temporal bone. Surg Neurol 8:363-391, 1977.

Parisier SC: The middle cranial fossa approach to the internal auditory canal. An anatomical study stressing critical distances between surgical landmarks. Laryngoscope 84: 1-20, 1974.

Paullus WC, Pait TG, Rhoton AL: Microsurgical exposure of the petrous portion of the carotid artery. J Neurosurg 47: 713-726, 1977.

Rhoton AL Jr: Acoustic neuromas and other tumors of the cerebellopontine angle. In: Kassell NF and Vollmer DG (eds). Advances in neurosurgery. Philadelphia: F. A. Davis Company, 1992.

Rhoton AL Jr: Meningiomas and other cerebellopontine angle tumors. In: Long D, ed. Current therapy in neurological surgery. Toronto: B.C. Decker Publishers, 14-19, 1989.

Rhoton AL Jr: Microsurgery of the internal acoustic meatus. Surg Neurol 2:311-318, 1974.

Rhoton AL Jr: Microsurgery of the temporal bone and of acoustic neuromas. Tryon, NC: Paul C. Bucy & Associates, 1977.

Rhoton AL Jr: Microsurgical anatomy of acoustic neuromas. Neurol Res 6:3-21, 1984.

Rhoton AL Jr: Microsurgical anatomy of the brainstem surface facing an acoustic neuroma. Surg Neurol 25:326-339, 1986.

Rhoton AL Jr: Microsurgical anatomy of the posterior fossa cranial nerves. Clin Neurosurg 26:398-462, 1979.

Rhoton AL Jr: Microsurgical removal of acoustic neuromas. Surg Neurol 6:211-219, 1976.

Rhoton AL Jr: Suboccipital-retrolabyrinthine removal of acoustic neuromas. J Fla Med Assoc 70:895-901, 1983.

Rhoton AL, Buza R: Microsurgical anatomy of the jugular foramen. J Neurosurg 42:541-550, 1975.

Rhoton AL: Microsurgical anatomy of the brainstem surface facing an acoustic neuroma. Surg Neurol 25: 326-339, 1986.

Shrontz C, Dujouny M, Ausman Jl, Diaz FG, Pearce JE, Berman SK, Hirsch E, Mirchandani HG: Surgical anatomy of the arteries of the posterior fossa. J Neurosurg 65/4: 540-544, 1986.

5

Anatomy of the paranasal sinuses

The paranasal sinuses are the following: the *ethmoid*, the *frontal*, the *maxillary*, and the *sphenoid sinuses* (Figs. 5-1, 5-2).

LATERAL NASAL WALL

On the lateral wall of the nasal fossa, we can recognize the inferior, middle, and superior turbinates, below which lie the respective meati. The turbinates are highly vascularized mucosal masses with an inner horizontal bony lamina: the superior, middle and inferior concha. The anterior wall of the sphenoid sinus is behind the tail of the superior and middle turbinates. Behind the tail of the superior turbinate there is the sphenoethmoidal recess, which presents the opening of the sphenoid sinus (Figs. 5-3, 5-4).

Superior meatus.

It is bounded by the superior nasal concha and bears the openings of the posterior ethmoidal cells.

Middle meatus.

The lower edge and the lateral surface of the middle concha are part of the middle meatus. It contains the openings of the anterior ethmoidal cells, the frontal sinus (frontonasal duct), the opening of the maxillary sinus.

Inferior meatus.

The lower edge of the lateral surface of the inferior concha are part of the inferior meatus, which contains the opening of the nasolacrimal duct.

If the vertical part of the middle turbinate is removed, the ethmoidal bulla and the uncinate process can be observed.

Ethmoidal bulla

The ethmoidal bulla is a large cell of the anterior ethmoid which adheres to the lamina papiracea. In rare instances, the bulla may be poorly pneumatized or absent.

The uncinate process

The uncinate process has a semilunar shape. Its superior boundary is under the insertion of the middle meatus, while its anterior margin connects to the lateral osseous nasal wall and may reach the lacrimal bone anteriorly. Its posterior margin is free and the ethmoidal bulla above borders the semilunar hiatus. Beyond the semilunar hiatus is a lateral space called the ethmoidal infundibulum.

ETHMOID BONE

Ethmoid bone is formed by a horizontal lamina, a medial lamina, and two lateral protuberances (Fig. 5-5).

The horizontal lamina, or cribriform plate, owes its name to the tiny holes all through it. The olfactory nerves pass through them. Its superior face is part of the anterior cranial fossa and accommodates the olfactory bulbs in two depressions beside a median osseous crest. A triangular, median bone, the crista galli, where the apex of the great falx cerebri attaches, projects up from this lamina.

The crista galli is the endocranial continuation of the perpendicular plate. The part of the perpendicular plate underlying the cribriform plate, along with the quadrangular cartilage and the vomer, makes up the nasal septum.

The lateral protruberances are the ethmoidal labyrinths.

The superior face relates to the frontal bone. The anterior and posterior ethmoidal canals are found here, reaching medially to the anterior cranial fossa, while laterally they enter the orbitary cavity.

Vessels and nerves are located here. Their presence influence the closure of CSF fistules.

The inferior face relates to the nasal surface of the maxillary bone.

The lateral face is very thin; hence its name, lamina papiracea. It makes up much of the medial wall of the orbit. Superiorly it is the line of suture with the frontal bone, site of the anterior and posterior ethmoidal foramina, where the anterior and posterior ethmoidal canals exit.

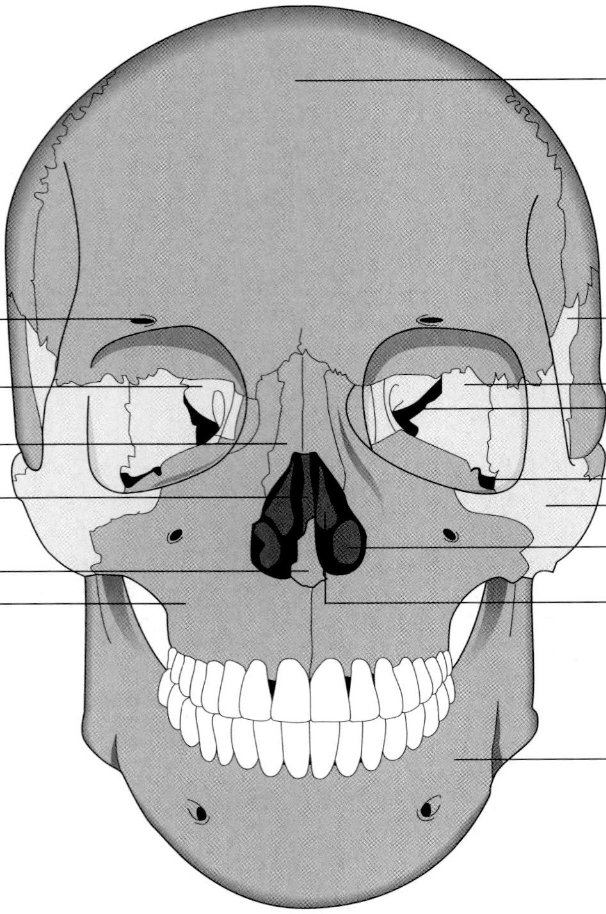

Fig. 5-1. Anterior aspect of the skull.

The medial face makes up much of the lateral wall of the nasal cavity.

The posterior face relates to the sphenoid body and the orbitary process of the palatine bone.

The anterior face relates to the medial surface of the lacrimal bone, and goes to the frontal process of the maxillary bone.

Inside, the ethmoidal labyrinth is partitioned by laminae outlining the ethmoidal cells.

The basal osseous lamina of the middle turbinate divides the ethmoidal cells into anterior and posterior ethmoid.

Anterior ethmoid

The orifice of these cells opens under the basal lamina, in the middle meatus. Only the ethmoid-ungueal cells, located anterior to the root of the bulla, communicate by means of a thin canal (the canal of Fiol or the maxillo-ethmoidal-frontal canal) in the canal uniting the maxillary sinus at the middle meatus.

Posterior ethmoid

The cells of the posterior ethmoid open over the basal lamina, in the superior meatus.

The anterior wall of the sphenoid sinus is generally behind the last posterior ethmoidal cells. Some cells, called Onodi cells, may surpass by up to 1.5 cm the anterior wall of the sphenoid sinus. The optic nerve and at times the internal carotid may thus enter in contact with the lateral wall of these cells. To open the anterior wall of the sphenoid sinus, it is thus advisable to go medially and inferiorly, to avoid the risk of injuring the optic nerve and the internal carotid artery.

Ethmoidal Infundibulum

The ethmoidal infundibulum is a space in the anterior ethmoid. Its medial wall is made up of the uncinate process. Its lateral wall consists of the lamina papiracea of the orbit and the frontal process of the superior maxillary bone.

Haller cells

Haller cells are cells that may occupy a lateral space in the ethmoid infundibulum. They occupy a space under the orbit. They may restrict transnasal access to the maxillary sinus and to the anterior ethmoidal cells.

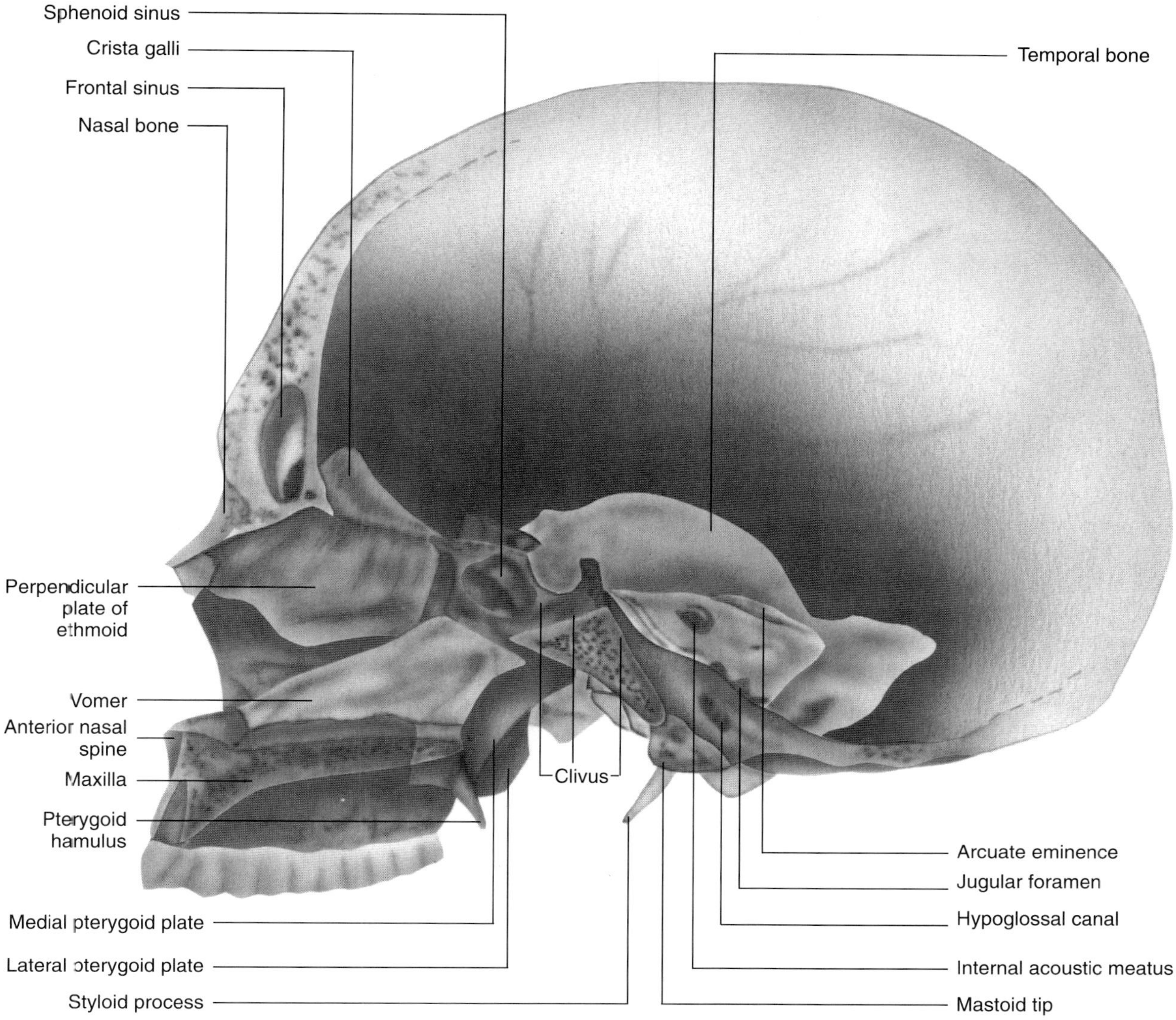

Fig. 5-2. The lower part of the skull. Sagittal section.

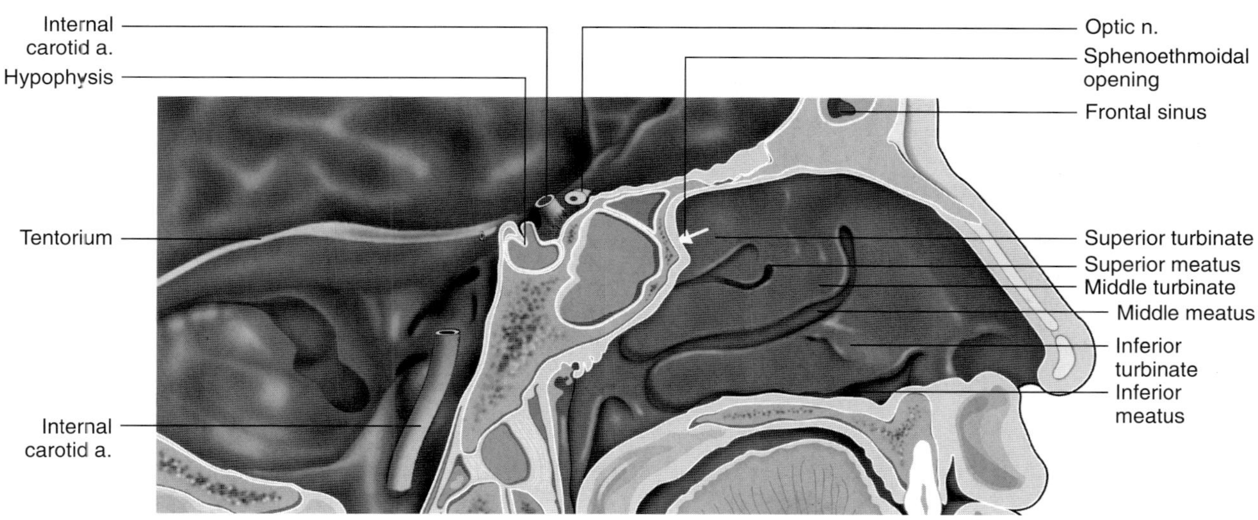

Fig. 5-3. The lateral wall of the left nasal cavity, the clivus and the tentorium. Sagittal section. (Adapted from Sobotta's anatomy).

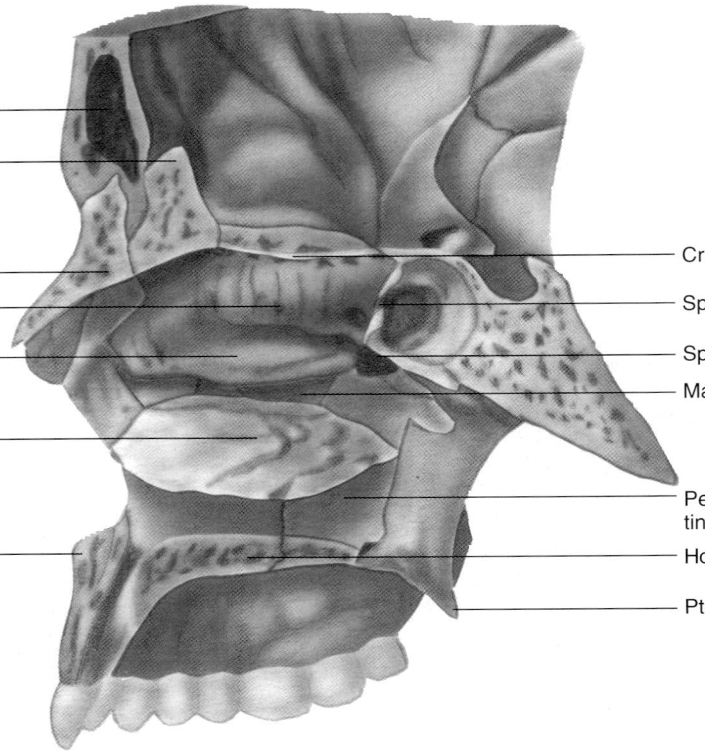

Fig. 5-4. The lateral wall of the right nasal cavity. The lateral concha has been removed.

Anterior ethmoidal artery

The anterior ethmoidal artery courses from the orbit to the olfactory fossa. It is important to know its pathway because it passes through less resistant areas, which are more exposed to traumas, dural lesions, and hemorrhaging.

The anterior ethmoid artery originates within the orbit, and enters the anterior ethmoid foramen. It transverses the anterior ethmoid run-

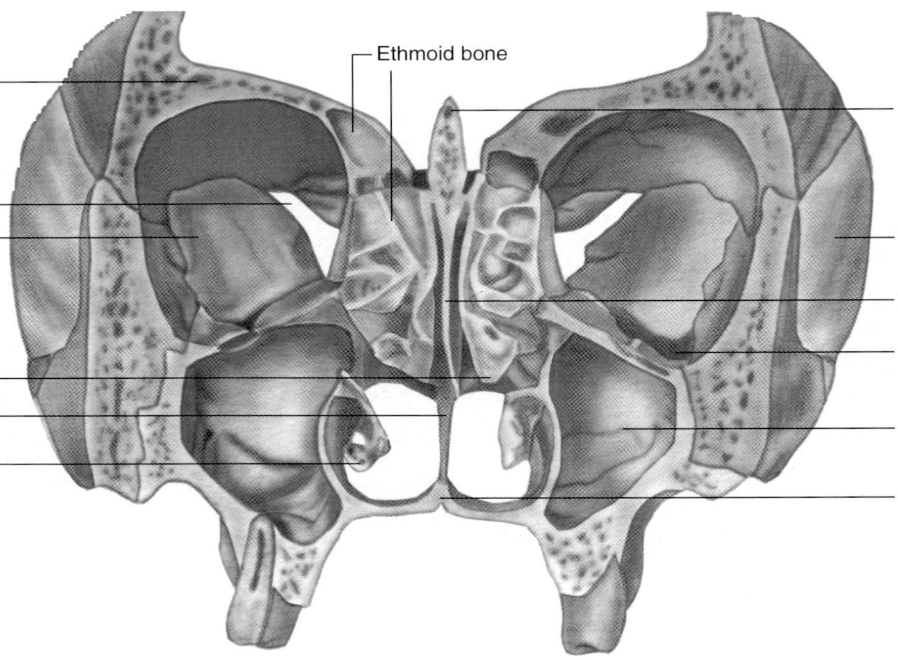

Fig. 5-5. Coronal section through the anterior part of the skull.

ning in an osseous canal, and enters the anterior cranial fossa through the lateral lamina of the cribriform plate. Here it reaches the olfactory fossa, and bends forward, to cross once again the cribriform plate. It enters the nasal cavity as the nasal artery and divides into a posterior and an anterior branch, and small meningeal branches.

FRONTAL SINUS

The two frontal sinuses are inside the frontal bone. The posterior wall is in contact with the frontal lobe. The inferior wall has a lateral (orbitary) part, and a medial (ethmoido-nasal) part. Some cells of the anterior ethmoid may elevate the floor of the frontal sinus (frontal bullae), or interpose between the roof of the orbit and the floor of the sinus (ethmoido-orbitary cells). The frontal sinus communicates with the middle meatus through the nasofrontal duct, which opens into the hiatus semilunaris two-thirds of the time. One third of the time it opens externally.

MAXILLARY SINUS

The two maxillary sinuses are shaped like a quadrangular pyramid, with five faces.
The inferior wall, or base, corresponds to the alveolar process of the superior maxillary bone.
The medial wall makes up much of the lateral wall of the nasal cavities. Centrally, an uneven-shaped aperture is found; this is the maxillary hiatus. Anterior to it is the nasolacrimal canal, which opens into the inferior meatus. Posterior to the hiatus is the pterygopalatine canal, formed due to the overlap of the palatine bone on the maxillary bone. A canal located in the superior margin connects the sinus to the middle meatus. This canal is found between the anterior third and the posterior two-thirds. The canal of Fiol opens into this canal. Within the meatus, the canal opens into the hiatus semilunaris.
The anterior wall corresponds to the canine fossa. Superior to the canine fossa is the infraorbital foramen, through which the infraorbital nerve exits (V2).
The superior wall forms the floor of the orbitary cavity. It is furrowed by the infraorbital canal, which accommodates the infraorbital nerve, opening onto the anterior face. The anterior alveolar canals depart from the anterior part of the canal. The anterior alveolar vessels and nerves (branches of V2) run in these canals to the incisor teeth and the superior canines.

The posterior wall is part of the infratemporal fossa and the pterygopalatine fossa. The apex of the pyramid is in contact with the zygomatic process. In the inferior part there are the alveolar foramina which give onto the posterior alveolar canals. In the posterior alveolar canals, the posterior alveolar nerves are found.
These are branches of V2 and go to the molar nerves.
In the maxillary sinus, four recesses may be observed: zygomatic, orbitary, palatine, and alveolar.

SPHENOID SINUS

The inside of the sphenoid body is occupied by two cavities: these are the sphenoid sinuses, separated by a middle septum.
The walls are as follows: superior, inferior, anterior, medial, and lateral.
The superior wall may bulge due to the presence of the sella turgica.
The floor of the sinus may have crests covering the vidian nerve.
The ostium of the sphenoid sinus is in the anterior wall, in the sphenoethmoidal recess, medial to the superior turbinate.
The medial wall is generally smooth.
On the lateral wall, there are two protruberances of variable size. These are formed by the optic nerve and the carotid artery. The osseous walls of these structures may at times produce dehiscences.
The sinus may be very pneumatized. Its pneumatization may also involve the clivus up to the foramen magnum, and may reach the foramen lacerum. In these instances, the maxillary nerve (V2) may be found covered by the pneumatization of the lateral wall and the vidian nerve by that of the sinus floor.

REFERENCES

Buschmann W, Linnert D: Wandel der Indikation und der technik in der chirurgie retrobulbarer orbitatumoren. Klin Monatsbl Augenheilkd 171:1-12, 1978.

Cope VZ: The internal structure of the sphenoid sinus. J Anat (Lond) 51:127-136, 1917.

Dietemann JL, Lang J, Francke JP, Bonneville JF, Clarisse J, Wackenheim A: Anatomy and radiology of the sellar spine. Neuroradiology 21:5-7, 1981.

Elwany S, Yacout YM, Talaat M, El-Nahass M, Gunied A: Surgical anatomy of the sphenoid sinus. J Laryngol 97:227-241, 1983.

Hammer G, Radberg C: Sphenoidal sinus. An anatomical and roentgenological study with reference to transsphenoid hypophysectomy. Acta Radiol. (Stockh) 56:401-422, 1961.

Jovanox S: Supernumerary frontal sinuses on the roof of the orbit. Their clinical significance. Acta Anat (Basel) 45:133-142, 1961.

Killian G: Zur anatomie der nase menschlicher embryonen. Arch Laryngol Rhin (Berl) 3:17-47, 1895/96.

Lang J, Kageyama I: Clinical anatomy of the ophthalmic artery and cavernous sinus. In: Samii M, ed. Surgery of the sellar region, vol 2. Springer 145- 148, 1991.

Lang J: Clinical anatomy of the head. Neurocranium-orbit-craniocervical regions. New York: Springer, 1983.

Lang J: Structure and postnatal organization of heretofore uninvestigated and infrequent ossifications of the sella turcica region. 99:121-139, 1977.

Maroon JC, Kennerdell JS: Lateral microsurgical approach to intraorbitaltumors. J. Neurosurg 44:556-561, 1976.

Montgomery WW: Cystic lesion of the petrous apex: transsphenoidal approach. Ann Otolaryngol 86: 429-435, 1977.

Pearson BW, MacKenzie RG, Goodman WS: The anatomical basis of the transantral ligation of the maxillary artery in severe epistaxis. Laryngoscope 79: 969-984, 1969.

Pickrell KL: Reconstructive plastic surgery of the face. In: Walton JH ed. Clinical symposia, vol 20. Canada: Ciba, 1968.

6

Pathways of the cranial nerves

The motor nerves are efferent, i.e. they originate in the central nervous system (CNS) and proceed peripherally. The sensory nerves are afferent, meaning they originate in cells outside the CNS and go towards it (Figs. 6-1, 6-2).

Olfactory nerve (I)

The olfactory nerve is a special afferent sensory nerve. Its task is to recognize smells.

The odorous substances inhaled by the nose reach the olfactory epithelium on the roof of the nasal cavity, on the superior nasal concha and the part adjacent the nasal septum. Here they blend with the secretion of the olfactory glands. The olfactory signal is then received by the primary olfactory neurons, which act as sensory receptors. The nervous fibers of these cells group together in approximately 20 bundles and transverse the cribriform plate of the ethmoid, synapsing with the secondary neurons located in the olfactory bulb. The post-synaptic fibers form the olfactory tract and the olfactory triangle, a branch of the anterior olfactory tract from the anterior perforated substance of the brain.

Most of the axons, upon reaching the olfactory tract, go through the lateral olfactory stria to the lateral olfactory area. Also called the pyriform area, this region includes the uncus, the entorhinal area, and the limen insulae.

Other axons transverse the medial olfactory stria to the medial part of the frontal lobe, into its subcallosa region. This is connected to the limbic lobe and has a role in emotional response to odors.

The intermediate olfactory stria goes to the olfactory area between the olfactory triangle and the optic tract. It has no importance in man.

The three olfactory areas are connected by the diagonal bands of Broca.

Olfactory sensation may provoke visceral responses, such as salivation or nausea, in response to pleasant or unpleasant stimuli. The autonomous centers for the visceral responses are the following: the hypothalamus, which receives information from the olfactory area through the medial fascia of the anterior brain; the epithalamus, which receives information through the stria medullaris thalami; the anterior hypothalamus and the preoptic region, which receive information from the amygdaloid body by means of the stria terminalis. The stimuli are then transmitted to the reticulated substance which in turn communicates with the cranial nerves to obtain the visceral response to the olfactory stimulus.

Optic nerve (II)

The optic nerve is a special sensory nerve (afferent). Its task is to transfer visual impulses from the retina to the visual cortex (Fig. 6-3).

The optic nerve originates in the retina, in the posterior part of the eye. Here the visual information are received by the photoreceptor layer, composed of rods and cones. The rods are more numerous periphericallly while the cones are more numerous centrally. The cones are responsible for color discrimination and for visual acuity. From here, the message is passed on to the bipolar cells, which are the primary neurons of the visual pathway, and then to the gangliar cells of the retina, secondary neurons. The fibers of the latter converge towards the optic disk, perforating the choroid and the perpendicular plate of the sclera, and forming the optic nerve which exits from the posterior part of the eye. The intraorbital part of the nerve is approx. 2.5 cm in length; the posterior half is transversed medially by the artery and by the central vein of the retina. The optic nerve runs in a posterior direction within the lesser wing of the sphenoid, in the optic canal (approx. 0.5 cm in length) (Fig. 6-4). The inferior branch of the oculomotor nerve is found inferiorly, while

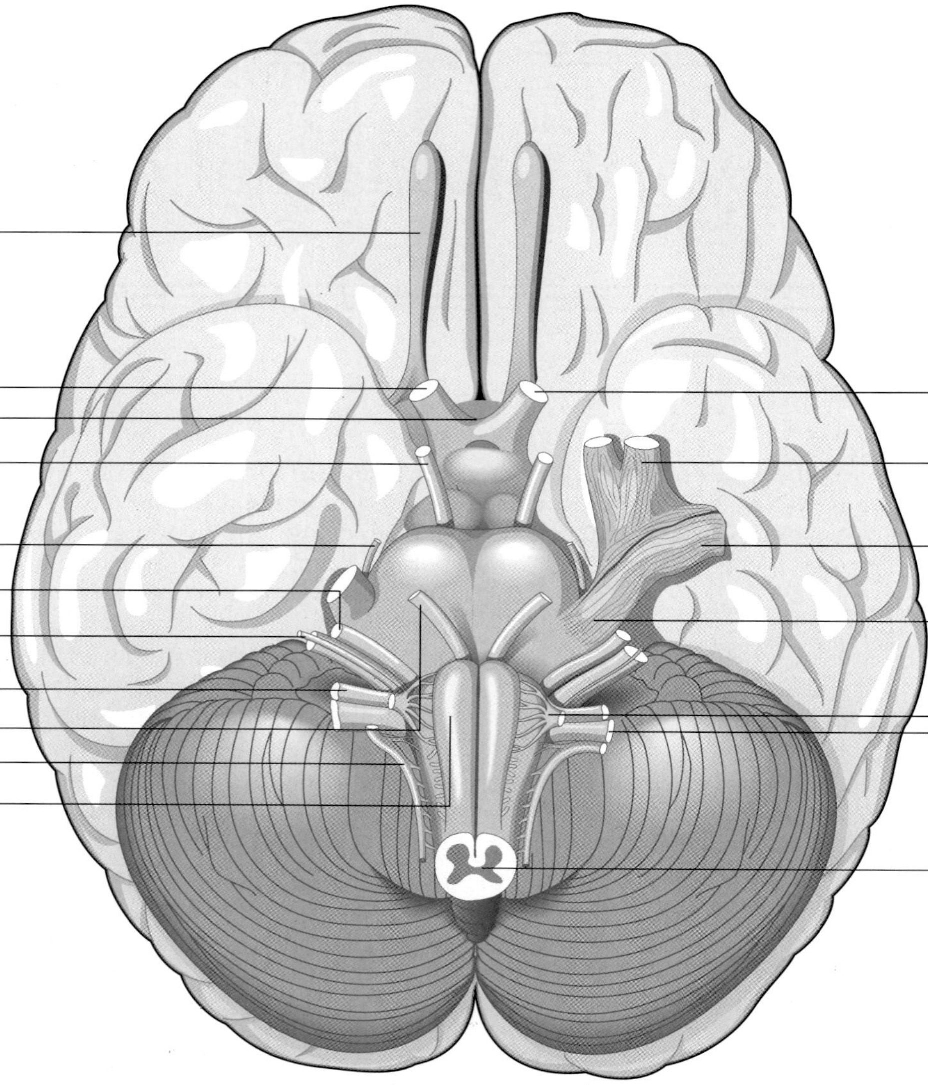

Fig. 6-1. The brain and the cranial nerves. Basal view.

the ophthalmic artery and the nasociliary nerve are found anteriorly. Medially, there are the posterior ethmoidal nerve and the ethmoid, under a thin bone plate. This goes to the middle cranial fossa where it runs for approx. 1 cm before forming the optic chiasma along with the contralateral optic nerve. Here, half of the axons cross the midline. Most of the fibers go to the homolateral lateral geniculate nucleus of the thalamus. Some reach the pretectal area and control the pupillary reflex. In the lateral geniculate nucleus are the bodies of the tertiary neurons. Their axons form the geniculocalcarine segment which goes to the occipital lobe and the primary visual cortex, around the calcarine fissure. The optic nerve is encased in three sheaths, external, medial, and internal, which are the anatomical-histological continuation of the dura mater, the arachnoid, and the pia mater.

Oculomotor nerve (III)

The oculomotor nerve has two components: the visceral and the somatic motor components.

- The somatic motor (efferent) component goes to the elevator muscle of the upper lid, as well as the superior, medial, and inferior recti (i.e. all the extraocular muscles with the exception of the lateral rectus (VI) and the superior oblique muscles (IV)).
- The visceral motor component (efferent) transverses the ciliary ganglion and provides the intraocular muscles with a parasympathetic contingent: the pupillary constrictor and the ciliary muscles.

The fibers of the oculomotor nerve arise from a nuclear complex located medially, on both sides of the midbrain, anterior to the cerebral aque-

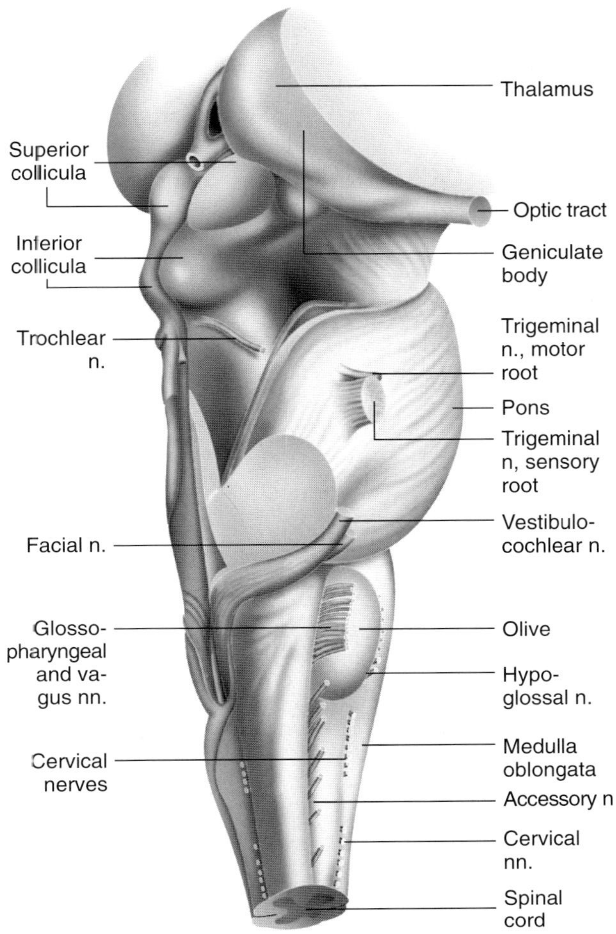

Fig. 6-2. Neural relationship on the brain stem. Lateral view.

duct. Here the bodies of the inferior motor neurons are located. Their axons descend into the midbrain through the red nucleus and the cerebral peduncles, and exit at the junction between the midbrain and the pons in the interpeduncular cistern. This forms the oculomotor nerve, which is covered by pia mater. Visceral motor fibers from the Edinger-Westphal nucleus join in forming nerve III.

The nerve passes between the posterior cerebral artery and the superior cerebellar artery, leaving the posterior communicating artery laterally. The nerve then perforates the dura and enters the cavernous sinus. It has the most cranial position in the sinus, superior to IV, V1, VI, and V2. The internal carotid runs medially, in the sinus. Medial to the cavernous sinus is the sphenoid sinus. The nerve proceeds to the superior orbitary fissure, transverses it, and enters the orbit. Here it divides into superior and inferior branches. The superior branch innervates the superior rectus and the elevator of the upper lid. The inferior branch divides into three parts: one part innervates the medial rectus, another the inferior rectus, and the third innervates the inferior oblique muscle (Fig. 6-5).

The pupillary constrictor muscle (which determines the pupil's size) and the ciliary muscles (which determine the lens curvature) are innervated by visceral motor fibers whose somas are located in the Edinger-Westphal nucleus. This nucleus is found in the midbrain, posterior to the

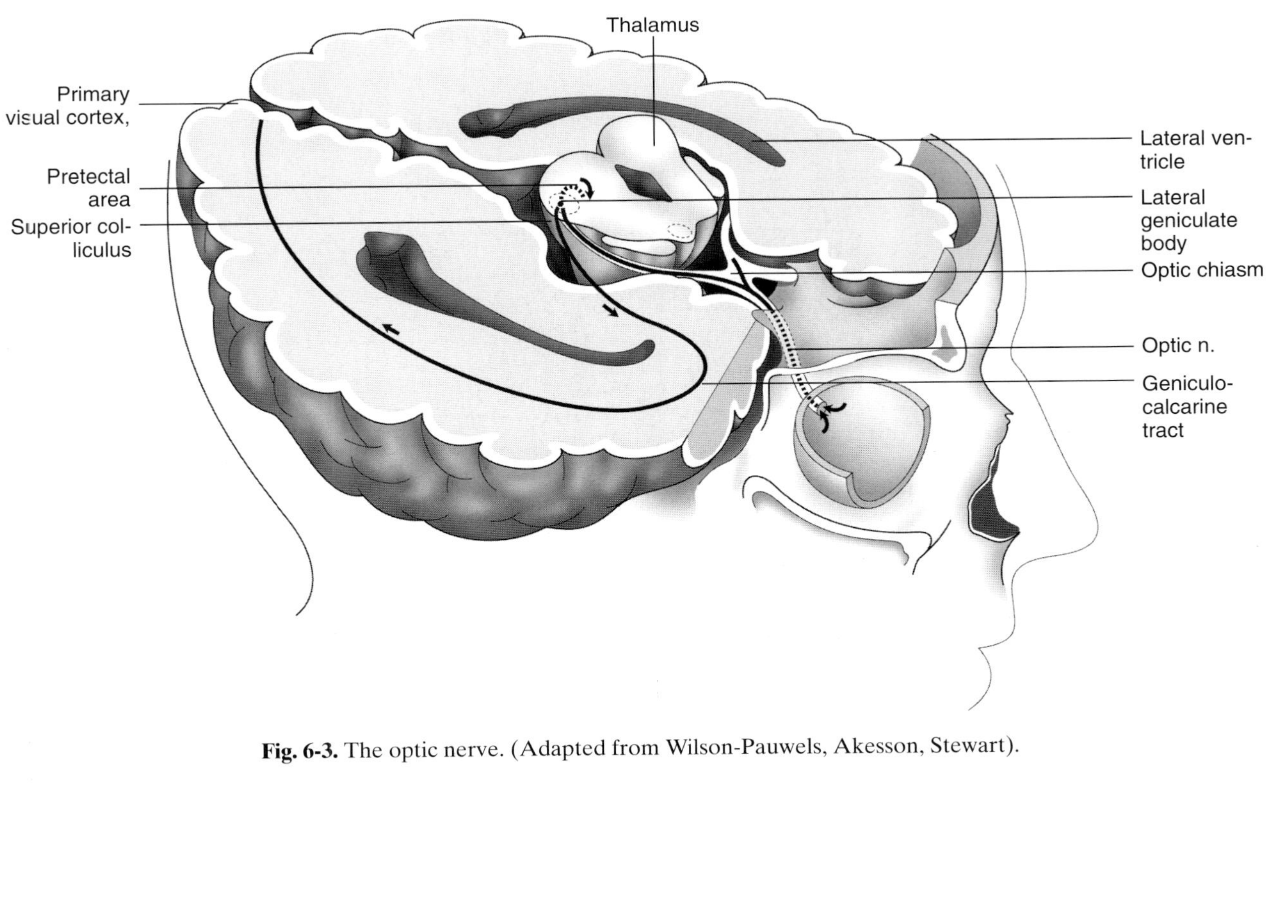

Fig. 6-3. The optic nerve. (Adapted from Wilson-Pauwels, Akesson, Stewart).

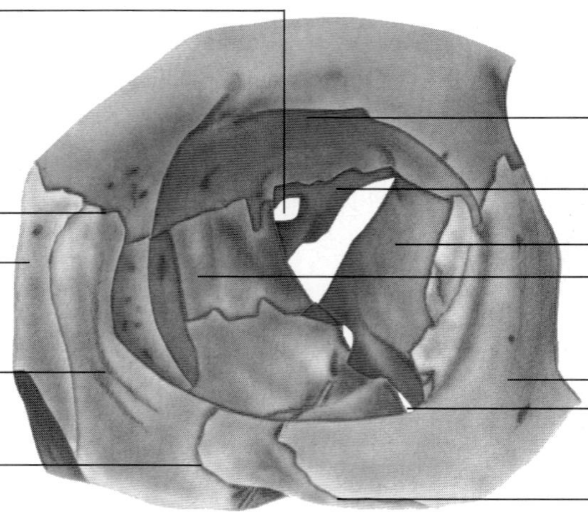

Fig. 6-4. The left orbit. Anterior aspect.

nucleic complex of the oculomotor nerve. Pregangliar fibers leave the nucleus and run with the oculomotor nerve to the superior orbitary fissure. They then enter the orbit and proceed to the ciliary ganglion. From here postgangliar fibers continue anteriorly, entering the ocular bulb, and running through sclera and choroid. They then reach the iris and the ciliated body.

Trochlear nerve (IV)

The trochlear nerve is a somatic motor nerve (efferent) which innervates the superior oblique muscle of the eye. This muscle moves the ocular bulb downward and laterally (Fig. 6-5).

The nucleus of V is found near the midline, at the level of the inferior colliculus, in the floor of the cerebral aqueduct. The fibers exit the nucleus in a posterior direction, decussate at the level of the anterior medullary velum, and emerge near the inferior colliculus, dorsal to the midbrain. In its anterior pathway, the nerve surrounds the cerebral peduncle over the pons, passes between the posterior cerebral and the superior cerebellar arteries, and perforates the dura under the free margin of the tentorium. It then enters the cavernous sinus, transverses the superior orbitary fissure, and enters into the orbit. It runs diagonally in the roof of the orbit, between the superior rectus muscle anteriorly and the levator palpebrae posteriorly, until it reaches the superior oblique muscle.

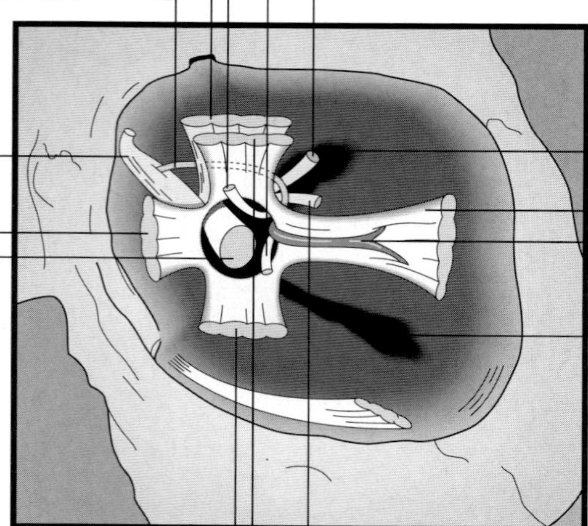

Fig. 6-5. Apex of left orbit. (Adapted from Wilson-Pauwels, Akesson, Stewart).

Trigeminal nerve (V)

The trigeminal nerve has two components: the branchial motor component and the general sensory component (Fig. 6-6).
The branchial motor component (efferent) innervates the anterior belly of the digastric and the mylohyoid muscles, the tensor veli palatini, the tensor tympani, and the masticator muscles.
The general sensory component (afferent) carries sensitivity from the meninges of the anterior and middle cranial fossa to the eye, the anterior half of the face, part of the tympanic membrane, and the lingual, oral, and sinusal mucosa.

The trigeminal nerve emerges laterally from the pons, in proximity to its superior border, with a larger sensory root and a smaller motor root. The fibers of the sensory root have their somas in the trigeminal ganglion (Meckel's cave), in a dural duplication approx. 1.5 cm from the apex of the petrous ridge.
Three roots detach from the trigeminal ganglion: the *ophthalmic, maxillary*, and *mandibular* roots.

THE OPHTHALMIC NERVE (V1)

In the cavernous sinus, the ophthalmic nerve divides into *frontal*, *lacrimal*, and *nasociliary branches*, and exits immediately from the cranium through the superior orbitary fissure.

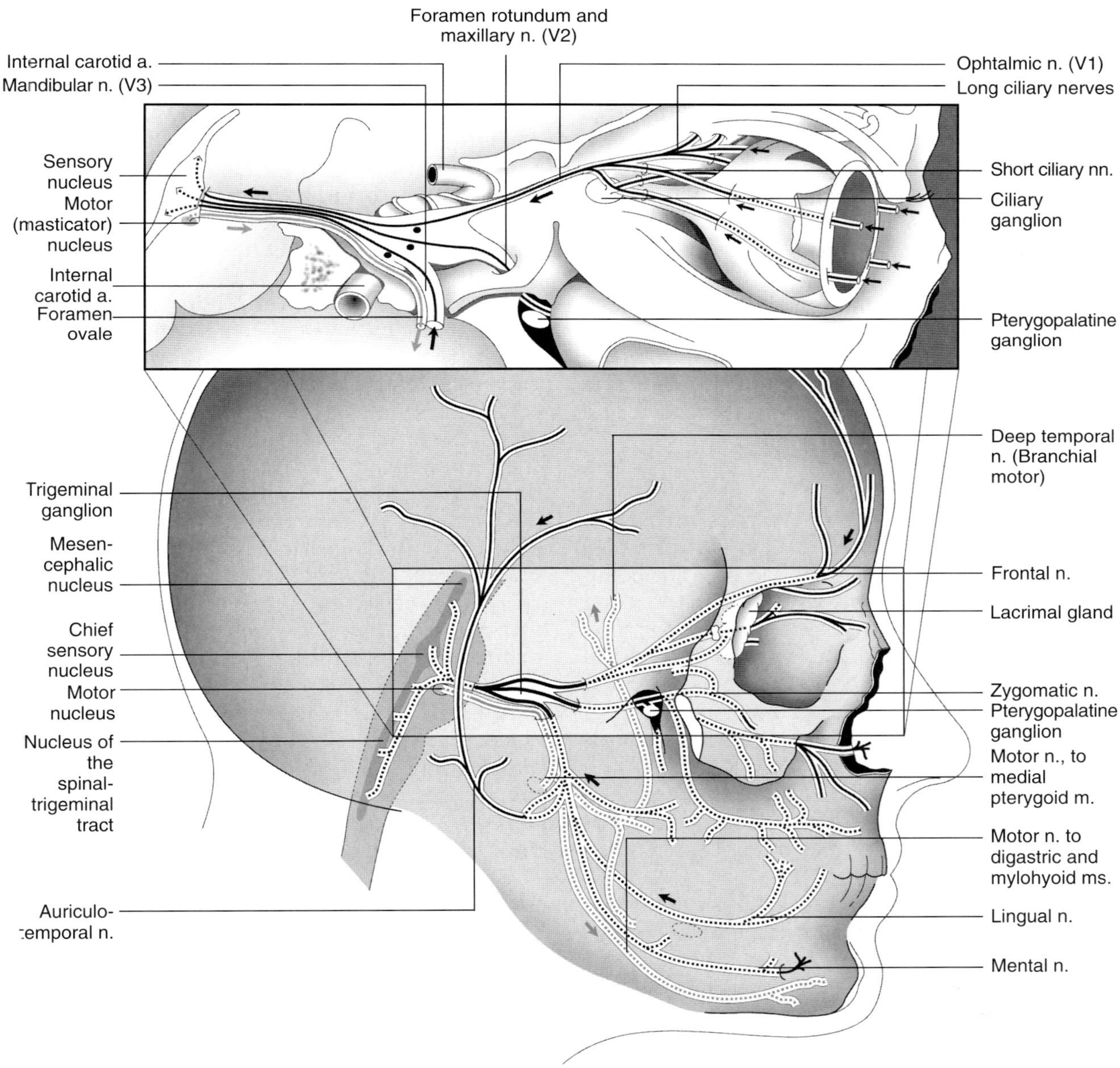

Fig. 6-6. The trigeminal nerve. (Adapted from Wilson-Pauwels, Akesson, Stewart).

The frontal nerve runs between the elevator of the upper lid and the periosteum. Halfway along its endoorbital pathway, it divides into the supratrochlear and supraorbital branches. The supratrochlear branch passes above the trochlea of the superior oblique muscle, emerges between the trochlea and the supraorbital foramen, and innervates the conjunctiva, the skin of the upper lid and the middle part of the lower forehead. The supraorbital nerve runs more superiorly, just under the roof of the orbit, through the supraorbital foramen, and innervates the upper lid, the conjunctiva and the skin of the forehead up to the lambdoid suture.

The lacrimal nerve runs in the orbit along with the lacrimal artery, along the superior surface of the lateral rectus. It then reaches the lacrimal gland and the conjunctiva.

The nasociliary nerve runs inferior to the other two branches. In the orbit, through the optic nerve and the ophthalmic artery, this nerve reaches the medial wall of the orbital cavity. It passes through the foramen and the ethmoidal canal to become the anterior ethmoidal nerve. It enters the cranium, runs over the cribriform plate of the ethmoid and descends beside the crista galli of the nasal cavity. Here it divides into a medial branch (for the mucosa of the septum) and a lateral branch. It exits at the inferior margin of the nasal bone and innervates the vestibule and the tip of the nose. A connecting branch goes from the nasociliary nerve to the ciliary ganglion, where the long ciliary branches and the infratrochlear and posterior ethmoidal nerves detach.

THE MAXILLARY NERVE (V2)

The maxillary nerve leaves the trigeminal ganglion, runs inferiorly into the cavernous sinus, crosses the foramen rotundum and exits the cranium. It then crosses the pterygopalatine fossa and enters the orbit through the inferior orbital fissure. Called the infraorbital nerve, it passes through the infraorbital canal in the orbital floor and exits the face through the infraorbital foramen.

The branches of the maxillary nerve are as follows:

The *meningeal nerve* leaves the nerve near the foramen rotundum to reach the dura mater of the middle cranial fossa, and part of the anterior cranial fossa.

The *ganglionic branches* reach the sphenopalatine ganglion in the pterygopalatine fossa. Sensory fibers run from here to the nose and the oropharynx, while motor fibers run to the lacrimal gland.

The *zygomatic nerve* goes from the pterygopalatine fossa to the orbit, where it divides into a zygomaticotemporal branch and a zygomaticofacial branch. The zygomaticotemporal nerve passes inferior to the orbit and enters the zygomatic bone. Upon reaching the temporal fossa and perforating the fascia of the temporalis muscle, it proceeds to innervate the skin of the temple. An anastomotic connection exists between the lacrimal nerve and the zygomaticotemporal nerve, which provides parasympathetic fibers to the lacrimal gland. The zygomaticofacial nerve passes inferolaterally to the orbit, transverses the zygomatic bone, and exits to innervate the cheek.

From the maxillary nerve, dental branches depart for the upper teeth. These are divided into posterior, medial, and anterior branches: the posterior branch goes to the molars, the gums, and the cheek; the medial branch goes to the premolars; and the anterior branch goes to the incisors, canines, and the lateral wall of the nose.

In the face, the maxillary nerve is divided into *palpebral, nasal* and *superior labial branches*.

The greater palatine nerve originates in the hard palate and the lesser palatine in the soft palate. They run through the pterygopalatine canal, are joined by nasal branches and a pharyngeal branch, pass through the pterygopalatine ganglion, join the maxillary nerve, traverse the foramen rotundum and enter the cranium.

THE MANDIBULAR NERVE (V3)

The mandibular nerve is composed of two roots: a sensory root, which leaves the gasserian ganglion to exit from the foramen ovale; and a motor root, which unites with the sensory root just after its exit from the foramen ovale.

It runs lateral and anterior to the tensor veli palatini muscle and the eustachian tube in the skull base, medially to the lateral pterygoid muscle. The otic nerve is located medially. Several branches exit the mandibular nerve as follows:

Meningeal nerve: exits the cranium through the foramen spinosum and reaches the dura mater of the middle cranial fossa.

Medial pterygoid muscle nerve: innervates the tensor tympani and the tensor veli palatini.

Buccal nerve: innervates the buccinator muscle and the mucosa of the gums. It runs medial to the masseter.

Masseter nerve: goes to the masseter and the temporomandibular articulation.

Deep temporal nerves: run to the medial face of the temporalis muscle.

Lateral pterygoid muscle nerve.

Auriculotemporal nerve: leaves the mandibular nerve posteriorly and divides into two branches which surround the middle meningeal artery. The branches unite once again in one single trunk, anterior to the ear. This runs under the lateral pterygoid muscle and the mandibular neck and emits di-

ramations for the external auditory meatus, the tympanic membrane (along with nerves VII and X) and the temporomandibular articulation.
Lingual nerve: The anterior two-thirds of the tongue are innervated by the lingual nerve, which runs alongside the tongue, superior to the submandibular gland. At the base of the tongue the nerve curves upward, ascends between the medial pterygoid muscle and the mandible, and reaches the mandibular nerve.
Mental nerve: The cheek and the lower lip are innervated by nerve branches that unite to form the mental nerve. The nerve enters the mandible through the mental foramen, runs in the mandibular canal where it receives nerve branches from the lower teeth, and forms the inferior alveolar nerve. This nerve exits the mandibular foramen to ascend, deep into the lateral pterygoid muscle, and reaches the mandibular nerve.

The sensory nucleus of the trigeminal nerve extends from the midbrain to the second cervical root of the bulb. It divides into three parts:
Mesencephalic nucleus.
Main sensitive nucleus.
Nucleus of the spinal tract.

The masticator nucleus (motor) is in the pons, medial to the principal sensory nucleus.

Abducens nerve (VI)

The abducens nerve is a somatic motor nerve (efferent). It innervates the lateral rectus muscle of the eye, which enables the eye to abduct (Fig. 6-5). The nucleus of VI is found in the pontine tegmen, proximal to the midline and anterior to the IVth ventricle. The nerve emerges from the brainstem at the junction between the medulla oblongata and the pons, and runs in the pontine cistern in a lateral and upward direction, generally posterior to the AICA. It perforates the dura lateral to the dorsum sellae of the sphenoid bone. It proceeds to the apex of the petrous bone, where it curves sharply and assumes an anterior direction. It enters the cavernous sinus and transverses it, inferior to III, IV, and VI and superior to V2. The internal carotid is located medially. The nerve then transverses the superior orbitary fissure, enters into the orbit, transverses the tendinous ring, and goes to the lateral rectus muscle.

Facial nerve (VII)

The facial nerve has various functions.

- A visceral motor function (efferent) which stimulates the secretion of the oral and nasal mucosal glands, the lacrimal glands, and the submandibular and sublingual glands.
- A branchial motor function (efferent) which innervates the occipital, buccinator, platysma, facial expression, stapedial, and stylohyoid muscles, and the posterior belly of the digastric muscle.
- A special sensory function (afferent) which carries taste sensation from the anterior two-thirds of the tongue and the hard and soft palates.
- A general sensory function (afferent), for the postauricular skin, the concha of the auricle, the walls of the auditory meatus and the external surface of the tympanic membrane (Fig. 6-7).

The motor impulse travels from the premotor cortex along axons in the corticobulbar tract and reaches the motor nuclei of the ipsilateral and contralateral nerves, in the lower part of the pons. The fibers innervating the muscles of the superior quadrants of the face are bilateral, while those of the inferior facial quadrants are contralateral. A supranuclear lesion thus manifests in a lower facial paralysis, while a subnuclear lesion is seen in a homolateral paralysis of the superior and inferior quadrants.
The *nervus intermedius* is a sensory root. The neuronal bodies are in the geniculate ganglion. The peripheral branches of these cells are taste fibers that run in the chorda tympani and greater petrosal nerve. The centripetal processes leave the trunk of the facial nerve in the IAC, entering the brainstem at the caudal limit of the pons.
There are connections with the sensory nucleus of the trigeminal nerve which is in the medulla, in the superior part of the nucleus of the tractus solitarius. Fibers innervate the cutaneous region, proceed to the geniculate ganglion (where they have their cell bodies) and join the sensory nucleus. The extensions of these unipolar cells cross the nervus intermedius to enter the pons and reach the trigeminal nucleus in the medulla. The secondary neurons continue to the contralateral thalamic nuclei. The tertiary neurons go to the postcentral gyrus.
The facial nerve emerges from the pons approx. 11 mm lateral to the midline. Its intracisternal length is approx. 15 mm. Its myelin sheath, approx. 2 mm from the brain, is made up of oligodendrocytes rather than Schwann cells. Direct or transmitted pressure finds less resistance in this area than the nerve, and may lacerate it. Neurovascular conflicts also have an immediate effect. The nerve enters the internal auditory canal at its porus and runs along its medial and superior wall. It is located above the transverse crest and medially to the vertical crest (see chapter 28). The nerve reaches the geniculate ganglion, where the

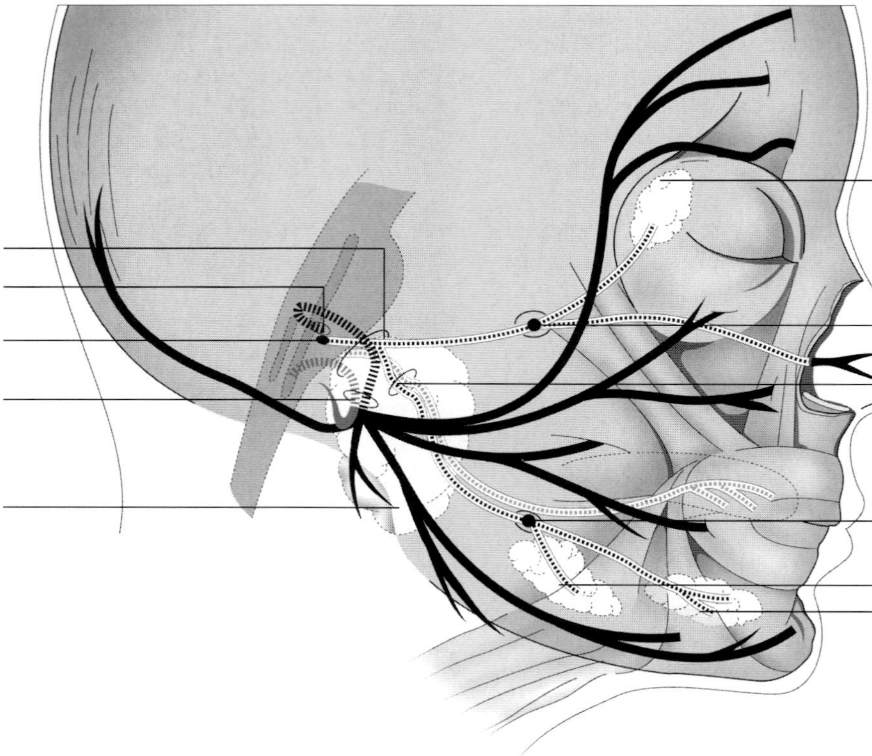

Fig. 6-7. The facial nerve. (Adapted from Wilson-Pauwels, Akesson, Stewart).

greater and lesser superficial petrosal nerves begin. Between the labyrinthine part of the nerve and that of the tympanic cavity, an approx. 70° angle is formed on a nearly horizontal plane. This is the first genu. The two arms are separated by a triangular area of compact bone, whose base rests on the vestibule and whose vertex projects like a cuneus into the genu.

The second tract, or tympanic segment, goes from the geniculate ganglion to the posterior wall of the tympanic cavity, running on its medial wall for 10-12 mm. Its pathway may be parallel to the horizontal semicircular canal, but usually it slopes downward and forms a 10° angle with the plane of this canal.

The angle formed by the second and third segments of the VII canal varies from 95-125°. Its curvature begins in the area posterior to the oval window, and terminates in the upper third of the vertical part of VII.

The third tract, or mastoid segment, runs from the second genu to the stylomastoid foramen. Its length is approx. 13 mm. It transverses the mastoid with a slight outward concavity. It then reaches the stylomastoid foramen, where it is more lateral compared to the level of the second genu.

The course of the facial nerve may be divided as follows (May):

Supranuclear
Cortex segment
Nuclear
Pons segment
Infranuclear
CPA segment
internal auditory canal segment
tympanomastoid segment
extracranial segment.

Two contingents of parasympathetic or motor fibers leave the superior salivary nerve. One part runs in the nervus intermedius, then in the greater petrosal nerve as it leaves the geniculate ganglion. It then unites with the deep petrosal nerve, enters the pterygoid canal, and becomes the pterygoid canal nerve. This nerve transverses the medial pterygoid lamina of the sphenoid and proceeds to the pterygopalatine ganglion, suspended from the maxillary branch of the trigeminal nerve, in the pterygopalatine fossa. The parasympathetic fibers synapse in the sphenopalatine ganglion and proceed along the zygomatic branch of the maxillary nerve to stimulate the nasal and oral mucous membrane and the lacrimal glands. The branches involved are the orbital branches, the greater palatine nerve (anterior), the lesser palatine nerves (medial and posterior) and the nasal branches.

Other parasympathetic fibers run along the nervus intermedius, enter the facial canal, and then pro-

ceed into the chorda tympani. The chorda tympani, which is just medial to the annulus tympanicus, transverses the tympanic cavity and then exits through the petrotympanic fissure. It joins the lingual branch of the mandibular nerve after its exit from the foramen ovale. The parasympathetic fibers synapse at the submandibular ganglion, suspended from V3 in the submaxillary region, inferior to the last molar. Postgangliar fibers runs from the ganglion to stimulate the submandibular and sublingual gland secretions.
Sympathetic fibers run from the cervical ganglion into the internal carotid plexus, then to the deep petrosal nerve and the pterygoid nerve.

Vestibulocochlear nerve (VIII)

The vestibulocochlear nerve is a special sensory (afferent) nerve. It carries acoustic stimuli from the cochlea and balancing signals from the maculae of the utricle, saccule and ampullas of the semicircular canals (see chapter 1).
The primary sensory neurons are located around the modiolus. Their somas form the cochlear (or spiral) ganglion. The axons make up the cochlear nerve which leaves the cochlea and enters with the vestibular nerve into the internal auditory canal (Fig. 6-8).
The internal auditory canal is divided by a crest, called the falciform or transverse crest. The latter divides the IAC into a superior and an inferior part. The facial nerve is thus anterior-superior, the cochlear nerve anterior-inferior, and the inferior vestibular nerve is posterior-inferior. At the

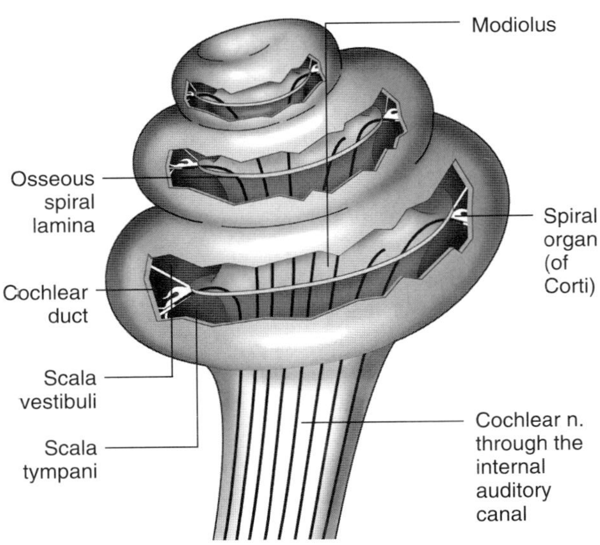

Fig. 6-8. Interior view of the cochlea.

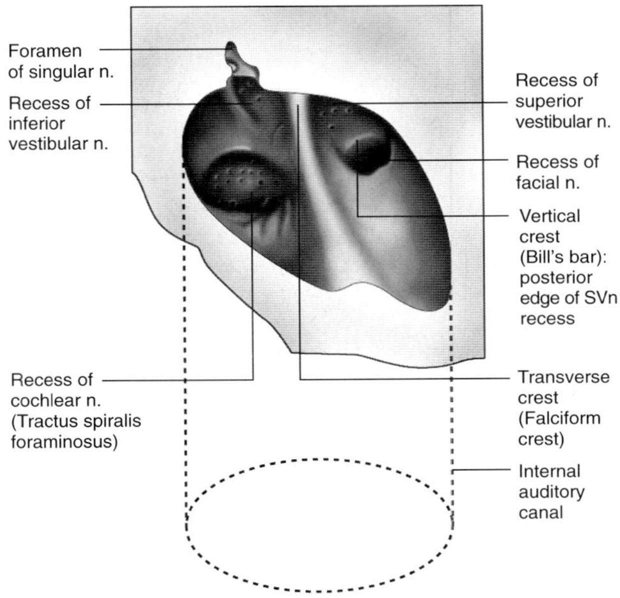

Fig. 6-9. The fundus of the internal auditory canal. (Adapted from Gray's anatomy).

internal auditory canal fundus, the vestibular nerve is separated from the facial nerve by a ridge called the vertical crest, or Bill's bar (name given it by colleagues of Dr. W. House, for his emphasis on its importance as a surgical landmark) (Fig. 6-9).
The *posterior ampullary nerve* (*singular nerve*) arises from the sensory cells of the posterior canal ampulla. It joins the inferior vestibular nerve in the IAC. The posterior ampullary nerve section has been proposed (Gacek) for the management of the benign paroxismal positional vertigo (cupulolithiasis) (see chapter 21).
The cochlear nerve exits the cochlea and unites with the vestibular nerve after approx. 2.3 mm, forming one single trunk. At its entrance into the junction of the medulla oblongata with the pons, the cochlear nerve is medial to the vestibular nerve. The facial nerve runs medial to the other two, whereas the labyrinthine artery runs between VII and VIII. The two nerves thus separate upon entering the brainstem, while the cochlear nerve runs lateral to the inferior cerebellar peduncle and the vestibular nerve medial (Fig. 6-10).
The primary acoustic neurons carry low frequency signals and synapse in the dorsal cochlear nucleus, at the bulbopontine junction, lateral to the entrance of the facial nerve. The vestibulocochlear nerve, in its intracisternal pathway, runs approx. 15 mm to enter the internal auditory meatus. For approx. 10 mm of its pathway from the brainstem to the internal auditory canal, this nerve has a myelin sheath made up of oligoden-

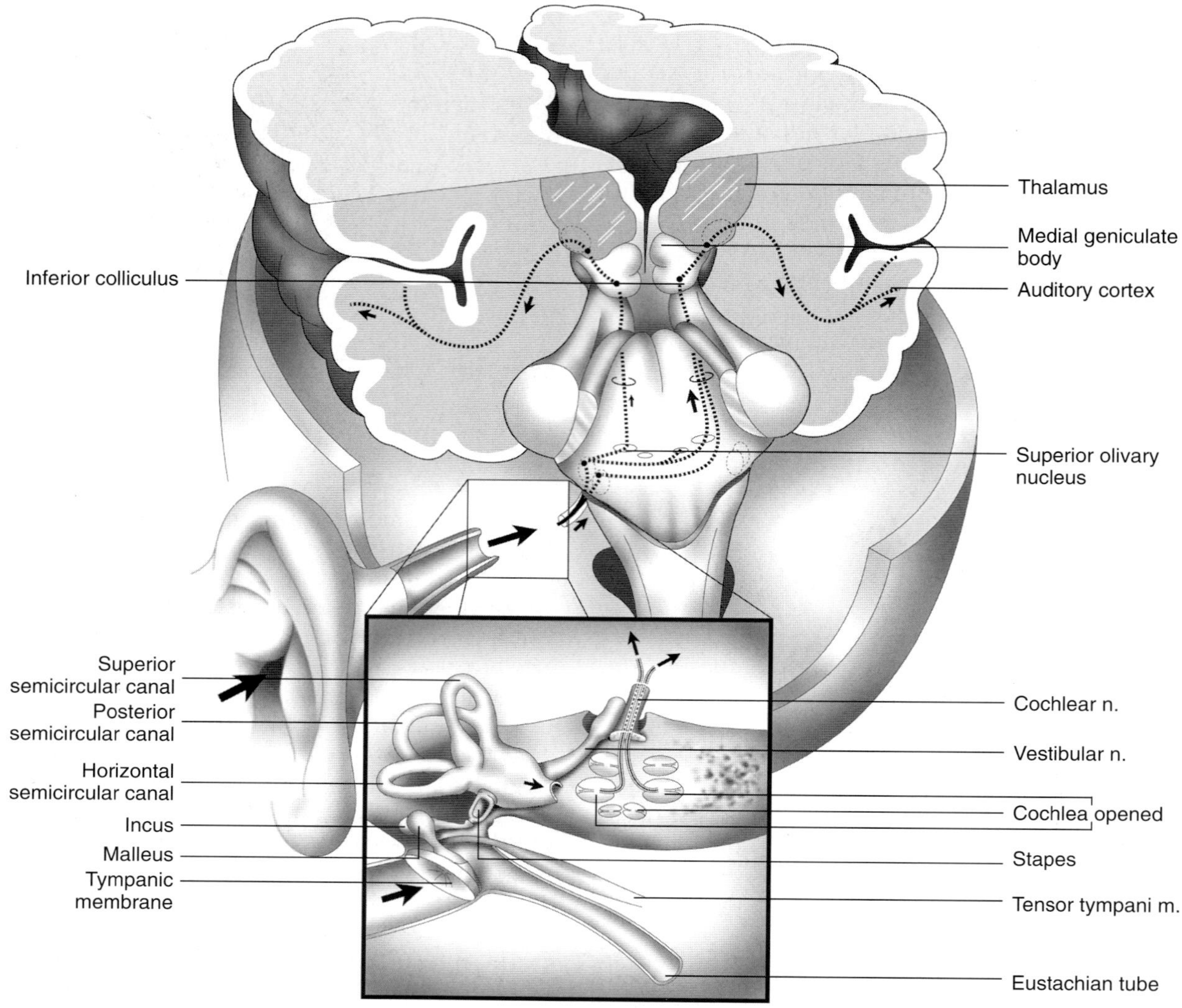

Fig. 6-10. The vestibulocochlear nerve.

drocytes, rather than Schwann cells (Lang). This explains its sensitivity to neurovascular conflicts.
The dorsal cochlear nucleus protrudes outside the brainstem with a bulge called the acoustic tubercle. The bodies of the secondary neurons are located here. Most of the secondary nerve fibers cross the midline and ascend the contralateral lateral lemniscus. The fibers originating from the ventral cochlear nucleus make up the trapezoid body. Both the trapezoid body and the superior olivary nucleus may be synapsing zones for the fibers, before they join in the lateral lemniscus. Some non-decussate fibers synapse in the superior olivary nucleus. Some fibers go directly from the superior olivary nucleus to the facial nucleus to activate the stapedial contraction, which acts in very intense sounds by diminishing the stapes' penetration into the labyrinth. The neurons grouped in the lateral lemniscus proceed in the ipsilateral lateral lemniscus across the pons and the midbrain to later synapse in the inferior colliculus.
The tertiary neurons ascend through the inferior branch and the medial geniculate body to the thalamus. Thalamo-cortical fibers go from the thalamus through the internal capsule, to reach the temporal transverse gyrus, where sound compression occurs.

THE VESTIBULAR NERVE

The superior vestibular nerve originates by the labyrinthine receptors in the ampulla of the superior and lateral semicircular canal and utricle. The inferior vestibular nerve originates by the receptors of the saccule and the posterior semicircular canal. Separated by a bony plate, the vertical or falciform crest, the two nerves unite after 2-3 mm in one single trunk, which also receives fibers from the cochlear nerve.

The cell bodies of the primary neurons form the vestibular ganglion or Scarpa's ganglion. The axons from diverse labyrinthine receptors separate into an ascending and a descending branch and terminate in the vestibular nuclei, in the floor of the fourth ventricle, where the nuclei of the secondary neurons are located.
The secondary neurons, where fibers from the cortex, cerebellum, brainstem, and reticular substance converge, send fibers to the nuclei of the oculomotor nerves (III, IV, VI) through the medial longitudinal fasciculus and the reticular formation. This causes reflex movements of the ocular bulbs. The secondary neurons also send fibers to the muscles of the limbs, the trunk, the neck, and the head, to maintain equilibrium.

AUDITORY PATHWAY

The spiral ganglion of Corti, located in the Rosenthal canal and contained in the modiolus, is made up of bipolar nerve cells. Its peripheral extensions transverse the osseous spiral lamina and distribute among the acoustic cells, whereas the central extensions form the cochlear branch of the acoustic nerve, and terminate in the dorsal and ventral cochlear nuclei.
Some fibers go from here to the lateral lemniscus, where they join the middle geniculate body. This may be direct or interrupted in the nucleus of the lateral lemniscus and the inferior quadrigeminal tubercle.
Other fibers proceed to the homolateral and contralateral superior olivary complexes, which connect with the nuclei of the cranial nerves to provoke acoustic-motor reflexes.
Some of these fibers go to the nuclei of V and VII and act on the tensor tympani muscle and the stapedius muscle.
Other (predominantly crossed) fibers enter the lateral lemniscus and go from the olivary complex to the quadrigeminal tubercle below and the geniculate body medially.
From the medial geniculate body, the last fibers reach the primary acoustic area, situated in the temporal lobe, in the internal two-thirds of the transversal gyrus of Heschl (Brodmann's area 40).
There are secondary areas (52 and 22) around the primary acoustic area with an associative function.
Centrifugal fibers leave these areas to cross the olivo-cochlear Rasmussen fibers and reach the acoustic cells, where they have a control function.

THE VESTIBULAR PATHWAY

The central vestibular extension of VIII reaches the medial vestibular nuclei (of Schwalbe), the lateral vestibular nuclei (of Deiters), and the superior vestibular nuclei (Bechterew) at the bulbopontine level.
The fibers go from here to the medial longitudinal fasciculus and the reticular formation. Some fibers run to the nuclei of the oculomotor nerves (III, IV, VI), at the base of the nystagmic reflex. Other fibers go to and from the brainstem, the cerebral cortex, and the cerebellum, determining the postural tone of the skeletal muscles.

Glossopharyngeal nerve (IX)

The glossopharyngeal nerve has various components.

- A visceral motor (efferent) component, which sends secretory fibers to the parotid glands.
- An efferent branchial motor component, which provides the stylopharyngeal muscle with a voluntary innervation.
- A visceral sensory component (afferent) which innervates the carotid sinus and body.
- A general sensory component (afferent) which innervates the posterior third of the tongue, the skin of the external ear and the internal mucosa of the tympanic membrane.
- A special sensory component (afferent) which has an excitatory function for the taste receptors in the posterior third of the tongue.

The nerve, in the form of three or four roots, exits the medulla oblongata between the olive and the inferior cerebellar peduncle (Fig. 6-11). These roots then converge to form the nervous trunk. The vagus nerve is below. This nerve, initially covered by the floccule, runs on the jugular tubercle of the occipital bone. It turns downward, crosses the jugular fossa and emits the tympanic nerve, before exiting from the jugular foramen. The jugular foramen is delineated by the jugular fossa of the petrous part of the temporal bone and by the occipital bone. The dura above the jugular foramen has two perforations: the glossopharyngeal meatus, where IX enters the nervous part; and the meatus vagalis, through which the vagus and the spinal accessory enter into the venous part. The glossopharyngeal meatus is found in the medial part anterior-superior to the jugular foramen.
The two meati are separated by a dural septum.
The jugular foramen is divided in two by a bridge, which is usually fibrous but may be osseous. There is a nervous part, which contains IX, and a venous part containing X, XI, and the jugular bulb. The inferior and superior ganglia pass through this foramen. The inferior ganglion,

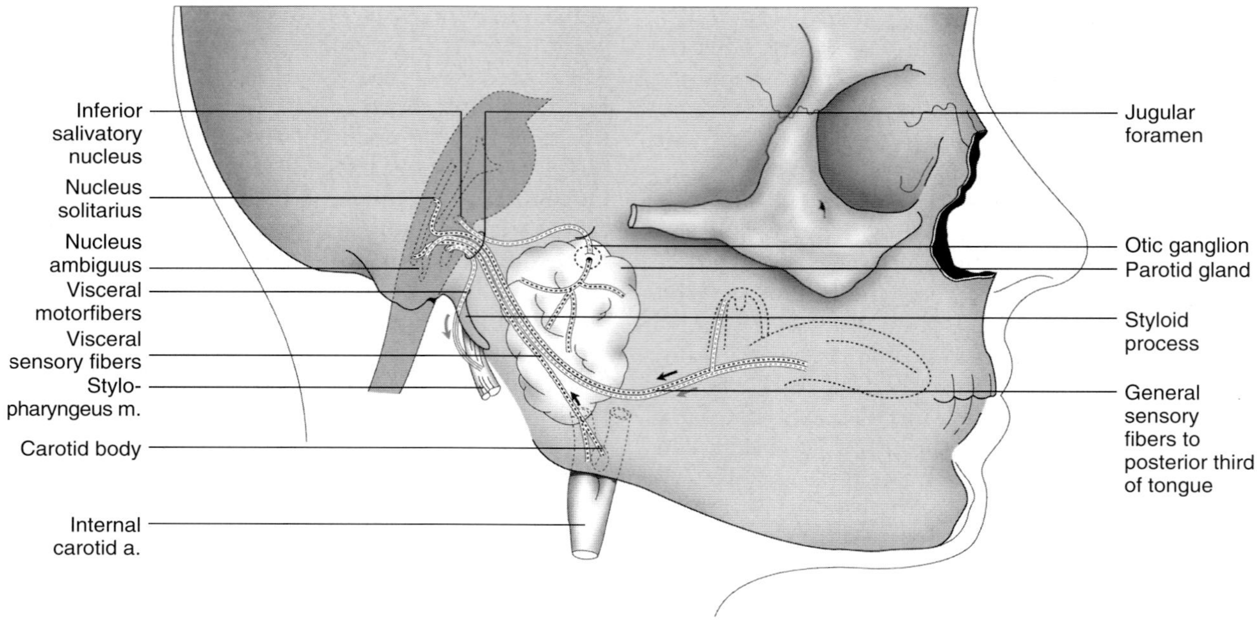

Fig. 6-11. The glossopharyngeal nerve. (Adapted from Wilson-Pauwels, Akesson, Stewart).

which is the larger of the two, is located below in the petrous part of the temporal bone. Branches from the posterior third of the tongue, the pharynx, the sinus and the carotid body join the unipolar cell bodies and carry general and visceral sensitivity.

The superior cervical ganglion does not send collateral branches and is considered part of the inferior ganglion.

The nerve exits the cranium, deeper than the styloid process, and runs first between the jugular vein and the internal carotid, and then in front of the carotid. Upon reaching the stylopharyngeal muscle, it curves anteriorly and passes above between the superior and middle constrictor muscles, reaching the mucosa of the pharynx and the posterior region of the tongue, the tonsils, and the buccal mucous glands.

The nerve communicates with the vagus and the facial nerve.

The superior cervical ganglion of the sympathetic nerve is connected to a branch leaving the inferior ganglion of IX.

Two branches exit the inferior ganglion to go to the auricular branch of the vagus nerve and its superior ganglion.

A branch of nerve IX runs inferior to the inferior cervical ganglion to the facial nerve near the stylomastoid foramen, after having perforated the posterior belly of the digastric nerve.

The following are branches of nerve IX: *tympanic*, *carotic*, *pharyngeal*, *muscular*, *tonsillar*, and *lingual*.

The *tympanic nerve* leaves the inferior ganglion, runs in the inferior tympanic canaliculus, and enters the tympanic cavity, running on the promontory where it forms the tympanic plexus. There are three branches of the tympanic plexus: the branch innervating the mucosa of the tympanic cavity; another for the greater superficial petrosal nerve; and one for the lesser petrosal nerve. The lesser petrosal nerve has a retrograde path, and emerges from a foramen lateral to the greater petrosal nerve. It then heads anteriorly, descends through the foramen ovale, and synapses with the otic ganglion. Fibers run from the otic ganglion to the auriculotemporal nerve, a branch of the V3 mandibular nerve (adjacent to the ganglion) and carry motor and secretory fibers to the parotid gland.

Chemoreceptive fibers of the carotic body and baroreceptors of the carotic sinus form the *carotic nerve*. Its task is to control arterial pressure and respiration. The nerve runs upward and reaches the inferior ganglion, where the cell bodies are located. The fibers pass from here to the brainstem, and descend into the tractus solitarius to the nucleus solitarius, where they connect with the reticular formation and the hypothalamus. The *carotid branch* descends along the internal carotid to reach the walls of the carotic body and the carotid sinus. In this area a nervous plexus is formed by IX and branches of the superior cervical ganglion and the sympathetic and vagus nerves.

The following are also found:
Pharyngeal branches which innervate the pharyngeal mucosa form the pharyngeal plexus along with the laryngopharyngeal branches of the sympathetic nerve.
Other branches go to the stylopharyngeal muscle, the tonsils, and the tongue.

Vagus nerve (X)

The vagus nerve contains sensory and motor fibers. It runs from the medulla oblongata to the splenic fissure of the colon. It exits the brainstem in multiple roots, which then form one single trunk which passes under the floccule and exits the jugular foramen. Surrounded by arachnoid and dura mater, the vagus runs beside the accessory nerve (just posterior) into the jugular foramen. A fibrous septum separates it from the more anteriorly located glossopharyngeal nerve. A widening in the foramen indicates the superior ganglion, with the inferior ganglion inferior to it. Thin collateral branches connect the superior ganglion to the inferior ganglion of nerve IX, the superior cervical ganglion of the sympathetic nerve, and to the facial nerve.
Cells with bodies in the superior ganglion have a somatic responsibility, while those in the inferior ganglion have the task of visceral sensitivity.
In its pathway below the inferior ganglion, the vagus nerve receives fibers from the nucleus ambiguus which run with the accessory nerve. The nerve enters the neck inside first the internal and then the common carotid sheath. It then runs from the carotid to the jugular, to the base of the neck. Here the nerves from the two sides take different pathways.

Right pathway

The nerve descends to the subclavian artery and transverses it. It then enters the thorax and penetrates the mediastinum lateral to the trachea, posterior to the brachiocephalic vein and superior cava vein. The nerve runs superior to the right pleura, with the interposition of the azygos vein. It then passes behind the right main bronchus. At the base of the right lung it divides into filaments which form the right posterior lung plexus together with the filaments from the thoracic ganglia II and IV. Descending branches unite with a branch of the left vagus on the esophagus, forming the posterior esophageal plexus. A branch (the posterior vagal trunk) exits to innervate the stomach and the abdominal viscera, up to the splenic flexure.

Left pathway

The left pathway descends between the carotid and the subclavian artery, posterior to the brachiocephalic vein. It then enters the mediastinum, where it runs posterior to the lung. It is crossed by the frenic nerve and passes the aortic arch. Here the intercostal superior vein crosses it superiorly. The left posterior pulmonary plexus forms analagously to the right. Two branches descend from here on the anterior esophagus and form the anterior esophageal plexus with a branch of the right posterior pulmonary plexus. The anterior vagal trunk exits and descends along the esophagus, entering the abdomen through the hiatus of the diaphragm. Branches then go to the heart, the liver, the pylorus, the duodenum, the pancreas, and the stomach.
The branches of the vagus nerve are as follows:
Meningeal and auricular branches in the jugular fossa.
Pharyngeal, superior laryngeal, right inferior laryngeal, cardiac in the neck.
Cardiac, left inferior laryngeal, pulmonary, esophageal in the thorax.
Gastrointestinal and hepatic in the abdomen.

The meningeal branch exits the superior ganglion and goes to the dura mater of the posterior cranial fossa.
The auricular branch begins at the superior ganglion of the vagus nerve. It then passes under the jugular vein, enters the mastoid canaliculus, transverses the facial canal 3-4 mm superior to the stylomastoid foramen, and sends a communicating branch with the facial nerve. It then passes through the tympanomastoid fissure and divides into the posterior auricular nerve and a branch for the skin of the auricle, the posterior and inferior external auditory canal, and the tympanic membrane.
The pharyngeal branch runs between the two carotid branches and divides into smaller branches. It joins with the glossopharyngeal, external laryngeal, and sympathetic nerves to form the pharyngeal plexus. Motor fibers run from here to the muscles of the pharynx and the soft palate.
The superior laryngeal nerve comes from the inferior ganglion of the vagus nerve. It descends lateral to the pharynx behind the internal carotid artery. It then proceeds medially and divides into two laryngeal nerves, the internal and the external.
The internal laryngeal nerve perforates the thyroid membrane and divides into a superior and an inferior branch. The superior branch goes to the pharynx and the supraglottic region, while the inferior branch goes to the arytenoid mucosa.
The external laryngeal nerve is smaller than the internal one. It runs to innervate the inferior pharyngeal constrictor. It then perforates it and distributes to the cricothyroid muscle, the pharyn-

geal plexus and enters in contact with the superior cardiac nerve and the superior sympathetic cervical ganglion.
The recurrent laryngeal nerve innervates all the muscles of the larynx with the one exception of the cricothyroid. Its pathway is different on each side.
To the left, it leaves the vagus at the aortic arch, passing under it. It then ascends into the tracheo-esophageal sulcus, in a deep or slightly anterior position. It then enters in contact with the thyroid laterally and with the thyroid artery inferiorly in a variable relationship. Posteriorly, it penetrates the larynx between the cricoid cartilage and the inferior horn of the thyroid cartilage, which it innervates. To the rigth the nerve may be posterior, anterior or intermingled with branches of the inferior thyroid artery, while on the left it is usually posterior.
The right recurrent laryngeal nerve originates anteriorly from the right vagus nerve. It passes below and ascends into the tracheo-esophageal sulcus, with relationships analogous to those of the recurrent contralateral nerve, behind the common carotid artery. It passes beside the inferior lobe of the thyroid, accompanied anteriorly by the inferior thyroid artery. The latter is rarely found in a posterior position, and continues to the larynx.
The cardiac branches leave the vagus superiorly at the level of the cardiac branches of the sympathetic nerve and inferiorly at the base of the neck, to reach the cardiac plexus.
The pulmonary branches separate into anterior and posterior branches. The anterior branches go to the anterior pulmonary plexus, while the posterior branches go to the posterior pulmonary plexus.
The gastric branches innervate the stomach.
The intestinal branches innervate the celiac plexus.
The hepatic branches innervate the hepatic plexus.
The renal branches innervate the renal plexus.

Accessory nerve (XI)

The accessory (motor) nerve innervates the sternocleidomastoid muscle and the trapezoid body (Fig. 6-12).
Axons descend from the motor cortex into the corticospinal tract, where they cross the posterior genu of the internal capsule. They then pass contralaterally into the decussation of the pyramids, descend into the corticospinal tract, and synapse in the accessory nucleus. The accessory nucleus is found at the level of the nucleus ambiguus, at the first 5-6 segments of the brainstem and lateral to their gray anterior column. Postsynaptic fibers emerge as small roots from the white matter of the brainstem, below the vagus nerve, to form the accessory nerve.
The roots form a trunk which exits posterior to the dentate ligament and ascends into the cranium through the foramen magnum, posterior to the vertebral artery. It then runs into the jugular foramen with an arachnoid fold which divides it from the contiguous nerve X.
As it exits the jugular foramen, the XI CN crosses the transverse process of the atlas, crossed by the occipital artery. It then passes posterior and medial to the styloid process and emerges halfway up the posterior margin of the sternocleidomastoid muscle. It then transverses the posterior triangle of the neck, in contact with the superficial lymph nodes. It runs posteriorly and encounters the anterior margin of the trapezoid muscle 4-5 mm above the clavicle. It penetrates the latter and innervates it, forming a plexus with the third and fourth cervical nerves.

Hypoglossal nerve (XII)

The hypoglossal is a motor nerve innervating the intrinsic and extrinsic muscles of the tongue, except for the palatoglossal muscle which is innervated by X (Fig. 6-13). The nucleus of the hypoglossal nerve is approx. 2 cm long and is located in the tegmen of the medulla. The cranial part of the nucleus forms the hypoglossal triangle in the floor of the fourth ventricle. The axons run in the medial lemniscus and emerge between the pyramid and the olive through the anterolateral sulcus in a series of small roots. The roots form the hypoglossal nerve which transverses the hypoglossal foramen in the posterior cranial fossa, then exits the cranium. The nerve becomes medial to the internal jugular vein, the internal carotid artery, and cranial nerves IX-X and XI. It runs between the jugular vein and the internal carotid and superiorly it is in contact with the inferior ganglion of the vagus. It loops at the level of the division of the common carotid and superior to the great horn of the hyoid bone. It enters in contact with the facial artery superiorly and the lingual artery inferiorly. It runs on the surface of the hyoglossal muscle, and enters in relationship with the lingual nerve, the submandibular gland and its duct. It then passes over the margin of the mylohyoid and goes on to innervate the lingual muscles.

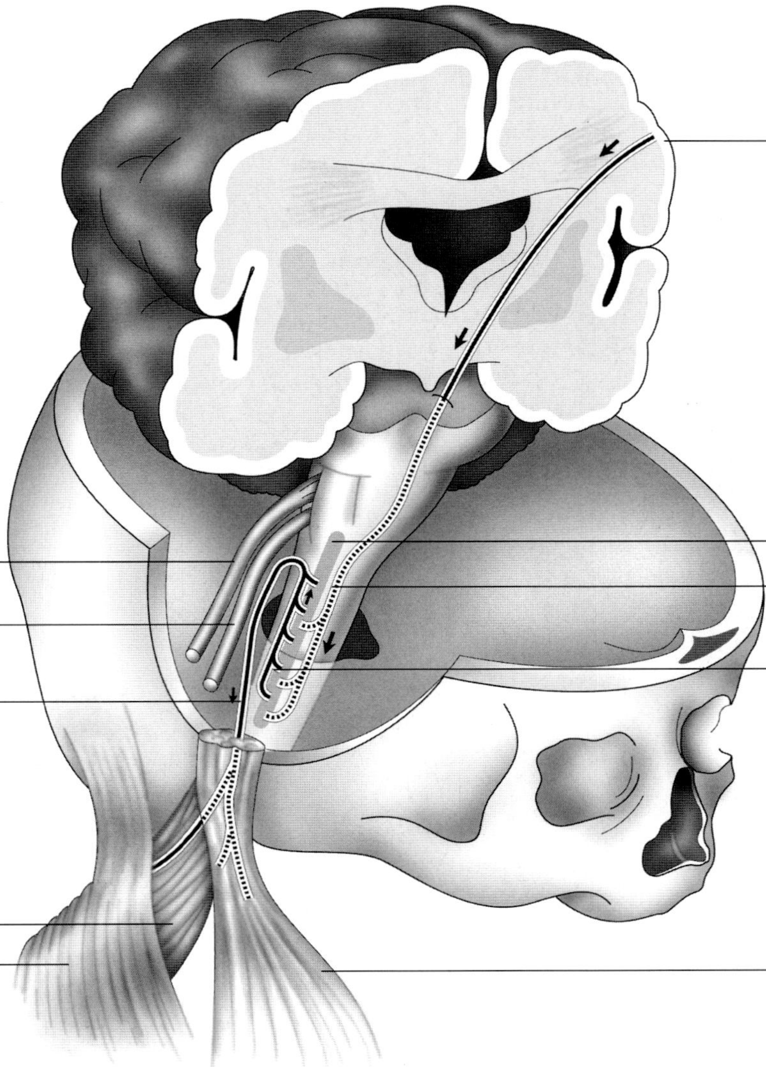

Fig. 6-12. The accessory nerve.

The nerve is in contact with the cervical sympathetic nerve: filaments from the superior cervical ganglion and the first and second cervical nerve run with XII and then separate and descend into the sternohyoid and sternothyroid muscles (superior root of the cervical loop).

The meningeal nerve is one of the branches of the hypoglossal nerve. The meningeal nerve leaves the nerve at its passage into the hypoglossal foramen; it goes to the dura of the posterior fossa and its venous structures.

Branches coming from the inferior vagal ganglion connect the hypoglossal nerve with the vagus nerve.

The geniohyoid and thyrohyoid are other branches of the hypoglossal nerve. They leave the nerve at its passage between the hyoglossal and the mylohyoid.

The descending branch, or the superior root of the cervical loop, is another of the hypoglossal's branches. From this branch the nerve departs for the superior belly of the homohyoid muscle. The descending branch then unites with the inferior root of the cervical loop to form the cervical, or hypoglossal, loop. Here branches leave for the sternohyoid and sternothyroid muscles and for the inferior belly of the homohyoid.

Arrangement and instrumentation

Following are drawings of the arrangement and proper use of surgical instruments (Figs. 6-14, 6-15, 6-16, 6-17, 6-18, 6-19, 6-20, 6-21, 6-22, 6-23, 6-24).

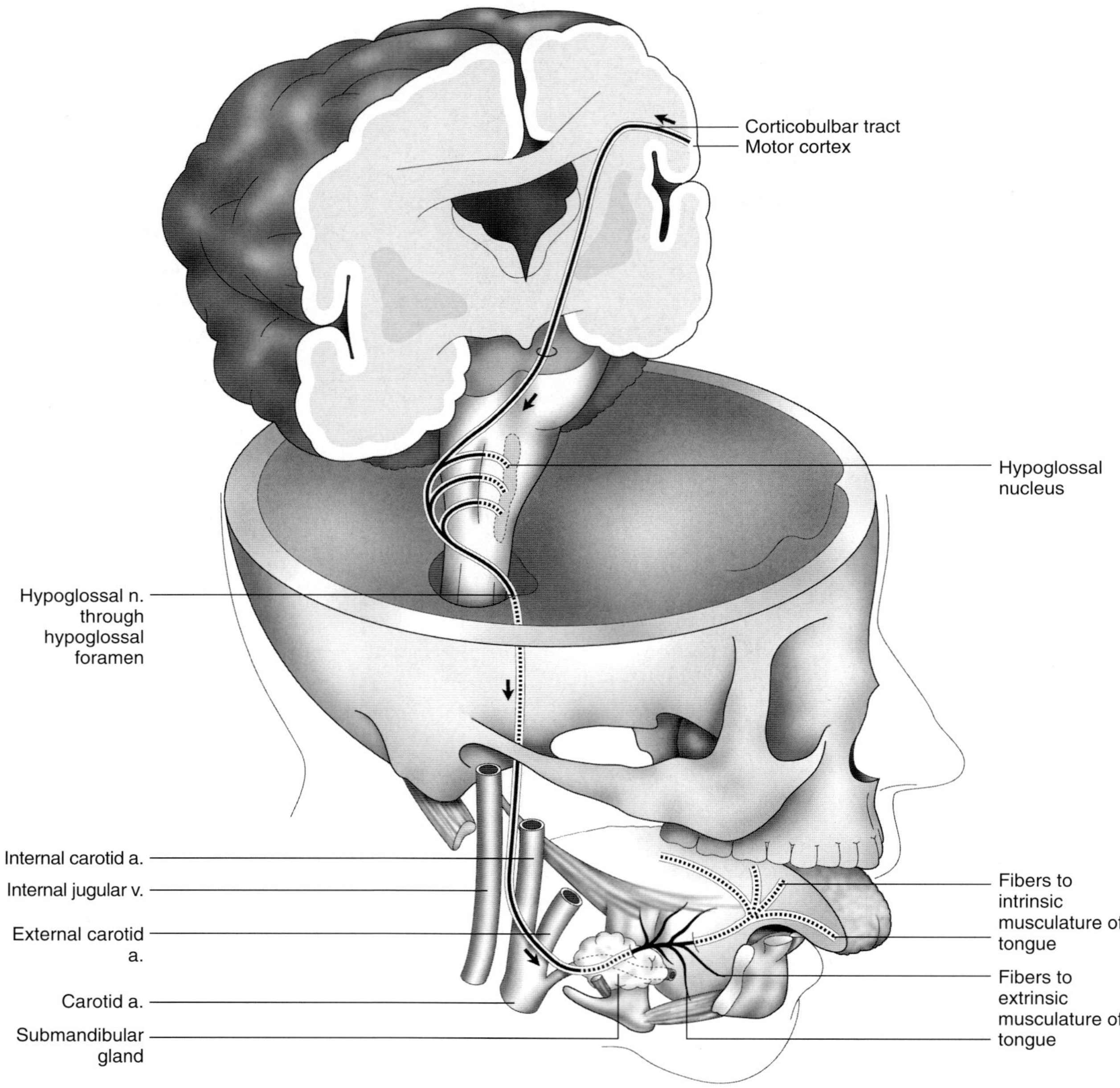

Fig. 6-13. The hypoglossal nerve.

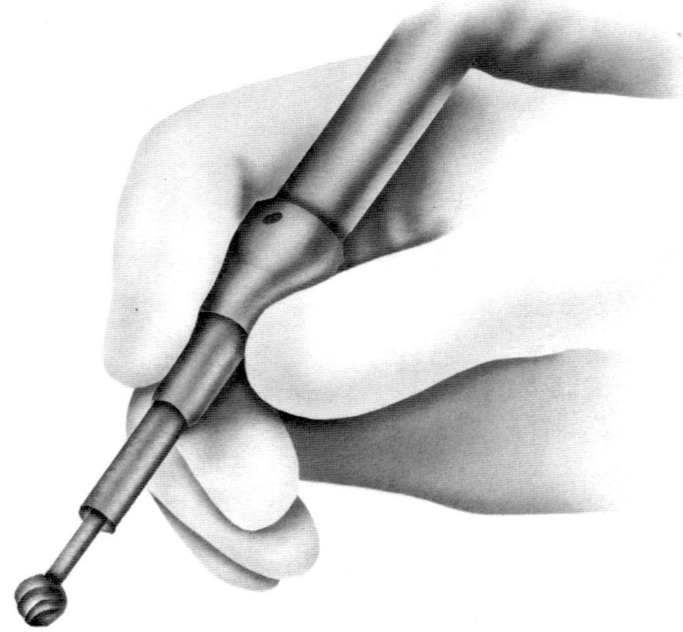

Fig. 6-14. Proper holding of drill.

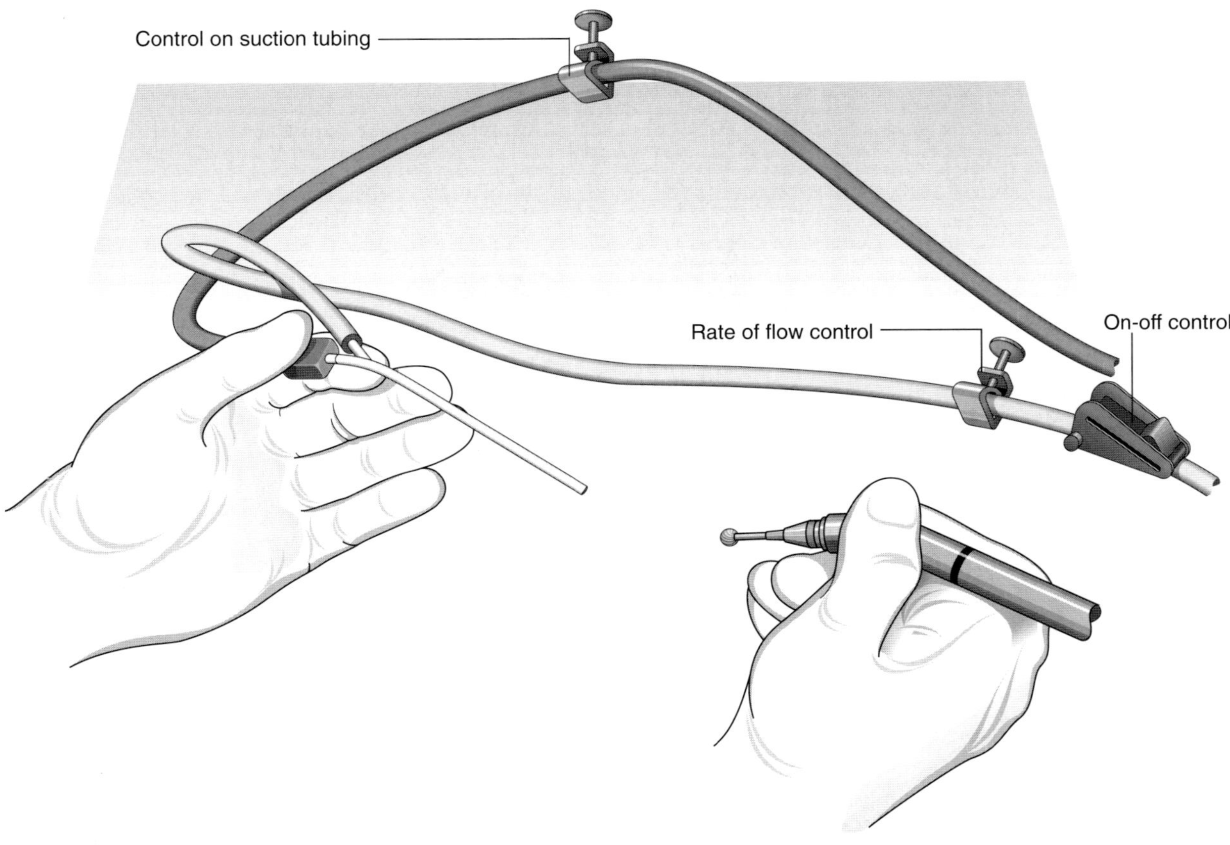

Fig. 6-15. Suction-irrigation controls. See chapter 28.

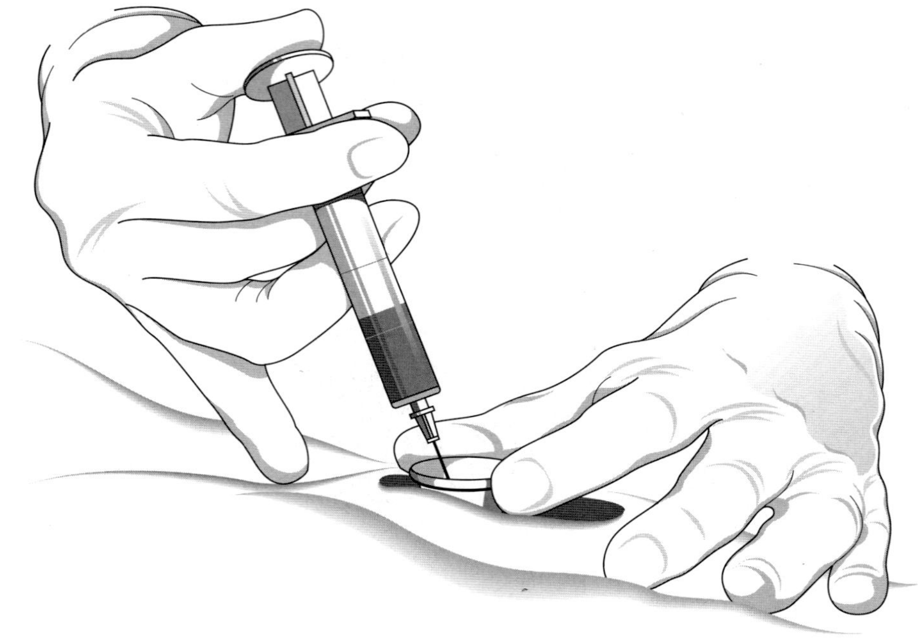

Fig. 6-16. Infiltration. In injecting the skin, note the bracing of the speculum in the usual manner with the syringe resting against the inner surface of the speculum. Note the small finger of the right hand being placed against the head as the injection proceeds.

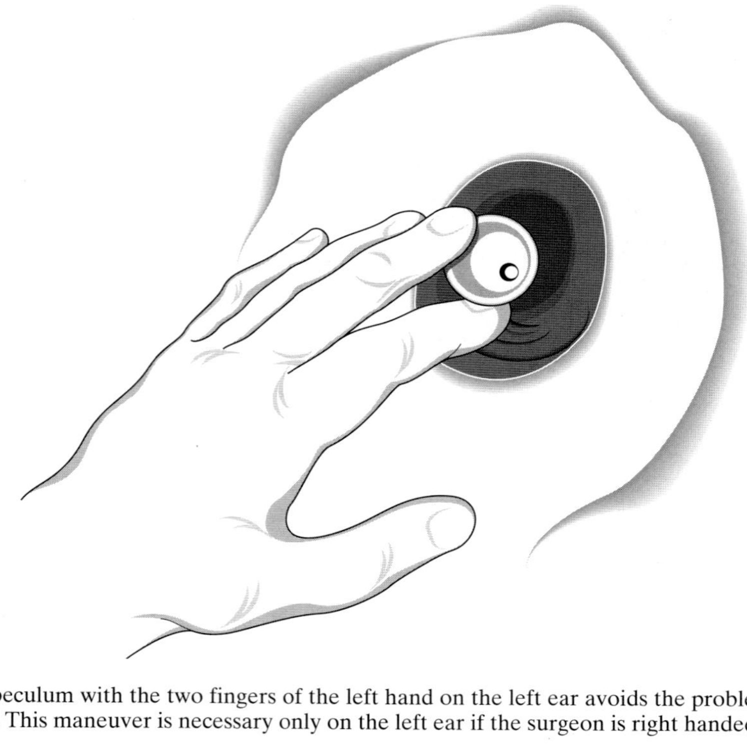

Fig. 6-17. Holding the speculum with the two fingers of the left hand on the left ear avoids the problem of the shoulder interfering with the positioning. This maneuver is necessary only on the left ear if the surgeon is right handed.

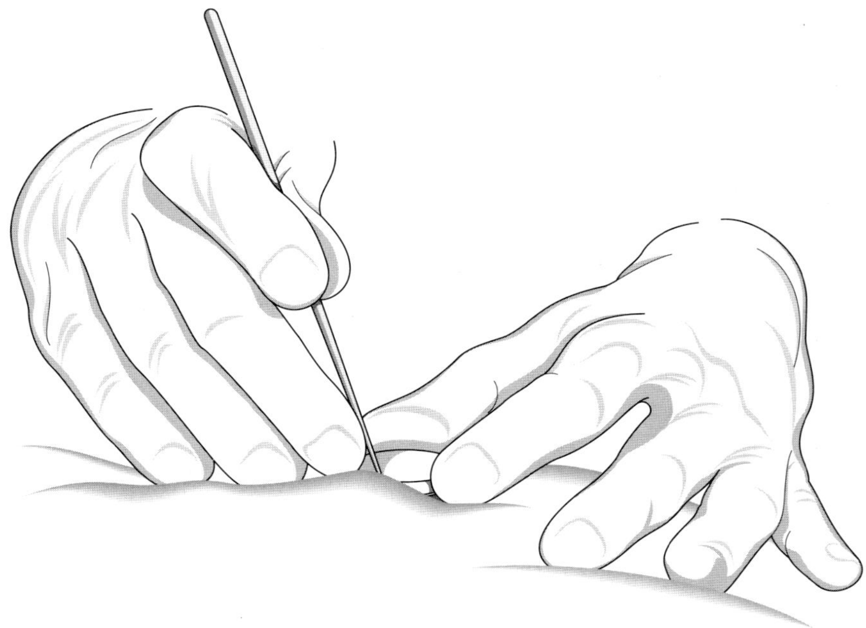

Fig. 6-18. Incision. Straight instrument. The speculum is being braced by the thumb and first finger of the left hand, using the third and fourth fingers to the left hand against the side of the second finger of the right hand. The third and fourth fingers are being used to steady the hand agaist the patient head.

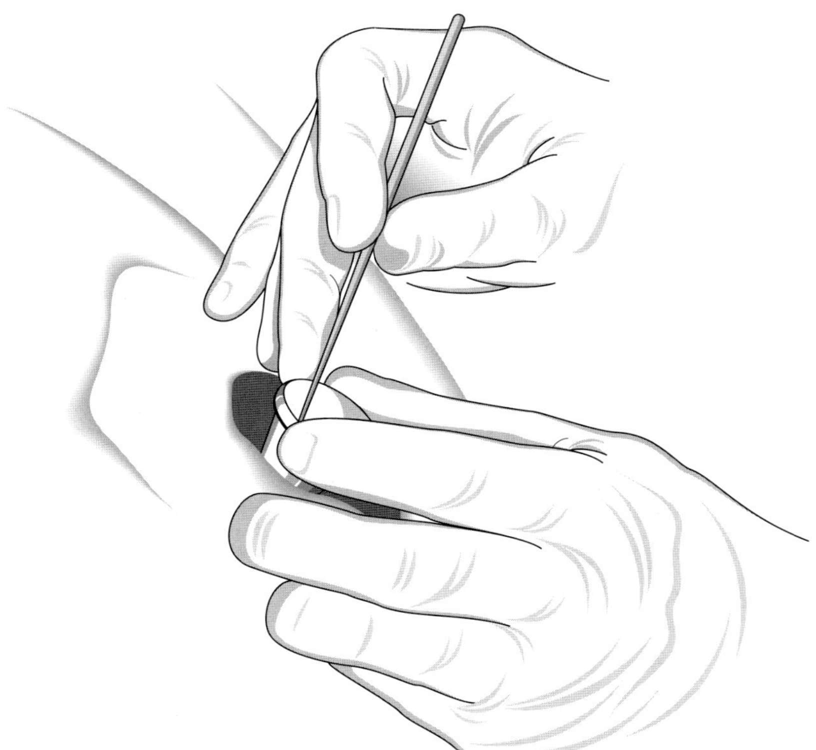

Fig. 6-19. Curetting. Note the steadying of the curette against the second finger. The second finger is also on the speculum. The third and fourth fingers are braced agaist the patient's head.

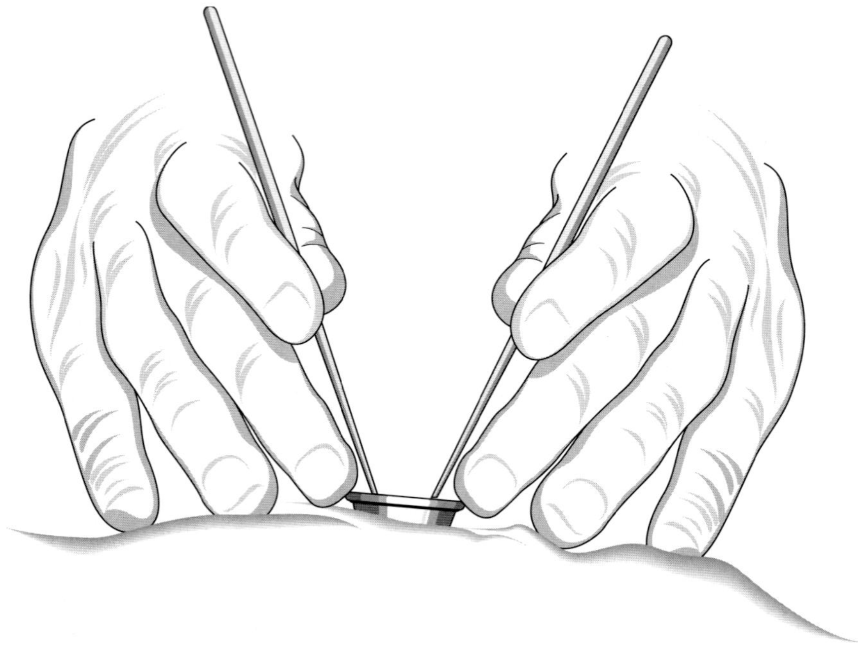

Fig. 6-20. Using both hands. This demonstrates the use of both hands manipulating instruments simultaneously and steadying both instruments against the fingers, as well as bracing the speculum against the patient's head.

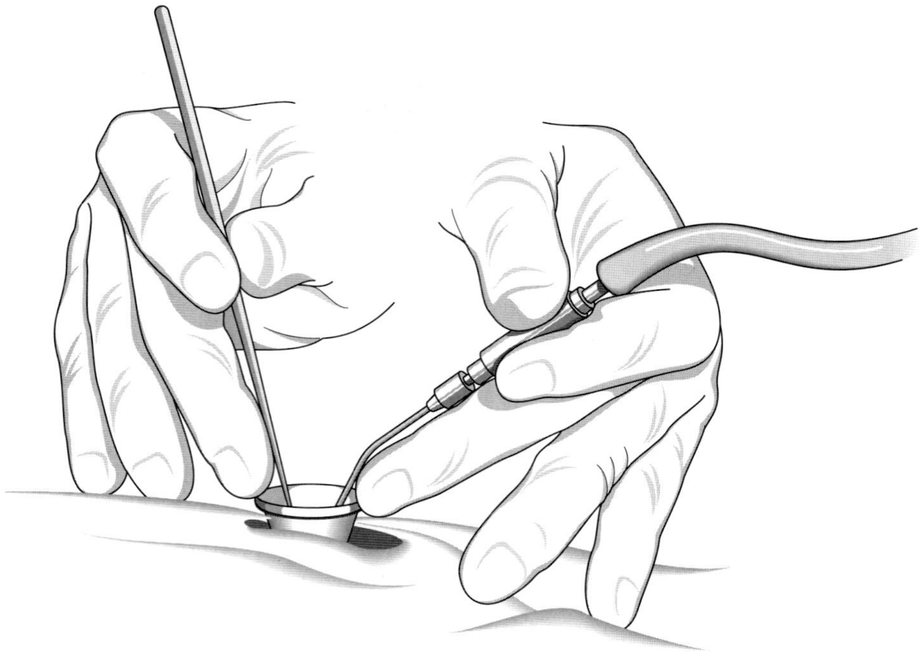

Fig. 6-21. Instruments in both hands and controlling speculum. Note the method of handling two instruments at one time, including steadying the speculum, steadying the two instruments against the second finger and using the third and fourth fingers to steady the two hands against the patient's head.

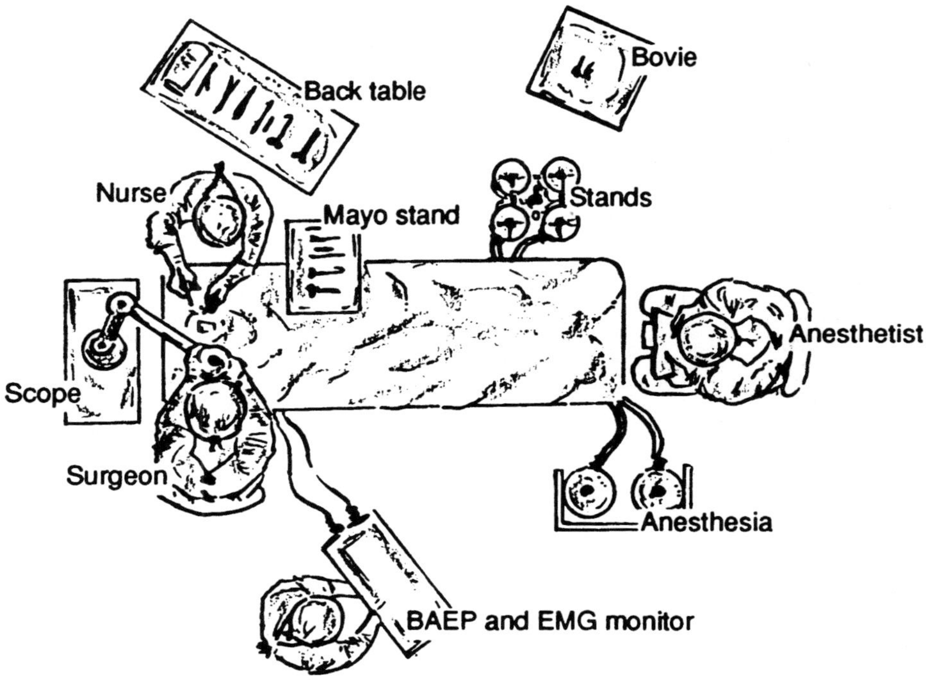

Fig. 6-22. OR setup for lateral skull-base approaches.

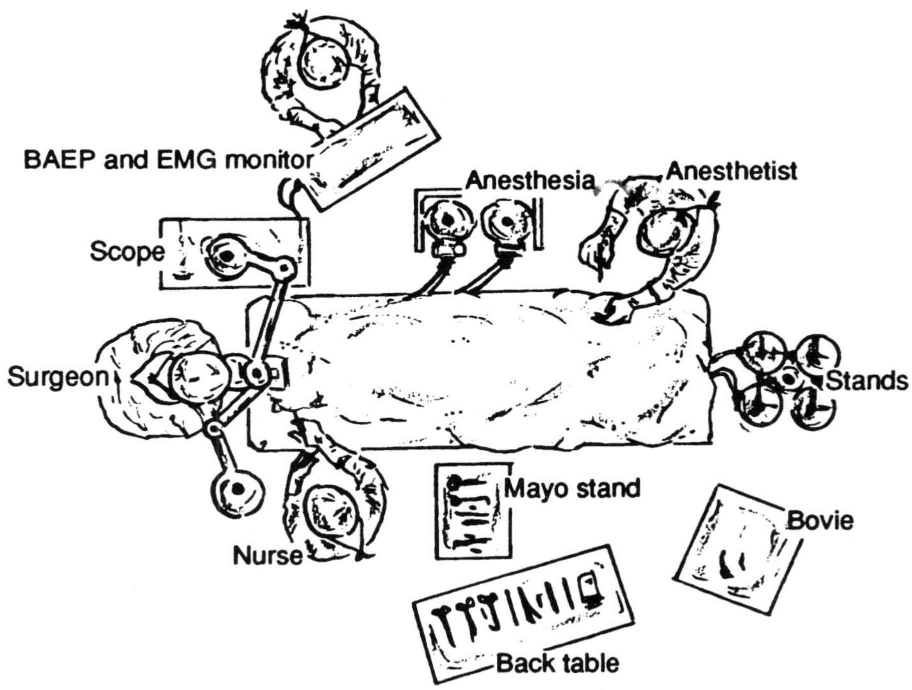

Fig. 6-23. OR setup for middle fossa surgery.

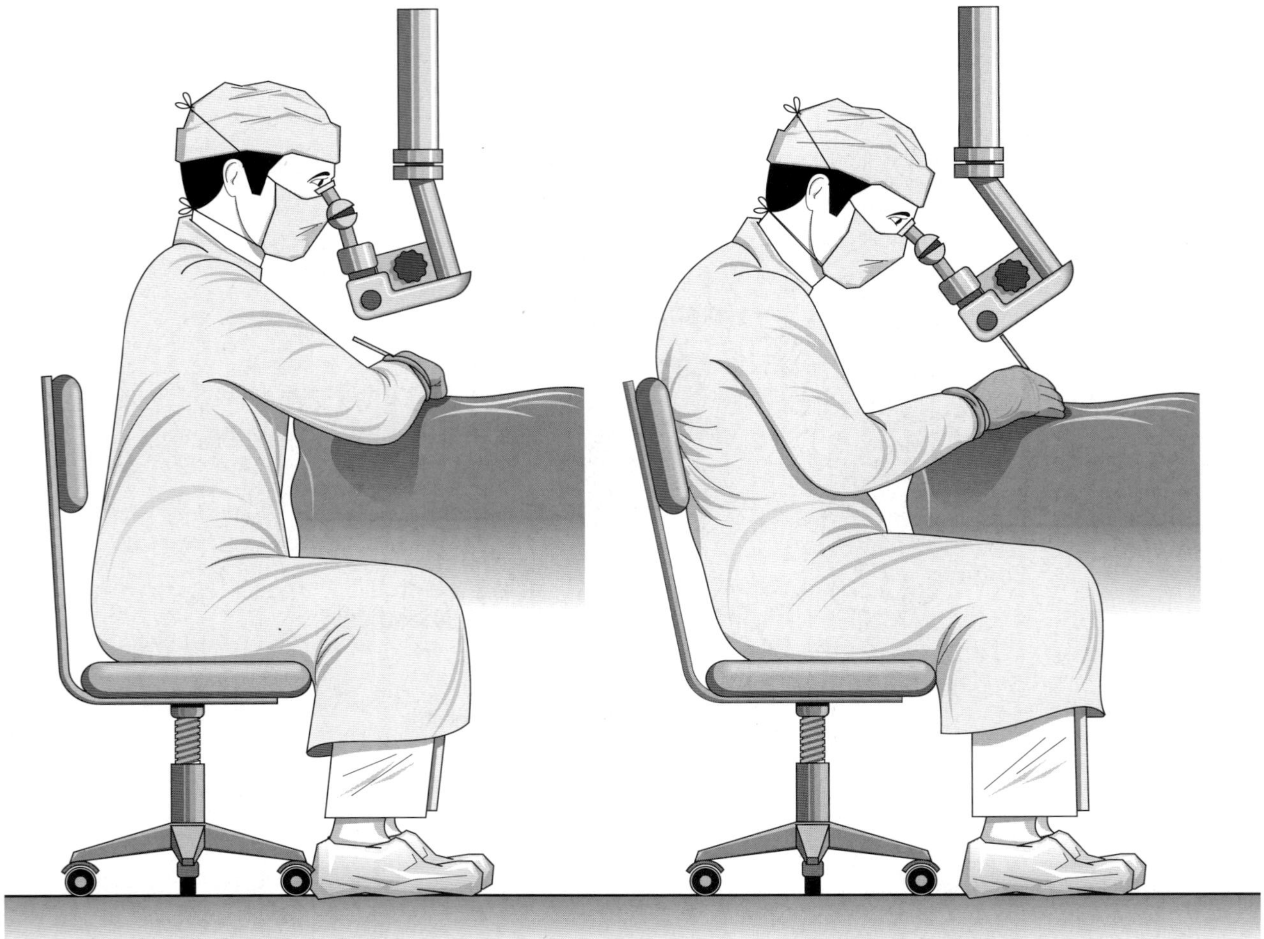

Fig. 6-24. Sitting positions at the operating table. The proper position is comfortable and muscles are relaxed.

REFERENCES

Barr ML, Kiernan IA: The human nervous system. 4th ed. Philadelphia: Harper Row, 1983.

Brodal A: Core textbook of neuroanatomy. 3rd ed. New York: Oxford University Press. 1981.

Carpenter MB: Core textbook of neuroanatomy. 3rd ed. Williams S Wilkins, 1985.

Chouard CH: Wrisberg intermediary nerve. In facial nerve surgery. Edit U Fisch-Kugler Med Pub Amstelveen. Aesculapius Pub; Comp Birmingham (Alab): 24-39, 1977.

Chusid IG: Correlative neuroanatomy and functional neurology. 19th ed. Los Altos: Lange Medical Publications, 1985.

Coates AE: A note on the superior petrosal sinus and its relation to the sensory root of the trigeminal nerve. J Anat 68: 428-430, 1934.

Fitzgerald MJT, Law ME: The peripheral connexions between the lingual and hypoglossal nerves. J Anat 92:178-199, 1958.

Gacek R: Surgical landmarks for the facial nerve in the epitympanum. Ann Otol Rhinol Laryngol 89:249-50, 1980.

Graham M. Surgical exposure of the facial nerve: contemporary transtemporal techniques. Am J Otol 1;137-46, 1980.

Guerrier Y: Surgical anatomy, particularly vascular supply of the facial nerve. In facial nerve surgery. Edit U Fisch. Kugler Med Pub (Amstelveen). Aesculapius Pub Comp Birmingham Alab: 13-23, 1977.

Hall GM, Pulec JL, Rhoton AL: Geniculate ganglion anatomy for the otologist. Arch Otolaryng 90: 568-571, 1969.

Lang J, Reiter U, Reiter W: Topographie des Orbitainhaltes. Teil II: Uber die Kammerung des Corpus adiposum orbitae. Neurochirurgia (Stuttg) 34:1-5, 1991.

Lang J, Reiter U: Uber den verlauf der hirnnerven in der seitenwand des sinus cavernosus. Neurochirurgia (Stuttg) 27:93-97, 1984.

Lang J, Schafer K: Uber Ursprung und Versorgungsgebiete der intracavernosen Strecke der A. carotis interna. Gegenbaurs Morphol Jahrb 122: 182-202, 1976.

Lang J, Schlehahn FA: Uber die postnatale entwicklung der fissurae orbitales. Gegenbaurs Morphol Jahrb 127:849-859, 1981.

Lang J: Uber die Pteriongegend und deren klinisch wichtigem Abstand zum Nervus opticus. 1. Pteriongegend. Neurochirurgia (Stuttg) 26:161-163, 1983.

Lazorthes G, Bimes C: Remarques sur la constitution du cavum de Meckel. CR Ass Anat 312-319, 1947.

Lowy R: Uber das topographische verhalten des nervus hypoglossus zur vena jugularis interna. Anat Anz 37:10-12, 1910.

Mercier Ph, Fardoun R, Cadou B, Le Patezour A, Guy G: Etude microchirurgicale du nerf facial intra-cranien. In diagnostic et traitement des neurinomes de l'acoustique. Lazorthes Y, Clanet M, Fraysse B Edit. Fournie Imp Toulouse: 61-70, 1983.

Mizuno N, Akimoto C, Mochizuki K, Matsuschima R: Experimental studies of efferent fibers in the hypoglossal nerve in the cat: a scanning electron microscopic observation in the lingual mucosa following transection of the nerve, and a degeneration study with silver impregnation methods. Arch Histol Jpn; 35: 99-113, 1973.

Moore K: Clinically oriented anatomy. 2nd ed. Baltimore: Williams S Wilkins, 1985.

Netter FH: The CIBA collection of medical illustrations. Vol. I Nervous System. Part I: Anatomy and physiology. New York: CIBA. 1983.

Paillas JE: Systeme nerveux central. Nerfs craniens. In: nouveau traite de technique chirurgicale. Tome VI. Masson Edit. 9, 1975.

Poritsky R: Neuroanatomical pathways. Philadelphia: WB Saunders. 1984.

Portmann M: Quelques observations sur la systematisation des nerfs transpetreux. Revue laryngol 76: 281-298, 1955.

Rasmussen AT: Studies of the VIIIth cranial nerve of man. Laryngoscope 50: 67-83, 1940.

Rougerie J, Guyot JF: Essai de conservation du nerf facial dans l'ablation des neurinomes de l'angle ponto-cerebelleux. Neuro-Chir (Paris) 10/1: 13-21, 1964.

Silverstein H, Norell H, Haberkamp, McDaniel AB. The unrecognized rotation of the vestibular and cochlear nerves from the labyrinth to the brainstem: its implications for surgery of the eighth cranial nerve. Otolaryngol Head Neck Surg 95:543-549, 1986.

Silverstein H, Norell H, Smouha A, Haberkamp T: The singular canal: a valuable landmark in surgery of the internal auditory canal. Otolaryngol Head Neck Surg 98:138-143, 1988.

Smith CG, Van der Kooy DL: Basic neuroanatomy. 3rd ed. Lexington: Collamore Press, 1985.

Sunderland S: Some anatomical and pathophysiological data relevant to facial nerve surgery and repair. In facial nerve surgery. U Fisch Edit Kugler Med Pub Amstelveen. Aesculapius Pub Comp Birmingham (Alab): 47-61, 1977.

Tator CH, Nedzelski IM: Preservation of hearing in patients undergoing excision of acoustic neuromas and other cerebellopontine angle tumors. J Neurosurg. 63:168-174. 1985.

Thompson IS: Core textbook of anatomy. Philadelphia: IB Lippincott. 1977.

Williams PL, Bannister LH, Berry MM, Collins P, Dyson M, Dussek JE, Ferguson MW: Gray's Anatomy. 38th ed. Edinburgh: Churchill Livingstone, 1995.

Wilson-Pauwels L, Akesson EJ, Stewart PA: Cranial nerves. Anatomy and clinical comments. Decker inc, Toronto, 1988.

Woodburne RL. Essentials of Human Anatomy. 7th ed. New York: Oxford University Press, 1983.

7

Surgical treatment of congenital malformations of the temporal bone

Reading books, rigorous training in basic microsurgery, an exquisite knowledge of skull base anatomy gained by repeated anatomic dissections, and observations of and training with individuals who are experienced in cranial base surgery are essential ingredients of the training process.

SEKHAR L.N., JANECKA I.P.

Congenital malformation of the temporal bone is characterized by aplasia or hypoplasia of the external auditory canal (EAC), often associated with absence or deformity of the auricle (microtia) and the middle ear, with occasional inner ear abnormalities. Aural atresia occurs in one in 10,000 to one in 20,000 live births, (Federspil; Granstrom) with unilateral atresia being three times more common than bilateral atresia (Federspil). This disorder occurs more commonly in males and on the right side (Federspil). EAC atresia is more often bony rather than membranous, and bony atresia is regularly accompanied by malformation of the middle ear cavity and structures of the middle ear (De La Cruz; Kelemen). More severe forms of congenital microtia are usually associated with EAC atresia; in rare instances, canal atresia may be seen in patients with a normal pinna (Harada). In general, a more severe external deformity implies a more severe middle ear abnormality (Harada; Hasso).

In 1883, Kiesselbach performed the first deep operation attempting to correct this malformation. Unfortunately, the procedure resulted in facial paralysis. Because of the lack of middle ear manipulation and the high complication rate, congenital aural atresia surgery was considered cosmetic at best, and dangerous and to be avoided in most cases. In 1914, Page reported hearing improvement in five of eight cases after surgery. In 1917, Dean and Gittens reported on an excellent hearing result in a patient and reviewed the various types of operations that had been tried by other surgeons. The prevailing attitude toward surgical correction in these cases remained generally pessimistic, despite these and other occasional reports of successful operations, until 1947. That year, Ombredanne, in France, and Pattee, in the United States each reported on a series of patients successfully operated on to improve hearing. Pattee's technique included removal of the incus to mobilize the stapes; Ombredanne added fenestration of the lateral semicircular canal (LSCC).

With the advent of tympanoplasty techniques in the 1950s, interest in atresiaplasty rose as the teachings of Wullstein and Zollner carried over into surgery of the congenital ear. Larger series with greater success rates were reported as surgeons attempted to improve their results, using LSCC fenestration, ossiculoplasty, differing degrees of bone removal, and different types and techniques of graft placement. Ombredanne went on to report on over 600 "aplasia" cases by 1971, and 1600 cases with major and minor malformations by 1976. Gill's series of 83 cases is a landmark paper. In the past two decades, Crabtree, Jahrsdoerfer, Marquet and De La Cruz have reported on large surgical series, with modifications of classification and operative techniques.

Although the techniques of canalplasty, meatoplasty, tympanoplasty, and ossiculoplasty have improved considerably, surgical correction of congenital aural atresia remains one of the most challenging operations performed by otologists. This is a complicated surgical problem, requiring application of all modern tympanoplasty techniques and a thorough knowledge of the surgical anatomy of the facial nerve, oval window, and inner ear, as well as their congenital variants.

The temporomandibular joint is displaced posteriorly by the lack of development of the EAC, narrowing the distance between the glenoid fossa and the anterior wall of the mastoid tip (Bellucci; Jahrsdoerfer). Fusion of the incus and malleus is common but because of its dual origin, the stapes footplate is usually normal (House; Ombredanne).

The timing of repair must take into account any planned auricular reconstruction procedures, as well as the degree of pneumatization of the temporal bone (De La Cruz). Criteria for patient selection must be stringent when closure of the air-bone gap to within 20 to 30 dB is attempted. Preoperative counseling and several postoperative visits are essential for optimal results. In this chapter, we discuss these issues and provide guidelines for patient evaluation and selection, surgical techniques, and postoperative management.

EMBRYOLOGY

Understanding the normal embryologic development of the ear aids in the understanding of the myriad of possible combinations of malformations encountered in congenital aural atresia. The inner ear, middle ear, and external ear develop independently and in such a way that deformity of one does not necessarily presuppose deformity of another (Kelemen; Aase). Most frequently, abnormalities of the outer and middle ear are encountered in combination with a normal inner ear structure (Sando; Van De Water).

- Microtia is a result of first branchial cleft and pouch anomalies. – Growth of mesenchymal tissue from the first and second branchial arches forms six hillocks around the primitive meatus that fuse to form the auricle (Table 7-1).
- By the end of the third month, the primitive auricle has been completed.
- The external auditory meatus develops from the first branchial groove. During the second month, a solid core of epithelium migrates inward from the rudimentary pinna toward the first branchial pouch. This core is the precursor of the EAC and starts to hollow out and take shape in the sixth month. It canalizes in the seventh month, causing the developing mastoid to become separated from the mandible. Its subsequent posterior and inferior development carries the middle ear and facial nerve to their normal positions (Federspil; Tjellstrom).
- The first branchial pouch grows outward to form the middle ear cleft. The plaque of tissue where this cleft meets the epithelium of the EAC forms the tympanic membrane. While the pouch is forming the eustachian tube, tympanic cavity, and mastoid air cells, Meckel's cartilage (first branchial arch) is forming the neck and head of the malleus and incus. Reichert's cartilage (second branchial arch) forms the remainder of the first two ossicles and the stapes superstructure. The footplate has a dual origin from the second arch and the otic capsule. The ossicles attain their final shape by the fourth month. By the end of the seventh or eighth month, the expanding middle ear cleft surrounds the ossicles and covers them with a mucous membrane (Federspil; Van De Water).
- The facial nerve is the nerve of the second branchial arch. At 4.5 weeks, this developing nerve divides the blastema, which is the condensation of the second arch mesenchymal cells, into the stapes, the interhyale (stapedius muscle precursor) and the laterohyale (precursor of the posterior wall of the middle ear). The nerve's intraosseous course is dependent on this bony expansion (Van De Water; Savic). The membranous portion of the inner ear develops during the third to the sixth week from an auditory placode on the lateral surface of the hindbrain. The surrounding mesenchyme transforms into the bony otic capsule (Melnick).

Table 7-1. Development of the Auricle.

First branchial arch	Second branchial arch
First hillock-tragus	Fourth hillock-antihelix
Second hillock-helical crus	Fifth hillock-antitragus
Third hillock-helix	Sixth hillock-lobule and lower helix

Knowledge of ear embriology has practical applications, because the different congenital anomalies depend on the arrest in development at a particular embryologic date. To know this date, which is also the date of the arrest in development of the facial nerve, allows the surgeon to reasonably predict the course of the VII nerve. For instance, a normal auricle, with a stenotic ear canal and a thick atretic plate is the consequence of an arrest in development after the 21st week. At this age, the facial nerve is fully developed, although more anterior and lateral then in normal adult patient (Bauer) (Fig. 7-1).

- Congenital aural atresia can therefore range in severity from a thin membranous canal atresia to complete lack of tympanic bone, depending on the time of arrest of intrauterine development (Federspil; Altmann; Bellucci). The usual finding of a normal inner ear is explained by the fact that the inner ear is already formed by the time of external/middle ear developmental arrest. Facial nerve course abnormalities are often seen. Only very severe congenital malformations of the external and middle ear are associated with inner ear deformations (Barrios-Montes; Gill; Melnick).

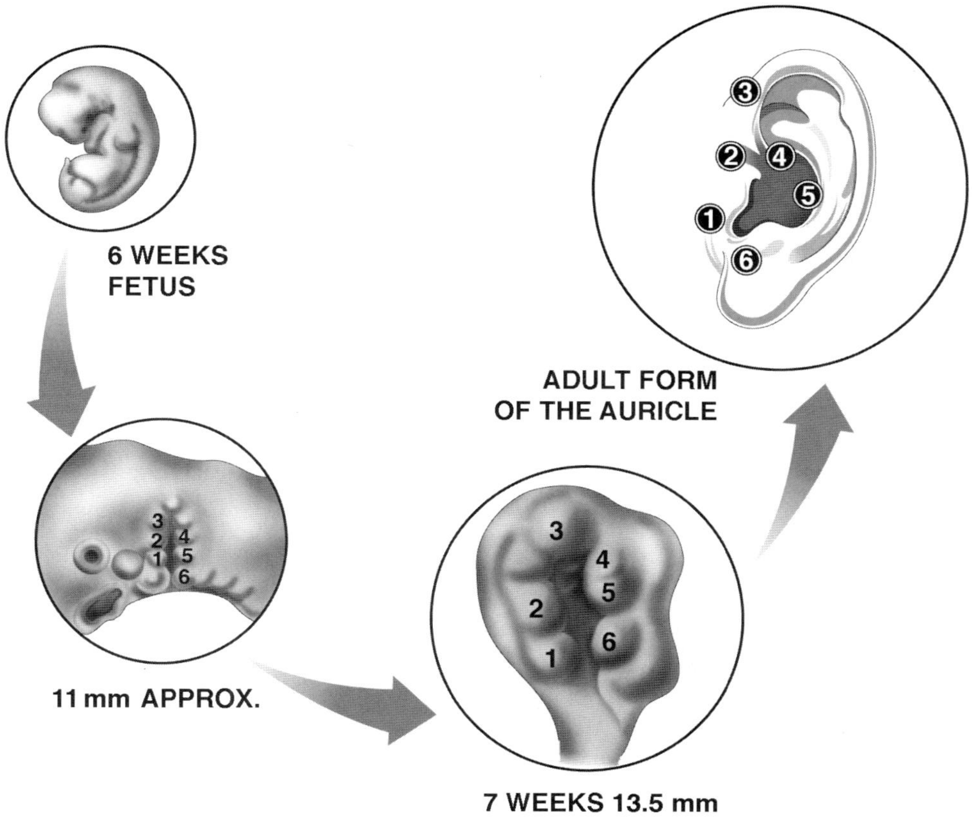

Fig. 7-1. Development of the auricle.

CLASSIFICATION SYSTEMS

A widely used classification system in congenital aural atresia was developed in 1955 by Altmann. In this system, atresias are categorized into three groups (Table 7-2).

Altmann's classification system is purely descriptive, and most surgical candidates fall into groups 2 and 3. De La Cruz has modified this system with more practical surgical guidelines. The De La Cruz modification involves only advanced Altmann groups 2 and 3 and divides abnormalities into "minor" and "major" categories (Table 7-3).

The clinical importance of this classification is that surgery in cases of minor malformations has a good possibility of yielding serviceable hearing, whereas cases of major malformations are frequently inoperable.

A point-grading system to guide surgeons in their preoperative assessment of the best candidates for hearing improvement has been developed by Jahrsdoerfer (Table 7-4). This system takes into account the parameters of mastoid pneumatization, presence of the oval and round windows, facial nerve course, status of the ossicles, and external appearance. Point allocation is based primarily on the findings on high-resolution computed tomography (HRCT).

Jahrsdoerfer proposes that when the preoperative evaluation of the patient is incorporated into this grading system, the best results (>80 per cent

Table 7-2. Altman's Classification of Atresia.

Group I:	Small external ear canal, hypoplastic tympanic bone and tympanic membrane with a normal or contracted middle ear space. Ossicles may be normal or malformed.
Group II.	The canal is absent, with an atretic plate present. The middle ear space is small. The malleus and incus are fixed and malformed.
Group III:	Includes those with absent external auditory canal with a contracted or absent middle ear space. The ossicles may be absent.

Table 7-3. De La Cruz's Classification of Atresia.

Minor Malformations
- Normal mastoid pneumatization.
- Normal oval window.
- Reasonable facial nerve-oval window relationship.
- Normal inner ear.

Major Malformations
- Poor pneumatization.
- Abnormal or absent oval window.
- Abnormal course of the horizontal portion of the facial nerve.
- Abnormalities of the inner ear, particularly the vestibule and semicircular canals.

Table 7-4. Grading System of Candidacy for Surgery of Congenital Aural Atresia.

Parameter	Points
Stapes present	2
Oval window open	1
Middle ear space	1
Facial nerve normal	1
Malleus-incus complex present	1
Mastoid well pneumatized	1
Incus-stapes connection	1
Round window normal	1
Appearance of external ear	1
Total available points	10

success) will be achieved with a score of eight or better. A score of seven implies a fair chance, six is marginal, and below this the patient becomes a poor candidate (Table 7-5).

Of note, Jahrsdoerfer credits presence of the stapes with two points. In our experience, this is less important than the presence of an oval window and a well pneumatized mastoid because:

1) with current ossiculoplastic tecniques, a good hearing result can be achieved with a footlate-to-drum prosthesis and

2) the new EAC is fashioned at the expense of the mastoid. A large, well pneumatized mastoid allows for greater ease of dissection with less risk to the facial nerve and inner ear structures, and also allows for the creation of a good-sized EAC.

Schucknecht's system of classification of congenital aural atresia is based on a combination of clinical and primarily surgical observations (Table 7-6).

In 1983, Chiossone presented a classification scheme based primarily on the location of the glenoid fossa

Table 7-5.

Rating	Type of candidate
10	Excellent
9	Very good
8	Good
7	Fair
6	Marginal
5	Poor

From Jahrsdoerfer RA, Yeakley JW, Aguilar EA, et al: Grading system for the selection of patients with congenital aural atresia. Am J Otol 13(1); 6-12, 1992.

Type I
The fossa is in the normal position.
Type II
The fossa is moderately displaced.
Type III
The fossa overlaps the middle ear
Type IV
In addition to the fossa overlapping the middle ear there is lack of mastoid pneumatization.

Cases with types I and II are ideal surgical candidates. Type III cases have a tendency toward graft lateralization. Type IV cases are not surgical candidates. In elective atresiaplasty surgery a classification scheme is useful for surgical planning, patient counseling and comparison of outcomes.

INITIAL EVALUATION AND PATIENT SELECTION

When aural atresia is noted in a newborn, several issues must be addressed. Where one congenital abnormality is found, others must be sought; a high-risk register for deafness is helpful in this regard (Sando). After the degree of aural deformity is assessed by physical examination, evaluation of auditory function in both unilateral and bilateral

Table 7-6. Schucknecht's Classification of Atresia.

Type A (meatal) atresia
It is limited to the fibrocartilaginous part of the EAC. Meatoplasty is the surgical procedure of choice and, when performed in a timely fashion, prevents formation of canal cholesteatoma and conductive hearing loss.

Type B (partial) atresia
There is a narrowing of both the fibrocartilaginous and bony EAC but a patent dermal tract allows partial inspection of the tympanic membrane. The tympanic membrane is small and partially replaced by a bony septum. Minor ossicular malformations exist, and hearing loss may be mild to severe.

Type C (total) atresia
Includes all cases with a totally atretic ear canal but a well-pneumatized tympanic cavity. There is a partial or total bony atretic plate, the tympanic membrane is absent, the heads of the ossicles are fused, there may be no connection to a possibly malformed stapes, and the facial nerve is more likely to have an aberrant course over the oval widow.

Type D (hypopneumatic total atresia)
It is a total atresia with poor pneumatization, common in dysplasias such as Treacher Collins syndrome. These patients with abnormalities of the facial nerve canal and the bony labyrinth are poor candidates for hearing improvement surgery.

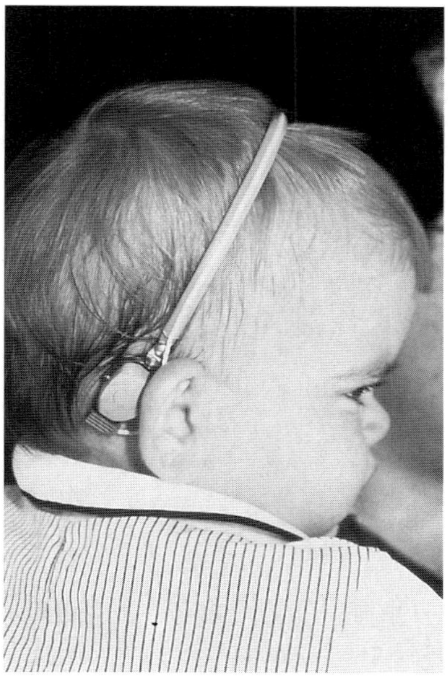

Fig. 7-2. In bilateral aural atresia, bone-conduction hearing aid should be applied as soon as possible.

atresia should be performed using auditory brainstem response audiometry with the first few days of life. The incidence of inner ear abnormality associated with congenital aural atresia is 11 per cent to 47 per cent (Hasso). In unilateral cases, a total sensorineural hearing loss may occur on the normal appearing ear (De La Cruz).

In bilateral cases, a bone-conduction hearing aid should be applied as soon as possible, ideally in the third or fourth week of life (Figs. 7-2, 7-3). In unilateral cases in which the opposite ear hears normally, a hearing aid is not necessary. We do not recommend implantable hearing aids in children because the surgical scars preclude future microtia repair. The syndromic child with aural atresia and associated cephalic abnormalities (e.g., Treacher Collins, Crouzon's, Rippel-Feil, Pierre Robin, and Goldenhar's syndromes, VATER, CHARGE, drug teratogenicity and hemifacial microsomia) should be recognized (Sando; Sanchez-Corona). In this subset, surgical correction yields poor results (Schuknecht) and long-term bone-conduction aiding is indicated.

Prompt and careful counseling of the parents of a child with sporadic (nonsyndromal) congenital aural atresia is necessary to alleviate concerns regarding possible occurrence in their subsequent children (no more than the general population), to answer questions regarding future auricular reconstruction, and, most important, to ensure that proper hearing amplification is instituted in a timely fashion. The child should be enrolled in special education at an early age to maximize speech and language acquisition, in preparation for mainstreaming at the preschool age. Radiologic and surgical evaluations are deferred until the child reaches age 6 and are discussed later in this chapter.

In the initial evaluation of an older individual with congenital aural atresia, the most crucial elements remain the functional and anatomic integrity of the inner ear. Audiometric and HRCT evaluation are necessary. Prognosis for hearing improvement is dependent on the presence and degree of malformations. Auricular reconstruction must be addressed prior to hearing restorative surgery to avoid alterations in the blood supply to the surrounding soft tissue that may compromise microtia repair.

A patient with congenital aural atresia may present with an infected or draining ear or acute facial palsy; 14% have congenital cholesteatoma (De La Cruz) (Figs. 7-4, 7-5). The priority in these cases is removal of the cholesteatoma and resolution of the infection; however, preoperative audiometry and HRCT scanning are necessary (De La Cruz; Schuknecht; Miyamoto) (Figs. 7-6, 7-7).

There are two indisputable requirements for surgery in congenital aural atresia: 1) radiographic evidence of an inner ear and 2) audiometric evidence of cochlear function. Other indications man-

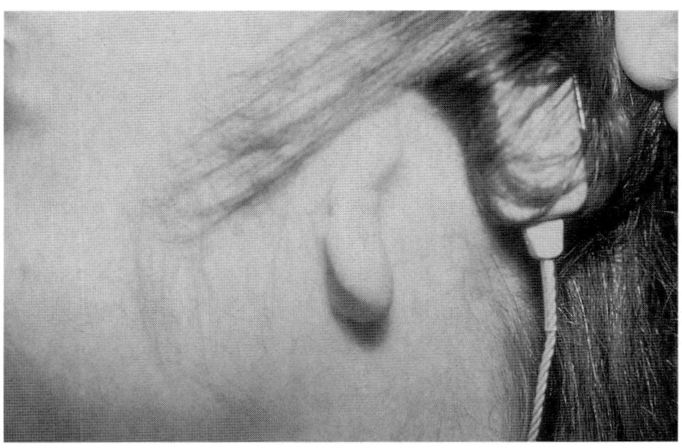

Fig. 7-3. CAA. Deformed auricle.

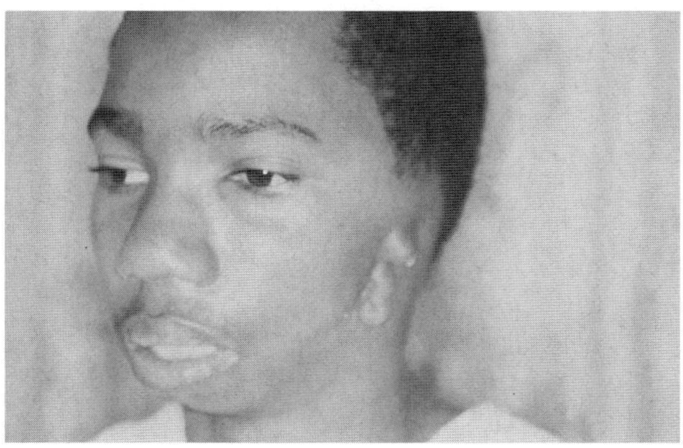

Fig. 7-4. An atretic ear can be affected by an otitis media, due to an infection spread via the eustachian tube.

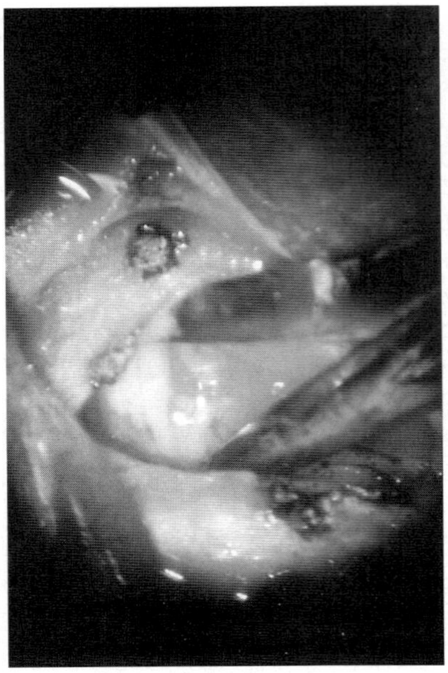

Fig. 7-5. Operation of the patient in Fig. 7-17. Drainage of an abscess.

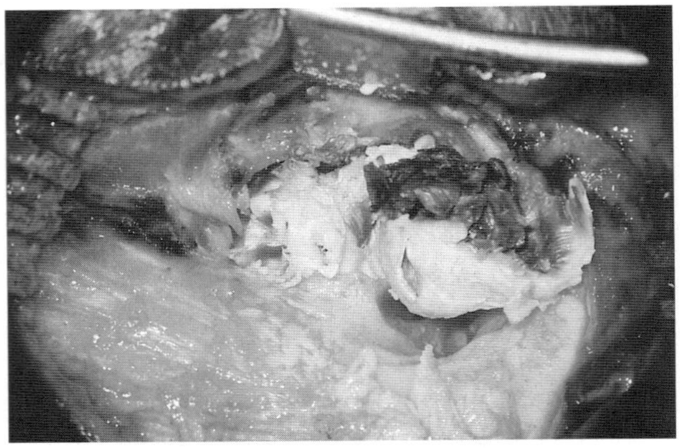

Fig. 7-7. CAA surgery. Removal of wide congenital cholesteatoma.

dating prompt surgical intervention are congenital cholesteatoma, a draining postoperative atretic ear, or acute facial palsy. The computed tomographic scan should always be reviewed for cholesteatoma, which necessitates surgery at any age (Schuknecht; Miyamoto, Jahrsdoerfer). Cholesteatoma is not included in any of the grading systems because these systems are used only for predicting hearing results in elective atresiaplasty surgery.

TIMING OF AURICULAR RECONSTRUCTION AND ATRESIAPLASTY

In binaural atresia, auricular reconstruction and atresiaplasty are recommended when the patient is 6 years of age, because:

- The costal cartilage has developed sufficiently to allow for harvesting and transplantation to the auricle. On the other side, when the child is small and the opposite normal ear is large, there may be not enough cartilage and the surgery must be postponed, even for years. In the opposite situation, when the child is large and the ear is small, the operation may begin at 5.5 years (Brent) .
- The mastoid has become as pneumatized as possible.
- The child is not yet traumatized by cruel teasing, which manifests at age 7-10.
- By age of six the child is cooperative regarding the surgery, because he is aware of the problem and wants it resolved.
- The microtia repair should be done first because the complex flaps and use of autologous rib graft demand excellent blood supply (Brent). (Of note, many surgeons will not perform atresiaplasty on an ear reconstructed with silicone sheeting stent) (Jahrsdoerfer).
- The hearing restoration surgery is then performed 2 months after the microtia repair. Rehabilitation of severe auricular defects using tissue-integrated percutaneous mastoid implant prostheses with and without bone conduction aids has also been described in the literature (Granstrom; Gates; Niparko).
- In unilateral atresia cases, atresiaplasty surgery is delayed until the patient is old enough to understand the significant risks to the cochlea, vestibular system, and facial nerve. The exception to this is the individual who has a very thin unilateral atresia plate with excellent pneumatization and normal middle ear, ossicles, and facial nerve. This deformity is a minor atresia. In these cases, surgery can be safely performed in childhood with the parents' consent (Molony). We often see older adults with unilateral atresia who request surgery when their normal ear begins having high-frequency hearing loss (presbyacusia) (Figs. 7-8, 7-9, 7-10, 7-11, 7-12).

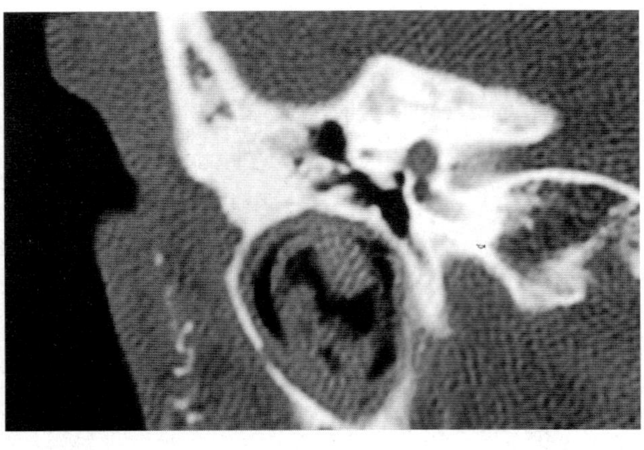

Fig. 7-6. CT. Congenital aural atresia, right ear. Congenital cholesteatoma. Wide osteolytic lesion in the mastoid, without involvement of the tympanic cavity.

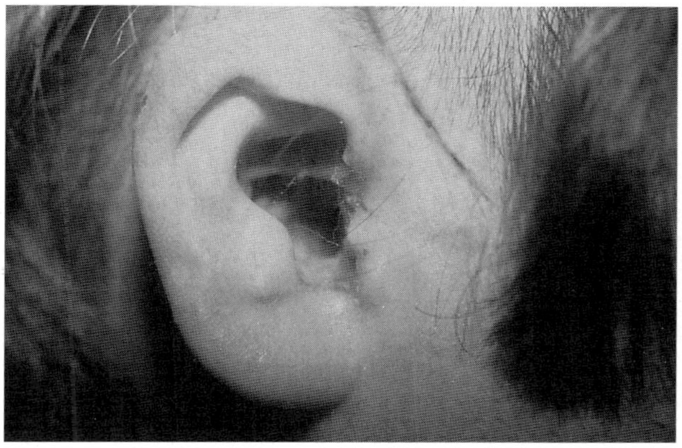

Fig. 7-8. CAA. Deformed auricle.

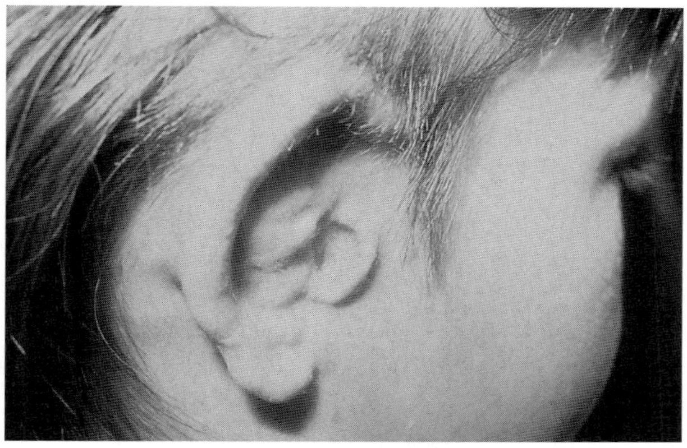

Fig. 7-10. CAA. Deformed auricle.

PREOPERATIVE EVALUATION AND PATIENT COUNSELING

Early diagnosis with auditory brainstem response audiometry and auditory enhancement with bone-conduction hearing aids in bilateral cases should be done in the first weeks of life (Sortini). Imaging is deferred until the child reaches age 6 years. The only imaging acceptable today for preoperative evaluation is HRCT scanning in both the axial and coronal planes. Three-dimensional reconstruction computed tomography is in its early stages of use for preoperative evaluation, but this new modality's utility is as yet unproven. The computed tomographic scan must be examined carefully by the otologic surgeon and the otoradiologist because one interpretation often does not provide all of the information necessary for operative planning (Figs. 7-13, 7-14).

The four important imaging elements that are most helpful to the surgeon planning reconstruction of a congenitally malformed ear are:

1. The degree of pneumatization of the temporal bone
2. The course of the facial nerve, both the relationship of the horizontal portion to the oval window and the location of the mastoid segment
3. The existence of the oval window and stapes footplate
4. The status of the inner ear (Mehra; De La Cruz).

- Computed tomography also provides information on thickness and form of the bony atretic plate, size and status of the middle ear cavity, existence of congenital cholesteatoma, and soft tissue contribution to the atresia (De La Cruz) but this information is less critical for the repair (Fig. 7-15).
- Sensorineural hearing loss is often caused by malformation of the membranous labyrinth, defects not seen on radiographic studies. Defects in the otic capsule visible radiographically range from complete lack of development of the inner ear structures, the Michel deformity, to the more common, less severe, deformity of the cochlea and vestibule, the Mondini deformity. The more severe congenital malformations of the external and middle ear are associated with inner ear deformities.
- Lack of pneumatization is the major cause of inoperability in congenital aural atresia (De La Cruz; Molony). Fortunately, normal pneumatization is present in most cases. Pro-

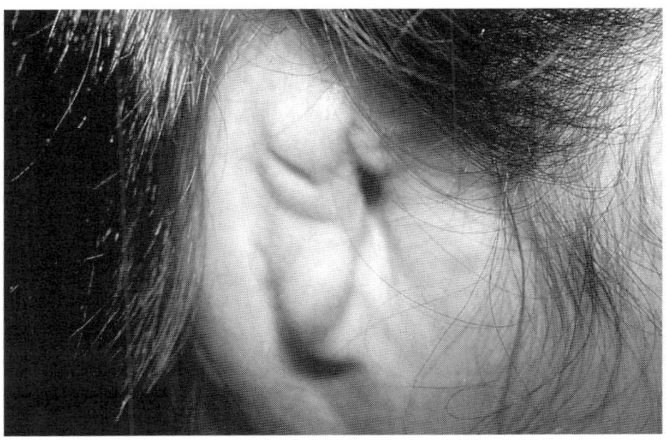

Fig. 7-9. CAA. Deformed auricle.

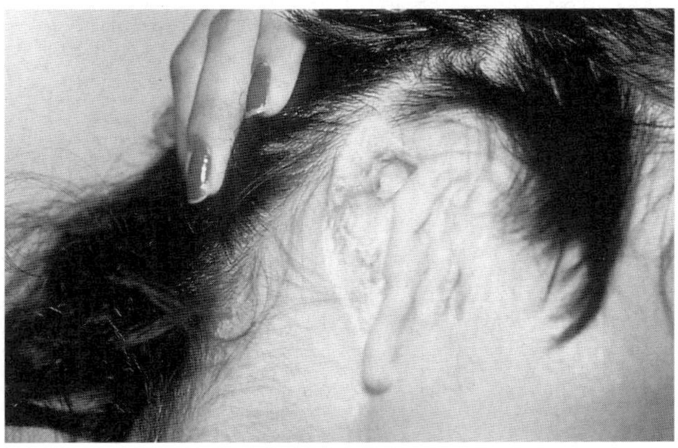

Fig. 7-11. CAA. Aspect of the right auricle after several attempts at microtia repair.

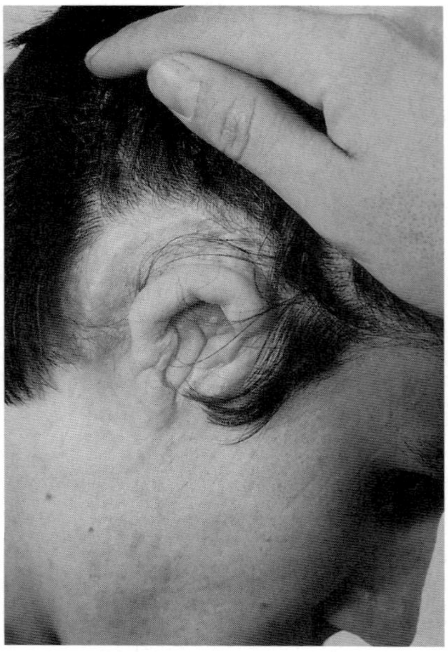

Fig. 7-12. Aspect of the right auricle after several attempts at microtia repair.

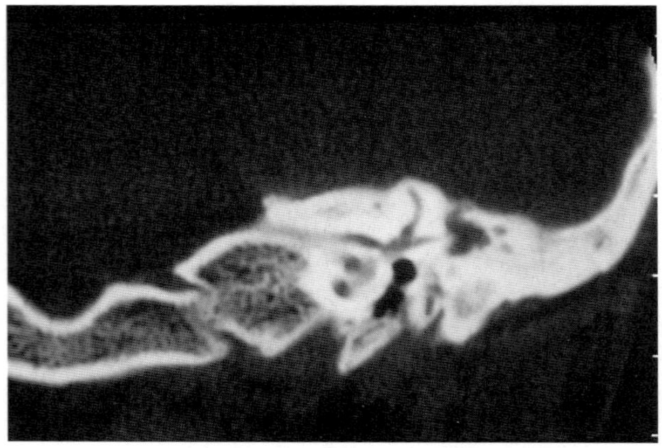

Fig. 7-14. CT. Atresia of the external ear and partial development of middle ear.

lapse of the facial nerve over the oval window may prevent ossiculoplasty and hearing improvement. If the oval window is absent, surgery with fenestration of the lateral semicircular canal or placement of a hearing aid is indicated. There is potential for facial nerve injury in atresia surgery (Crabtree). The nerve may describe a more acute angle rather than its usual 120 degrees at the second genu and often lies more lateral than usual. On HRCT, it is important not to mistakenly identify the vertical line of the facial nerve to the marrow bone of the styloid process (Chandrasekhar). Even in atretic ears in which the facial nerve does not have an abnormal course, a significantly reduced distance is found between the facial canal and the temporomandibular joint (Jahrsdoerfer) and the facial canal and the posterior wall of the cavum tympani (Savic) (Figs. 7-16, 7-17).

- Jahrsdoerfer suggest the routine use of three-dimensional imaging of the CT scan, that alerts the surgeon preoperatively to potential intraoperative problems and clearly shows the relationship of the zygomatic arch to the temporal bone and to the temporomandibular joint.

An estimate of the size of the mastoid can be determined by palpation of the mastoid tip, suprameatal spine of Henle (if present), condyle, and zygomatic arch. This measure is useful because the new ear canal will be constructed at the expense of the mastoid air cell system (De La Cruz).

To be considered a surgical candidate, the patient must have:

- Sufficient cochlear function by auditory brainstem response audiometry or on routine audiometry.
- A normal-appearing inner ear on computed tomographic scan.
- Preferably, a well developed mastoid and a good oval window-facial nerve relationship.

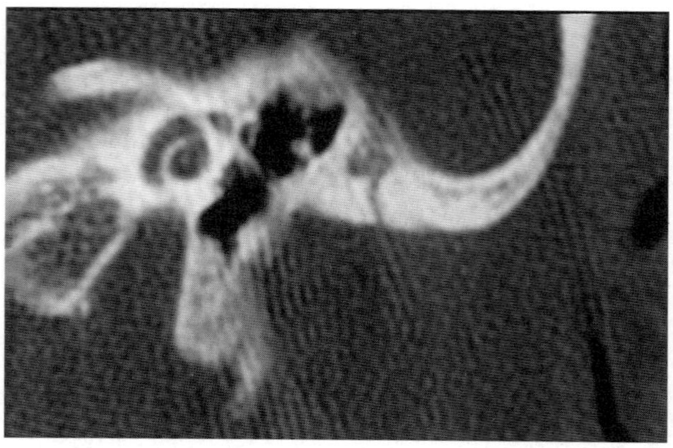

Fig. 7-13. CT. Atretic ear. Absence of external auditory canal. Antrum and epitympanum well pneumatized, deformed ossicles in situ.

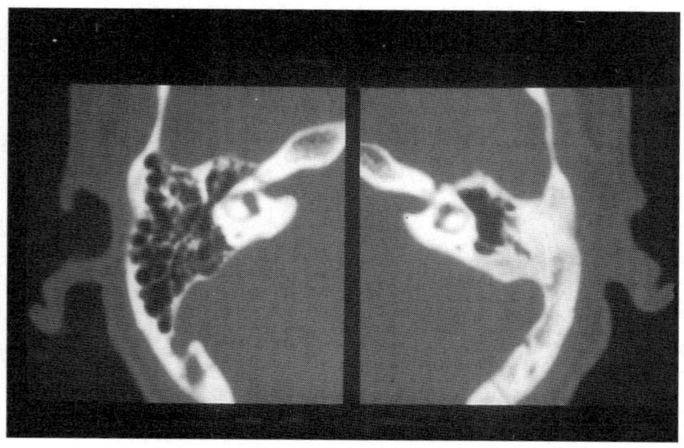

Fig. 7-15. CT. Normal left ear, atretic right ear.

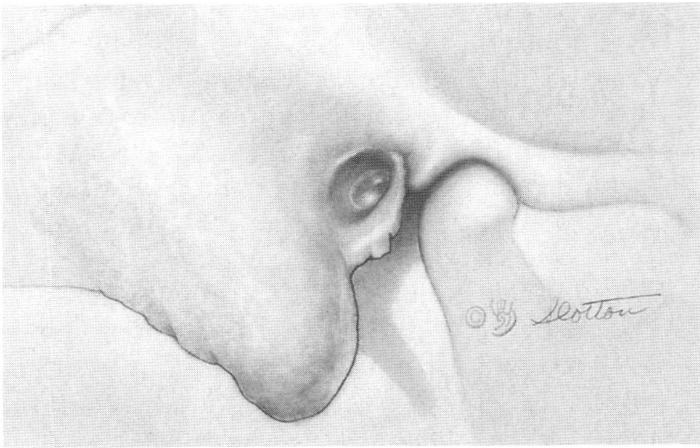

Fig. 7-16. Right ear. Normal aspect of tympanic ring and mastoid. Normal location of glenoid fossa.

Patient counseling integrates all of these issues. Patients with a degree of malformation equivalent to a seven or better on the Jahrsdoerfer grading scale are given a greater than 75 per cent chance of hearing improvement. The risk to the facial nerve is small and further reduced by the use of the facial nerve monitor (Molony; Linstrom). Patients are informed that a split-thickness skin graft from the hypogastrium will be used to line the new EAC. Initially, frequent postoperative visits are necessary.

The risks:

- Graft lateralization: 26 to 28 per cent.
- Sensorineural hearing loss: 2 per cent.
- Facial nerve palsy: 1 per cent.
- Otherwise, the risks and complications are similar to those for other mastoidectomy procedures.

SURGICAL TECHNIQUE

Auricular Repair

This is performed by the plastic surgeon, at least two months before the hearing restoration surgery. Here are some indications**:**

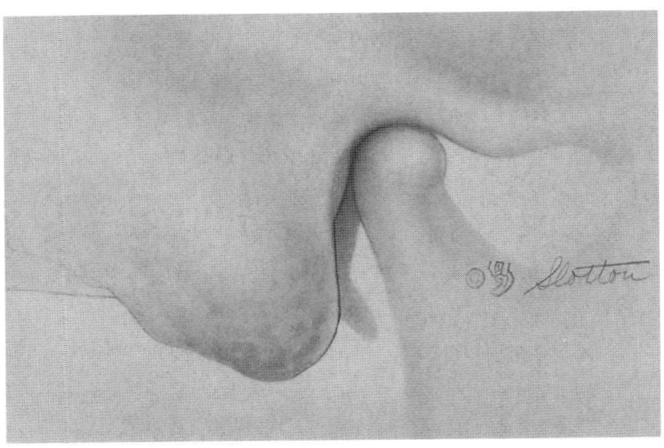

Fig. 7-17. Congenital aural atresia (CAA). Right ear. Partial development of the tympanic ring and mastoid. Posterior positioning of the glenoid fossa.

- To reconstruct the ear, autologus cartilage is the primary material, whereas homologous cartilage absorbs and silicone frameworks may be lost to even minor trauma.
- The grafting of the cartilage framework must be done first, to deal with good circulation and skin elasticity. Several months after this procedure, if successful, secondary procedures, like tragus construction, lobule rotation and sulcus grafting may take place. "First the house foundation, then the ornaments".
- The rib cartilage is harvested from the first free floating cartilage to form the helix and from the synchondrotic region of sixth and seventh ribs to form the framework. The shape of the cartilage framework is predetermined, thanks to reversed film patterns, similar to the normal ear, and a template is used. The cartilage is harvested, sculptured with a wider concha to allow the confection of the future ear canal, and inserted in the same procedure. The cartilage is inserted below a cutaneous pocket; skin tensions and blanching must be avoided. Petrolatum gauze and dressing is used.
- When reconstructing the ear, one must try to match the opposite side, since an ear constructed from autogenous rib cartilage grows at the same rate as the normal ear (Tanzer).
- Secondary procedures takes place several months after (Brent) (Figs. 7-18, 7-19).

Hearing Restoration Surgery

The repair of the atretic ear is a difficult otologic surgery, due to particular features that hinder the

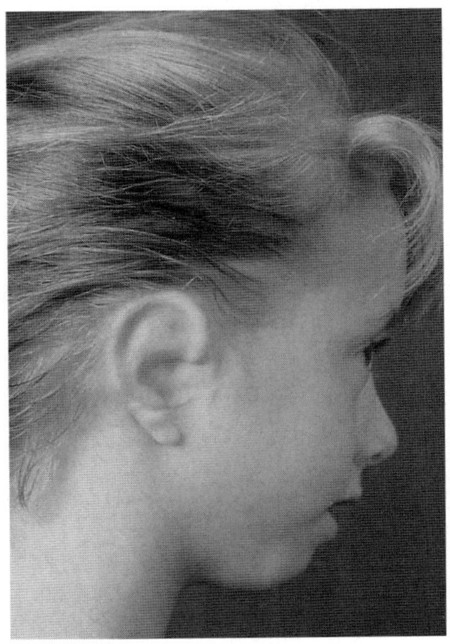

Fig. 7-18. Right microtia repair. Auricular reconstruction is done first, because the complex flaps and use of autologus rib graft demand excellent blood supply.

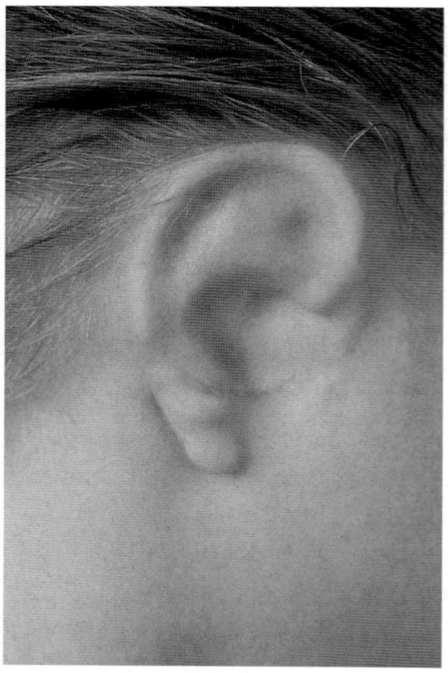

Fig. 7-19. Close-up view of Figure 7-18.

goal of restoring hearing and put the middle ear structures at risk:

- Lack of landmarks.
- Altered anatomy of the seventh nerve and middle ear.
- Limited space for middle ear reconstruction.
- Failure of the healing process (Bauer).

The first atresiaplasty operations failed because of poor tympanoplasty technique (Pattee); as this was improved, hearing restoration was added through lateral semicircular canal fenestration (Bellucci; Woodman; Altmann). Simultaneously, advances in meatoplasty added to the success rate of atresiaplasty surgery (Bellucci; Chole). Although fenestration remains an option in congenital absence of the oval window, modern methods of ossiculoplasty are used preferentially and yield superior results. There has been debate in the literature over techniques of tympanoplasty and ossiculoplasty in atresia repair. Many materials have been used, including acrylic stents, full-thickness skin grafts, fascia and homografts, the intact (deformed) ossicular mass, stapes (with and without stapedectomy or mobilization), and ossicular replacement prostheses.

- We use general endotracheal anesthesia and avoid using muscle relaxants. Facial nerve monitoring is used in all cases. The patient is in the otologic position, and the head is turned away. A large shave of the postauricular area is done, and the auricle and postauricular area are prepared with povidone-iodine (Betadine) and draped. Additionally, the lower abdomen is shaved, prepared, and draped for the skin graft donor site. Perioperative antibiotics are used routinely.
- A postauricular temporo-occipital incision is made. In cases in which microtia repair has been done, care is taken not to expose the grafted costal cartilage. Subcutaneous tissue is elevated anteriorly to the temporomandibular joint. A T-shaped incision is made in the periosteum, which is elevated , exposing the mastoid cortex and, anteriorly, the temporomandibular joint space. Care is taken to avoid injury to an anomalous facial nerve exiting the temporal bone in this area. A large piece of temporalis fascia is harvested, trimmed of excess soft tissue if needed, and placed aside to dry (Fig. 7-20). The temporomandibular joint space is explored to verify that the facial nerve or tympanic bone is not lying within it (Fig. 7-21).

The literature has fostered the belief that there are separate and distinct approaches to the bony work necessary in atresiaplasty: the anterior approach, the transmastoid approach, and modification of the anterior approach. We feel that this strict distinction between these surgical approaches is unnecessary, as each can be used alone or in combination to facilitate the atresiaplasty. For purposes of discussion, however, each technique will be elucidated in detail.

Anterior Approach

- If a remnant of tympanic bone is present, the new ear canal is begun either through it or at the level of the middle fossa dura. If no such remnant is present, drilling begins at the level of the linea temporalis, just posterior to the glenoid fossa (Figs. 7-22, 7-23).

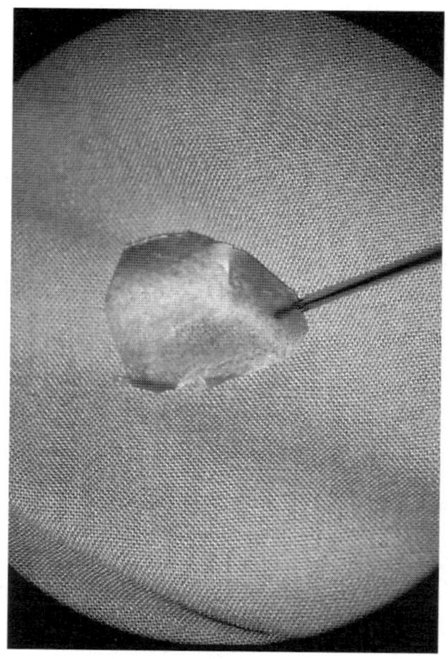

Fig. 7-20. Temporalis muscle fascia graft.

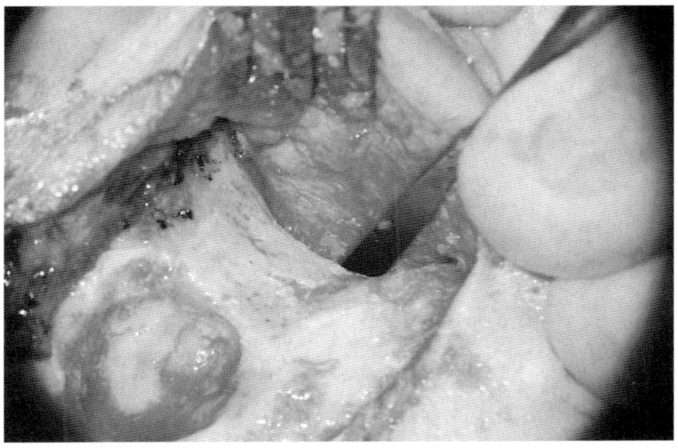

Fig. 7-21. The glenoid fossa is located with a dissector.

- *There are few landmarks through atretic bone.* By use of cutting and diamond burrs, the dissection is carried anteriorly and medially. The middle fossa plate is identified and followed to the epitympanum, where the fused malleus head-incus body mass is identified (Figs. 7-24, 7-25).
- Care is taken not to drill on the ossicular mass because the incudostapedial joint is presumed intact, and transmission of high-speed drill energy to the inner ear can result in sensorineural hearing loss. The epitympanic ossicular mass in the epitympanum is meticulously dissected free of the atresia plate and is left intact. This action helps protect the horizontal facial nerve, which lies medial to these structures.

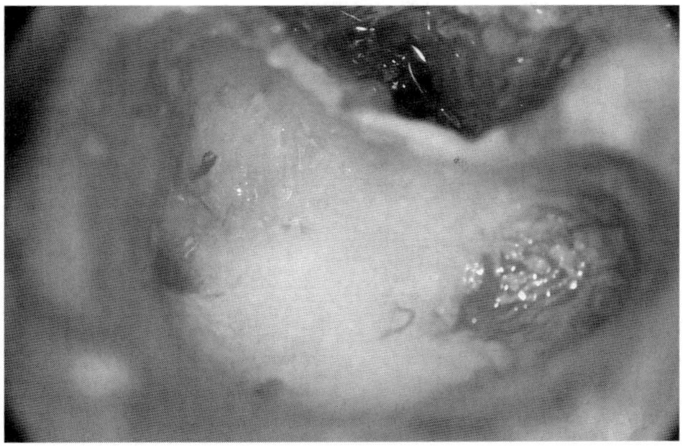

Fig. 7-23. Initial dissection of the mastoid air cell system.

- The atresia plate is removed with diamond microdrills and curettes to completely expose the ossicles. While the inferior and posterior aspects are dissected, an aberrant facial nerve may be encountered as it passes laterally through the atresia plate in this area. Although deformed, if the ossicular chain is felt to be complete, it is left in place (Figs. 7-26, 7-27, 7-28).
- The ever-present fibrous ligaments and adhesions are better vaporized with a carbon dioxide laser in the final phases of ossicular dissection, to avoid delayed refixation of the ossicles.
- Ossicular reconstruction with the patient's intact ossicular chain is preferred to the use of

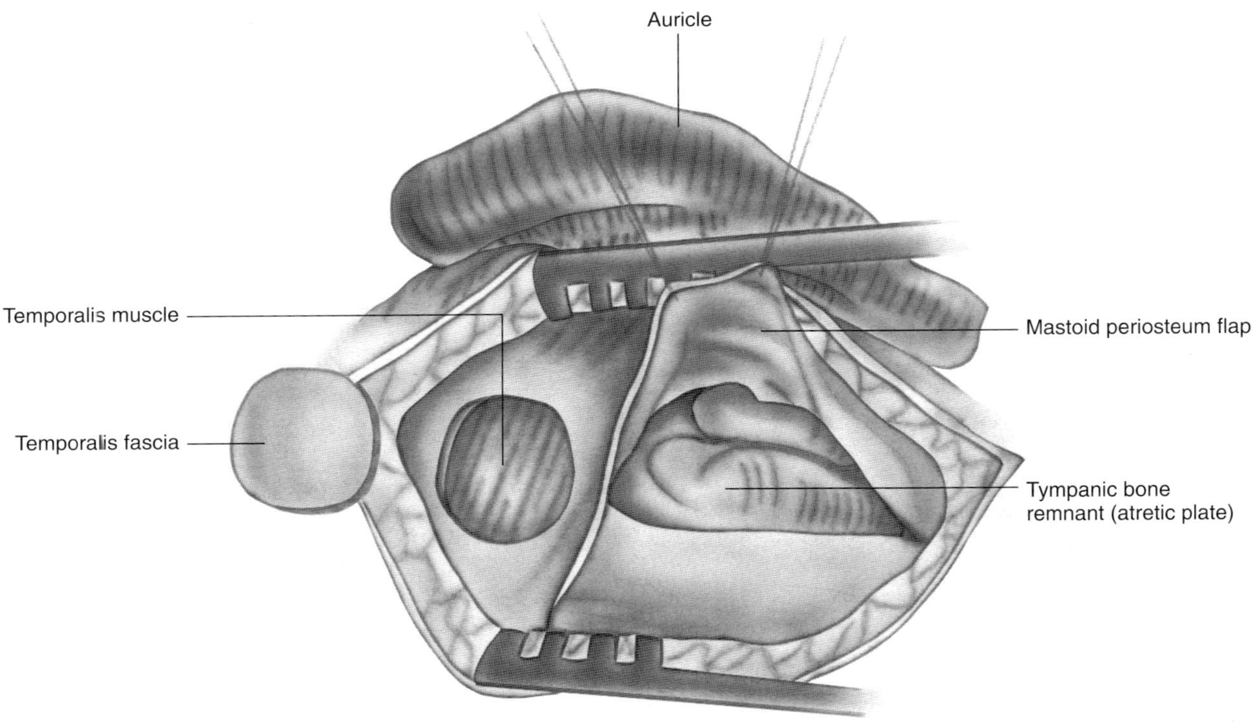

Fig. 7-22. Incision and harvesting of temporalis fascia.

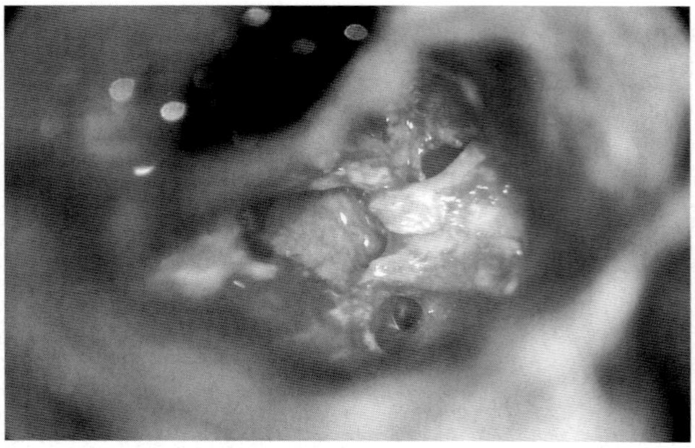

Fig. 7-24. CAA, left ear. The ossicular chain is exposed.

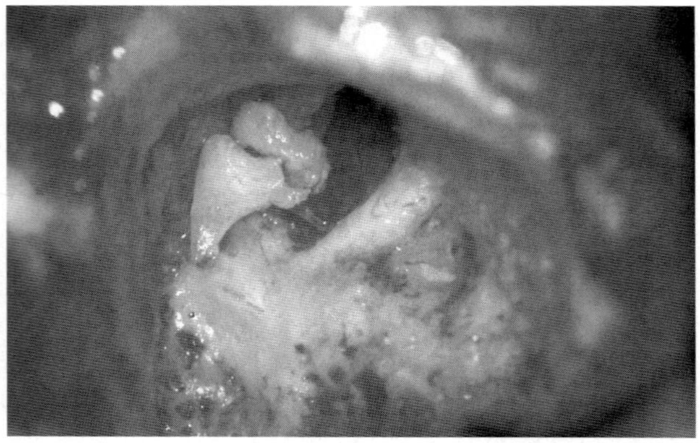

Fig. 7-25. CAA, right ear. The facial nerve describes a more acute angle than its usual 120 degrees at the second genu.

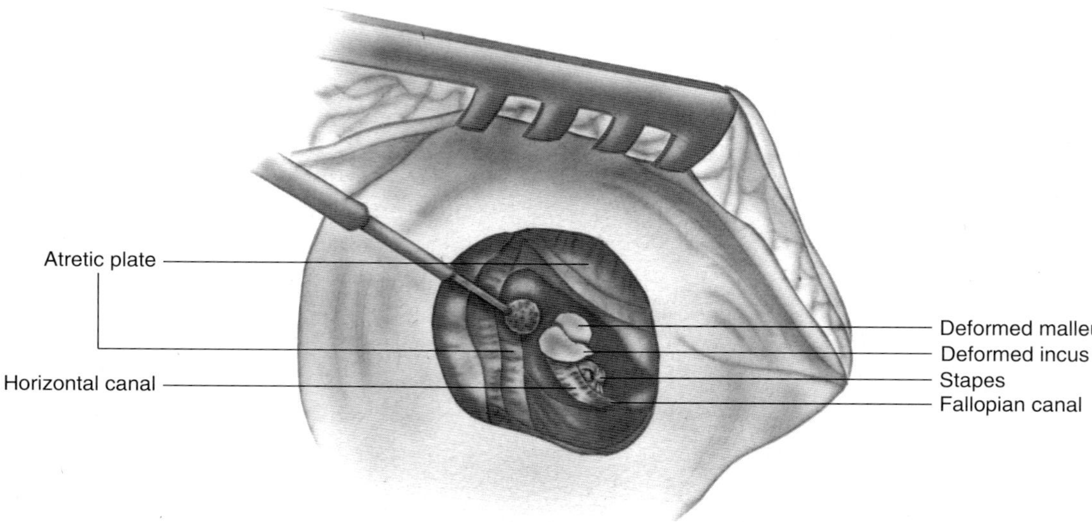

Fig. 7-26. Mastoidectomy has been completed.

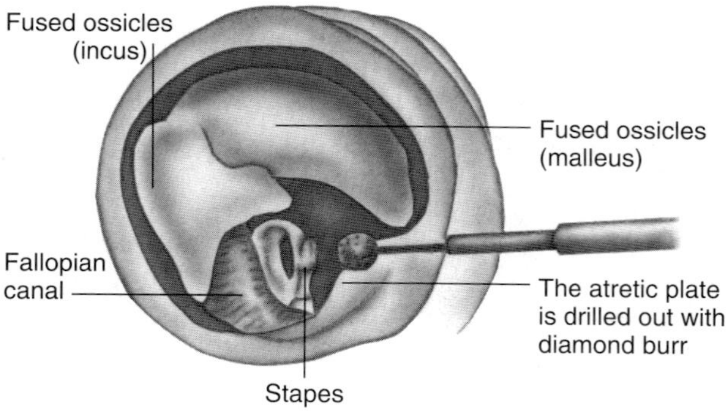

Fig. 7-27. Initial exposure of the ossicles. The external diameter of the cavity should be at least 14 mm.

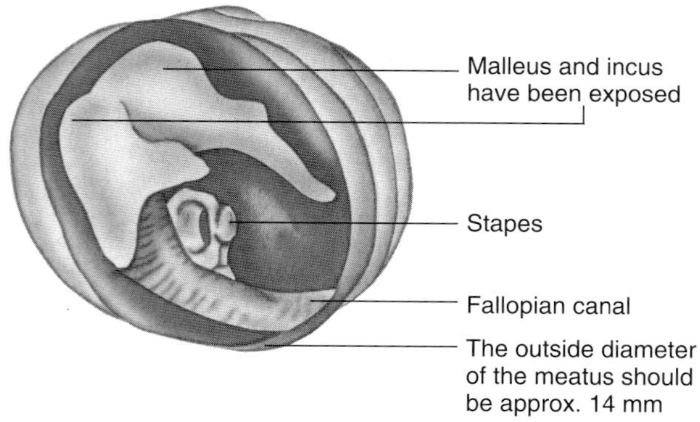

Fig. 7-28. The ossicles are completely exposed. In this case the incudo-stapedial joint is missing.

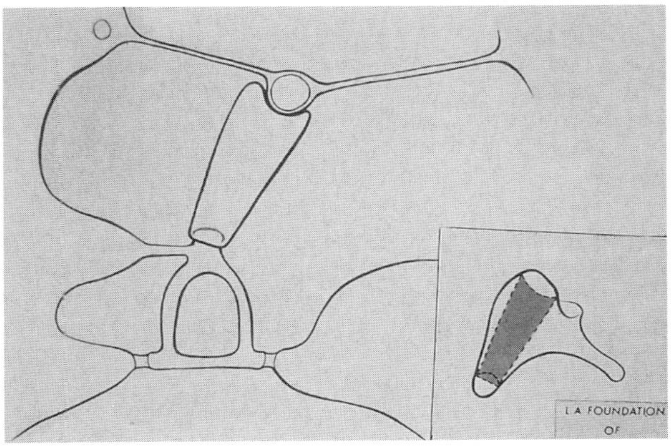

Fig. 7-29. When the ossicular chain is not complete, ossiculoplasty is performed with a partial (PORPE)(Fig. 7-29) or total ossicular reconstruction prostheses (TORPE) (Fig. 7-30).

prostheses. When the ossicular chain is not complete, ossiculoplasty is performed by use of a total or partial ossicular reconstruction prosthesis to either a mobile footplate or to the stapes head (Figs. 7-29, 7-30, 7-31). Infrequently, it is necessary to drill out an obliterated oval window (Ombredanne). The prosthesis is covered with cartilage prior to the grafting of the new drum. On occasion, the stapes footplate may not be seen well because of anomalous facial nerve anatomy, making placement of an ossicular prosthesis difficult or dangerous. In these instances, hearing restoration can be accomplished with LSCC fenestration, or the patient can be counseled to use a hearing aid. Drilling is continued to create a new ear canal measuring about 1.5 times the normal size, with the surgeon being careful not to violate the temporomandibular joint space or to expose an excessive number of mastoid air cells.

- The previously prepared skin graft donor site is exposed. A 0.012-inch thick, 6 cm × 6 cm split-

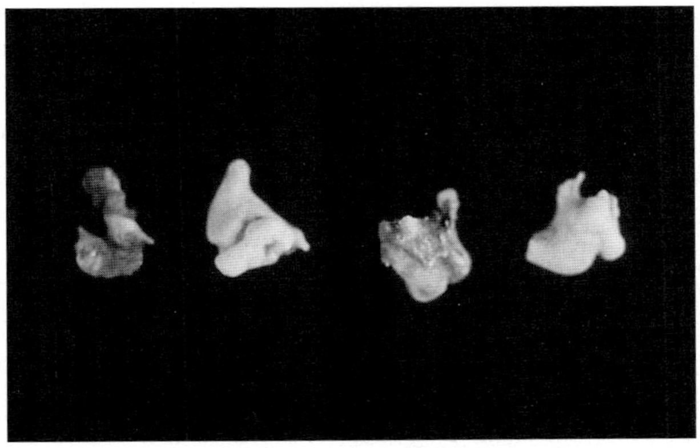

Fig. 7-31. Deformed ossicles.

thickness graft is obtained by use of a Brown dermatome. Hemostasis of the donor site is accomplished by pressure with a gauze sponge wet with 1 per cent lidocaine with epinephrine 1:100,000U and thrombin solution. When the donor site is dry, a sterile Op-Site dressing is applied (Weymuller). One edge of the skin graft is cut in a zigzag fashion such that four or five triangular points are created. The points of the zigzag are colored with a skin marker, as are the two points on the other edge. This marking allows for easy inspection in the final stages of the procedure. The skin graft is kept moist and set aside (Figs. 7-32, 7-33).
- The now-dry temporalis fascia is inspected and trimmed to size, ideally a 20 mm × 15 mm oval. Small 3 mm × 6 mm tabs are cut into the anterior and superior aspects of the fascia to prevent lateralization of this tympanic membrane graft (Sheehy) (Fig. 7-34). Lateralization is the most common delayed cause of a poor hearing outcome, occurring in 22 per cent of patients (De La Cruz; Molony). Nitrous oxide, if used by the anesthesiologist, must be discontinued 30 minutes before grafting begins.

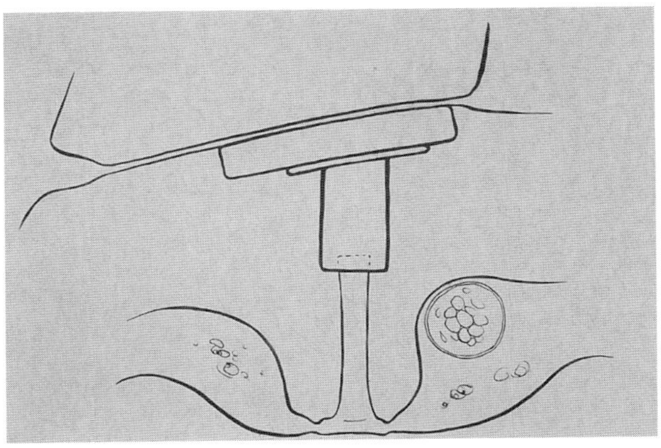

Fig. 7-30. Ossiculoplasty performed with a TORPE.

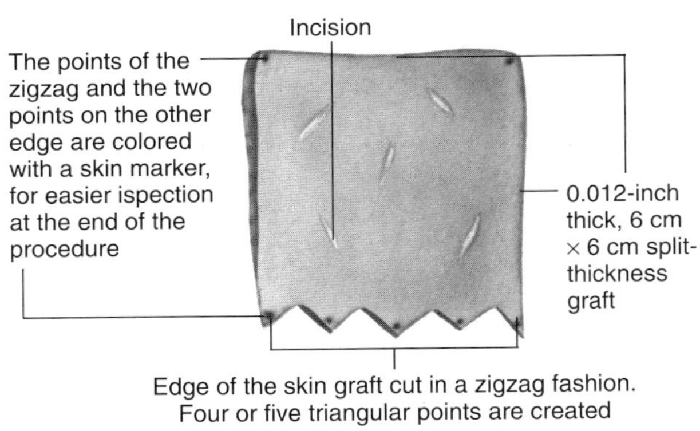

Fig. 7-32. The 0.012- inch thick, 6 cm × 6 cm split-thickness skin graft used to line the new EAC.

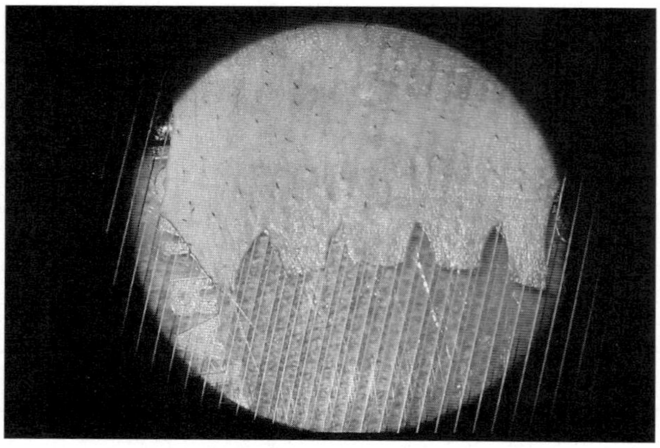

Fig. 7-33. A 0.012-inch thick, 6 cm × 6 cm split-thickness graft is harvested. One edge of the skin graft is cut in a zigzag fashion.

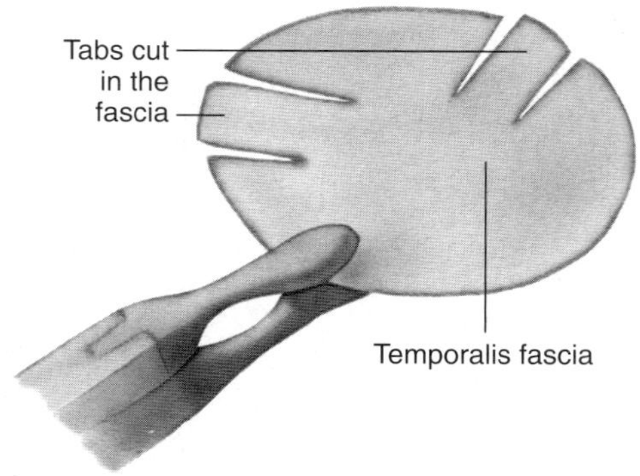

Fig. 7-34. When malleus is absent, the fascia is prepared with tabs tucked medially into the protympanum and epytimpanum, to prevent lateralization.

- The fascia is placed over the ossicular chain, medial to the malleus or, when ossicular reconstruction is needed, over the cartilage covering the prosthesis (Figs. 7-35, 7-36). The tabs are placed medially into the protympanum and epitympanum in an attempt to prevent lateralization of the new tympanic membrane (Fig. 7-37). The new ear canal is circumferentially lined with the split-thickness skin, and the zigzags are placed medially and partially overlap the fascia (Fig. 7-38). All bone of the EAC is covered (Mehra; Jahrsdoerfer). The colored points allow the surgeon to be sure that no skin lies folded on itself, and that the entire width of the graft is being used (the number of points seen matches the number of points created). Two centimeters to 3 cm of (apparent) excess skin remains laterally, to be tacked down later. A single layer of antibiotic-soaked absorbable gelatin sponge (Gelfoam) is used to hold the fascia and skin of the new ear drum in place. A disk of 0.020-inch reinforced silicone sheeting is placed over the tympanic membrane to reproduce the anterior tympanomeatal angle. A large Merocel wick is placed over this medial canal wall packing, and attention is then turned to meatoplasty.
- A 14 mm meatus is created, as 30 per cent of the diameter will eventually reduce as a result of the normal healing process (Figs. 7-39, 7-40). We avoid denuding or otherwise damaging the cartilage of the microtia repair. Skin, subcutaneous tissue, and cartilage are re-

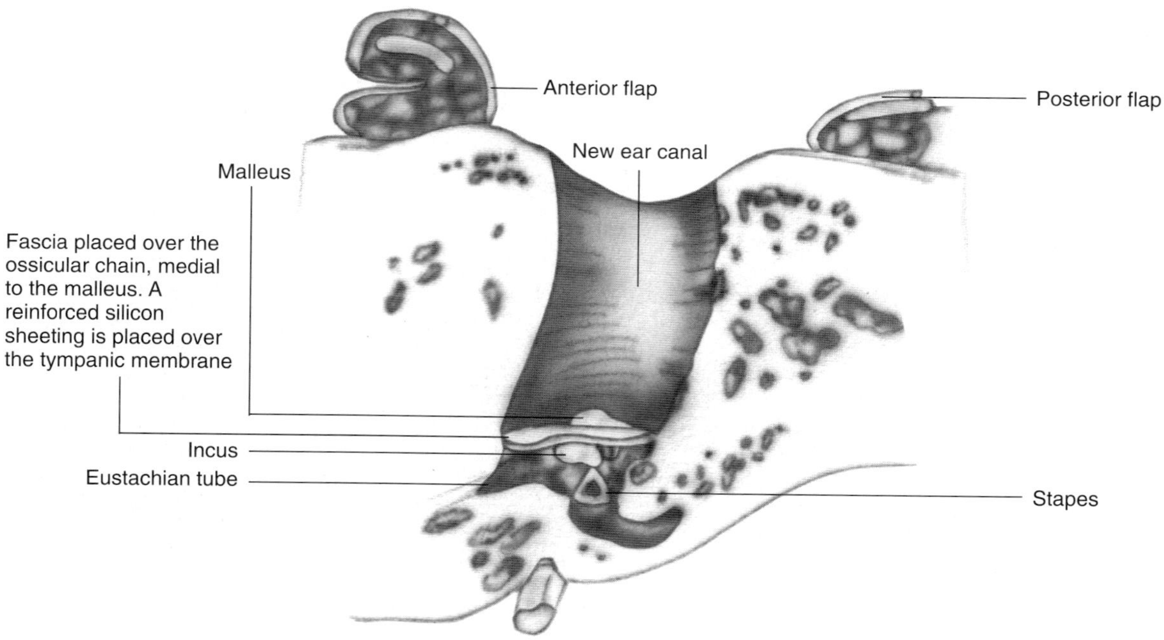

Fig. 7-35. The fascia is placed over the ossicular chain, medial to the malleus, to prevent lateralization.

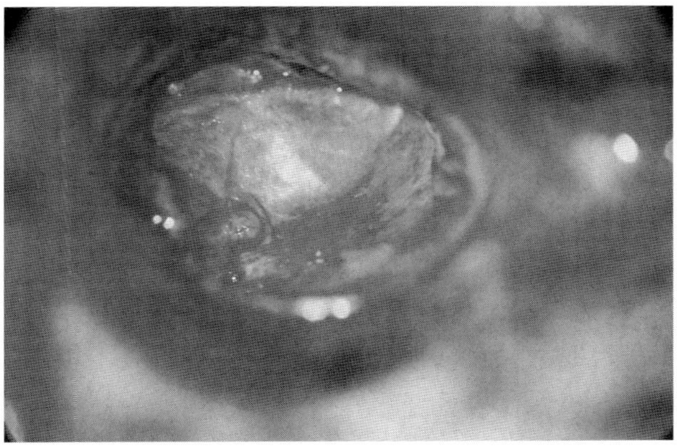

Fig. 7-36. The fascia is positioned.

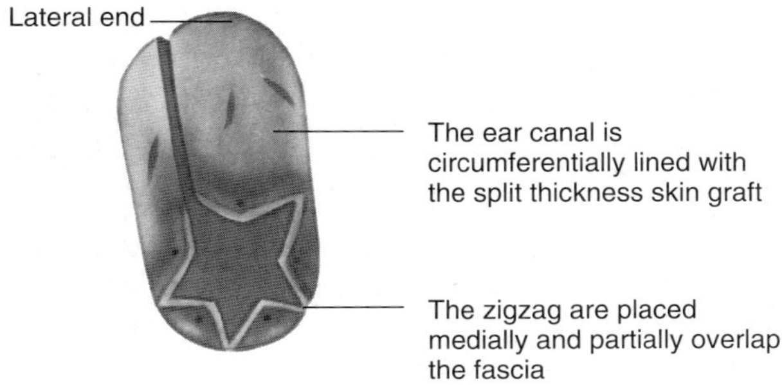

Fig. 7-38. Shape of split-thickness skin graft in the new EAC.

moved in a 1.4 cm diameter core over the new meatus (Figs. 7-41, 7-42). The ear is turned, and the excess canal skin graft is brought through the meatoplasty (Figs. 7-43, 7-44).

- With one or two absorbable sutures bringing the periosteum back in place over the mastoid cortex, the pinna and meatus are stabilized. Six or seven tacking sutures of 5-0 Ti-Cron attach the lateral edge of the skin graft circumferentially to the meatal skin. Next, absorbable suture (6-0 fast absorbing plain gut) is used in a running fashion between each Ti-Cron suture (Fig. 7-45). The lateral portion of the EAC and the meatus are packed. We prefer to use the large Ambros Merocel ear wick, divided longitudinally as necessary for diffuse pressure over the entire lateral skin graft and for wide packing of the meatus (Figs. 7-46, 7-47).
- The periosteum is sutured back into position. This action allows additional insurance that the meatus will heal wide open. The postauricular incision is closed with absorbable sutures (3-0 Dexon). Steri Strips cover the incision, a mastoid dressing is applied, anesthesia is reversed, monitoring equipment is removed, and the patient leaves the operating room.

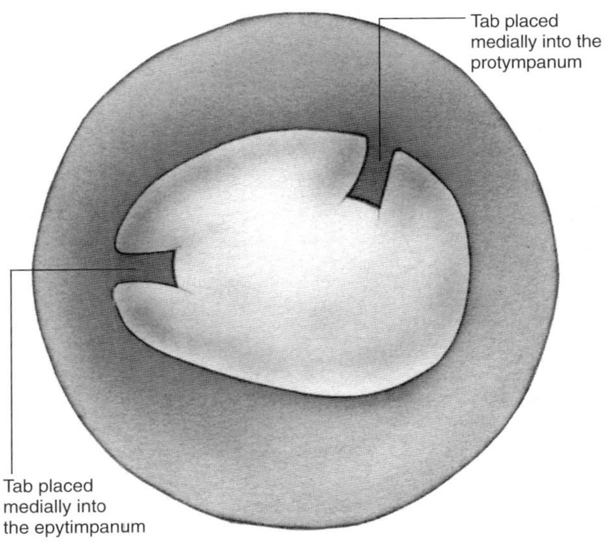

Fig. 7-37. Tabs are placed medially into the protympanum and epitympanum, to prevent lateralization.

Transmastoid Approach

The authors have not used the transmastoid approach in over 10 years.

- Exposure of the mastoid cortex and glenoid fossa is obtained as for the anterior approach. Dissection is then begun at the level of the linea temporalis, well posterior to the temporomandibular joint.
- The sinodural angle is identified and followed medially to the antrum. Bone paté is obtained during drilling.
- The lateral semicircular canal, the malleus-incus complex, and the atresia plate are identified, and the atresia plate is removed carefully with microdrills to avoid inner ear acoustic trauma.
- Mastoid air cell exenteration and lowering of the facial ridge to the facial nerve allow access

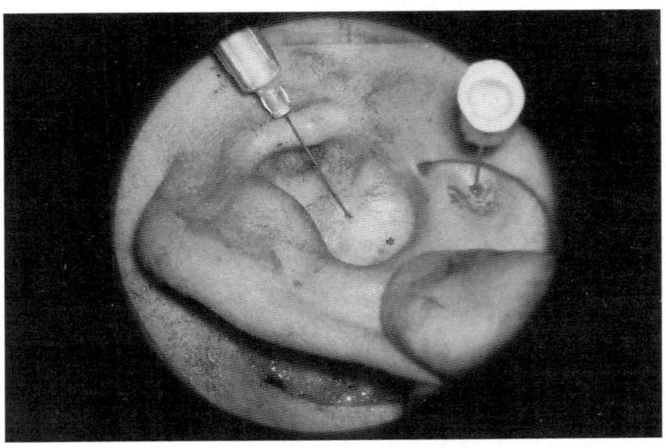

Fig. 7-39. A 14 mm meatus is created, as the diameter will eventually be reduced by 30% as a result of the normal healing process. Needles are inserted to mark the limits of meatoplasty, when the auricle is turned anteriorly.

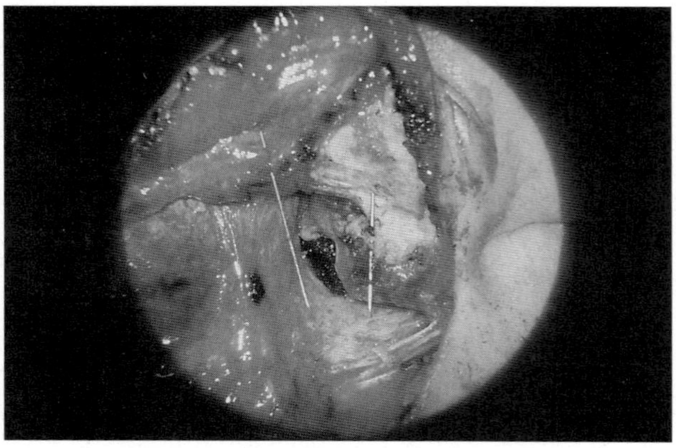

Fig. 7-40. Needles mark the medial limits of the meatoplasty.

and creation of an EAC with a canal wall down technique.

- The remainder of the operation (ossiculoplasty, timpanoplasty) proceeds as outlined earlier. The only additional step is bone paté or soft tissue obliteration of the large mastoid cells before meatoplasty and canal skin grafting is performed (Fig. 7-48).

Modified Anterior Approach

In patients with thick, bony atresia plates, orientation may be difficult during the medial dissection. These patients typically have few air cells, making this approach particularly challenging. Dissection too far in either the inferior or the posterior direction risks inadvertent carotid, lateral canal or facial nerve injury.

- Orientation is achieved in these cases with initial posterior dissection and limited posterior antrotomy at the sinodural angle only, enabling identification of the levels of the lateral semicircular canal and the ossicular mass.
- A new ear canal is then created in a method similar to that used for the anterior approach by drilling just posterior to the glenoid fossa and following an intact canal wall mastoidectomy approach. The lateral canal can be used repeatedly as a landmark to indicate depth and anteroposterior and superoinferior directionality, thus making the dissection safer.
- An intact canal wall-like procedure is then carried out. The remainder of the surgery proceeds as described earlier.

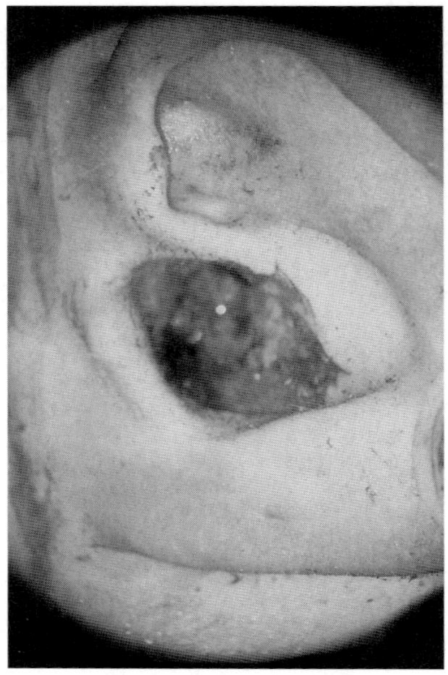

Fig. 7-42. Meatoplasty completed.

POSTOPERATIVE CARE

- The mastoid dressing is removed on the first postoperative day and the Steri-Strips are left in place over the postauricular incision for 7 days.
- The patient is counseled to keep the operative site dry and to change the cotton ball over the canal-meatus packing once or twice daily. The Op-Site over the skin graft donor site is left on

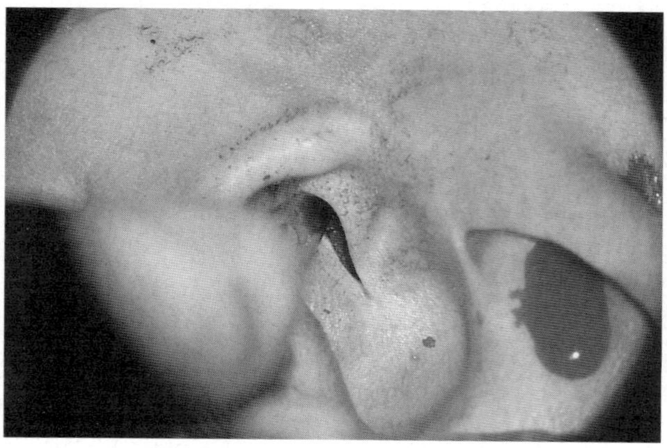

Fig. 7-41. Meatoplasty. Skin, subcutaneous tissue and cartilage are removed.

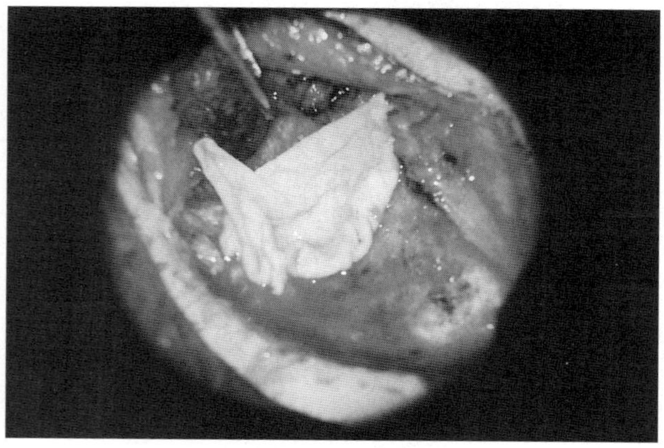

Fig. 7-43. The new ear canal is circumferentially lined with the split-thickness skin graft, and the zigzags are placed medially and partially overlap the fascia.

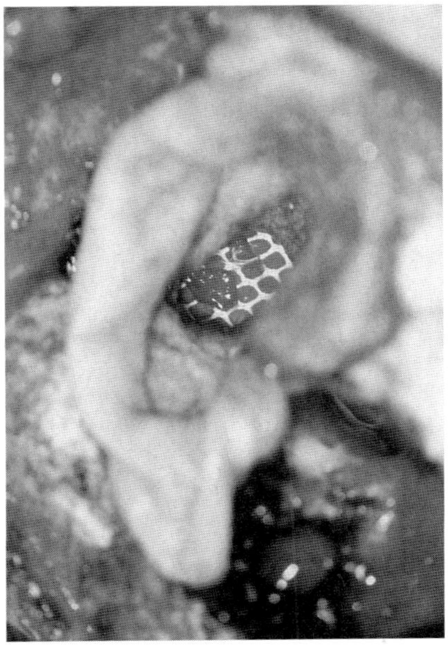

Fig. 7-44. The excess canal skin graft is brought through the meatoplasty.

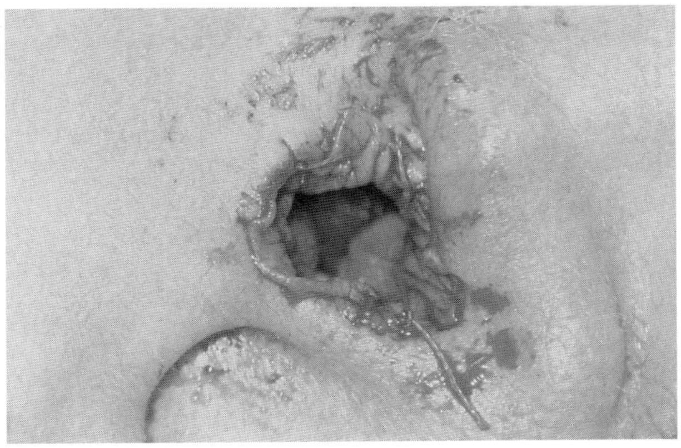

Fig. 7-45. Tacking sutures of 5-0 Ti-Cron attach the lateral edge of the skin graft circumferentially to the meatal skin. Next, absorbable suture (6-0 fast absorbing plain gut) is used in a running fashion between each Ti-Cron suture.

for at least 3 weeks and requires no special attention. Epithelization occurs under the plastic, and the typical pain associated with older methods of donor site dressing is absent (Weymuller). The patient is given a 5 day course of oral anfistaphylococcal antibiotics.

- The patient is seen 1 week after surgery, at which time the postauricular strips are removed, the tacking Ti-Cron sutures at the meatus are removed, and the dried and crusted lateral end of the meatus pack is trimmed off. The donor site is inspected. The postauricular site can now be washed, but water precautions continue to apply to the canal.
- We see the patient again after 2 weeks, and at this time the dried portion of the Merocel pack is removed. The meatus is repacked with an-

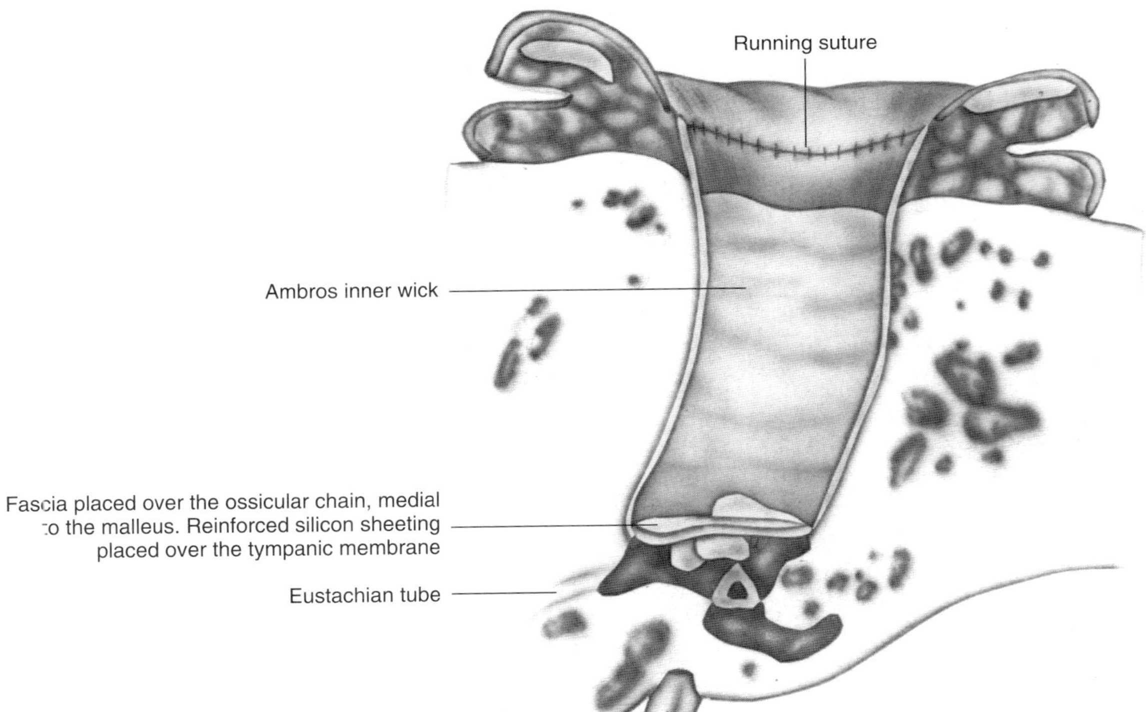

Fig. 7-46. STSG is in place, over fascia. An inner Merocel wick is placed in the canal. A reinforced silicon sheeting is placed over the tympanic membrane, to reproduce the anterior tympano-meatal angle.

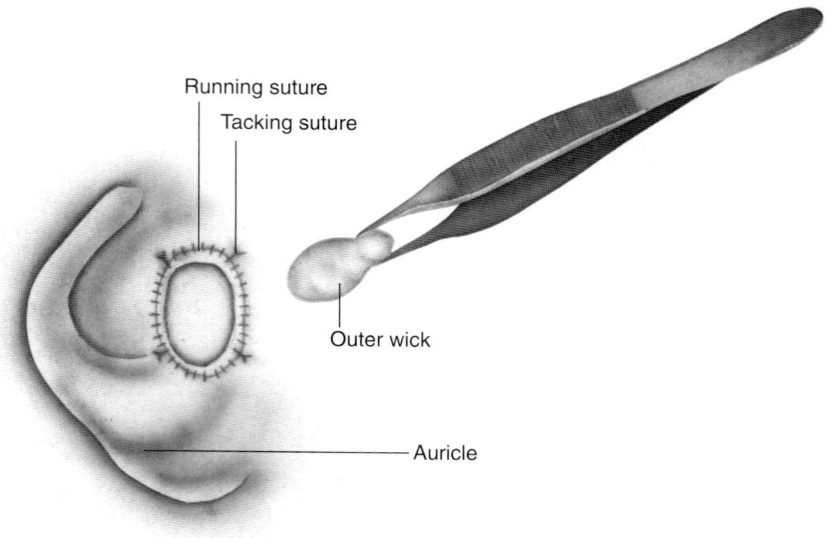

Fig. 7-47. STSG is sutured to the new EAC. The lateral portion of the EAC and the meatus is packed with a large Ambros Merocel ear wick.

tibiotic soaked gelatine sponge. At this point, the patient is instructed to begin applying antibiotic suspension to the packing in the EAC twice a day. By this time, also, the Op-Site has peeled off and the donor site has completed the initial hearing phase. At the third postoperative week, the gelatin sponge and silicone sheeting disk are removed. The patient continues to use the drops for 8 to 12 weeks.

The first postoperative audiogram is obtained at 6 to 8 weeks, when nearly all of the gelatin sponge is gone and the canal is healing well. Audiograms are then obtained at 6 month, 1 year, and yearly thereafter.

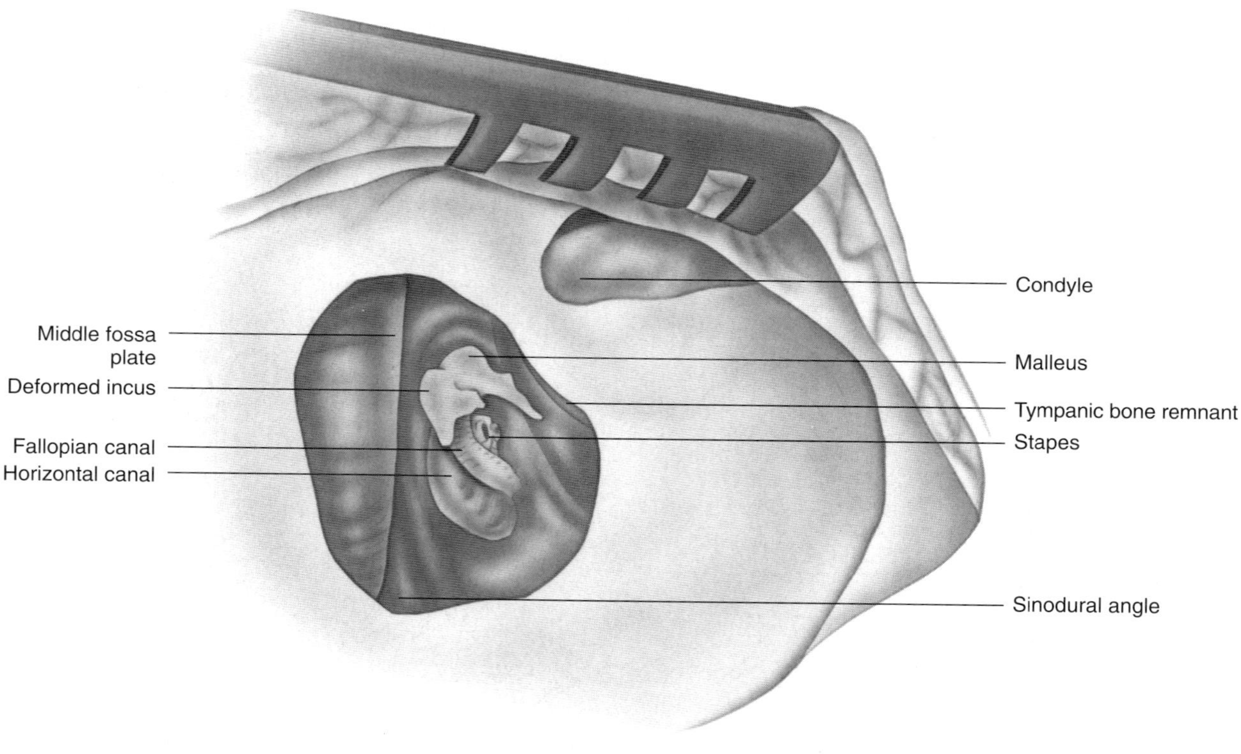

Fig. 7-48. Transmastoid approach.

TIPS AND PITFALLS

- In all cases, we prefer and often begin with an anterior approach; however in atretic bone often no clearly identifiable landmark exist. The only "knowns" are the middle fossa plate or the sinodural angle, and the occasional atresiaplasty surgeon can follow these forward to reach the epitympanum.

- Complete communication between the surgeon and the anesthesiologist will ensure that the patient is not paralyzed during the procedure because facial nerve monitoring is essential in these cases. When the monitor is off transiently because of the use of electrocautery, we monitor the facial nerve manually with a hand on the patient's face. In poorly pneumatized mastoids, the otic capsule may be difficult to distinguish, resulting in blue lining, or worse, of the semicircular canals. In these cases, we recommend the modified anterior approach. We do not use the transmastoid approach.

- Postoperative office care is important. Patients should know beforehand that they must precisely follow the instructions given and that they must keep all scheduled postoperative office visits. An infected graft in a patient who has missed appointments for a month is a serious and difficult problem. We recommend checking the circumference of the pack each week to ensure that there is no ingrowth of grafted skin into the pack, although we have not seen this problem with the Ambros packs. If the meatus appears to be narrowing, usually at the third month, it can be dilated every 2 weeks and restented effectively with the large Merocel wick and gelatin sponge for 12 to 24 months.

RESULTS

At the House Ear Clinic, a review of 302 atretic ears in 239 patients was done by De La Cruz et al. in 1985. The results are summarized in the Table 7-7.

The treatment of congenital aural atresia requires:

- Early identification, amplification, and speech and language therapy are crucial in bilateral cases.
- Cooperation with the auricular reconstruction surgeon allows for both esthetic and functional success, and the use of strict radiologic and clinical criteria for operative candidates is necessary.
- Patients whose disorders are classified into categories of "minor" and "major" malformations should understand the prognosis for hearing improvement and the risks and results of surgery.

The treatment of congenital aural atresia is a challenging surgery, but a thorough understanding of embryologic maldevelopment and rigorous adherence to the surgical principles of mastoidectomy, facial nerve dissection, and tympanoplasty enable us to offer our patients optimal hearing restoration. Diligent postoperative office care is vital to maintaining the good results obtained at surgery.

COMPLICATIONS AND THEIR MANAGEMENT

Complications of atresiaplasty include:

- Lateralization of the tympanic membrane in up to 26 per cent.
- Stenosis of the external auditory meatus in 8 per cent.
- Sensorineural hearing loss in 2 per cent.
- Facial nerve palsy in 1 per cent.

Care taken at the time of surgery can help minimize the incidence of lateralization.

- The anesthesiologist should be alerted to shut off any nitrous oxide 30 minutes before grafting is begun.
- The graft should be anchored medially to the malleus, and the tabs placed into the hypotimpanum and epitympanum.
- Use of an accurately sized silicone sheeting disk will help reform an anterior timpanomeatal angle and keep the graft in position.
- The patient must be followed up carefully for at least 12 to 16 months because lateralization has been known to occur up to 12 months postoperatively.
- The incidence of stenosis has been reduced with the use of large, split thickness skin grafts. Careful inspection of the meatus at frequent intervals and early stenting with Merocel wicks can obviate reoperation. The importance of early identification and treatment of infection to prevent graft failure and stenosis can not be overemphasized.
- With better imaging techniques, oval window problems can be identified preoperatively and problems of sensorineural hearing loss due to oval window drill-out can be avoided. Likewise, patients with computed tomographic evidence of severe malformations in whom surgery would be fraught with problems can be counseled against surgical intervention and fitted with hearing aids instead. The facial nerve can be imaged preoperatively. Along with intraoperative facial nerve electromyo-

Table 7-7. HEC: A Review of 1985. 302 Atretic ears in 239 Patients.

Male	141	(59%)
Female	98	(41%)
Unilateral cases	169	
• Either nonhearing ear or cholesteatoma in the normal appearing ear	5	
Bilateral cases	70	
Associated anomalies	30	
• Congenital ipsilateral facial anomaly -either microtia or paralysis	11	
• Mondini's inner ear deformity	7	
• Treacher Collins	6	
• Cleft palate	5	
• Stenotic internal auditory canal	1	
Cholesteatoma in the atretic ear	9	
Nonhearing ears before surgery	2	
Surgery		
Primary atresiaplasty	65	
Hearing results		
Conductive deficit <10 dB		(16%)
<20 dB		(53%)
<30 dB		(73%)
Patients with poorer auditory outcomes		
• No hearing restoration attempted for the severity of malformation and poor mastoid pneumatization	6	
• NSHL with preservation of the low tones	1	
• Development of a nonhearing ear following a LSCC fenestration procedure	1	
• Facial nerve injuries	No	
Revision Surgery	20	
• Lateralization of the tympanic membrane, usually within 12 months after surgery	14	(22%)
• Canal stenoses		
• Persistent drainage	5	
• No. of patients were was used a full-thickness skin graft at the first operation	1	
• The change to split-thickness skin graft has reduced the incidence of stenosis and the need for revision surgery	18	
	2	
Hearing results		
Conductive deficit <10 dB	2	(10%)
<20 dB	12	(60%)
Profound SNHL following a drill out for an absent oval window	1	
24 Atresiaplasty from the HEC (1984-1988)		
Similar rates of air-bone gap closure		
Sensorineural hearing loss	No	
Success rate		
• Anterior approach		(79%)
• Transmastoid approach		(60%)
Failure		
• Anterior approach (it has the only case of recurrent drainage)	4	
• Posterior approach	3	

graphic monitoring, this preoperative imaging will serve to reduce even further the incidence of facial nerve injury.

ALTERNATIVE TECHNIQUES

Patients with bilateral atresia must have auditory amplification. Initially as we have discussed, newborns receive bone-conduction aids. At age 6, if evaluation reveals a high surgical risk or poor predicted outcome, a bone conduction aid is a good option. In patients with unilateral atresia and contralateral normal auditory function, no intervention is mandatory but implantation of a bone-conduction hearing aid can be considered. These aids can also anchor synthetic auricular prostheses (Granstrom; Niparko). They are osseointegrated titanium devices that are implanted into the mastoid. Experience in the United States with these devices is limited. We do not recommend implantable bone-conduction hearing aids in children, because surgical scarring and disruption of vascular planes preclude future auricular reconstruction.

The two types of implantable bone aids available for clinical use are the bone-anchored hearing aid (BAHA), introduced in 1977 in Sweden, and the Audiant, introduced in 1984 and manufactured in the United States (Granstrom; Tjellstrom). Surgery for the BAHA is a two-stage procedure with an interval of 3 to 4 months between operations, allowing for osseointegration to start before a load is applied. The first stage is implantation of the fixture into the mastoid cortex. Following implantation, the skin flap is replaced, and healing is allowed to take place. At the second stage, a skin penetrating abutment is secured to the fixture, reducing the amount of subcutaneous tissue and eliminating hair follicles in the site. Often, this step necessitates a hairless skin transplant. The aid is first useable 3 to 5 weeks following the second stage. Clinical trials are at present underway to convert the insertion of the BAHA into a one-stage procedure. The Audiant has two parts: an internal magnet housed in a titanium disk and coated with medical-grade silicone attached to the skull through an orthopedic screw, and an external device, which is the sound processor, which includes a second rare earth magnet and an induction coil. Transmission is transcutaneous through a thickness of 4mm to 6mm of skin and subcutaneous tissue.

For use of the Audiant, a bone conduction hearing threshold of better than 25dB for the speech frequencies is recommended. For the BAHA, 45dB or better bone thresholds result in subjective improvement in 90 per cent of patients. Further comparisons between the two types of devices are available in the literature (Gates; Håkansson).

REFERENCES

Aase, JM: Microtia-clinical observations. Birth Defects 16(4): 289-297, 1980.

Altmann F: Congenital atresia of the ear in man and animals. Ann Otol Rhinol Laryngol 64: 824-858, 1955.

Andrews JC, Anzai Y, Mankosich NJ, et al: Three-dimensional CT scan reconstruction for the assessment of congenital aural atresia. Am J Otol 13(3): 236-240, 1992.

Barrios-Montes JM: Malformaciones auriculares. Acta Otorrinolaringol Esp 27(1): 17-46,1976.

Bellucci RJ: Congenital aural malformations: diagnosis and treatment. Otolaryngol Clin North Am 14(1): 95-124, 1981.

Bellucci RJ: Congenital auricular malformation: indications, contraindications, and timing of middle ear surgery: an otologist's viewpoint. In Converse JM (ed): Reconstructive Plastic Surgery, Vol 3. Philadelphia, WB Saunders, 1977, pp 1719-1724.

Bellucci RJ: The problem of congenital auricular malformation. 1. Construction of the external auditory canal. Trans Am Acad Ophthalmol Otolaryngol 64: 840 852, 1960.

Brent B: Auricular repair with autogenous rib cartilage grafts: two decades of experience with 600 cases. Plast Reconstr Surg 90: 355-374, 1992.

Brent B: The correction of microtia with autogenous cartilage grafts: 1. The classic deformity. Plast Reconstr Surg 66(1): 1-12, 1980.

Chiossone E: Surgical management of major congenital malformations of the ear. Read at the Politzer Society International Conference. Montreux, Switzerland, September 1983.

Chole RA: Meatoplasty using inferiorly based island pedicle flap for congenital aural atresia. Laryngoscope 93 (7): 954-955, 1983.

Colman BH: Congenital malformations of the ear -aspects of management. J Otolaryngol Soc Aust 4(3): 197-200, 1978.

Crabtree JA: Congenital atresia: case selection, complications, and prevention. Otolaryngol Clin North Am 15(4): 755-762, 1982.

Crabtree JA: The facial nerve in congenital ear surgery. Otolaryngol Clin North Am 7(2): 505-510, 1974.

Crabtree JA: Tympanoplastic techniques in congenital atresia. Arch Otolaryngol Head Neck Surg 88: 89-96, 1968.

De La Cruz A, Linthicum FH Jr, Luxford WM: Congenital atresia of the external auditory canal. Laryngoscope 95: 421-427, 1985.

Dean LW, Gittens TR: Report of a case of bilateral, congenital osseous atresia of the external auditory canal with an exceptionally good functional result following operation. Trans Am Laryngol Rhinol Otol Soc 296 309, 1917.

Federspil P, Delb W: Treatment of congenital malformations of the external and middle ear. In Ars B (ed): Congenital External and Middle Ear Malformations: Management. Amsterdam, Kugler Publications, 1992, pp 47-70.

Fernandez AO, Ronis ML: The Treacher Collins syndrome. Arch Otolaryngol Head Neck Surg 80: 505-520, 1964.

Gates GA, Hough JV, Gatti WM, Bradley WH: The safety and effectiveness of an implanted electromagnetic hearing device. Arch Otolaryngol Head Neck Surg 115: 924-930, 1989.

Gill NW: Congenital atresia of the ear—a review of the surgical findings in 83 cases. J Larvngol Otol 83: 551-587, 1969.

Gill NW: Congenital atresia of the ear. J Laryngol Otol 85: 1251-1254, 1971.

Granstrom G, Bergstrom K, Tjellstrom A: The bone-anchored hearing aid and bone-anchored epithesis for congenital ear malformations. Otolaryngol Head Neck Surg 109: 46-53, 1993.

Grundfast KM, Camilon F: External auditory canal stenosis and partial atresia without associated anomalies. Ann Otol Rhinol Laryngol 95: 505-509, 1986.

Hakansson Bt, Liden G, Tjellstrom A, et al: Ten years of experience with the Swedish bone-anchored hearing system. Ann Otol Rhinol Laryngol (Suppl) 151: 1-16, 1990.

Harada O, Ishii H: The condition of the auditory ossicles in microtia: findings in 57 middle ear operations. Plast Reconstr Surg 50(1): 48-53, 1972.

Hasso AN, Broadwell RA: Congenital anomalies. In Som PM, Bergeron RT (eds): Head and Neck Imaging. St. Louis, CV Mosby, 1991, 960-966.

Hiraide F, Nomura Y, Nakamura K: Histopathology of atresia auris congenita. J Laryngol Otol 88: 1249-1256, 1974.

House HP: Management of congenital ear canal atresia. Laryngoscope 63(10): 916-946, 1953.

Jahrsdoerfer RA, Cole RR, Gray LE: Advances in congenital aural atresia. Adv Otolaryngol Head Neck Surg 5: 1-15, 1991.

Jahrsdoerfer RA, Garcia ET, Yeakley JW, Jacobson JT: Surface contour three-dimensional imaging in congenital aural atresia. Arch Otolaryngol Head Neck Surg 119: 95-99, 1993.

Jahrsdoerfer RA, Hall JW: Congenital malformations of the ear. Am J Otol 7(4): 267-269, 1986.

Jahrsdoerfer RA, Yeakley JW, Aguilar EA, et al: Grading system for the selection of patients with congenital aural atresia. Am J Otol 13(1): 6-12, 1992.

Jahrsdoerfer RA, Yeakley JW, Hall III JW, et al: High-resolution CT scanning and auditory brain stem response in congenital aural atresia: patient selection and surgical correlation. Otolaryngol Head Neck Surg 93: 292-298, 1985.

Jahrsdoerfer RA: Clinical aspects of temporal bone anomalies. AJNR 13: 821-825, 1992.

Jahrsdoerfer RA: Congenital atresia of the ear. Laryngoscope 88(9 Suppl) 13: 1-48, 1978.

Kelemen G: Aural participation in congenital malformations of the organism. Acta Otolaryngol Suppl (Stockh) 321: 1-35, 1974.

Linstrom CJ, Meiteles LZ: Facial nerve monitoring in surgery for congenital auricular atresia. Laryngoscope 103: 406-415, 1993.

Linthicum FH Jr: Surgery of congenital deafness. Otolaryngol Clin North Am 4(2): 401-409, 1971.

Marquet J, Declau F, De Cock M, et al: Congenital middle ear malformations. Acta Otorhinolaryngol Belg 42: 117-302, 1988.

Marquet J: Homogreffes tympano-ossiculaires dans le traitement chirurgical de l'agenesie de l'oreille; rapport preliminaire. Acta Otorhinolaryngol Belg 25(6): 885-897, 1971.

Mehra YN, Dubey SP, Mann SBS, Suri S: Correlation between high-resolution computed tomography and surgical findings in congenital aural atresia. Arch Otolaryngol Head Neck Surg 114: 137-141, 1988.

Melnick M: The etiology of external ear malformations and its relation to abnormalities of the middle ear, inner ear, and other organ systems. Birth Defects 16(4): 303-331, 1980.

Meurman Y: Congenital microtia and meatal atresia. Arch Otolaryngol Head Neck Surg 66(4): 443-463, 1957.

Minatogawa T, Nishimura Y, Inamori T, Kumoi T: Results of tympanoplasty for congenital aural atresia and stenosis, with special reference to fascia and homograft as the graft material of the tympanic membrane. Laryngoscope 99: 632-638, 1989.

Miyamoto RT, Fairchild TH, Daugherty HS: Primary cholesteatoma in the congenitally atretic ear. Am J Otol 5(4): 283-285, 1984.

Molony TB, De La Cruz A: Surgical approaches to congenital atresia of the external auditory canal. Otolaryngol Head Neck Surg 103: 991-1001, 1990.

Nager GT: Aural atresia: anatomy and surgery. Postgrad Med 29(5): 529-541, 1961.

Niparko JK, Langman AW, Cutler DS, Carroll WR: Tissue-integrated prostheses in the rehabilitation of auricular defects: results with percutaneous mastoid implants. Am J Otol 14(4): 343-348, 1993.

Ombredanne M: Absence congenitale de fenetre ronde dans certaines aplasies mineures. Ann Otolaryngol (Paris) 85(5): 369-378, 1968.

Ombredanne M: Chirurgie de la surdite: fenestration dans les aplasies de l'oreille avec imperforation du conduit. Resultats. Otorhinolaryngol Int 31: 229-236, 1947.

Ombredanne M: Chirurgie des surdites congenitales par malformations ossiculaires. Acta Otolaryngol Belg 25: 837 869, 1971.

Ombredanne M: Malformations des osselets dans les embryopathies de l'oreille. Acta Otorhinolaryngol Belg 20(6): 623-652, 1965.

Ombredanne M: Transposition d'osselets dans certaines "aplasies mineures." Ann Otolaryngol (Paris) 83(45): 273-280, 1966.

Page JR: Congenital bilateral microtia with total osseous atresia of the external auditory canals, operation and report of cases. Trans Am Otol Soc 13: 376-390, 1914.

Pattee GL: An operation to improve hearing in cases of congenital atresia of the external auditory meatus. Arch Otolaryngol Head Neck Surg 45(5): 568-580, 1947.

Patterson ME, Linthicum FH Jr: Congenital hearing impairment. Otolaryngol Clin North Am 201-219, 1970.

Rapin I, Ruben RJ: Patterns of anomalies in children with malformed ears. Laryngoscope 86: 1469-1502, 1976.

Ruben RJ, Toriyama M, Dische MR, et al: External and middle ear malformations associated with mandibulo-facial dysostosis and renal abnormalities: a case report. Ann Otol Rhinol Laryngol 78: 605-624, 1969.

Ruben RJ: Management and therapy of congenital malformations of the external and middle ears. In Ruben RJ, Alberti PW (eds): Otologic Medicine and Surgery. New York, Churchill Livingstone, 1988, pp 1135-1154.

Ruedi L: The surgical treatment of the atresia auris congenita: a clinical and histological report. Laryngoscope 64: 666-684, 1954.

Sanchez-Corona J, Garcia-Cruz D, Ruenes R, Cantu JM: A distinct dominant form of microtia and conductive hearing loss. Birth Defects 18(3B): 211-216, 1982.

Sando I, Shibahara Y, Takagi A et al: Congenital middle and inner ear anomalies. Acta Otolaryngol Suppl (Stockh) 458: 7678, 1988.

Sando I, Suehiro S, Wood RP II: In Bluestone CD, Stool SE (eds): Congenital anomalies of the external and middle ear. Pediatric Otolaryngology. Philadelphia, WB Saunders, 1983, pp 309-326.

Savic D, Jasosric A, Djeric D: The relations of the mastoid segment of the facial canal to surrounding structures in congenital middle ear malformations. Int J Pediatr Otorhinolaryngol 18: 13-19, 1989.

Scheer AA: Correction of congenital middle ear deformities. Arch Otolaryngol Head Neck Surg 85(3): 269-277, 1967.

Schuknecht HF: Congenital aural atresia and congenital middle ear cholesteatoma. In Nadol JB Jr, Schuknecht HF (eds): Surgery of the Ear and Temporal Bone. New York, Raven Press, 1993, pp 263-274.

Schuknecht HF: Reconstructive procedures for congenital aural atresia. Arch Otolaryngol Head Neck Surg 101: 170-172, 1975.

Shambaugh Jr GE: Developmental anomalies of the sound conducting apparatus and their surgical correction. Ann Otol 74: 873-887, 1952.

Sheehy JL: Surgery of chronic otitis media. In English GE (ed): Otolaryngology, Vol 1. Harper & Row, 1977.

Sortini AJ: Hearing aids for children with bilateral congenital ear canal atresia. Hear Instrum 6: 20-23, 1981.

Tjellstrom A, Bergstom K: Bone-anchored hearing aids and prostheses. In Ars B (ed): Congenital External and Middle Ear Malformations: Management. Amsterdam, Kugler Publications, 1992, pp 1-9.

Van De Water TR, Maderson PFA, Jaskoll TF: The morphogenesis of the middle and external ear. Birth Defects 16(4): 147-180, 1980.

Weymuller EA Jr: Dressings for split thickness skin graft donor sites. Laryngoscope 91: 652-653, 1981.

Wigand ME: Tympano-meatoplastie endaurale pour les atresies congenitales severes de l'oreille. Rev Laryngol 99 (1-2): 14-28, 1978.

Woodman DG: Congenital atresia of the auditory canal. Arch Otolaryngol Head Neck Surg 55: 172-181, 1952.

Zalzal GH, Shott SR, Towbin R, Cotton RT: Value of CT scan in the diagnosis of temporal bone diseases in children. Laryngoscope 96: 27-32, 1986.

8

Cochlear implant surgery

I can never go into a dissection laboratory without learning something new. House W.F., at the age of 60.

The U.S. Food and Drug Administration has approved the Nucleus 22-channel device manufactured by the Cochlear Corporation for use in adults (18 years or over) and children (2-17 years) (Staller). Other devices, such as the San Francisco (Claryon) Device, manufactured by MiniMed and the Ineraid device (Richards), can be used in adults and are undergoing FDA controlled clinical tests in children.

SELECTION CRITERIA

Some basic selection criteria are always observed:

- Bilateral profound-to-total sensorineural hearing loss (three-frequency average 500-1000-2000 Hz).
- Pure tone audiometric threshold in the better ear equal to or greater than 95 dB.
- Unable to benefit or insufficient benefits from conventional hearing aids.
- Good psychological and physical health.
- Motivation and consistency in attending a rehabilitation program (Luxford). In children, these requirements must also be fulfilled by the parents or guardians.

ADULTS

The following audiological tests are performed:

- Unaided and aided warble tone. Speech detection thresholds. Speech discrimination test. Environmental sound tests.
- Performance in the weaker ear with appropriate, powerful hearing aids is compared to that of the patient with a cochlear implant (see selection criteria). Recruitment and discomfort are also taken into account.

Potential candidate for a cochlear implant:

- Unable to obtain aided speech detection threshold of 70 dB SPL and hearing level of approx. 53 dB HL or better.
- Poor performance on the discrimination test with conventional amplification, with scores of less than 10 % on the W-22 word list.
- Electrical stimulation test at either the promontory or the round window membrane (Waltzman) is not critical in candidate selection. It is often useful, however, to reassure the patient that hearing can be restored in the other ear.

CHILDREN

- Children must fulfill the same criteria as adults. There are also more specific requirements:
- Tympanometry rules out otitis media with effusion.
- Behavioral audiometry or play audiometry is used.
- The child must have used an appropriate hearing aid for at least 6 months, with inadequate results.

General criteria

The child's language skills are completely developed by five years of age.

- Children with an onset of acquired hearing impairment before 1 year of age are defined prelingual. One to five year-olds with acquired hearing loss are called perilingual, and children over five years of age are termed postlingual.
- No correlation between age and performance has been observed.
- The best results are obtained in postlingual hearing impaired children, who have an auditory memory. The prelingual hearing impaired children are more likely to benefit from a cochlear implant than the prelingual hearing impaired adult, who is more likely to simply not use the device.
- The greater the duration of the profound hearing impairment, the worse the patient's performance (this may be due to a loss in central auditory processing) (Dowell).
- Teenagers are usually poor candidates: nonusers advocate mostly peer pressure and cosmetic issues (Luxford).

Physical and Radiological Evaluation

- Any active infection of the external and/or middle ear or eardrum perforations must be treated before inserting a cochlear implant.

High resolution computed tomography may demonstrate:

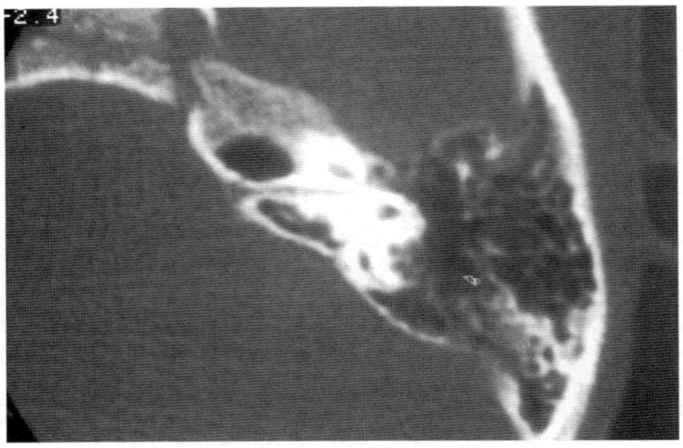

Fig. 8-1. CT. Hypoplasia of the internal auditory canal. Absent or abnormal acoustic nerve is a contraindication for cochlear implant placement.

- Agenesis of the cochlea: absolute contraindication.
- Reduction of IAC diameter -1-2 mm - synonym of acoustic nerve aplasia: absolute contraindication (Fig. 8-1).
- Fibrous and/or osseous occlusion of the cochlea: relative contraindication (Fig. 8-2).
- The outcome may be poorer than normal because of partial insertion of the electrode array. The use of both Gd-enhanced T1-weighted MR images and additional gradient-echo images (0.7 mm thick) enables a certain definition of the extent of cochlear fibrosis. The high signal intralabyrinthine fluid (white in these images) is replaced by the low signal fibrous tissue.
- Cochlear hypoplasia (Mondini's deformity): no contraindication (Figs. 8-3, 8-4).

Cochlear implants may be distinguished by several features:

- *The insertion site*: in extracochlear devices, the electrode array is placed outside the cochlea, on the promontory or the round window. In intracochlear devices, the electrode array is placed in the cochlea.

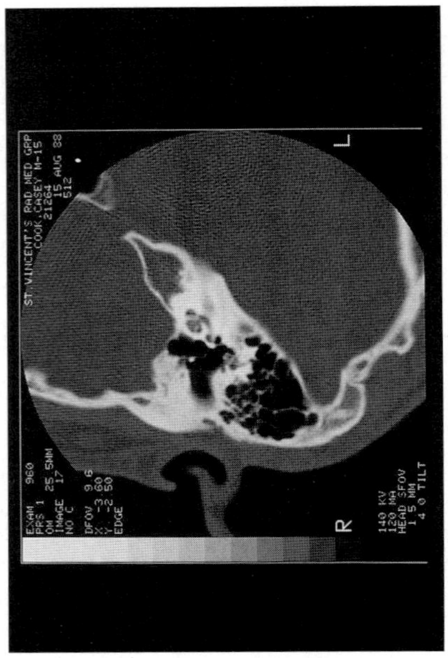

Fig. 8-2. CT. Ossification of the round window. Ossification of the round window or ossification of the cochlea does not exclude a patient from implantation, but it may influence the outcome.

- *Number of electrodes*: There are monochannel and multichannel devices.
- *Other features* are monopolar or bipolar electrodes, pulsating or continuous transmission, and different means of sound transmission through the skin.

EXTRACOCHLEAR SINGLE CHANNEL IMPLANTS

London

Designed by Douek et al., this device consists of a round electrode connected to an auricular plug. It

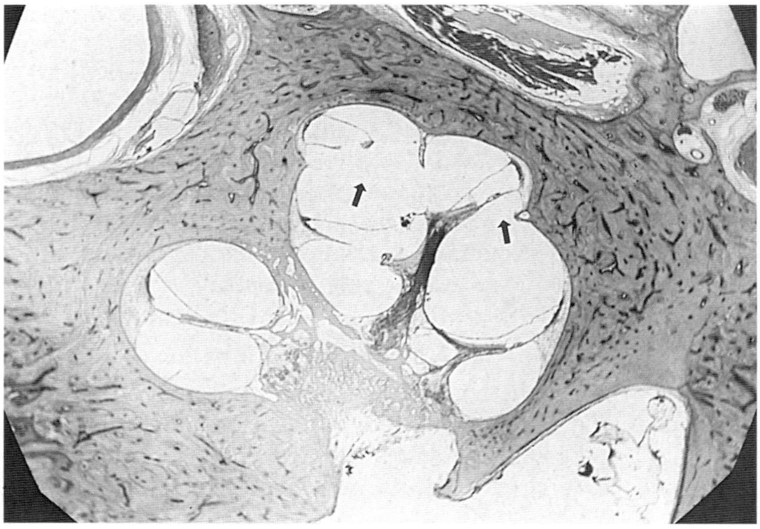

Fig. 8-3. Courtesy of Linthicum FH. Mondini dysplasia. Interscalar septi are missing between the apical and middle turns (arrows). ×15.

Fig. 8-4. Courtesy of Linthicum FH. Cochlear saccular degeneration (Sheibe deformity). The organ of Corti is represented by a clump of cells. There are no dendrites in the osseous spiral lamina. The saccular macula has degenerated (large arrow). Some ganglion cells remain (small arrow). × 56.

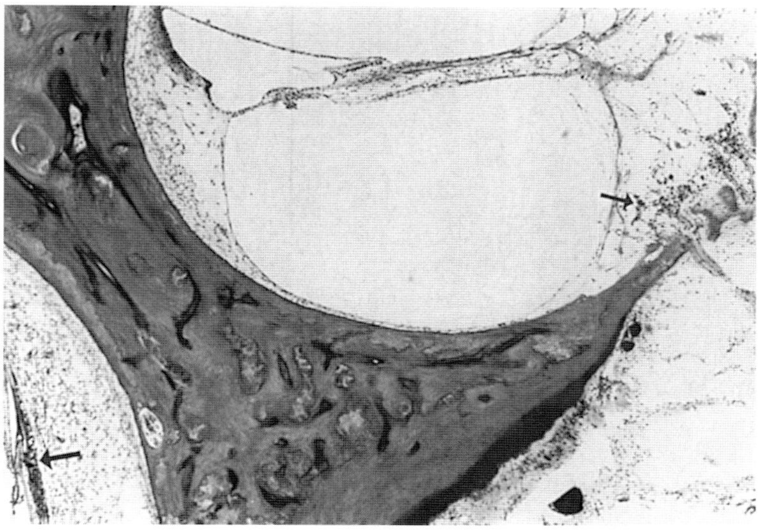

must rest on the promontory, which makes it indicated in subjects operated with a radical mastoid cavity. It may be used by performing a miringopexy of the promontory membrane.
It is mobile, so it can be inserted or removed by the patient at will.

Vienna
Designed by E.S. Hochmair and I.H. Hochmair, it has an electrode which is positioned in contact with the membrane of the round window.

EXTRACOCHLEAR MULTICHANNEL IMPLANTS

Cologne
Developed by Banfai et al, this has a monopolar electrode which is positioned on the promontory.

INTRACOCHLEAR SINGLE CHANNEL DEVICES

Los Angeles
The House-3M was the first to be approved by the FDA and is the most widely used today. It consists of a platinum wire electrode inserted 6 mm into the scala tympani. If the cochlea is obliterated by bone or fibrous tissue, the electrode may be inserted through an hole drilled in the promontory.

Vienna
Designed by E.S. Hochmair and I.H. Hochmair, this device consists of a 4-channel wire inserted up to 22 mm into the scala tympani. According to the patient's preferences, only one of these electrodes is stimulated.

Stanford
Developed at Stanford University, the only place where it has been tried, this device consists of a single-channel and a multichannel implant.

INTRACOCHLEAR MULTI CHANNEL DEVICES

Utah
This device has a series of 6 electrodes, 4 mm apart, for a total length of 24 mm. It is inserted into the scala tympani. Four of the six electrodes are active.

San Francisco
This device has an array of 16 electrodes and eight channels. It is inserted 25 mm into the scala tympani. Each canal is independent and enables a complete and simultaneous stimulation.
It is very widely used. The external receiver is very thin and may be inserted below the temporalis muscle, without needing to prepare an osseous niche in the squama of the temporal bone.

Paris
This is a 12-electrode system developed by Chouard. It calls for a radical mastoidectomy, drilling of the windows, and the positioning of individual isolated Silastic electrodes in the cochlea.

Melbourne
The House Ear Institute has used the House/3M system from the beginning, and has recently begun using the Nucleus 22 channel (Fig. 8-5).
The Nucleus Mini-22 implant system consists of an array of 22 electrodes which are surgically implanted in the cochlea for up to 23 mm, and is connected to a small receiver-stimulator unit placed under the skin behind the ear. An external speech processor determines which electrodes are to be stimulated, based on incoming sounds picked up by a directional microphone worn at ear level. This information is passed on to the implanted stimulator by a transmitter coil, which is held against the skin above the stimulator by a magnet. The transmitter coil is electromagnetically linked to a coil in the implanted receiver, and

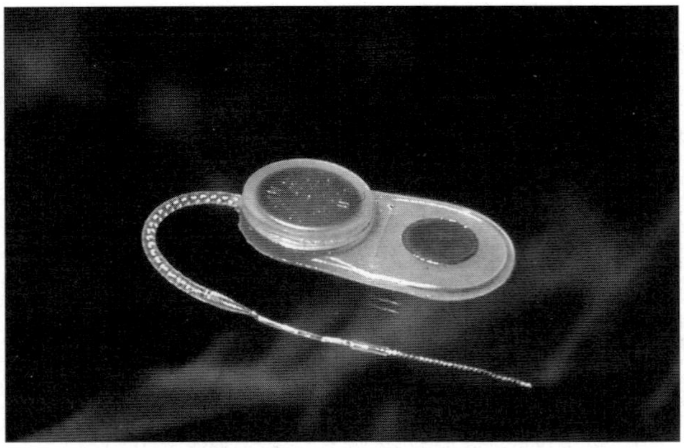

Fig. 8-5. Cochlear implant. The internal receiver.

this link is also used to provide the power needed by the receiver. The speech processor is programmed by a computer-based diagnostic programming system. This system allows the clinician to set individual electrodes to match the specific requirements of each patient, and thus accommodate any changes in electrical requirements that may occur in a given patient over time.

A candidate has been selected.
Which side to implant?

- When a symmetric hearing loss is seen in both ears, we prefer to implant the ear with the shortest history of hearing impairment. This is because the longer the duration of hearing impairment, the higher the loss of central auditory processing (Fig. 8-6).
- Likewise, when the hearing loss is chronologically and audiometrically similar in both ears, but one ear has used a prosthetic device until hearing became unusable, this ear is implanted. The patient is informed that he will lose residual hearing following implantation, and may need to use a hearing aid even for sound awareness.
- In two identical ears, the one with the least caloric response is chosen.
- When no acoustic differences exist, HRTC and Gd-enhanced T1-weighted MR images and very thin gradient echo images are used to determine which ear to implant. As a rule, the better mastoid pneumatization, the lesser the cochlear ossification or fibrosis.

POSITION

The patient's hair is shaved as in a translabyrinthine approach.
The patient is placed under general anesthesia.
The patient is in a supine position with his head turned away from the surgeon.
The electrodes for monitoring the facial nerve are put in place.

- Before cutting, the model is placed on the skin and the outlines are drawn with a dermographic pencil (Fig. 8-7). The flap must be large enough to cover the receiver-stimulator with a surplus of at least 1 cm, to avoid problems in the recovery of the limbs and possible extrusion of the implant (Fig. 8-8).
- In adults and older children, the cutaneous and subcutaneous flaps are elevated by sliding along the avascular plane of the temporalis muscle fascia (Fig. 8-9).
- Part of the temporalis muscle is removed to expose the bone in the squamous temporal bone, where a niche is prepared with a cutting burr to accommodate the internal receiver, in the position planned (Fig. 8-10).
- In smaller children, the flap is elevated up to the bone, since it is not thick enough to cover the implant. It is important to keep in mind that the implant is identical for adults and children.
- The niche is drilled in the squama of the temporal bone. In children around two years of age, the structures of the cavum tympani are almost as large as those of adults, but the squama of

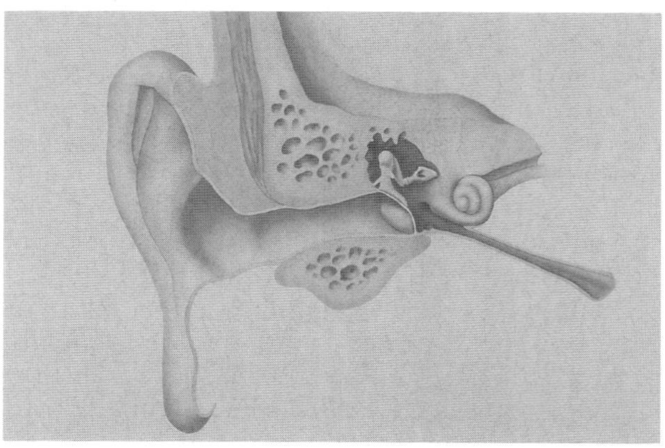

Fig. 8-6. Sagittal cut of the right ear.

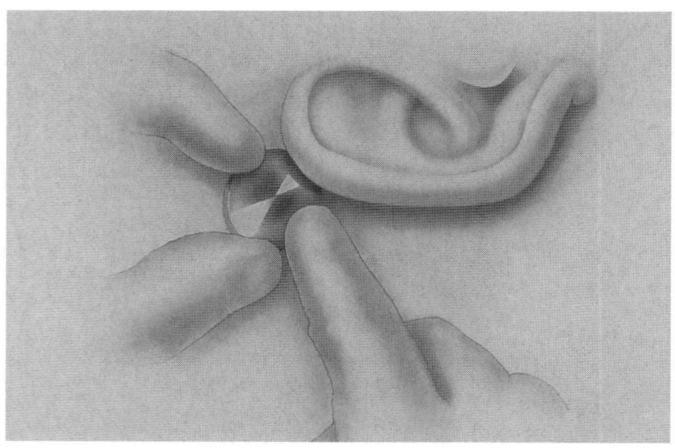

Fig. 8-7. The site for the internal receiver in the skull is previously determined.

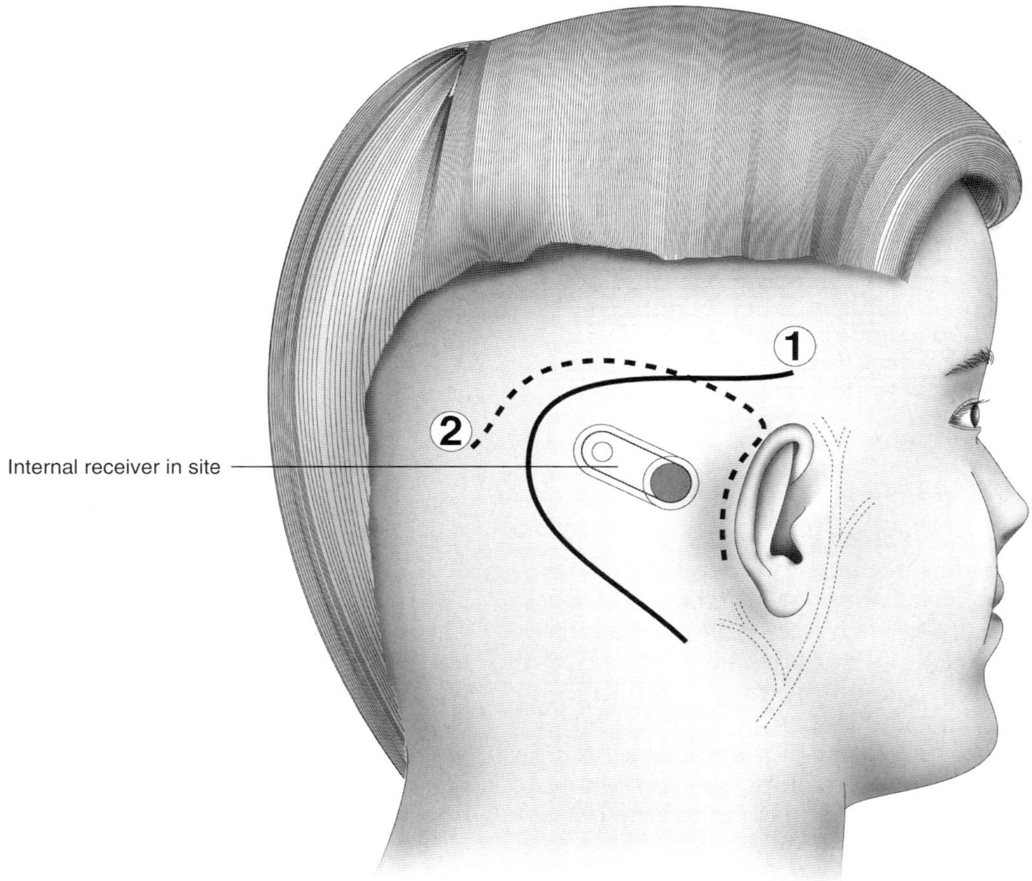

Fig. 8-8. Two different incisions for cochlear implantation.**1:** C incision. **2:** Inverted U incision.

the temporal bone is very thin (less than 3 mm), as is the scalp.

- It is preferable to leave at least a plate of bone underneath, without exposing the dura (Figs. 8-11, 8-12, 8-13, 8-14, 8-15).

MASTOIDECTOMY

- A simple mastoidectomy is performed with aspiration-irrigation as usual (Fig. 8-16). It is pointless to smooth the margins, since the rough bone helps to prevent migration of the implant.
- The mastoidectomy is extended posteriorly to the sigmoid sinus, which need not be decompressed.
- The posterior bone canal is thinned with a cutting burr, to facilitate the view of the round window, which lies on the same projection line as the IAC.

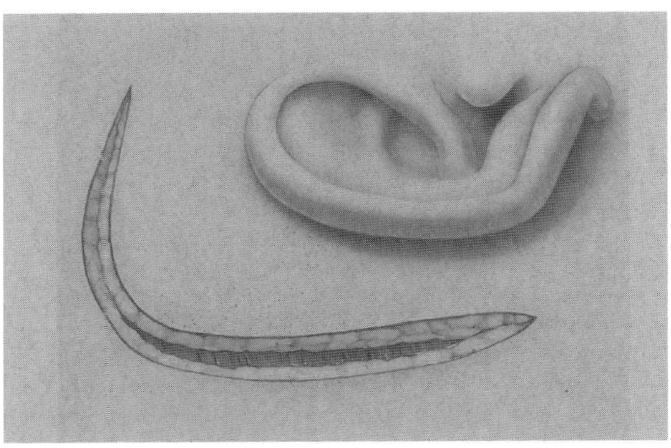

Fig. 8-9. Skin incision (C incision).

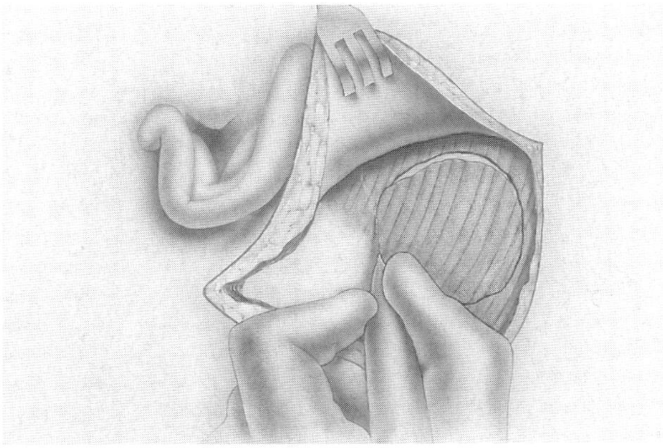

Fig. 8-10. The temporalis muscle is cut or preferentially elevated off the parietal portion of the skull.

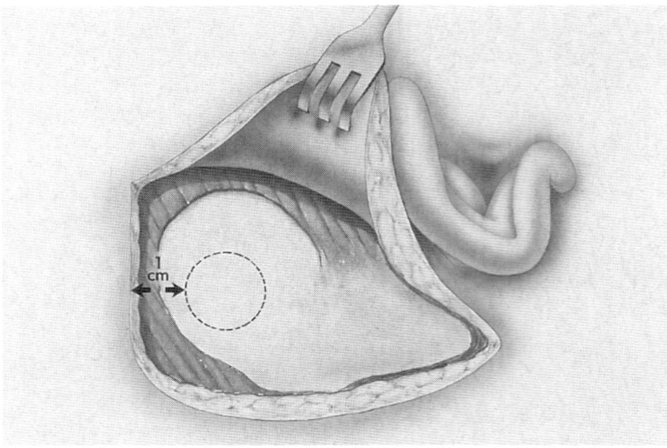

Fig. 8-11. The site for the internal receiver in the skull is previously determined.

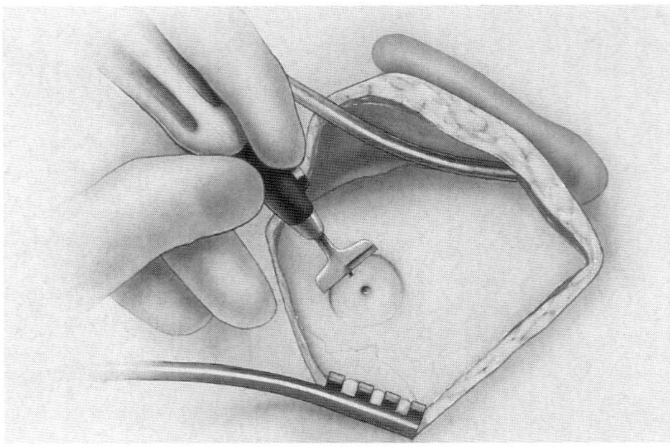

Fig. 8-13. The tip of a butterfly burr is inserted in the hole previously drilled and the site for the internal receiver is created.

- Cells are removed from the attic, until the body of the incus has been exposed. To identify the body of the incus when the attic bone still obstructs the surgical view, the following manoeuvre can be used. Under increased magnification, a copious amount of fluid is used to remove bone dust and is then left in the surgical cavity. The water reflects the light of the microscope and acts as a refracting lens, thus allowing the surgical view to arrive behind the bone, where the direct observation can not.
- The incus need not be dislodged, since no more space would be gained.
- The facial recess is opened (see chapter 16) with a 1 mm cutting burr or a diamond burr. The facial recess lies on the projection line of the short process of the incus and the facial nerve need not be exposed. If it is, it is preferable to leave a thin sheet of bone on the nerve (Figs. 8-17, 8-18).
- The recess has a right triangular shape and the most space is gained on its short side. Thus it is enlarged proceeding toward the attic. The spur of bone separating the incus from the facial recess is thinned as much as possible, but without breaking it, so that the incus is not dislodged. Thus the upper limit near the attic is reached. The medial limit is the facial nerve, and the lateral limit is the chorda tympani. The chorda tympani may be exposed, but it is important not to ascend superiorly, since the chorda tympani lies on the same level as the annulus. To create more space in the facial recess, the chorda may be removed.
- The round window is inferior to the stapes tendon and the head of the stapes. The anterior margin of bone covering the round window niche is removed with a 1 mm diamond burr (Figs. 8-19, 8-20).
- It is not unusual to find an ossification of the round window and its membrane during surgery, particularly in patients with a history of

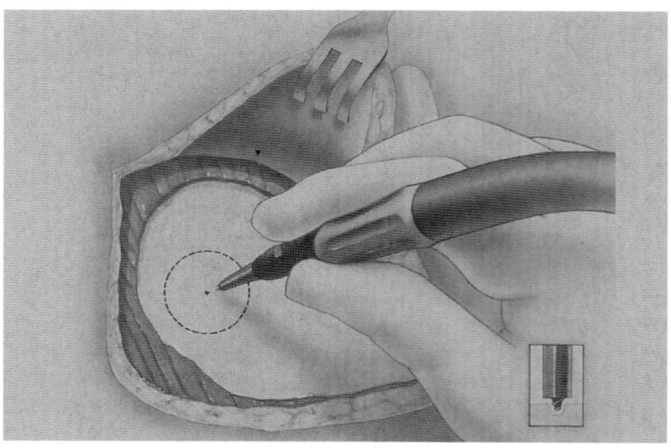

Fig. 8-12. A hole is created with a guarded burr at the center of the site for the internal receiver.

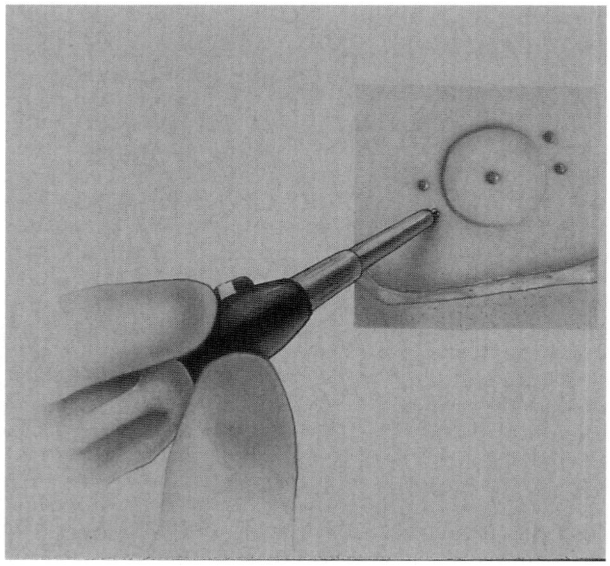

Fig. 8-14. Suture tunnel holes are created with a guarded burr.

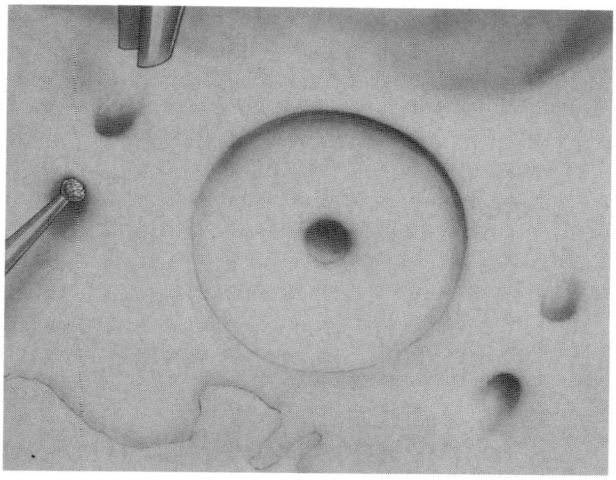

Fig. 8-15. The site for the internal receiver is completed.

meningitis. In this case the newly formed bone must be removed. Its whitish color distinguishes it, until the permeable scala tympani is reached. If the scala tympani is not found, the electrode may be inserted into the scala vestibuli. The complete ossification of the cochlea is a contraindication to surgery. If it is discovered intraoperatively, the operation may proceed by closing the IAC a cul-de-sac, and a canal wall down mastoidectomy is performed. A hole is made around the modiolus and the electrode is put into place (Figs. 8-21, 8-22, 8-23).

- The anatomical limits in the middle ear do not vary significantly from child to adult. It has been observed that after 24 months of life the anatomy of the cochlea and the facial recess have the same dimensions as that of an adult.

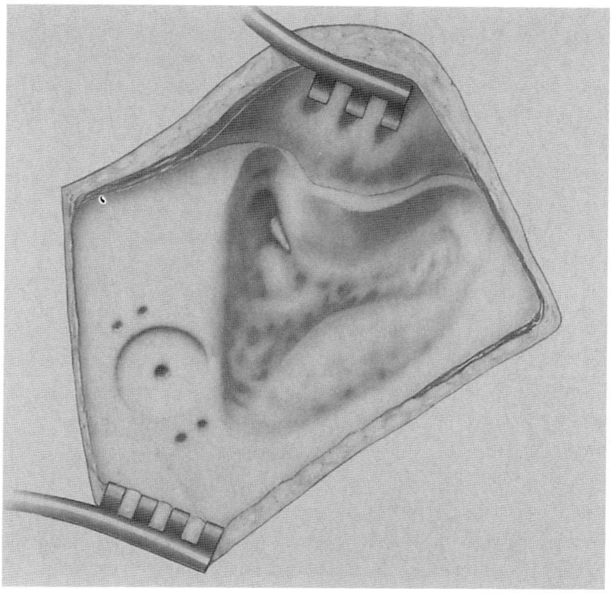

Fig. 8-16. Mastoidectomy.

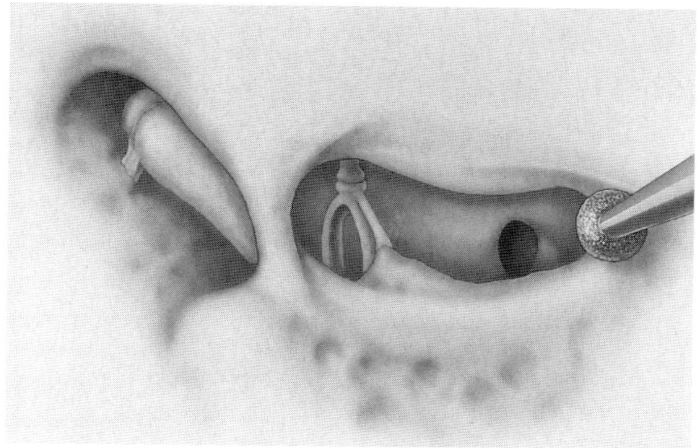

Fig. 8-17. The facial recess is opened.

The antrum and the mastoid cells are also well developed by that age.

- The implant must not come in contact with the external ear before implantation. This prevents the risk of bringing skin into the middle ear and causing the formation of an iatrogenous cholesteatoma.
- The internal receiver is placed in its niche and the electrodes are introduced and advanced through the oval window, into the scala tympani. The electrode array may be also inserted through a fenestration of the promontory, which limits direct damage to the inner ear in an area of approx. 0.75 mm (Figs. 8-24, 8-25, 8-26, 8-27, 8-28).

It is not necessary to insert the entire array into the cochlea; the last 10 bands serve to strengthen and mark the depth and do not provide functional stimulation to the cochlear nerve (Fig. 8-29).

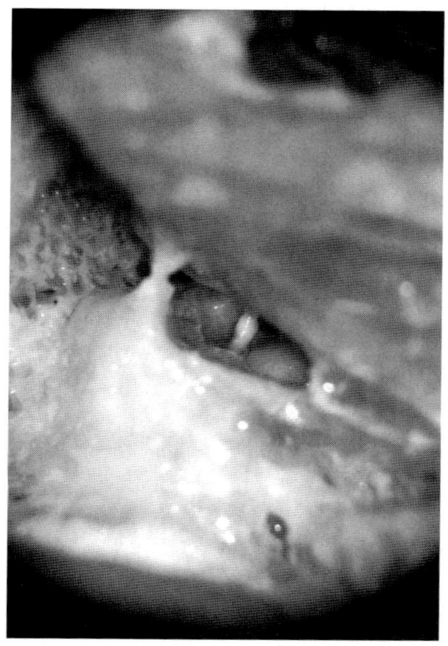

Fig. 8-18. The facial recess. The facial nerve, the chorda, and the stapedius tendon are visible.

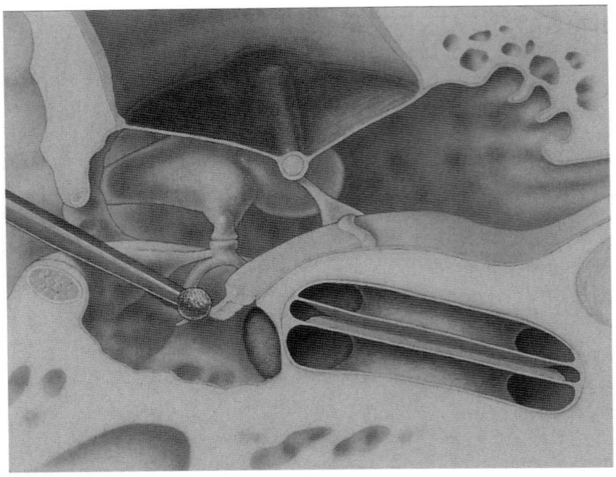

Fig. 8-19. The lip of the niche is removed, until the round window membrane comes into clear view: lateral drilling.

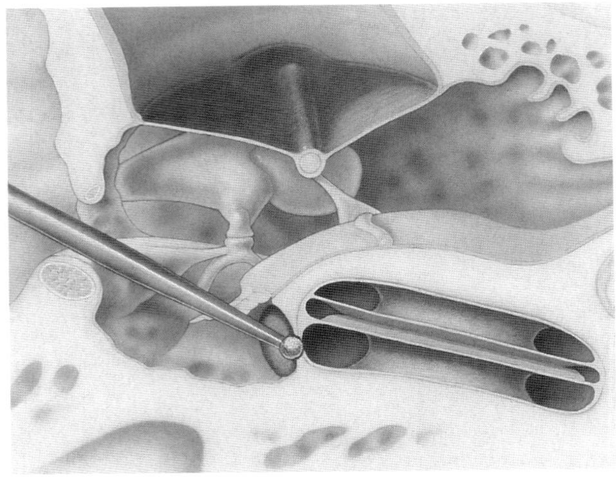

Fig. 8-20. The lip of the niche is removed, until the round window membrane comes into clear view: medial drilling.

- It is essential not to force the electrode, which must be introduced without trauma. In children, the excess electrode is positioned in the mastoid, so that it is not dislodged by the growth of the cranium.
- Muscle or fascia is positioned around the oval window to immobilize the electrode and to prevent the formation of perilymphatic fistulas. Muscular tissue is put in place to close the facial recess. The electrode can be also stabilized with ionomeric cement over the facial recess. Holes are made near the receiver, which is anchored with prolene thread (Figs. 8-30, 8-31, 8-32). The silk must be tight because otherwise the implant may rub against the skin, causing pressure atrophy and delayed necrosis of the overlying postauricular skin.

COMPLICATIONS

- After placement of the internal receiver, no electrocautery should be used. If needed, bipolar electrocautery reduces the possibility of the current damaging the receiver.
- The elastic memory of the cavum, wrapped under tension from the mastoid, may lead to a sudden exit of the electrodes from the scala tympani.
- Mesh tie-downs have been suggested to control extrusion of the electrode(s) in the mastoid, while ligation with platinum ribbon has been suggested for the middle ear, along with modifications in the cavum tympani's thickness to reduce its mass and its elasticity.
- Another proposal has been to divide the bridge joining the incus and the facial recess, using a 0.7 mm diamond burr for the Nucleus Mini-22 and a 1mm diamond burr for the Clarion Mini-Med. This bridge is located between the short process of the incus and the horizontal semicircular canal. A Rosen needle is used to check the aperture, and the implant proceeds normally.

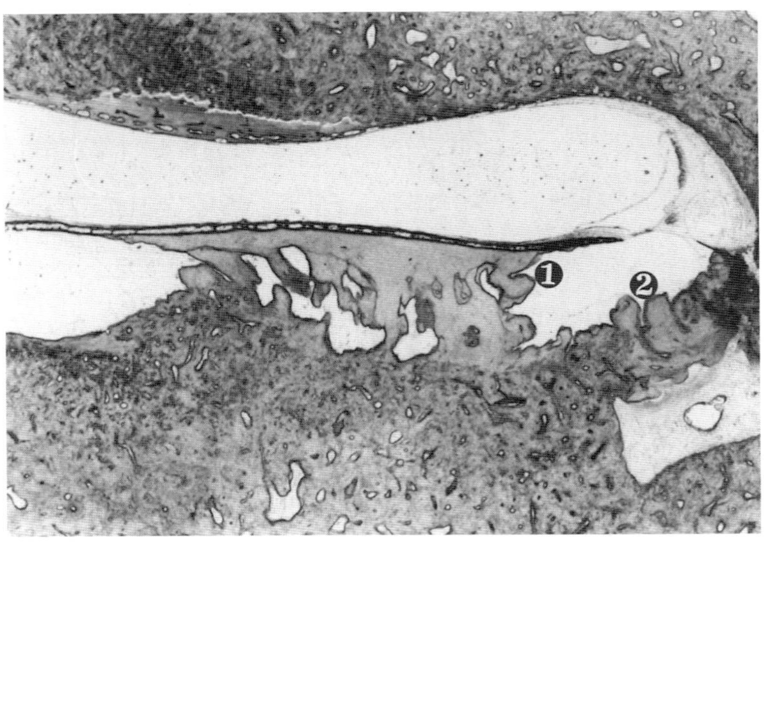

Fig. 8-21. Courtesy of Linthicum FH. Ossification of the scala tympani in the basal turn of the cochlea in a patient with cochlear otosclerosis (1). Obliteration of the round window by otosclerosis (2). × 70.

Fig. 8-22. Courtesy of Linthicum FH. Ossification of the basal turn of the cochlea and the round window area postmeningitis. × 30.

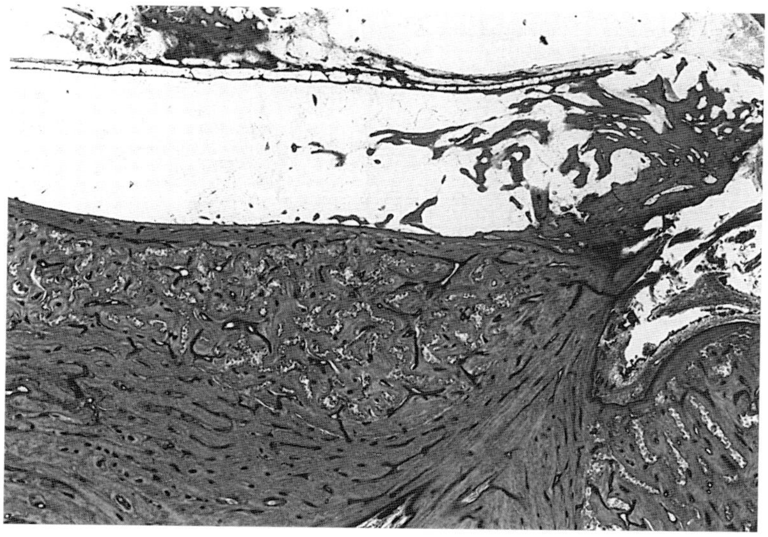

- Before closing the cochleotomy with connective tissue, the cavum is gently pushed through the gap created in the bridge of the incus. Extreme care must be taken not to injure the lining of the cavum. In our experience, this technique is effective in preventing partial acute extrusion of the cavum tympani.
- The most frequent complications in cochlear implant procedures are related to the postauricular flap. Among the most commonly reported problems in literature are necrosis of the flap, hematoma, sieroma, and infection.
- Cases of extrusion have been seen due to the implantation being made too close to the wound, or the excessive thinness of the flap (under 6 mm). On the other hand, an overly thick flap decreases transcutaneous transmission.
- Alterations in the facial nerve are rare and have the same incidence as in middle ear surgery. It is important to avoid drilling near the nerve without adequate irrigation; otherwise overheating may occur. The bit of the burr, when inserted in the facial recess to drill the osseous crest overlying the oval window, may damage nerve VII. This risk may be avoided by using the same drill as is utilized for otosclerosis surgery. It has a longer and thinner bit, and has a protective covering.
- In patients with a congenital deformation of the cochlea, the danger of injuring the facial nerve is greater. The facial nerve stimulator helps, as in surgery of the atresia auris.
- Cerebral-spinal fistulas are avoided by closing the oval window with muscle or temporalis fascia fragments.
- No increase in the incidence or degree of otitis media has been observed in implanted subjects.
- A simple chronic otitis or cholesteatoma does not constitute a contraindication to a cochlear

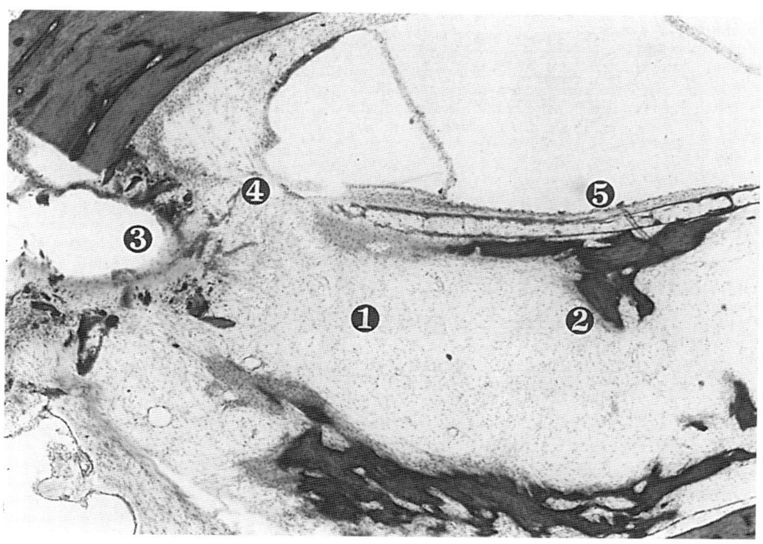

Fig. 8-23. Courtesy of Linthicum FH. Fibrosis (1) and ossification (2) occurring in the basal turn of the round window area in a cochlear implant patient. The path of the electrode is visible at (3). The organ of Corti and basilar membrane have disappeared adjacent to the electrode path (4). The osseous spiral lamina is still present (5). × 46.

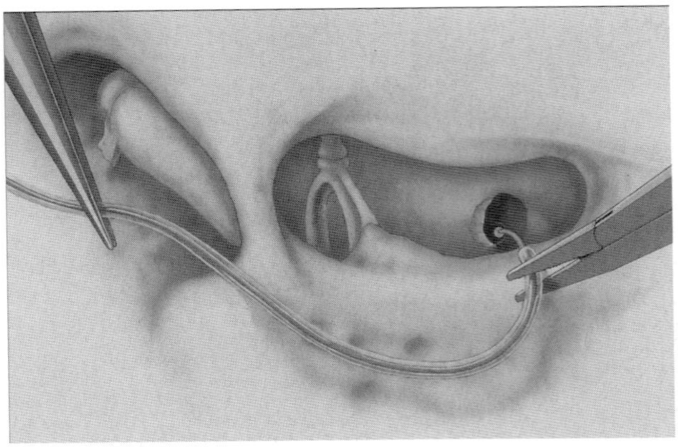

Fig. 8-24. Electrode is advanced carefully into the scala tympani, either with smooth thumb forceps or small two-prong guides.

implant. A radical mastoidectomy is the treatment preferred. This is because the reconstruction of the ossicular chain is not as important as the complete eradication of the infection. The cavity is obliterated. The tube is closed, to avoid the spreading of possible retrograde infections in the nose. A cul-de-sac closure is performed of the external auditory canal. After 8-12 months, a new operation is performed, which gives more control over the situation in the cavity. In the absence of recurrence of the original disease, the implant may be put in place. If not, the cavity is disinfected and the operation is reconsidered after 8-12 months.

- The danger of lesions to the facial nerve is greater in repeated operations, since previous radical pathologies may have caused dehiscence of the nerve. When the objective is the implant's substitution due to malfunction or for an upgrade, the connective tissue placed in the facial recess at the first operation may remain adherent to a dehiscent nerve. Its sudden removal may be damaging.

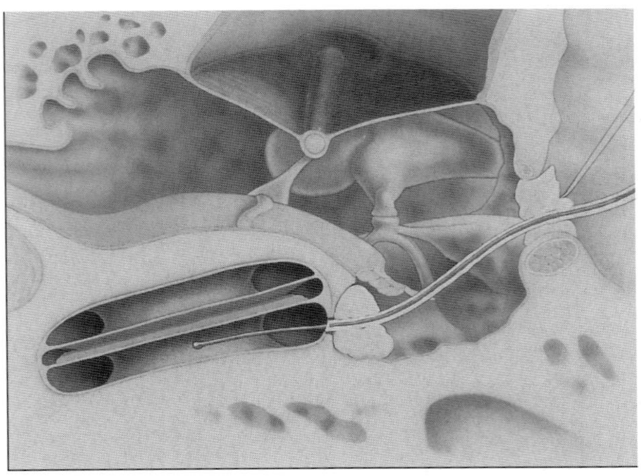

Fig. 8-25. The electrode is advanced carefully into the scala tympani.

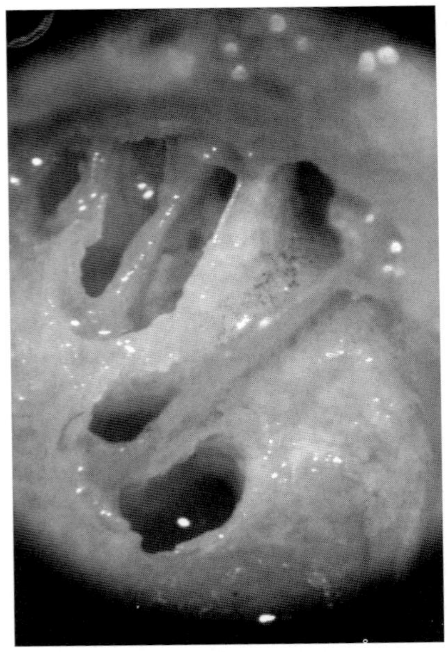

Fig. 8-26. Temporal bone dissection. Middle fossa approach. The cochlea has been opened to show the turns, the osseous spiral lamina, the helicotrema.

- **Facial nerve stimulation by cochlear implant**
Cochlear implants, when activated, generate electrical fields which produce a flow of regional current. Accidental stimulation of the nervous structures adjacent to the cochlea may take place, when the flow of extracochlear current surpasses their threshold (Parkins).
The experience of the VA Study group on Cochlear Implants has revealed facial movements in 12 patients implanted out of 82. The patients had undergone implants with the Nucleus, the Ineraid or the 3M/Vienna single-channel device.
In four patients implanted with the Nucleus, the problem was resolved by deactivating the apical electrodes in two patients, and the basal electrodes in two others.
Two patients implanted with Ineraid showed a facial nerve stimulation which was spontaneously resolved after 3 months.
With the 3M/Vienna, stimulation of the facial nerve disappeared spontaneously in two cases, and in two cases facial stimulation was eliminated, reducing the protruberance of the language processor, but inadequate hearing sensation was obtained. In two other cases, despite the appropriate positioning of the electrodes, the problem was resolved only with the alternative positioning of a multichannel Nucleus implant.

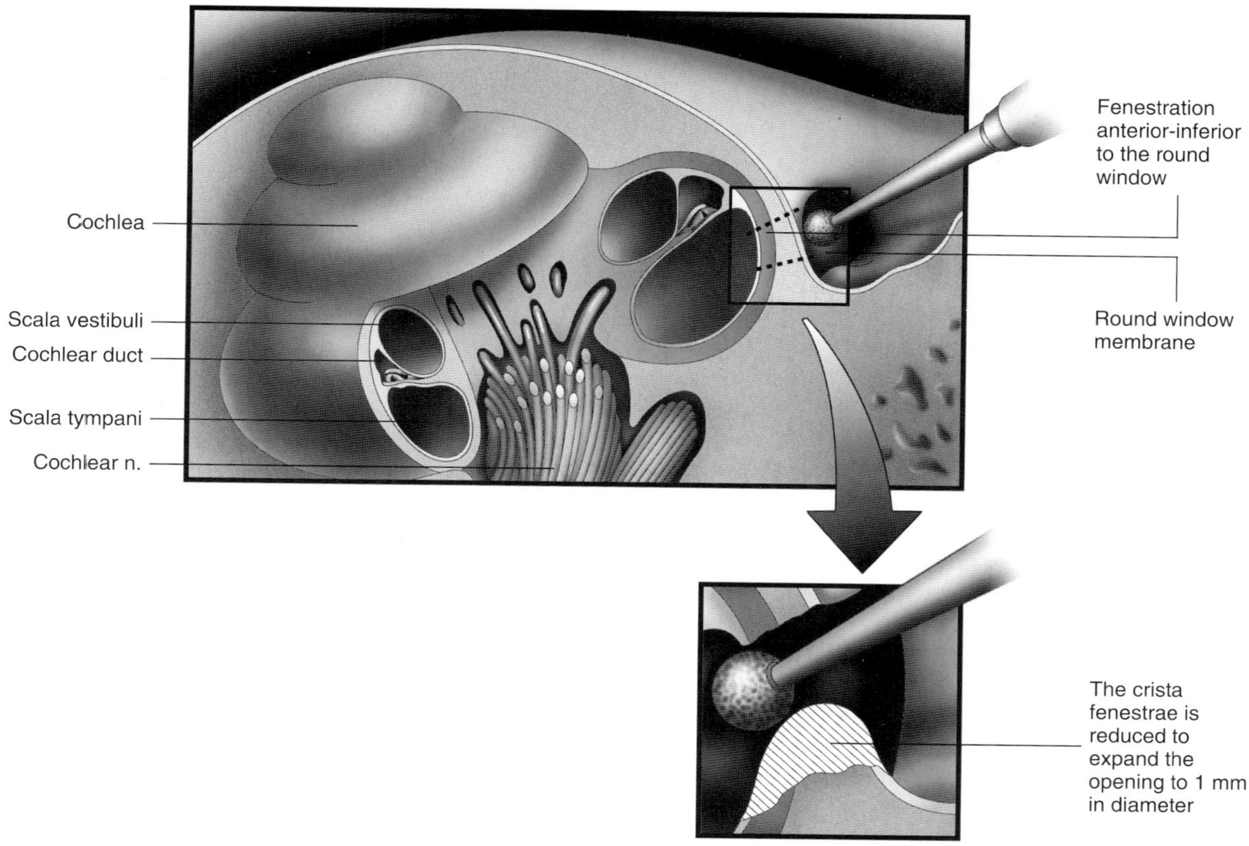

Fig. 8-27. Access to the scala tympani can be achieved either directly through the round window or via a fenestration anterior and inferior to the round window.

According to this study the 3M/Vienna, of simple construction, requires a low intensity of current for nerve stimulation and has a relatively large current field of distribution, and is at any rate more inclined to spread current to the facial nerve (Niparko).

REVISION SURGERY

Revision surgery may be necessary to substitute an altered implant or to utilize a more modern one.

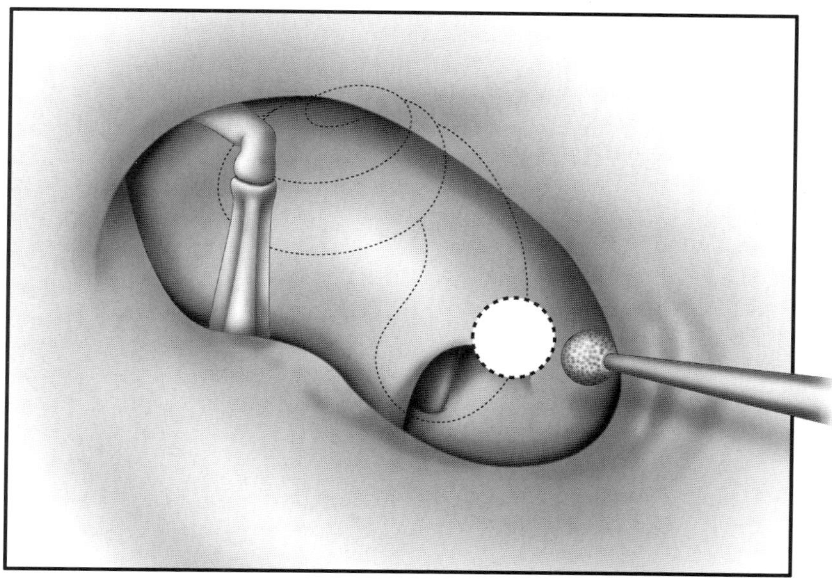

Fig. 8-28. Fenestration anterior and inferior to the round window.

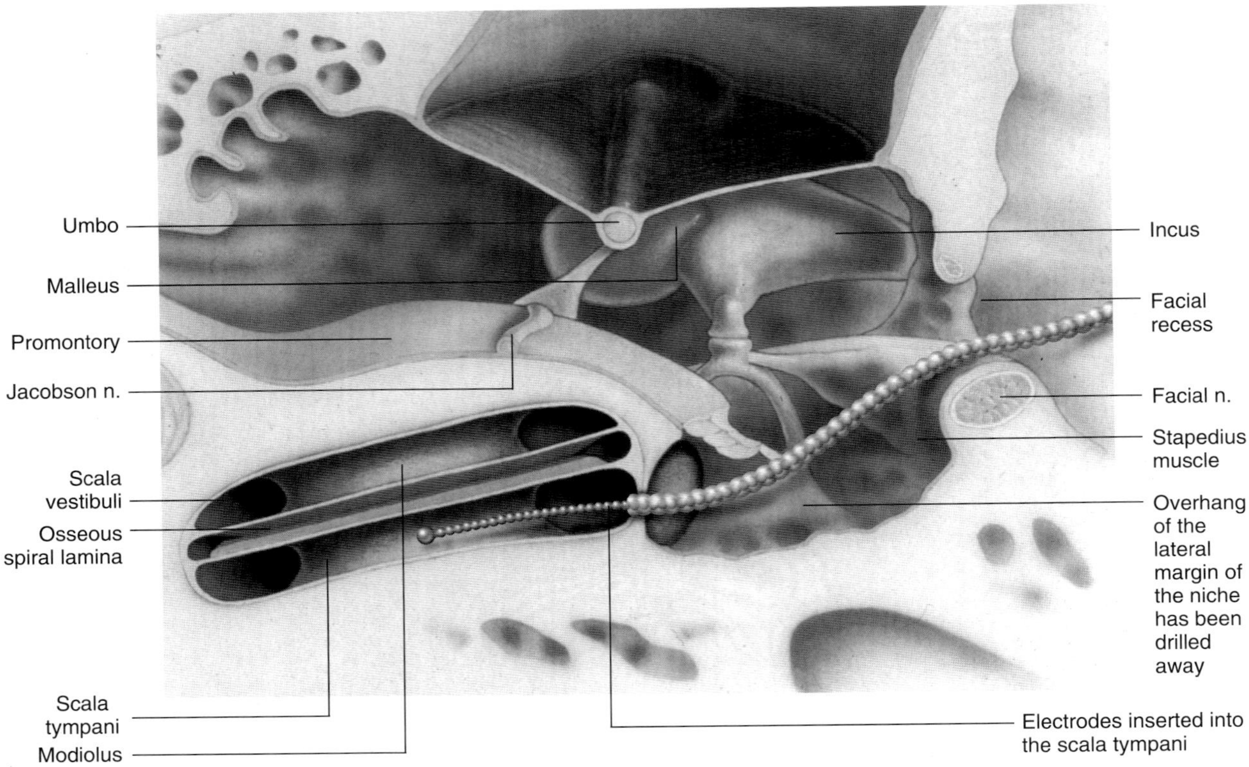

Fig. 8-29. The electrode is advanced carefully into the scala tympani.

Substitution of an altered implant
The substitution of the external parts of the implant such as the microphone, the cables, and the language processor does not require surgery. No particular difficulty is found in the second operation. In the experience of the House Ear Clinic, no problems due to mechanical trauma, osteogenosis, nervous tissue degeneration from electrical stimulation, or the spread of infection from the middle ear to the inner ear and the brain have been seen.

Substitution with an updated implant
The possibility of an "upgrade" should always be kept in consideration, especially in children, who have the longest life expectancy and can benefit from technological progress. This is why the implant is performed in one ear at a time.

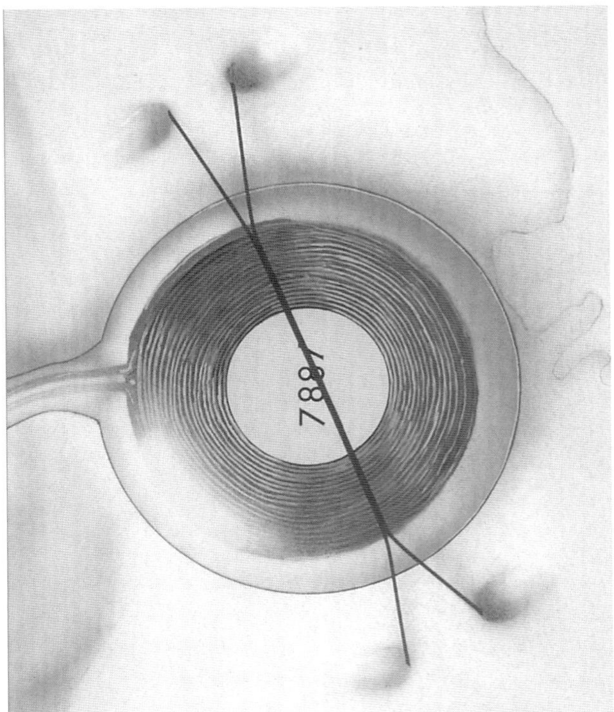

Fig. 8-30. After electrode placement, the internal receiver is fixed in its seat with non-absorbable sutures.

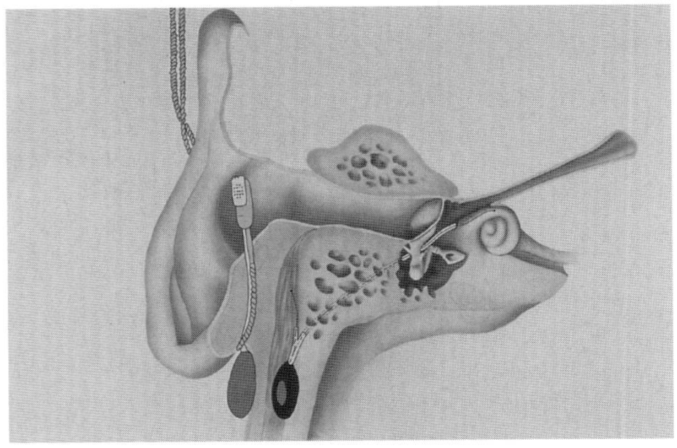

Fig. 8-31. Cochlear implant in site.

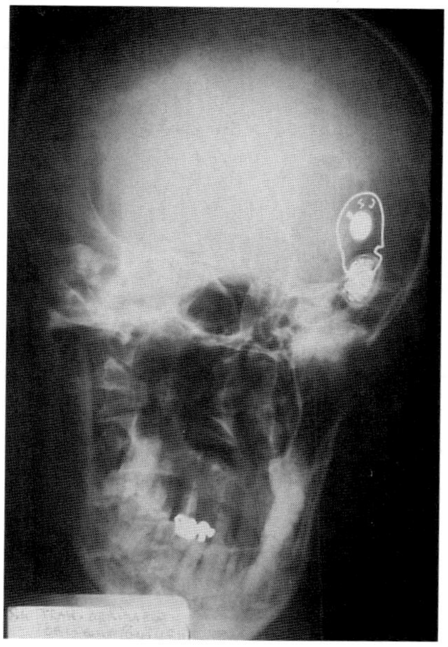

Fig. 8-32. Anteroposterior transorbital plain film of the skull: cochlear implant in site.

When the upgrade is performed, we prefer to implant the controlateral ear, unless some radiological alterations appear in this ear to contraindicate surgery. In this way, a secure source of hearing is maintained in the operated ear while pursuing an improvement in the ear still to be operated. If this improvement becomes reality, another upgrade will be possible in future, in the ear with poorer hearing.

RESULTS

- Cochlear implantation is the gold standard rehabilitative approach for patients with profound hearing losses, who are unable to benefit from conventional hearing aids. It provides auditory threshold to detect speech and environmental sounds, as well as timing and intensity information.
- Postlingually deafened adults with a short duration of deafness are excellent candidates (Luxford).
- Postlingually deafened children have the potential to derive maximal use from the implant (significant and continuous improvements in speech production, as well as improvements over time of auditory discrimination test scores).
- Prelingually deafened children, altough not the best candidates, have substantial benefit that are likely to increase in future, with improved devices and better speech processing strategies.

REFERENCES

Balkany T, Cantz B, Nadol JB Jr: Multichannel cochlear implants in partially ossified cochleas. Am Otol Rhinol Laryngol Suppl 135: 3-7, 1988.

Balkany T, Telischi F: Fixation of the electrode cable during cochlear implantation: The split bridge technique. Laryngoscope 105: 217-218, 1995.

Beiter AL, Staller S, Dowell R: Evaluation and device programming in children. Ear and Hearing, 12, 4 (Suppl.), 25-33, 1991.

Bergeron F, Ferron P, Gbeil S, Desgagne M: Multielectrode cochlear implantation in children: the Quebec experience. J Otolaryngol, 19, 5, 324-330, 1990.

Boothroyd A, Geers A, Moog J: Practical Implications of cochlear implants in children. Ear and Hearing, 12, 4, 81-89, 1991.

Boothroyd A: Auditory capacity and the generalization of speech skills. In: Lauter J, Ed. Speech planning and production in normal and hearing impaired children. ASHA Reports 15: 8-14, 1985.

Clopton B, Spelman F: Neural mechanisms relevant to the design of an auditory prosthesis: location and electrical characteristics. Ann Otol Rhinol Laryngol 91:9-14, 1982.

Cohen NL, Hoffman L: Complications of cochlear implant surgery in adults and children. Am Otol Rhinol Laringol 100(9Pt) 708-711, 1991.

Daspit CP: Meningitis as a result of a cochlear implant: Case report. Otolaryngol Head Neck Surg 105(1): 115-116, 1991.

Dosvell RC, Mecklenburg DC, Clark GM: Speech recognition for 40 patients receiving multi-channel cochlear implants. Arch Otolaryngol Head Neck Surg 112: 1054-1059, 1986.

Edgerton BJ, House WF, Hitselberger W: Hearing by cochlear nucleus stimulations in humans. Ann Otol Rhinol Laryngol 91 (Suppl. 91), 117-124. 1982.

Eisemberg LS, Kirk KI, Thielemeir MA. et al: Cochlear implants in children: speech production and auditory discrimination. Otolaryngol Clin North Am, 19 (2), 409-421, 1986.

Eisemberg LS, Maltan AA, Portillo F, Mobley JP, House WF: Electrical stimulation of the auditory brainstem structures in defined adults. J Rehabil Res Dev 24, 9-22, 1987.

Eisemberg LS: Use of the cochlear implant by the prelingually deaf. Ann Otorhinolaryngol, 91, 62-66, 1982.

Cohen NL, Hoffman R.A, Stroschein M: Medical or surgical complications related to the nucleus multichannel cochlear implant. Ann Otol Rhinol Laryngol 97 (Suppl. 135): 8-13, 1988.

Finley C, Wilson B, White M: Models of neural responsiveness to electrical stimulation. In: Miller J, Spelman F, eds. Cochlear implants: models of the electrically stimulated ear. New York: Springer-Verlag. 1989:55-96.

Fretz R, Fravel R: Design and function. A physical and electrical description of the 3M/House cochlear implant system. Ear and Hear, 6 (Suppl.), 145-195, 1985.

Gantz BJ, Tyler RS, Knutson JF, Woodworth et al: Evaluation of five different cochlear implant designs: audiological assessment and predictions of performance. Laryngoscope, 98, 1100-1106, 1988.

Gantz BJ: Cochlear implants: an overview. In: Myers E. Bluestone C, Brackmann D, Krause C, eds. Advances in Otolaryngology Head and Neck Surgery. Chicago: Year Book Medical Publishers, 171-196, 1987.

Gantz BJ, McCabe BF, Tyler RS: Use of multichannel implants in obstructed and obliterated cochleas. Otolaryngol Head Neck Surg 98(1): 72-81, 1988.

Geers AE, Moog JS: Evaluating the benefits of cochlear implants in an education setting. Am J Otol. 12 (Suppl), 116-125, 1991.

Geers AE, Moog JS: Predicting long-term benefits of cochlear implants in profoundly hearing impaired children. Am J Otol 9,169-176, 1988.

Gray RF, Evans RA, Freer CEL, et al: Radiology for cochlear implants. J Laryngol Otol 105: 85-88, 1991.

Green JD Jr, Marion MS, Hinojosa R: Labyrinthine ossification: Histopathologic consideration for cochlear implantation. Otolaryngol Head Neck Surg 104(3): 320-326, 1991.

Haberkamp TJ, Schwaber MK: Management of flap necrosis in cochlear implantation. Am Otol Rhinol Laryngol 101(1) 38-41, 1992.

House JR, Luxford WM: Facial nerve injury in cochlear implantation. Presented at the Southern Section, Triological Society, Boca Raton, FL, January 1993.

House WF, Berliner KL, Luxford WM: Cochlear implants in deaf children. Curr Probl Pediatr 176 (6): 345-388, 1987.

Jackler R, Luxford W, House W: Sound detection with the cochlear implant in five ears of four children with congenital malformations of the cochlea. Laryngoscope 97:15-7, 1987.

Jackler RK, Luxford WM, Scindler RA et al: Cochlear patency problems in cochlear implantation. Laryngoscope, 97, 801-805, 1987.

Lambert PR, Ruth RA, Hodges AV: Multichannel cochlear implant and electrically evoked auditory braistem responses in a child with labyrinthitis ossificans. Laryngoscope 101 (1Pt) 14-19, 1991.

Luxford WM, Brackmann DE: The history of cochlear implants. In Gray RF (ed): Cochlear Implants. London, Croom Helm, 1985, pp 1-26.

Luxford WM, House WF, Tonokawa LL, Berliner Kl, Martin E: Experiences with the nucleus multichannel cochlear implant in children. Ann Otol Rhinol Laryngol, 98: 2-7, 1988.

Luxford WM: Cochlear implant indications. Am J Otol 10(2): 95-98, 1989.

Luxford WM: Surgery for cochlear implantation. In Brackmann DE, Shelton C, Arriaga MA (eds): Otologic Surgery, 426-436, 1995.

Mangham CA, Luxford WM: Cochlear prosthesis surgery in children. In: Mecklemburg DJ, Ed. Cochlear implants in children: Proceedings from a multidisciplinary colloquium. Semin Hear,7 (4): 361-369, 1986.

Marks DR, Jackler RK, Bates GJ, Greenberg S: Pediatric cochlear implantation: Strategies to accommodate for head growth. Otolaryngol Head Neck Surg 101(1): 38-46, 1989.

Naggar ME, Hawthorne M: Delayed extrusion of a cochlear implant: a case report of an implant extruding 21 months after the original operation. The Journal of Laryngology and Otology, 109, 56-57, 1995.

Niparko D, Oviatt J, Newton C, Sutton L, Waltzman S, Cohen NL, and the VA Cooperative Study Group on Cochlear Implantation: Facial Nerve Stimulation with Cochlear Implantation. Otolaryngol Head Neck Surg 104: 826-830, 1991.

Niparko JK, Oviatt DL, Coker NJ, et al: Facial nerve stimulation with cochlear implantation. A cooperative study group on cochlear implantation. Otolaryngol Head Neck Surg 104, 826-830, 1991.

Novak MA, Fifer RC, Barkmeier JC, Firszt JB: Labyrinthine ossification after meningitis: Its implications for cochlear implantation. Otolaryngol Head Neck Surg 103(3) 351-356, 1990.

O'Donoghue GM, Jackler RK, Jenkins WM, et al: Cochlear implantation in children: The problem of head growth. Otolaryngol Head Neck Surg 94: 78-81, 1986.

Otto SR, House WF, Brackmann DE, Hitselberger WE, Nelson RA: Auditory brainstem implant: effect of tumor size and preoperative hearing level on function. Ann Otol Rhinol Laryngol 99, 789-799, 1990.

Parisier SC, Chute PM, Weiss MH, et al: Results of cochlear implant reinsertion. Laryngoscope 101(9):1013-1015, 1991.

Parkin JL, Randolph LJ: Auditory performance with simultaneous intracochlear multichannel stimulation. Laryngoscope 101: 379-383, 1991.

Parkin JL: Percutaneous pedestal in cochlear implantation. Am Otol Rhinol Laryngol 99(10Ptl) 796-800, 1990.

Parkins C: The bionic ear: principles and current status of cochlear prostheses. Neurosurgery 16:6, 853-65, 1983.

Patrick JF, Graeme MC: The Nucleus 22-Channel Cochlear Implant System. 12, 4, Supplement, 3-9, 1991.

Rosen S: Cochlear implants: some consensus at last? Br J Audiol 24. 361-366. 1990.

Schindler RA, Jackler RK, Kessler DK, Merzenich MM: Multichannel cochlear implants: Current status and future directions. In Johnson J, et al. (eds): Instructional Courses, Vol I. St. Louis, CV Mosby Company, 1988, pp 195-218.

Shelton C, Luxford WM, Tonokawa LL, et al: The narrow internal auditory canal in children: A contraindication to cochlear implants. Otolaryngol Head Neck Surg 100(313): 227-331, 1989.

Silverstein H, Smouha E, Morgan N: Multichannel cochlear implantation in a patient with bilateral Mondini deformities. Am J Otol 9(6): 451-455, 1988.

Spelman F, Clopton B, Pfingst B, Miller J: Design of the cochlear prosthesis: effects of the flow of current in the implanted ear. Ann Otol Rhinol Laryngol 89:8-10, 1980.

Staller SJ, Beiter AL, Brimacombe JA, et al: Pediatric performance with the Nucleus 22-channel cochlear implant system. Am J Otol 12(Suppl): 126-136, 1991.

Steenerson RL, Gary LB, Wynens MS: Scala vestibuli cochlear implantation in labyrinthine ossification. Am J Otol 11, 360-363, 1990.

Thielemeir MA, Tonokawa LL, Peterson et al: Audiological results in children with cochlear implant. Ear and Hearing, 6 (Suppl. 3), 275-355,1985.

Waltzman SB, Cohen NL, Shapiro WH, Hoffman RA: The prognostic value of round window electrical stimulation in cochlear implant patients. Otolaryngol Head Neck Surg 103(1) 102-106, 1990.

Wang RC, Parisier et al: Cochlear implant flap complications. Ann Otol Rhinol Laryngol 99, 791-795. 1990.

Webb RL, Lehnhardt E, Clark CM, et al: Surgical complications with the cochlear multiple-channel intracochlear implant: Experience at Hannover and Melbourne. Am Otol Rhinol Laryngol 100(2): 131-136, 1991.

Webb RL, Lehnhardt E, Clark GM, Laszig R, Pyman BD, Franz BH: Surgical complications with the cochlear multiple-channel intracochlear implant: experience at Hannover and Melbourne. Ann. Otol. Rhinol. Laryngol, 100, 131-136. 1991.

9

Drainage of petrous apex lesions

See anatomy of petrous apex, chapter 1.
Petrous apex lesions are rare lesions. They may be cholesterol granuloma, cholesteatoma, mucocele, aneurysm of the ICA, chordoma, chondroma, chondrosarcoma, or metastatic lesions (Fig. 9-1). There may be also trigeminal, facial, acoustic and jugular foramen neuromas.

Symptomatology

Hearing loss and vestibular disorders.
These symptoms are seen in large lesions that compress the VIII nerve in the internal auditory canal. There can be sensorineural or mixed hearing loss.
Pain
This symptom is more frequent in malignant lesions.
- Retro-orbital pain: V nerve involved: superior petrosal and middle fossa lesions.
- Neck pain: IX nerve involved: mastoid lesions.
- Pain in the area of distribution of IX-X CNs and I-III CNs: posterior fossa lesions.
- Other possible symptoms can be otalgia, aural pressure, diplopia, facial paralysis.

Symptoms may be present together in the Gradenigo syndrome: Otorrhea, VI and VII nevralgia and VI n. paresis.

Diagnosis
CT is the radiographic first choice in the diagnosis of petrous apex lesions. It shows the bone structure, the normal or pathologic air cells, and the vascular and bony structures of petrous bone. In malignant lesions, bone destruction and calcification are evident, as well as indistinct borders of metastatic lesions.
Benign lesions such as retained mucus, mucocele and cholesteatoma do not enhance in a CT, while cholesterol granuloma may show occasional rim enhancement. Vascular and neural abnormalities -trigeminal, facial, acoustic and jugular foramen neuromas, aneurysm of ICA- enhance.
MRI is useful for characterizing the substance of the lesions. One way to remember MRI images is:
- Chondroma has the radiologic appearance of a malignant lesion.
- Benign lesions (mucus, mucocele, cholesteatoma) do not enhance, while malignant lesions enhances.
- Cholesteatoma, retained mucus and mucocele are all hypointense in T1 and hyperintense in T2. Asymmetric pneumatization is the opposite. Cholesterol granuloma is hyperintense in both T1 and T2.

The most common lesion of the petrous apex is cholesterol granuloma. It is indeed very rare: 1/3,000,000 a year (Fig. 9-2).
It develops in a well pneumatized petrous bone when the aeration is compromised by eustachian tube obstruction, mucosal edema, temporal bone fracture, or cholesteatoma.
Surgery is performed when the symptoms appear. Surgery of cholesteatoma and tumors of the temporal bone is indicated as soon as the diagnosis is made, since these pathologies tend to grow.
Treatment is based on aeration and re-establisment of normal aeration. A complete removal is not necessary.
MRI is useful in the follow-up. Since the goal of the operation is not total removal, a retained mucus cyst, hypointense in T1 and hyperintense in T2, will appear. A recurrence will be signalled by hyperintensity in T1.

INFRALABYRINTHINE DRAINAGE

- Preparation and retroauricolar incision is similar to mastoid surgery.
- A mastoidectomy is performed.
- Skeletonization of the anterior part of lateral canal and identification of the third part of facial nerve.
- Following the sigmoid sinus, skeletonization of jugular bulb is performed. The JB becames evi-

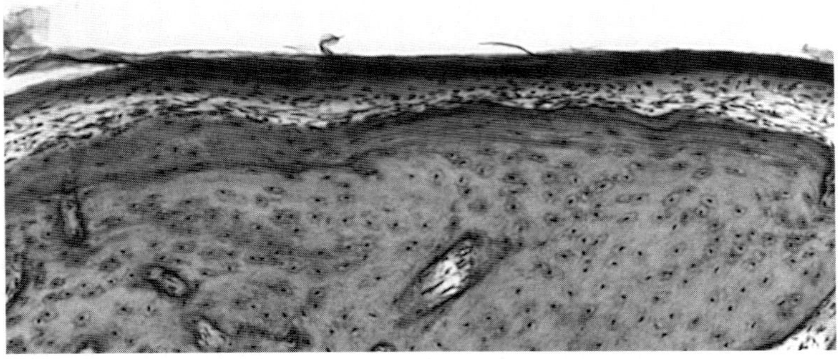

Fig. 9-1. Courtesy of Linthicum FH. Primary (congenital) cholesteatoma matrix with no evidence of inflammation. Desquamation is visible on left side of picture. ×117.

dent as a blue image under a thin plate of bone, which is left undisturbed.

- The lateral canal is followed posteriorly to expose the posterior canal, whose anterior tip points to the VII nerve.
- The posterior semicircular canal superiorly, the jugular bulb inferiorly, the sigmoid sinus posteriorly and the facial nerve anteriorly delineate a space: this is the path to the petrous apex.
- The bone is removed with a curette or a diamond burr, passing medially to the facial nerve. It is important not to disrupt the endolymphatic sac or duct. This is easily done by leaving a thin sheet of bone over the area of the sac. Lesioning of the sac may lead to postoperative endolymphatic hydrops. The lesion is reached, opened and drained with suction irrigation as much as possible, although the complete removal of the lesion's sheath is not possible with this method.
- A large silicone sheeting catheter is inserted to maintain the opening patent. Disadvantages of the drainage are possible occlusion and drainage into the mastoid, far from Eustachian tube.
- The closure is as usual in mastoid surgery.
- Complications: semicircular canals, jugular bulb, and facial nerve injuries are possible (see chapter 11).

This approach is more suitable for large cysts whose limits are easily reached, while difficulties may arise in the treatment of small cysts, medially based.

A high jugular bulb can impede a propitious path to the petrous apex and contraindicate this operation.

TRANSCANAL INFRACOCHLEAR APPROACH

A transcanal approach for treatment of small hypotympanic tumors was presented by Farrior J.B. in 1984. Ghorayeb and Jahrsdoerfer described a

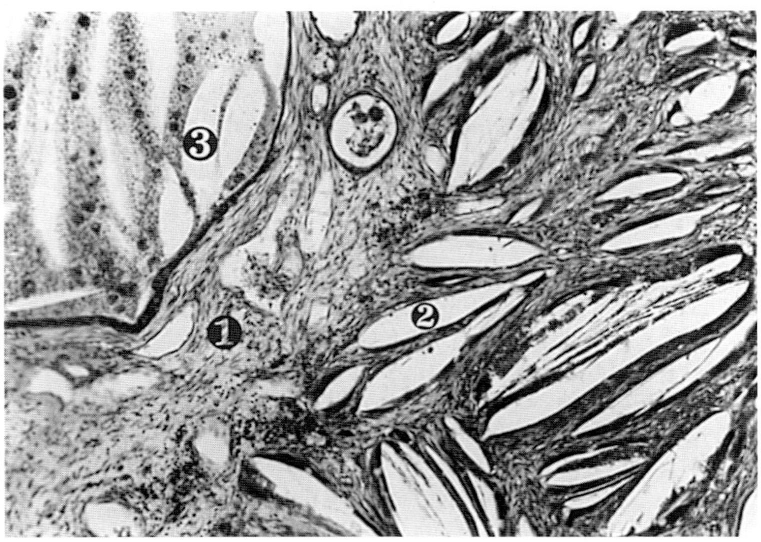

Fig. 9-2. Courtesy of Linthicum FH. Cholesterol granuloma showing granulation tissue (1) containing cholesterol clefts lined with foreign body giant cells (2). Loculated cyst (3) also contains cholesterol clefts and macrophages. ×117.

subcochlear approach in 1989. Giddins, Brackmann and Kwartler J. presented a transcanal infracochlear approach to the petrous apex in 1990, which is a combination of the two techniques. This approach has become the treatment of choice in the HEC group, for cystic lesions of the petrous apex.

- Postauricular incision.
- Complete transection of membranous external auditory canal (see chapter 16).
- A semicircular incision is made.
- A tympanomeatal flap is raised from inferior to superior, leaving the tympanic membrane attached to the malleus handle. A semicircular space of bone, almost 1 cm deep, is stripped of epithelium (Fig. 9-3).
- The chorda tympani is followed posteriorly up to the facial nerve, to define the posterior limit of dissection.
- The EAC is enlarged to visualize the hypotympanum. The bone can be drilled out anteriorly without major risks: the first structure encountered is the temporomandibular joint. A diamond burr is preferable inferiorly, due to the risk of injuring the jugular bulb.
- The dissection is carried medially with a small diamond burr, in the hypotympanic space. The jugular bulb is outlined posteriorly and the internal carotid artery anteriorly. The superior limit of the dissection is the round window and the basal turn of the cochlea, which bulges in the medial wall of the tympanic cavity. There is only one millimeter of bone between the basal turn of cochlea and ICA, anteriorly. The area of drilling must be maintained in a triangular shape, with the vertex between the carotid and the jugular bulb, in the so called "crotch", to avoid injury to the vascular or inner ear structures. When going deeper, smaller diamond burrs are used (Fig. 9-4).
- The lesion is reached, opened, and drained with suction irrigation. A complete removal of the lesion's sheath is not possible by this route. The curette is also useful.
- A silicone sheeting catheter is placed to mantain areation of the cavity.
- The ear drum and the external auditory canal skin are returned to their normal positions. The deficit between the external auditory canal skin and the bone is filled with previously obtained bone patè.

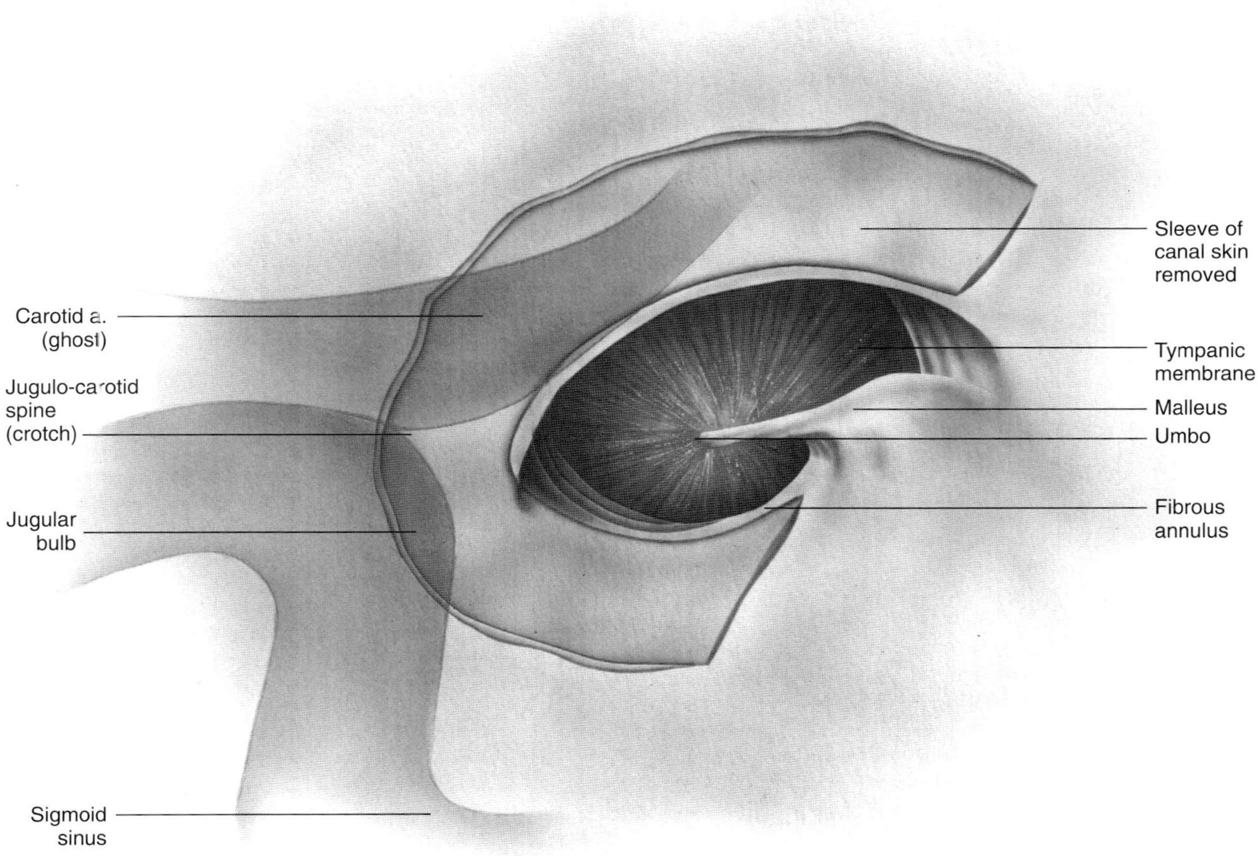

Fig. 9-3. The skin from the inferior bony canal is removed, from two o'clock to ten o'clock.

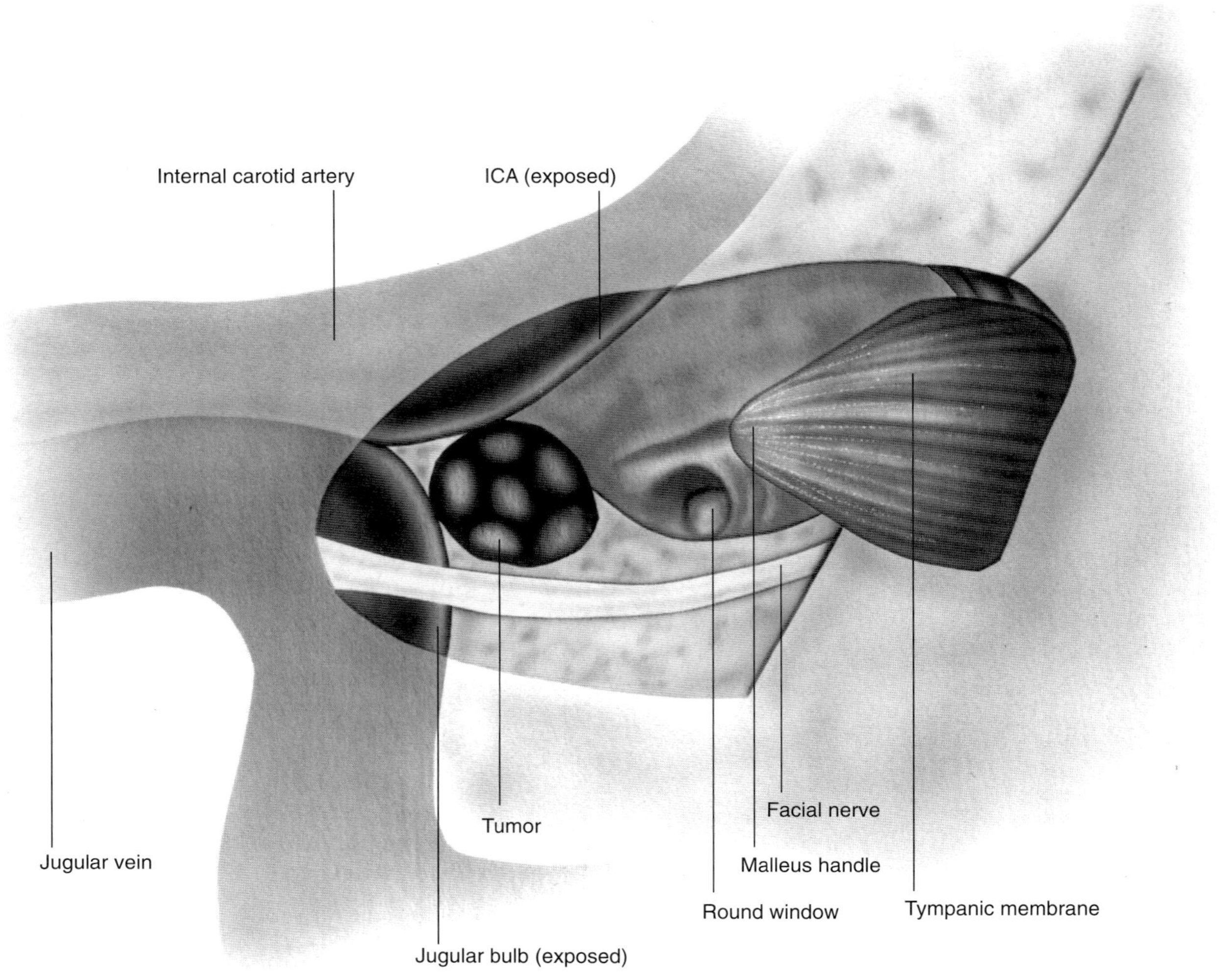

Fig. 9-4. The area of drilling is maintained between the carotid and the jugular bulb.

- Gelatin sponge (Gelfoam) is used to pack the tympanic membrane and the external auditory canal skin. The membranous external auditory canal and the auricle are repositioned and gelfoam is left inside.
- A mastoid pressure dressing closes the ear for one day. The second day the dressing is removed and the patient is dismissed. The patient is advised to begin instillation of antibiotic drops two weeks after the operation, until the packing has melted.

Complications

- Jugular bulb injury is treated as explained in chapter 28 (see complications).

  Injury of the basal turn of the cochlea is treated like lesions of the semicircular canals, but the hearing preservation prognosis is much poorer.
- The most serious complication is injury to the internal carotid artery. This is a life threatening lesion and the manipulation for the closure, even in the best cases, involves the risk of cerebral infarct. While working in close proximity to the ICA, 1x enlargement is to be used at least. The first barrier not to cross is a thin plate of bone that must be left to protect the vessel. If this barrier is broken, the adventitia is felt under the burr as an elastic membrane that must be kept intact. If the ICA is opened, it can be temporarily occluded proximally and distally with two kocher clamps with pusher sponges (Fisch).The perforation is closed with 5-0 vascular nylon suture. When the perforation is close to the crotch or is large, distal control is obtained with an intra-arterial catheter threaded past the opening, while proximal control is obtained by ligating the ICA in the neck. The perforation is then closed with 5-0 vascular nylon sutures.

  In the postoperative period a 1 cm long Pope Ear Wick (Merocel) is positioned in the external auditory canal to prevent stenosis, due to its previous complete transection. The packing is changed in the third postoperative day and mantained up to the eighth day.

SUBTOTAL PETROSECTOMY

This approach has been proposed by Fisch and Mattox. It permits the complete removal of cystic lesions of petrous apex. The price to pay is a total sensorineural hearing loss due to the complete removal of the otic capsule

- Postauricular skin incision (see chapter 16).
- Closure of external auditory canal (see chapter 16).
- Subtotal petrosectomy. Skeletonization of the third part of the facial nerve.
- Section of middle meningeal artery. If the lesion has an anterior extent, the section of V3 may be necessary.
- Removal of the bone around the ICA.
- Removal of the bony labyrinth and cochlea.
- The ICA is elevated from the carotid canal with an umbilical tape.
- The cyst wall can be peeled away from posterior fossa dura.
- The membranous ET is closed with 4.0 Vicryl sutures passed through a fragment of muscle. In this way the ET is closed and the muscle fragment goes to fill the residual opening, if present.
- The cavity is closed with abdominal fat and the temporalis muscle is rotated to cover the fat.
- Closure of the incision in layers.

REFERENCES

Al-Mefty O, Fox JL, Smith RR: Petrosal approach for petroclival meningiomas. Neurosurgery 22: 510-517, 1988.

Beaumont GD: Cholesterol granuloma. J Otolaryngol Soc Aust 2: 28-35, 1967.

Behneke EE, Schindler RA: Dermoid of the petrous apex. Laryngoscope 94: 779-783, 1984.

Bourgouin PM, Tampieri D, Robitaille Y, et al: Low-grade myxoid chondrosarcoma of the base of the skull: CT, MR, and histopathology. J Comput Assist Tomogr 16: 268-273, 1992.

Brackmann DE, Hitselberger WE, Beneke JE, House WF:Acoustic neuromas: middle fossa and translabyrinthine removal. In: Rand RW, ed. Micro Neurosurgery. St. Louis: Mosby, 311-334, 1985.

Chole RA: Petrous apicitis: surgical anatomy. Ann Otol Rhinol Laryngol 94:251-57, 1985.

Congdon E: The distribution and mode of origin of septa and walls of the sphenoid sinus. Anat Rec 18: 97, 1920.

Davis AE, Robin PE: Transpalatal approach to the petrous apex. J Laryngol Otol 103: 94-96, 1989.

Dearmin RM: A logical approach to the tip cells of the petrous pyramid. Arch Otolaryngol Head Neck Surg 26: 314-320, 1937.

Domb GH, Chole RA: Anatomical studies of the posterior petrous apex with regard to hearing preservation in acoustic neuroma removal. Laryngoscope 90: 1769-1776, 1980.

Eagleton WP: Unlocking the petrous apex for localized bulbar (pontile) meningitis secondary to suppuration of the petrous apex. Arch Otolaryngol Head Neck Surg 13: 386-422, 1931.

Farrior JB: Anterior hypotympanic approach for glomus tumor of the infratemporal fossa. Laryngoscope 94: 1016-1020, 1984.

Fisch U, Mattox D: Microsurgery of the Skull Base. New York, Thieme Medical Publishers, 1-655, 1988.

Fisch U, Pillsbury HC: Infratemporal fossa approach to lesions in the temporal bone and base of the skull. Arch Otolaryngol 105:99-107, 1979.

Flood LM, Kemink JL: Surgery in lesions of the petrous apex. Otolaryngol Clin North Am 7:565-75, 1984.

Frenckner P: Some remarks on the treatment of apicitis (petrositis) with or without Gradenigo's syndrome. Acta Otolaryngol (Stockh) 17: 97-120,1932.

Gacek R: Evaluation and management of petrous apex cholesteatoma. Otolaryng Head Neck Surg 88: 519-523, 1980.

Gherini SG, Brackmann DE, Low WW, Solti-Bohman LG: Cholesterol granuloma of the petrous apex. Laryngoscope 95: 659-664, 1985.

Ghorayeb BY, Jahrsdoerfer RA: Subcochlear approach for cholesterol granulomas of the inferior petrous apex. Otolaryngol Head Neck Surg 103: 60-65, 1990.

Gianoli-GJ, Amedee RG: Hearing results in surgery for primary petrous apex lesions. Oto-Laryngol-Head-Neck-Surg. 111(3 Pt 1): 250-7, 1994.

Giddings NA, Brackmann DE, Kezartler JA: Transcanal infracochlear approach to the petrous Apex. Otolaryngol Head Neck Surg 104: 29-36, 1991.

Glasscock ME, Harris PF, Newsome G: Glomus tumors: diagnosis and treatment. Laringoscope 84, 2006-2032, 1974.

Graham MD, Kemink JL, Latack JT, Kartush JM: The giant cholesterol cyst of the petrous apex: A distinct clinical entity. Laryngoscope 95: 1401-1406, 1985.

Hendershot EL, Wood JW: The middle fossa approach in the treatment of petrositis. Arch Otolaryngol Head Neck Surg 98: 426-427, 1973.

Hollinshead WH: The ear. In Anatomy for Surgeons, Vol 1. Philadelphia, Harper & Row, 1982, pp 159-221.

House JL, Brackmann DE: Cholesterol granuloma of the cerebello-pontine angle. Arch Otolaryngol 108: 504-506, 1982.

Jackler RK, Parker DA: Radiographic differential diagnosis of petrous apex lesions. Am-J-Otol 13(6): 561-74, 1992.

Lempert J: Complete apicectomy (mastoidotympanoapicectomy). Arch Otolaryngol Head Neck Surg 25: 144-177, 1937.

Lipper MH, Cail WS: Chordoma of the petrous bone. South Med J 84: 629-631, 1991.

Lo WW, Solti-Bohmann LG, Brackmann DE, Grunskin P: Cholesterol granuloma of the petrous apex: CT Diagnosis. Radiology 153: 705-711, 1984.

Main TS, Shimada T, Lim DJ: Experimental cholesterol granuloma. Arch Otolaryngol 91: 356-359, 1970.

Mawson SR: Complications of otitis media. In Ludman H (ed): Mawson's Diseases of the Ear. Baltimore, William & Wilkins, 1963, pp 347-352.

Myerson MC, Rubin J, Gilbert JG: Anatomic studies of the petrous portion of the temporal bone. Arch Otolaryngol Head Neck Surg 20: 195-210, 1934.

Nager GT, Vanderveen TS: Cholesterol granuloma involving the temporal bone. Ann Otol Rhinol Laryngol 85: 204-209, 1976.

Osborn AG, Parkin JL: Mucocele of the petrous temporal bone. Ann J Radiol 132: 680-681, 1979.

Pellet W, Valenzuela S, Malca S, Cannoni M, Perez-Castillo-AM: Les kystes a cholesterine geants de l'apex petreux. Neurochirurgie. 38(5): 267-80; 1992.

Ramadier J: Exploration de la pointe du rocher par la voie du canal carotidien. Ann Otolaryngol 4: 422-444, 1933.

Rand RW, Kurze T: Micro neurosurgical resection of acoustic tumors by a transmeatal posterior fossa approach. Bull Los Angeles Neurol Soc 30:17-20, 1965.

Roland PS, Meyerhoff WL, Judge LO, Mickey BE: Asymmetric pneumatization of the petrous apex. Otolaryngol Head Neck Surg 103: 80-88, 1990.

Sakaki S, Takeda S, Fujita H, Otita S: An extended middle fossa approach combined with a suboccipital craniectomy to the base of the skull in the posterior fossa. Surg Neurol 28:245-252, 1987.

Samii M: Micro surgery of acoustic neuromas with special emphasis on preservation of seventh and eighth cranial nerves and the scope of facial nerve grafting. In: Rand RW, ed. Micro neurosurgery. St. Louis: Mosby, 1985.

Sanna M, Zini C, Gamoletti R, Frau N, Taibah A, Russo A, et al: Petrous bone cholesteatoma. Skull Base Surgery 3:201-213, 1993.

Sekhar LN, Estonillo R: Transtemporal approach to the skull base: an anatomical study. Neurosurgery 19:799-808, 1986.

Sekhar LN, Jannetta PJ, Maroon JC: Tentorial meningiomas: surgical management and results. Neurosurgery 14:268-275, 1984.

Sekhar LN, Pomeranz S, Janecka IP, et al: Temporal bone neoplasms: A report on 20 surgically treated cases. J Neurosurg 76: 578-587, 1992.

Sterkers JM, Corlieu P, Viala P, Riviere F, Chobaut JC: Les petrosites actuelles. Ann Oto-Laryng Paris 103: 515-521, 1986.

Thedinger BA, Nadol JB, Montgomery WW, et al: Radiographic diagnosis, surgical treatment, and long term follows-up of cholesterol granulomas of the petrous apex. Laryngoscope 99: 896-907, 1989.

Van Alyea OE: Sphenoid sinus: Anatomic study, with consideration of the clinical significance of the structural characteristics of the sphenoid sinus. Arch Otolaryngol Head Neck Surg 34: 225, 1941.

Yasargil MG, Mortara RW, Curcic M: Meningiomas of basal posterior cranial fossa. In: Krayen BH, ed. Advances and technical standards in Neurosurgery vol 7. Wien: Springer Verlag, 1-115, 1980.

10

Malignant tumors of the temporal bone

Nothing is accomplished by proving that the impossible is impossible. The only real discovery is to prove the impossible, possible.

Malignant tumors of the temporal bone are rare. Basal cell carcinomas are seen primarily in the external ear, while squamous cell carcinomas may appear in other parts of the temporal bone. Other malignant lesions are adenoid cystic carcinoma and ceruminous adenocarcinoma.
These tumors tend to have regional invasions and rarely metastasize.

- Basal cell carcinoma manifests a surface crust that tends to reappear after removal, and may pass undiagnosed for long periods of time.
- Squamous cell carcinoma is lighter in appearance, with granulation tissue or ulcer. Though it can be mistaken for an external otitis, errors may be prevented by using more detailed criteria in diagnosis.
- Lack of response to medical therapy in patients over 60 suggests a biopsy.
- The neck is examined, to evaluate parotid and/or cervical lymph node involvement.
- The function of nerves VII, IX, X, and XI is assessed.
- High resolution axial and coronal CT's permit the assessment of temporal bone involvement, whereas an MRI investigates intracranial spreading.
- Angiography, as well as temporary balloon occlusion of the ICA and cerebral blood flow measurements, are useful when the ICA is involved.

Tumor spread
A tumor of the external ear may invade the bony part of the external auditory canal and extend:

- Anteriorly to involve the glenoid fossa and the condyle of the mandible.
- Inferiorly to the crotch to involve the carotid and/or jugular vein.
- Superiorly to the dura of the middle fossa, involving the middle meningeal artery and V3.
- Posteriorly to the posterior fossa dura.
- Medially to the skull base (Fig. 10-1).

Surgical treatment is based on partial or total temporal bone resection.

PARTIAL TEMPORAL BONE RESECTION

SECTION OF THE LATERAL TEMPORAL BONE
This procedure aims at total gross tumor removal. It involves removing the tympanic ring: the skin of the auditory canal, the bony canal walls, the tympanic membrane, and the malleus and incus all at once. This operation is indicated in cases of carcinoma of the conchal area of the ear or the external auditory canal.
The resection of the lesion "en bloc" is not possible, unlike in total temporal bone resection, but the morbidity and mortality rates are lower.

- Postauricular incision (Fig. 10-2).
- Tragal-conchal incision and cartilage removal.
- The external canal is everted and cul-de-sac sutured to prevent medial diffusion of tumor cells.
- The flap is elevated (Fig. 10-3).
- Postauricular mastoidectomy.

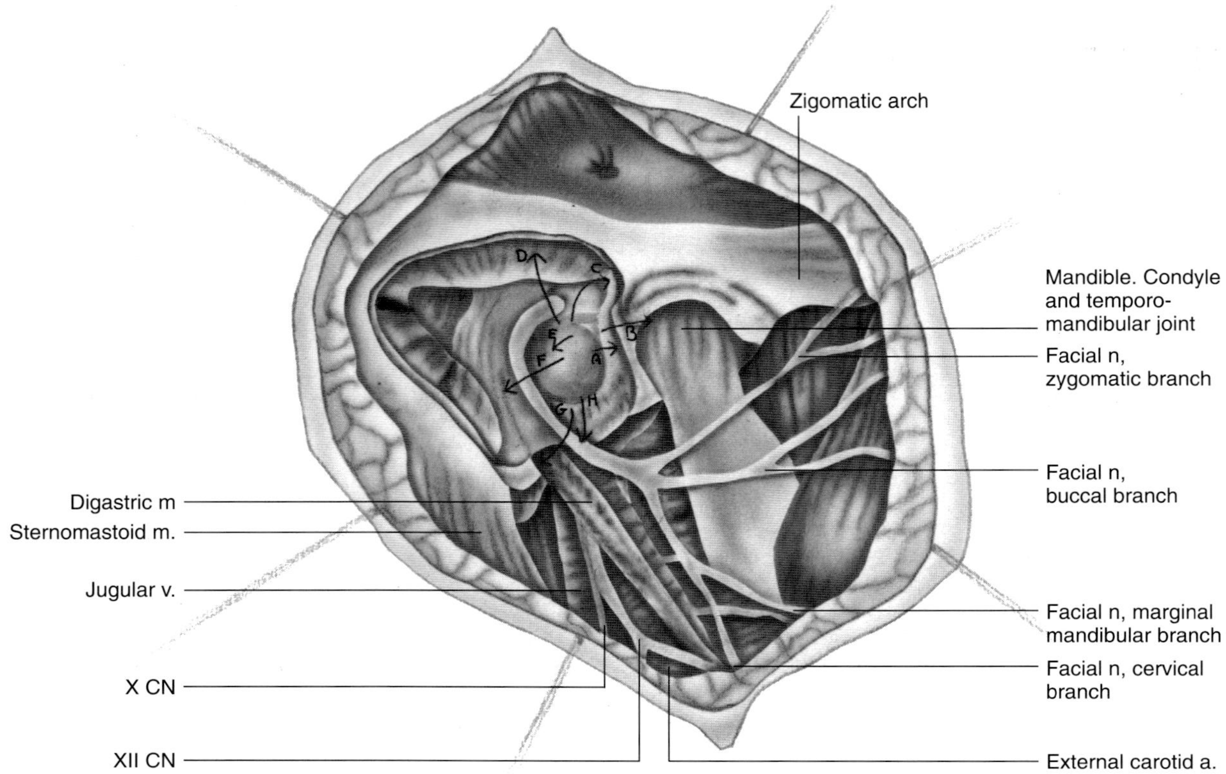

Fig. 10-1. The tumor can extend in various directions. **A:** To the soft tissue of the temporo-mandibular joint. **B:** To the glenoid fossa. **C:** Along the middle fossa dura, to the petrous apex. **D:** To the middle fossa dura. **E:** To the cochlea or semicircular canals. **F:** To the posterior fossa dura. **G**: To the stylomastoid foramen. **H:** To the carotid jugular spine.

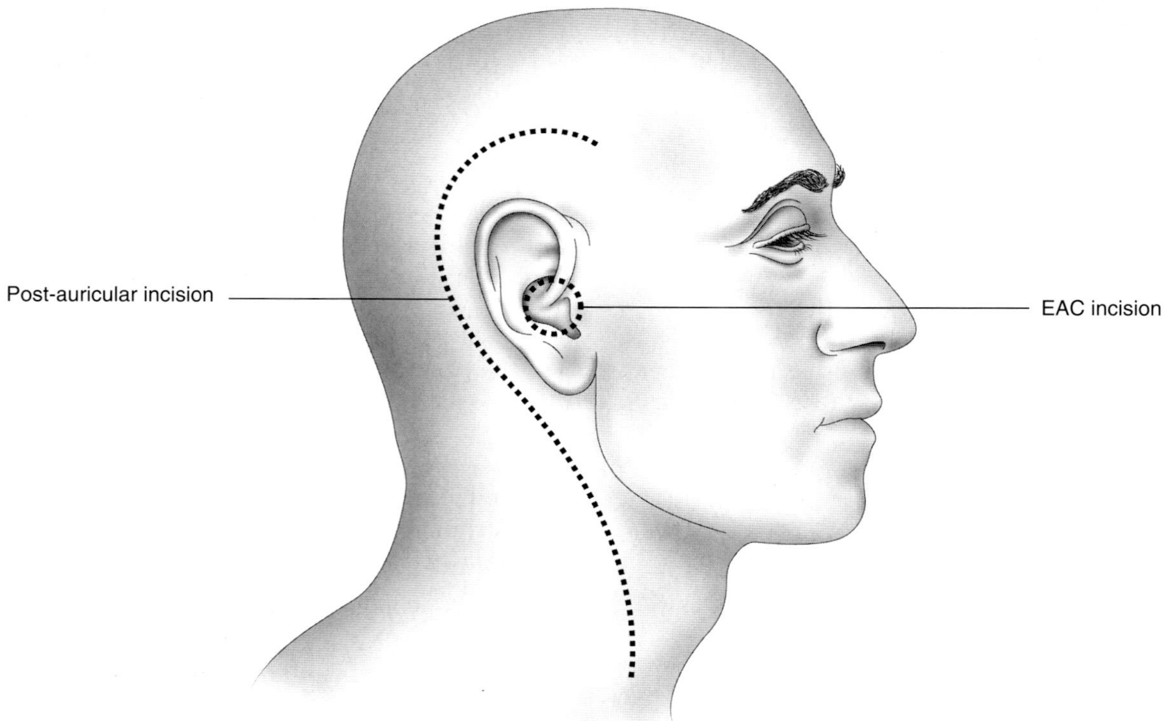

Fig.10-2. Skin incision and tragal-conchal incision.

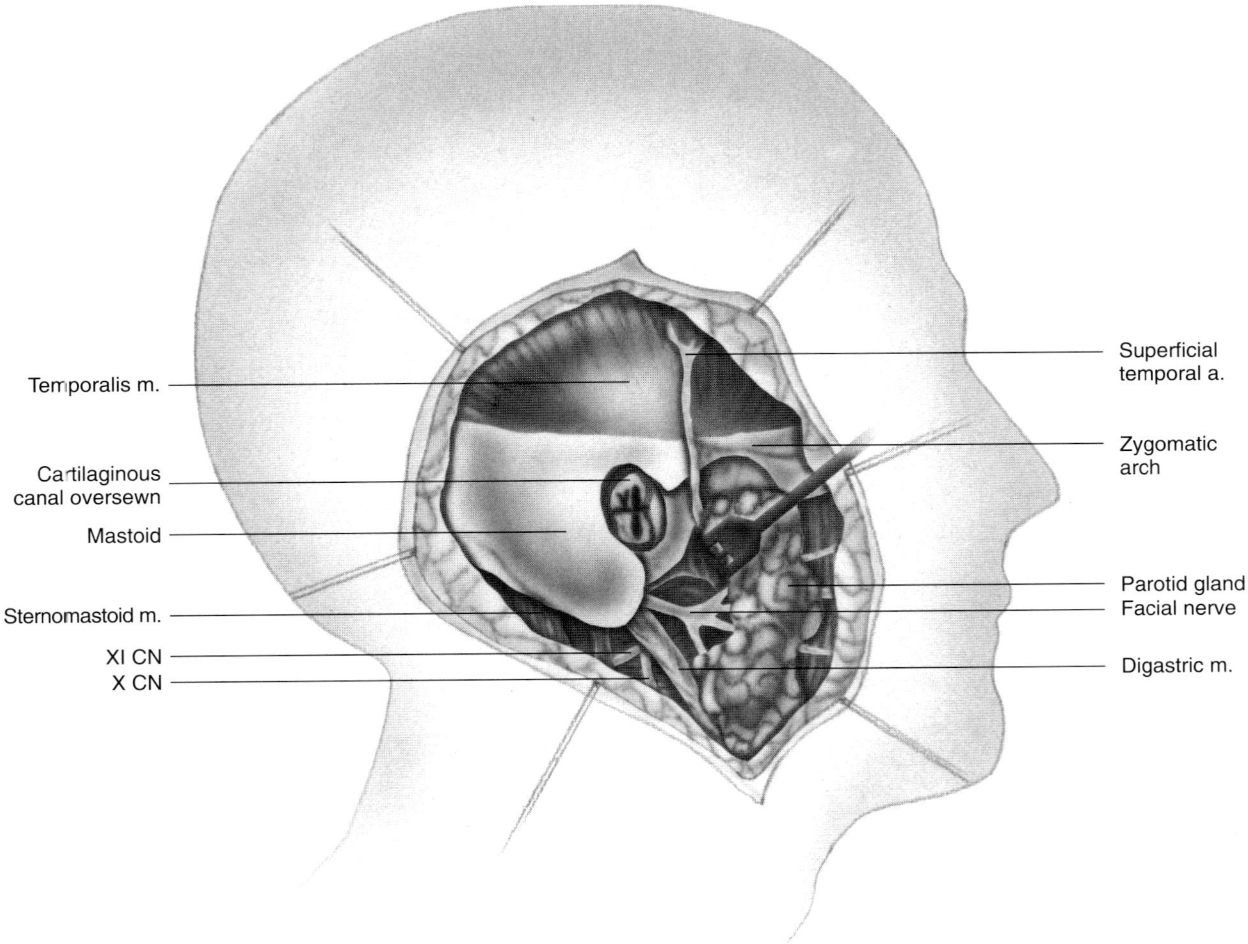

Fig. 10-3. The external auditory canal is transected. The skin of EAC is everted and sutured with 4-0 nylon sutures. The parotid gland is exposed. (Adapted from Kinney SE).

- Enlarged facial recess. The lateral part of the jugular bulb and the posterior wall of the ICA in the hypotympanum represent the medial-most part of the dissection.
- Superiorly, the dissection goes from the antrum, through the epitympanum and the zygomatic root below the dura of the middle fossa to the temporomandibular joint.
- Section of the remaining connection between the lateral part of the ear to the cavum tympani.
- Identification of the facial nerve at its exit from the stylomastoid foramen. It is easier for the otologic surgeon to follow the mastoid part of the facial nerve, identify the digastric fibers at the stylomastoid foramen, obtain an indication of the level of nerve VII in the parotid gland, and finally expose the nerve along its path into the gland.
- The auditory canal is removed along with the superficial parotid gland (Fig. 10-4).
- Surgical removal is extended as needed.
- A split-thickness skin graft may be placed over the incision, to cover the defect of the ear.
- The temporalis muscle is turned to cover the defect and protect the underlying bone from radionecrotization, in case of postoperative irradiation. Other flaps can be obtained from the superior two-thirds of the sternocleidomastoid muscle and the pectoralis muscle.
- The eustachian tube is sealed with bone wax and muscle, to prevent retrograde infection or rhynoliquorrea, if the dura is lacerated.
- Postoperative radiotherapy is planned in all cases. Some authors (S. Kinney) do not plan postoperative radiation therapy in T1 lesions of the external auditory canal, since the survival rate at five years is reported to be almost 95%. The average dosage of radiation therapy is 6000 rads.

According to the literature, the T2 five-year survival rate is 85%, while T3 is 55% and T4 is 40%.

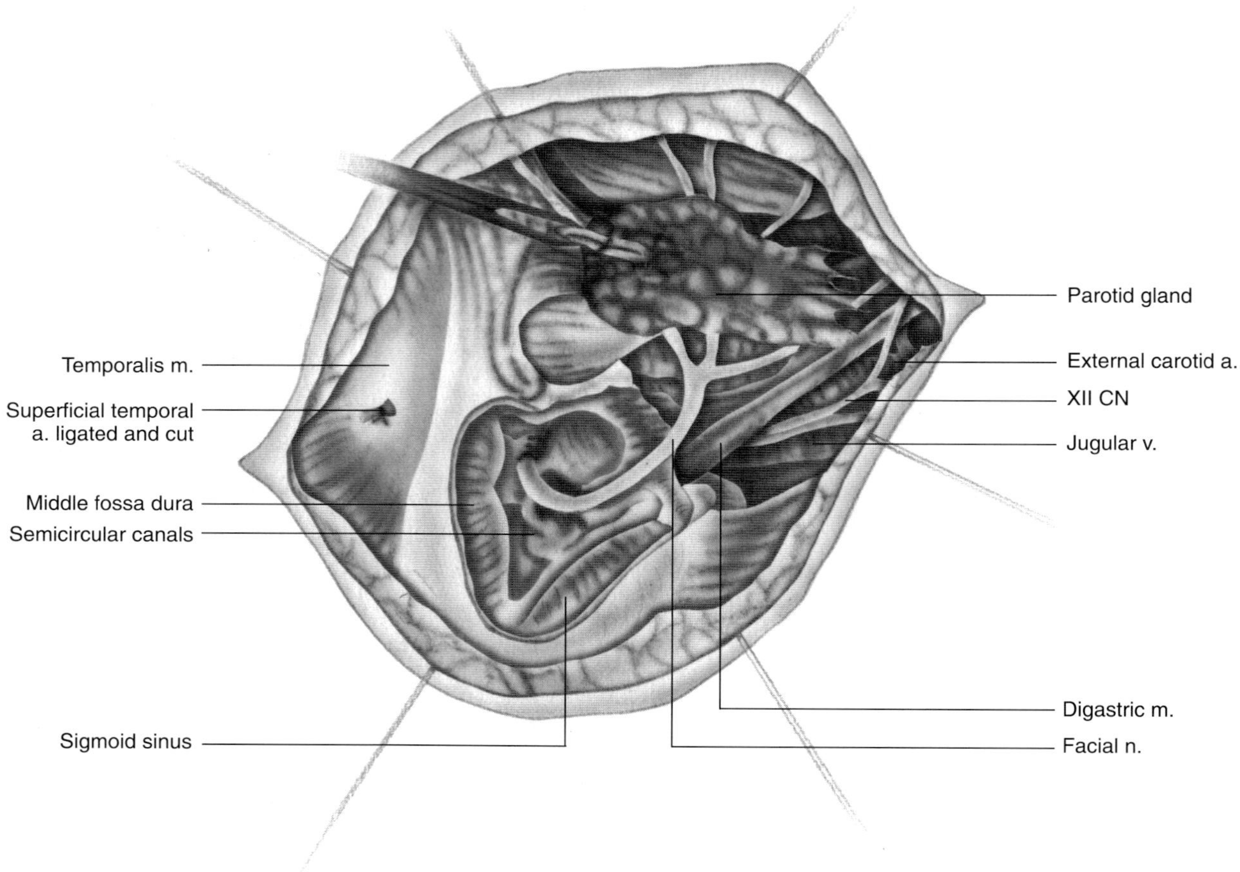

Fig. 10-4. A complete mastoidectomy is performed. The mastoid bony tip is removed. The external canal together with the superficial lobe of the parotid gland are removed, then the deep lobe is removed. (Adapted from Kinney SE).

REFERENCES

Adams WS, Morfison R: On primary carcinoma of the middle ear and mastoid. J Laryngol Otol 69: 115-131, 1955.

Arena S, Keen M: Carcinoma of the middle ear and temporal bone. Am J Otol A 351-356, 1988.

Arena S, Keen M: Carcinoma of the middle ear and temporal bone. Am J Otol 9 (5): 351-356, 1988.

Arriaga M, Curtin H, Takahashi H, et al: Staging proposal for external auditory meatus carcinoma based on preoperative clinical examination and computed tomography findings. Ann Otol Rhinol Laryngol 99(9.1), 714-721, 1990.

Benecke JE Jr, Noel FL, Carberry JN, et al: Adenomatous tumors of the middle ear and mastoid. Am J Otol 11(1): 20-26, 1990.

Conley T, Schuller DE: Malignancies of the ear. Laryngoscope 86: 1147-1163, 1976.

Coodman ME: Middle ear and mastoid neoplasms. Ann Otol Rhinol Laryngol 80: 419-424, 1971.

Crabtree JA, Britton BH, Pierce MK: Carcinoma of the external auditory canal. Laryngoscope 86: 405-415, 1976.

Eby TL, Makek MS, Fisch U: Adenomas of the temporal bone. Ann Otol Rhinol Laryngol 97(6.1): 605-612, 1988.

Gacek RR: Management of temporal bone carcinoma. Trans Penn Acad Otolaryngol Ophthalmol 32: 67-71, 1978.

Greer JA, Body DTR, Weitland LH: Neoplasms of the temporal bone. J Otolaryngol 5: 391-398, 1978.

Howard JD, Elster AD, May JS: Temporal bone: Three-dimensional CT. Part II, Pathologic alterations. Radiology 177(2): 427-430, 1990.

Johns ME, Headington JT: Squamous cell carcinoma of the external auditory canal: A clinicopathologic study of 20 cases. Arch Otolaryngol Head Neck Surg 100: 45-49, 1974.

Kinney SE, Wood BG: Malignancies of the external ear canal and temporal bone: Surgical techniques and results. Laryngoscope 97: 158-164, 1987.

Kinney SE: Tumors of the external auditory canal, middle ear, mastoid and temporal bone. In Thawley SE, Panje WR, Batsakis TG, Lindberg RD (eds): Comprehensive Management of Head and Neck Tumors. Philadelphia, WB Saunders, 1987, p 182.

Lewis JS: Temporal bone resection. Arch Otolaryngol 101: 23-25, 1975.

Mafee MF, Valvassori GE, Kumar A, et al: Tumors and tumor-like conditions of the middle ear and mastoid: Role of CT and MRI. An analysis of 100 cases. Otolaryngol Clin North Am 21(2): 349-375, 1988.

Meyerhoff WL, Mickey BE, Roland PS, Drummond JE: Magnetic resonance imaging in the diagnosis of temporal bone and skull base lesions. Am J Otol 10(2): 121-137, 1989.

Sataloff RT, Roberts BR, Myers DL, Spiegel JR: Total temporal bone resection. A radical but life-saving procedure. AORN J 48(5): 932-948, 1988.

Wiatrak BJ, Pensak ML: Rhabdomyosarcoma of the ear and temporal bone. Laryngoscope 99(11): 1188-1192, 1989.

TOTAL TEMPORAL BONE RESECTION

Subtotal temporal bone resection involves the removal of the tympanic ring (as performed in temporal bone resection) and the otic capsule. Total temporal bone resection is extended to the petrous apex.

SURGICAL TECHNIQUE (proposed by Sekhar, Janecka, Prasad, Hirsch).

- Incision (Fig. 10-5).
- The external canal is everted and cul-de-sac sutured to help prevent the medial spread of tumor cells.
- Elevation of skin flaps. Temporal arteries are ligated.
- If the parotid gland is involved by the tumor, the peripheral branches of the facial nerve are sacrificed and the gland is elevated posteriorly while maintaining contact with the area of the tumor (the external auditory canal).
- If the parotid gland is thought not to be involved by the tumor, the facial nerve is cut 1 cm beyond the stylomastoid foramen and the gland is reflected anteriorly.
- A few lymph nodes of the upper neck are sent for pathological analysis; if positive, a functional neck dissection is performed.
- The neurovascular structures of the neck are exposed. Nerves are harvested for facial nerve repair (greater auricular nerve or cervical cutaneous nerve or sural nerve...).
- The sternocleidomastoid, the digastric, and the masseter muscles are detached from their superior connection.
- The temporomandibular joint is opened, the meniscus is dissected inferiorly and mandibular and zygomatic osteotomies are performed (Fig. 10-6).
- The temporalis muscle is elevated. Resection of the lateral and medial pterygoid muscles is performed (Fig. 10-7).
- The infratemporal fossa is exposed. Vessels in the foramen spinosum and the foramen ovale are exposed.
- Separation of the styloglossus, stylopharingeus and stylohyoid muscles from the styloid process. Removal of the styloid process.
- The internal maxillary artery is preserved whenever possible.
- The ascending and transverse segments of the ICA are unroofed. The vessels are anteriorly mobilized (Fig. 10-8).
- A temporal craniotomy is performed. Some structures are sacrificed, such as the greater petrosal nerve with the petrosal artery, the lesser petrosal nerve and the superior tympanic artery. The membranous eustachian tube is ligated.

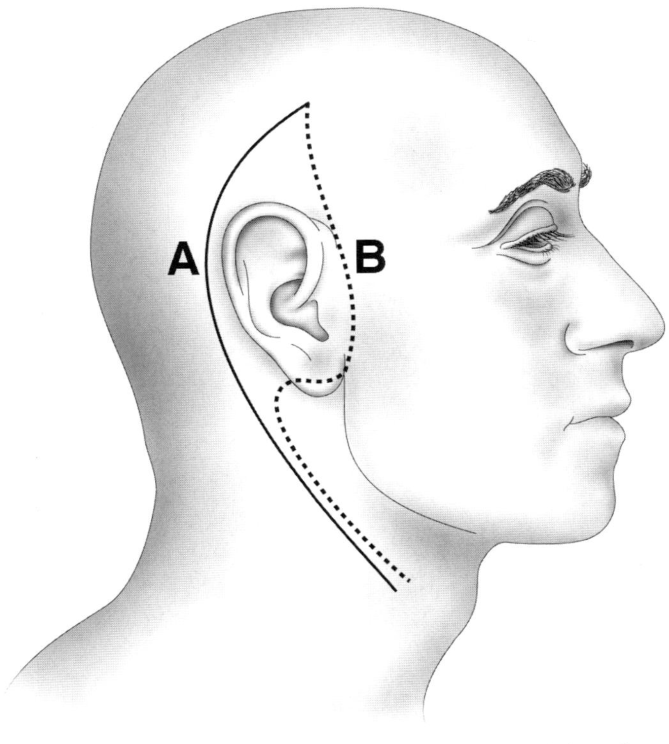

Fig.10-5. Skin incision. A: Lesions within the temporal bone. B:Lesions close to conchal cartilage or periauricular skin. (Adapted from Prasad S, Janecka IP).

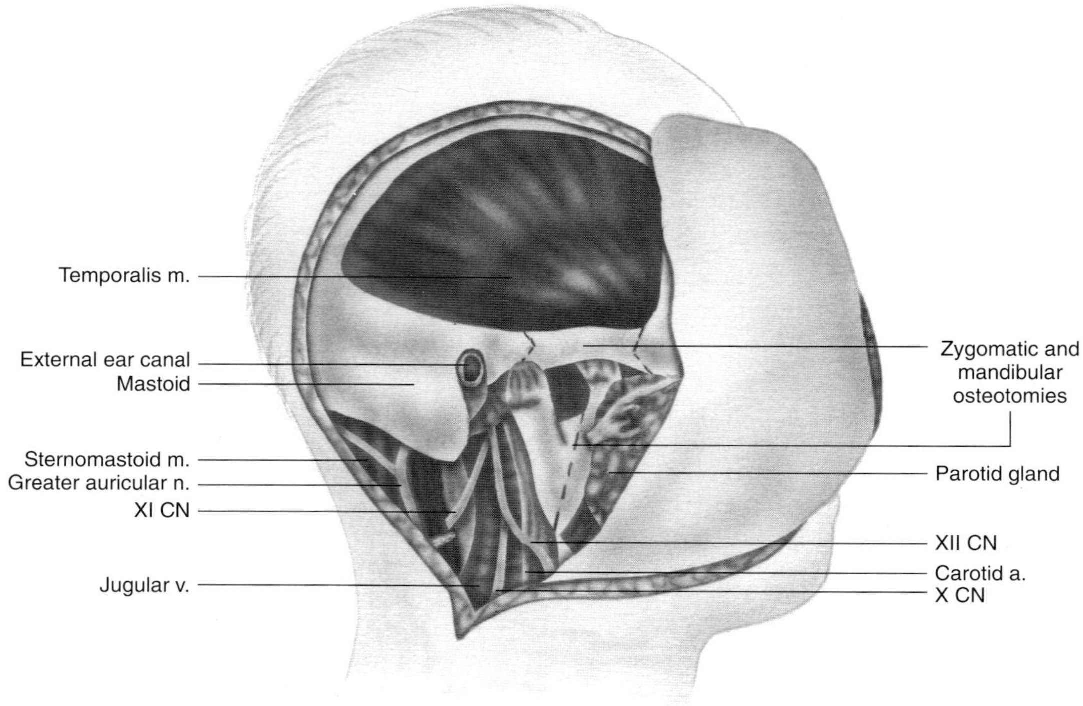

Fig. 10-6. The masseter is dissected from the zygomatic arch. Zygomatic and mandibular osteotomies (dotted lines) are performed. (Adapted from Prasad S, Janecka IP).

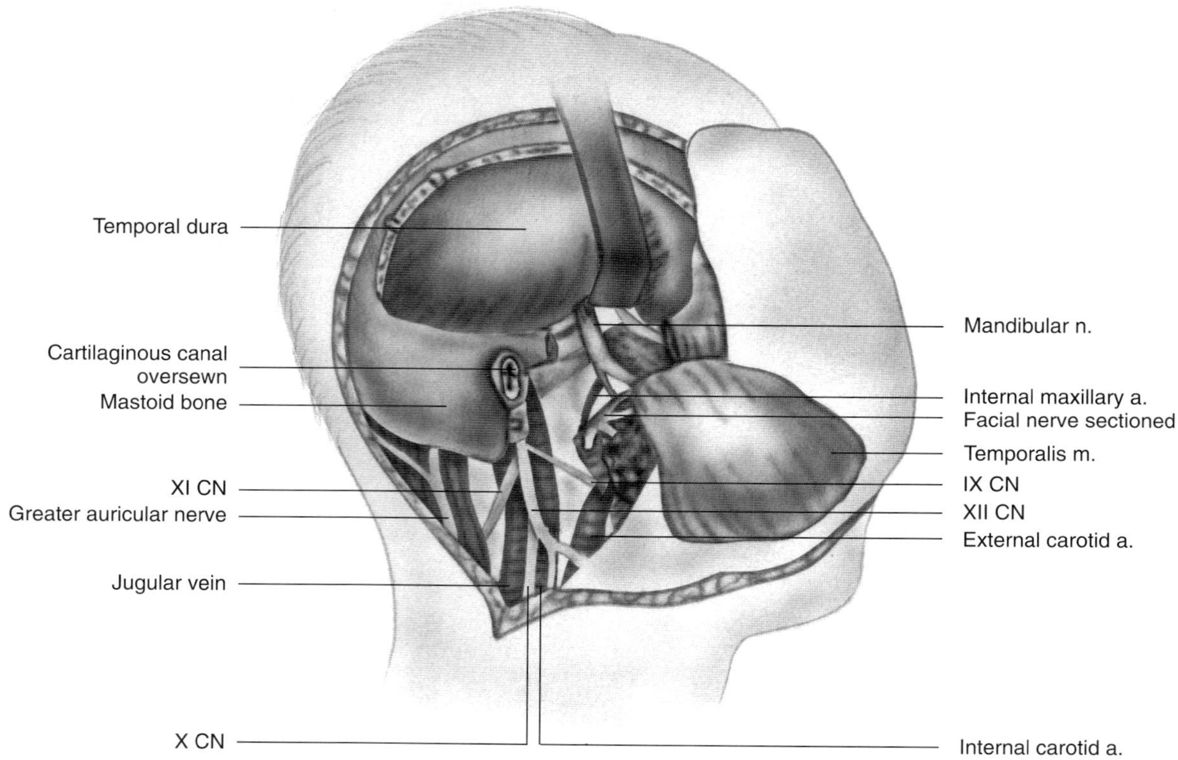

Fig. 10-7. Blind sac closure of the EAC. Temporal craniotomy. Dissection in the infratemporal fossa.

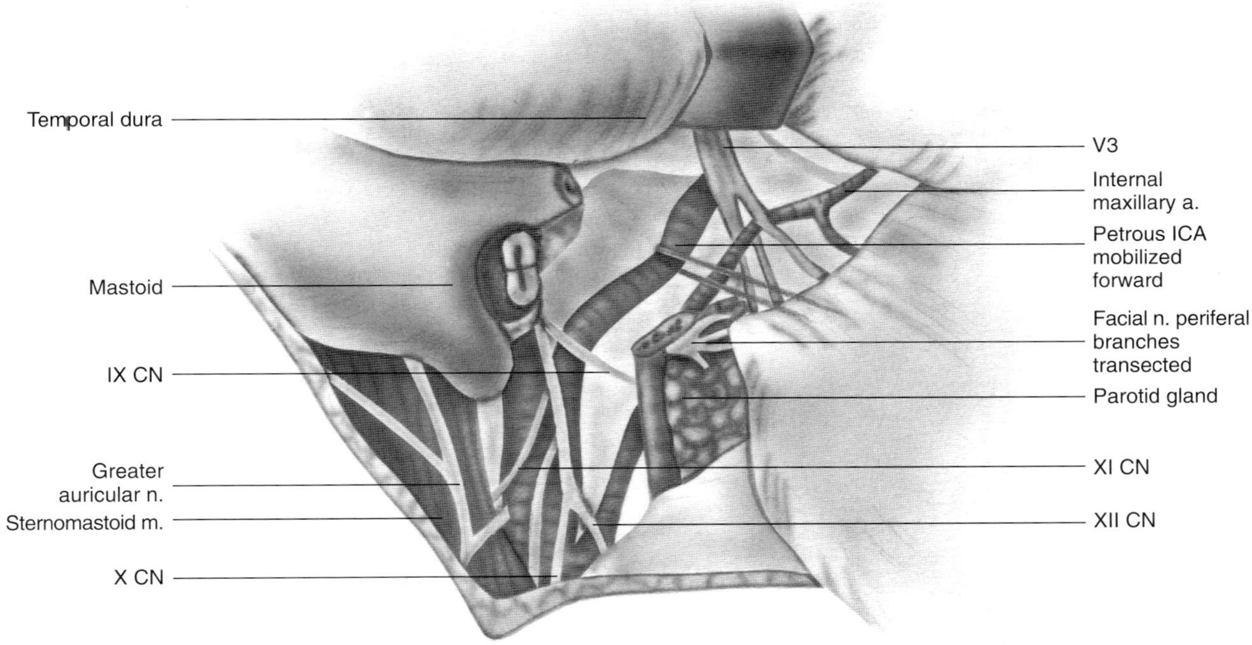

Fig. 10-8. Temporal craniotomy. The petrous internal carotid artery is displaced anteriorly. (Adapted from Seckar LN).

- A translabyrinthine approach to the internal auditory canal is performed if the mastoid is not involved by the tumor; if involved, a retrosigmoid or presigmoid approach to the tumor is performed (Figs. 10-9, 10-10).
- The acoustic facial nerve bundle is divided.
- The ICA is mobilized anteriorly and the temporal bone is released all at once, dividing the petrous bone of the carotic canal from the occipital bone and clivus with an osteotome or a drill (Fig. 10-11).
- When the tumor involves the venous system and the sigmoid sinus is not dominant, the jugu-

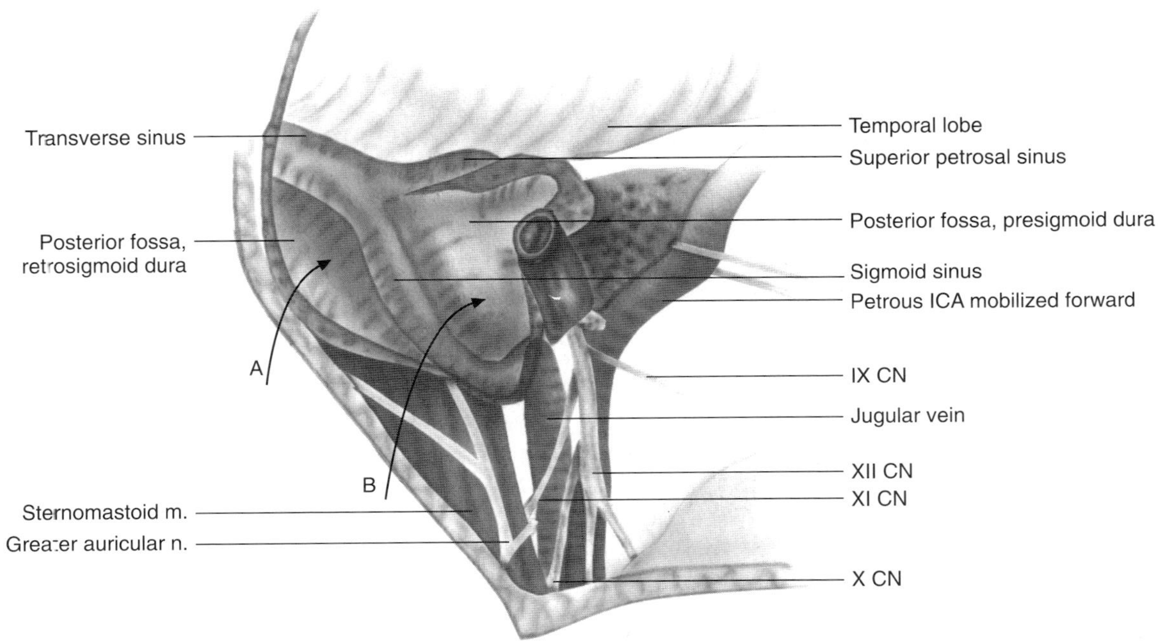

Fig. 10-9. When the mastoid is thought to be free of tumor, a translabyrinthine approach (A) is used. When the mastoid is thought to be involved by tumor, a presigmoid or retrosigmoid (B) intradural approach can be used.

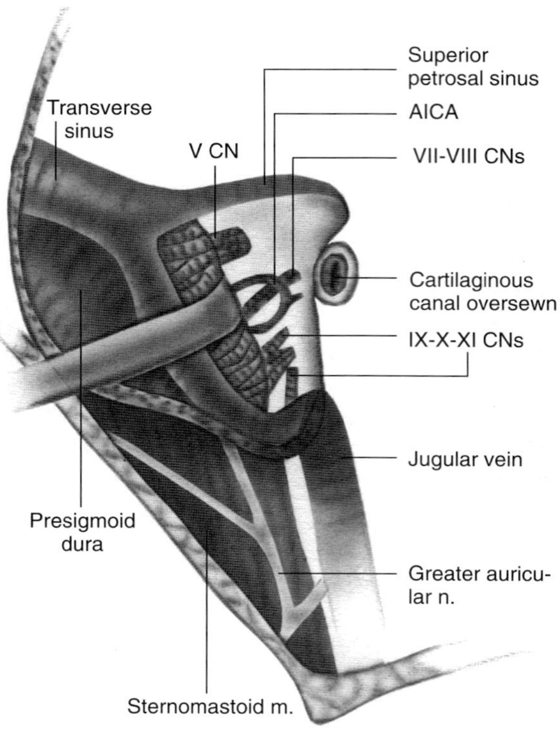

Fig. 10-10. A presigmoid (Figure) a retrosigmoid or a translabyrinthine approach can be used to expose the CPA and the porus acousticus.

lar bulb is ligated in the upper part of the neck and the sigmoid sinus is occluded with oxidized cellulose, without injuring Labbé's vein (see chapters 2, 34, 35, 36).

- In malignant tumors, the goal is en bloc resection of infiltrated petrous bone (Fig. 10-12 and Table 10-1).
- When the tumor involves the ICA, the surgical procedure depends on the preoperative ICA occlusion test (see chapter 16).
- When the dura of the middle and/or posterior fossa is involved, it is resectioned, and a limited resection of the temporal lobe and cerebellum may be performed. The dural defect is repaired with a fascia lata patch.
- The facial nerve is repaired with a graft (see chapters 13, 14). If the IX, XI, and XII cranial nerves have been injured during dissection, they are repaired with a neural graft (Fig. 10-13).
- The sternocleidomastoid, temporalis, splenius capitis and semispinalis muscles are sutured together to fill the defect and protect the dural closure (Fig. 10-14).
- Superior and inferior drains are positioned.

A lumbar drain is positioned and kept in place to reduce CSF pressure with intermittent drainage for almost two days.

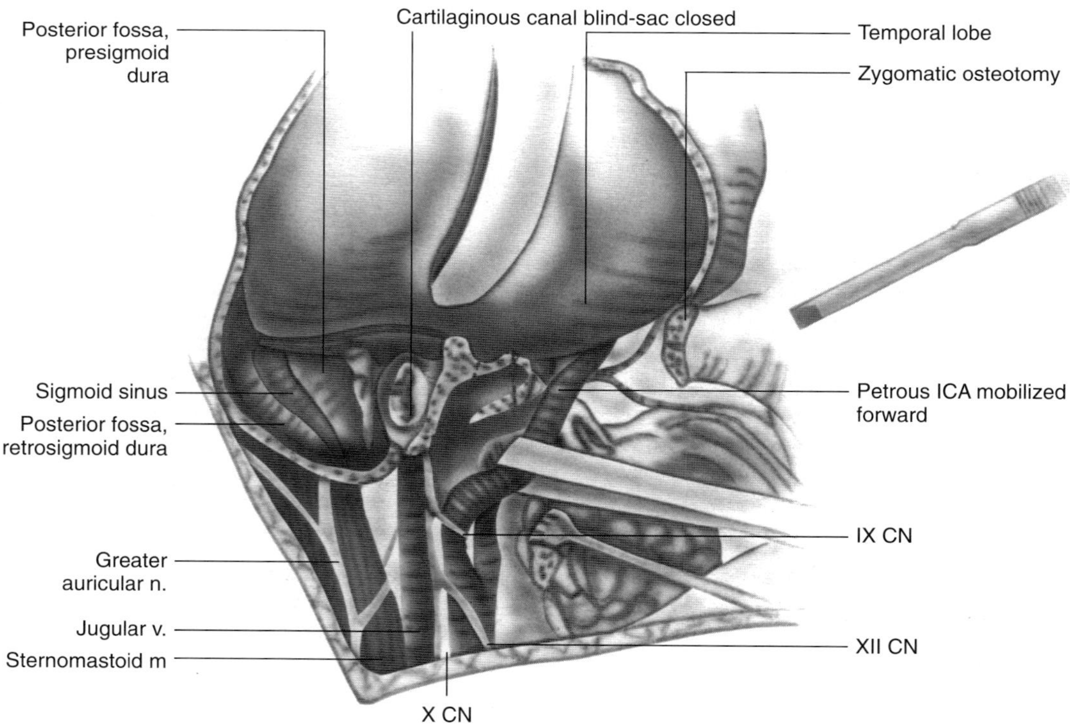

Fig. 10-11. The internal carotid artery is mobilized. An osteotome is used to remove the horizontal petrous carotid canal so as to release the temporal bone specimen. (Adapted from Prasad S, Janecka IP).

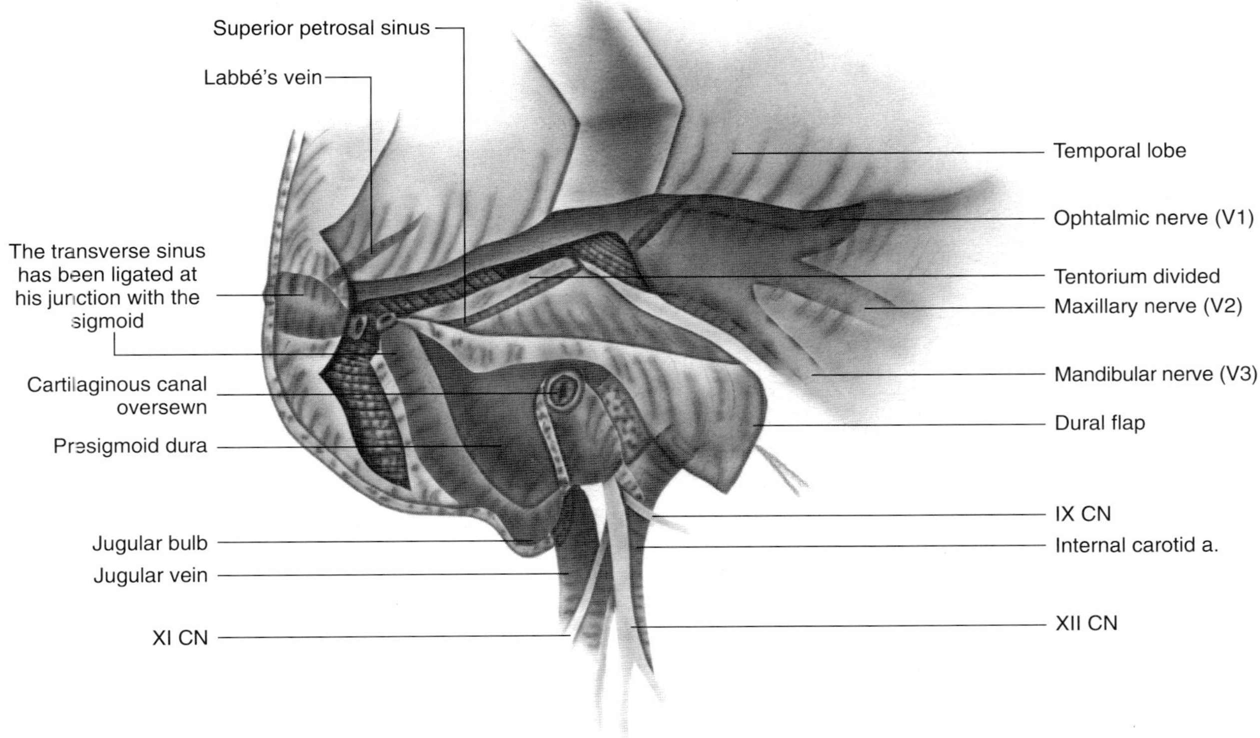

Fig. 10-12. A suboccipital craniotomy is performed. If needed, all the presigmoid dura can be exposed. The transverse sinus is ligated. The temporal and retrosigmoid dura are opened. The tentorium is opened along the inferior edge of V3. The superior petrosal sinus is cut, when needed. When the SPS is not involved, it may be preserved by changing the dural incisions. (Adapted from Sekhar LN).

POSTOPERATIVE MANAGEMENT

After surgery, the patient is transferred to the intensive care unit. If a serious paresis of the IX and X cranial nerve becomes evident, a tracheostomy and/or gastrostomy may be required, especially in older patients. During the time needed for the facial rehabilitation to become effective, the eye is protected with a tarsorrhaphy (see chapter 15). Antibiotic treatment is prolonged for a week, and anticonvulsant therapy is prolonged for 7 months. External beam radiation treatment follows the operation.

Based on radiological and intraoperative evidence, the following classification of petrous bone tumors was proposed by Sekhar, Janecka, and Hirsch, following the proposal of Arena; Lederman; Ariyan; Goodwin and Jesse (Table 10-1).

Table 10-1. Degrees of Petrous Bone Tumors.

Grade 1	Tumor infiltrates only part of the petrous bone.
Grade 2	Tumor infiltrates the entire petrous bone.
Grade 2a	Tumor infiltrates the petrous ICA.
Grade 3	Tumor extends beyond the petrous temporal bone and infiltrates the adjacent cranial base (3a), the dura (3b), the infratemporal upper cervical soft tissue (3c) and the cavernous sinus (3d).

CONCLUSIONS

Once a no man's land, surgery of temporal bone malignant tumors still defies definitive statements. Lateral temporal bone resection (LTBR)

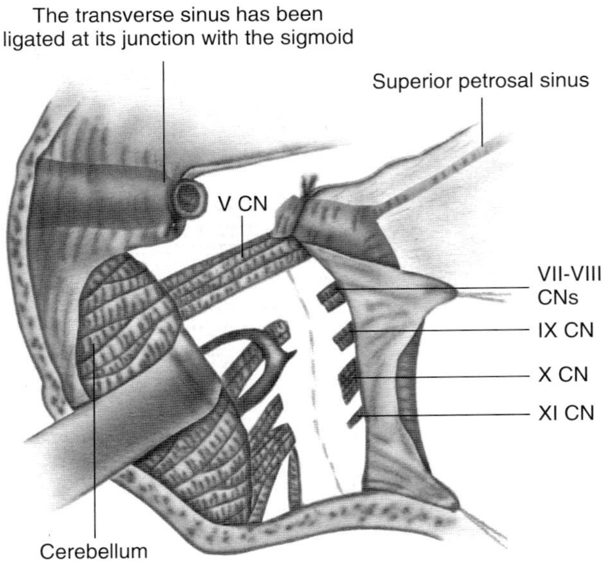

Fig. 10-13. At the end of the procedure, CNs VII-XI have been transected. They will be grafted with the greater auricular nerve or the sural nerve. (Adapted from Sekhar LN).

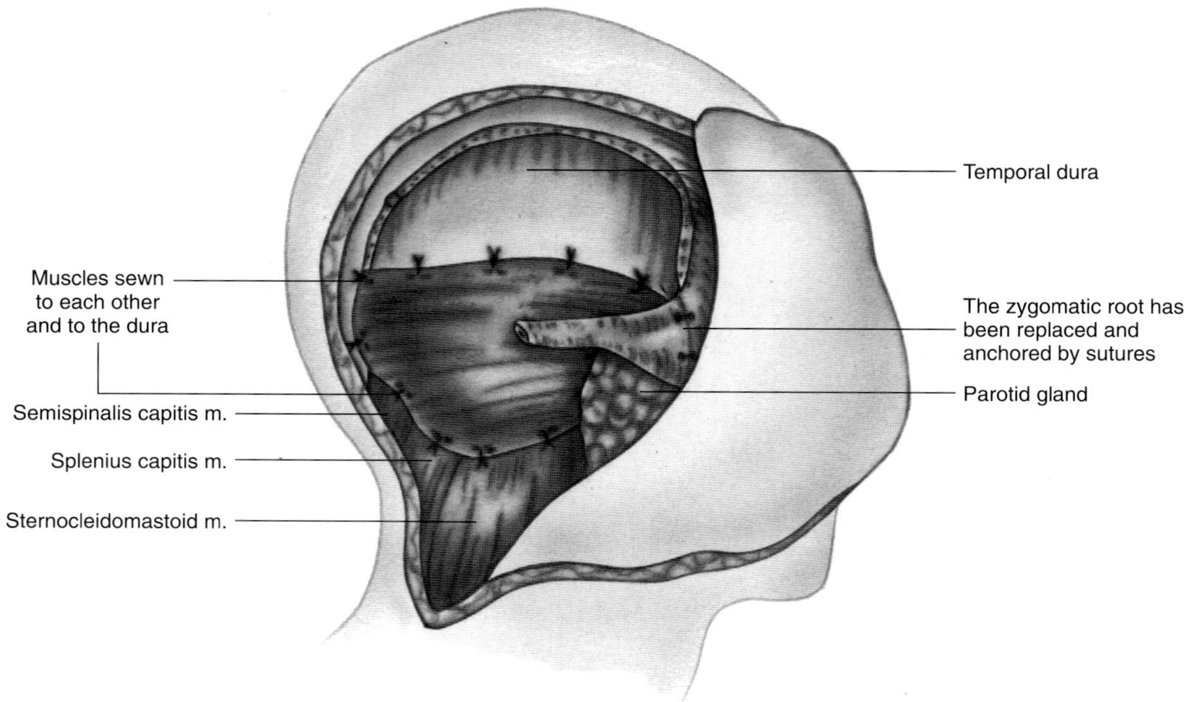

Fig. 10-14. Muscles are rotated and sutured to each other and to the dura to seal the surgical defect. (Adapted from Sekhar LN).

is preferable to subtotal temporal bone resection (STBR) for malignant tumors of the external ear, since it obtains the same 5-year survival rate (around 50%) with lower morbidity. The STBR, on the other hand, provides better results in tumors extended to the middle ear (40%).

In tumors spread to the petrous apex and even outside the temporal bone, the benefits of surgery are still questionable. It could prolong life, though not for more than two years, and the quality of life must also be taken into account. We owe a debt of gratitude to the pioneers (Sekhar, Janecka, Sen, Prasad, and others) who led the way to the present and future treatment of once inoperable tumors.

REFERENCES

Adams CL, Paparella MM, Fiky FM: Primary and metastatic tumors of the temporal bone. Laryngoscope 81: 1273-1285, 1971.

Adams WS, Morfison R: On primary carcinoma of the middle ear and mastoid. J Laryngol Otol 69: 115-131, 1955.

Arena S, Keen M: Carcinoma of the middle ear and temporal bone. Am J Otol 9: 351-356, 1988.

Arena S: Tumor surgery of the temporal bone. Laryngoscope 84: 645-670, 1974.

Ariyan S, Sasaki CT, Spencer D: Radical en-bloc resection of the temporal bone. Am J Surg 142: 443-447, 1981.

Arriaga M, Curfin H, Takahashi H, et all: Staging proposal for external auditory meatus carcinoma based on preoperative clinical examination and computed tomography findings. Ann Otol Rhinol Laryngol 99: 714-721, 1990.

Arriaga M, Hirsch BE, Kamerer DB, Myers EN: Squamous cell carcinoma of the external auditory meatus (canal). Otolaryngol Head Neck Surg 101: 330-337, 1989.

Arthur K: Radiotherapy in carcinoma of the middle ear and auditory canal. J Laryngol Otol 90: 753-762, 1976.

Barnes EB: Carcinoma of the ear. Proc R Soc Med 23: 1231-1234, 1930.

Beal DD, Lindsay JR, Ward PH: Radiation-induced carcinoma of the mastoid. Arch Otolaryngol Head Neck Surg 81: 9-16, 1965.

Bergetedt HF, Lind MG: Temporal bone scintigraphy. Acta Otolaryngol (Stockh) 89: 465-473,1980.

Boland J: The management of carcinomas of the middle ear. Radiology 80: 285, 1963.

Bradley WH, Maxwell JH: Neoplasms of the middle ear and mastoid. Report of 54 cases. Laryngoscope 54: 533-556, 1954.

Brooker GB: Bilateral middle ear carcinomas associated with Waldenstrom's macroglobulinemia. Ann Otol Rhinol Laryngol 91: 299-303, 1982.

Buckmam W, Barre W: Carcinoma of the middle ear and mastoid. Ann Otol Rhinol Laryngol 52: 194-201, 1943.

Campbell E, Volk BM, Burkland CW: Total resection of the temporal bone for malignancy of the middle ear. Ann Surg 134: 397-404, 1951.

Clairmont AA, Conley JJ: Primary carcinoma of the mastoid bone. Am Otol Rhinol Laryngol 86: 306-309, 1977.

Clark LJ, Narola AA, Morgan DAL, Bradley PJ: Squamous carcinoma of the temporal bone: A revised staging. J Laryngol Otol 105: 346-348, 1991.

Coleman CC, Khuri A: A rational treatment for advanced cancer of the external ear and temporal bone. VA Med Monthly 86: 21-24, 1959.

Coleman CC: Removal of the temporal bone for cancer. Am J Surg 112: 583-590, 1966.

Colledge L: Two cases of malignant disease of the temporal bone. J Laryngol Otol 58: 251-254, 1943.

Conley J: Cancer of the middle ear and temporal bone. NY State J Med 1575-1579, 1974.

Conley J, Nosrack AJ: The surgical treatment of malignant tumors of the ear and temporal bone. Arch Otolaryngol Head Neck Surg 71: 635-652, 1960.

Conley J, Schuller DE: Malignancies of the ear. Laryngoscope 86: 1147-1163, 1976.
Conley J, Novack N: Surgical treatment of cancer of the ear and temporal bone. Trans Am Acad Ophthalmol Otolaryngol 64: 83-92, 1960.
Coodman ME: Middle ear and mastoid neoplasms. Ann Otol Rhinol Laryngol 80: 419-424, 1971.
Coodwin WJ, Jesse RH: Malignant neoplasms of the external auditory canal and temporal bone. Arch Otolaryngol Head Neck Surg 106: 675-679, 1980.
Corey JP, Nelson E, Crawford M, et al: Metastatic vaginal carcinoma to the temporal bone. Am J Otol 12: 128-131, 1991.
Crabtree JA, Britton BH, Pierce MK: Carcinoma of the external auditory canal. Laryngoscope 86: 405-415, 1976.
Cundy RL, Sando I, Hemevay WG: Middle ear extension of nasopharyngeal carcinoma via the eustachian tube. Arch Otolaryngol Head Neck Surg 98: 131-133, 1973.
Figi FA, Weisman PA: Cancer and chemodectoma in the middle ear and mastoid. JAMA 156: 1157-1162,1954.
Frazer JS: Malignant disease of the external acoustic meatus and middle ear. Proc R Soc Med 23: 1235-1244, 1930.
Frew I, Finney R: Neoplasms of the middle ear. J Laryngol Otol 77: 415-421, 1963.
Gacek RR, Goodman M: Management of malignancy of the temporal bone. Laryngoscope 87: 1622-1634, 1977.
Gacek RR: Management of temporal bone carcinoma. Trans Penn Acad Otolaryngol Ophthalmol 32: 67-71, 1978.
Graham MD, Sataloff RT, Kemink J, McGillicuddy JF: En bloc resection of the temporal bone and carotid artery for malignant tumors of the ear and temporal bone. Laryngoscope 94: 528-533, 1984.
Greer JA, Body DTR, Weitland LH: Neoplasms of the temporal bone. J Otolaryngol 5: 391-398, 1978.
Grossman AA, Domelly WA, Smithan MF: Carcinoma of the middle ear and mastoid process. Ann Otol Rhinol Laryngol 56: 709-721, 1947.
Hahn SS, Kim JA, Goodchild N, Constable WC: Carcinoma of the middle ear and external auditory canal. Int J Rad Oncol Biol Phys 9: 1003-1007, 1983.
Hanna DC, Richardson GS, Caisford JC: A suggested technique for resection of the temporal bone. Am J Surg 114: 553-558, 1967.
Haughey BH, Gates GA, Skerhut HE, Broztn WE: Cerebral shift after lateral craniofacial resection and flap reconstruction. Otolaryngol Head Neck Surg 101: 79-86, 1989.
Hilding DA, Selker R: Total resection of the temporal bone for carcinoma. Arch Otolaryngol Head Neck Surg 89: 98-107, 1969.
Hiraide F, Inouye T, Ishii T: Primary squamous cell carcinoma of the middle ear invading the cochlea: A histopathologic case report. Ann Otol Rhinol Laryngol 92: 290-294,1983.
Holmes KS: The treatment of carcinoma of the middle ear by the 4MV linear accelerator. Proc R Soc Med 53: 242-244, 1960.
Hutcheon JR: Experiences with aural carcinoma over the past six years. Med J Aust 2:406-407, 1966.
Jahn AF, Farkashidy J, Berman JM: Metastatic tumors in the temporal bone. A pathophysiologic study. J Otolaryngol 8: 85-95,1979.
Janecka IP, Sekhar LN, Horton JA, Yonas H: Cerebral blood flow evaluation. In Cummings CW, Frederickson JM, Harlor LA, et al. (eds): Otolaryngology Head and Neck Surgery Update II. St. Louis, Mosby Year Book, 1990, pp 54-63.
Johns ME, Headington JT: Squamous cell carcinoma of the external auditory canal: A clinicopathologic study of 20 cases. Arch Otolaryngol Head Neck Surg 100: 45-49, 1974.
Katsarkas A, Seemayer L: Bilateral temporal bone metastases of a uterine cervix carcinoma. J Otolaryngol 5: 315-318, 1976.
Kenyon GS, Marks PV, Scholts CL, Dhillon R: Squamous cell carcinoma of the middle ear: A 25 year retrospective study. Ann Otol Rhinol Laryngol 94: 273-277, 1985.
Kinney SE, Wood BG: Malignancies of the external ear canal and temporal bone: Surgical techniques and results. Laryngoscope 97:158-164, 1987.
Kinney SE: Squamous cell carcinoma of the external auditory canal. Am J Otol 10: 111-116, 1989.
Kinney SE: Tumors of the external auditory canal, middle ear, mastoid and temporal bone. In Thawley SE, Panje WR, Batsakis TG, Lindberg RD (eds): Comprehensive Management of Head and Neck Tumors. Philadelphia, WB Saunders, 1987, p 182.
Lederman M: Malignant tumors of the ear. J Laryngol Otol 79: 85-119, 1965.
Lessor RW, Spector GJ, Diviens VR: Malignant tumors of the middle ear and external auditory canal. A 20 year review. Otolaryngol Head Neck Surg 96: 43-47, 1987.
Lewis JS, Page R: Radical surgery for malignant tumors of the ear. Arch Otolaryngol Head Neck Surg 83: 56-61, 1966.
Lewis JS, Parsons H: Surgery for advanced ear cancer. Ann Otol Rhinol Laryngol 67: 364-399, 1958.
Lewis JS: Squamous carcinoma of the ear. Arch Otolaryngol Head Neck Surg 97: 41-42, 1973.
Lewis JS: Surgical management of tumors of the middle ear and mastoid. J Laryngol Otol 97: 299-311, 1983.
Lewis JS: Temporal bone resection: Review of 100 cases. Arch Otolaryngol Head Neck Surg 101: 23-25, 1975.
Liebeskid MM: Primary carcinoma of the external auditory canal, middle ear and mastoid. Laryngoscope 61: 1173-1187, 1951.
Lindahl JWS: Carcinoma of the middle ear and meatus. J Laryngol Otol 69: 457-467, 1955.
Lodge WO, Jones HM, Smith MEN: Malignant tumors of the temporal bone. Arch Otolaryngol Head Neck Surg 61: 535-541, 1955.
Mattick WL, Mattick JW: Some experience in management of cancer of the middle ear and mastoid. Arch Otolaryngol Head Neck Surg 53: 610-621, 1951.
McCrea RS: Radical surgery for carcinoma of the middle ear. Laryngoscope 82: 1514-1523, 1972.
Mems RG, Gersten J: Primary carcinoma of the mastoid process. Am Otol Rhinol Laryngol 62: 93-100, 1953.
Meyerhoff WL, Mickey BE, Roland PS, Drummond JE: Magnetic resonance imaging in the diagnosis of temporal bone and skull base lesions. Am J Otol 10(2): 121-137, 1989.
Michaels L, Wells M: Squamos cell carcinomas of the middle ear. Clin Otolaryngol 5: 235-248, 1980.
Miller D, Silverstein H, Gacek RR: Cryosurgical treatment of carcinoma of the ear. Trans Am Acad Ophthalmol Otolaryngol 76: 1363-1367, 1972.
Miller D: Cancer of the external auditory meatus. Laryngoscope 65: 448-461, 1955.
Nadol JB, Schukecht HE: Obliteration of the mastoid in the treatment of tumors of the temporal bone. Ann Otol Rhinol Laryngol 93: 6-12, 1984.
Newhart H: Primary carcinoma of the middle ear: Report of a case. Laryngoscope 27: 543-555, 1917.
Parsons H, Lewis JS: Subtotal resection of the temporal bone for cancer of the ear. Cancer 7: 995-1001, 1954.
Peele JC, Hauser GH: Primary carcinoma of the external auditory canal and middle ear. Arch Otolaryngol Head Neck Surg 34: 254-266, 1941.
Prasad S, Janecka IP: Efficacy of surgical treatments for squamous cell carcinoma of the temporal bone. Otol Head Neck Surg 110:270-280, 1994.
Ramsden M, Bulman CH, Lorigan BP: Osteoradionecrosis of the temporal bone. J Laryngol Otol 89: 941-955, 1975.
Robison GA: Malignant tumors of the ear. Laryngoscope 41: 467-473, 1931.

Rosenwasser H: Neoplasms involving the middle ear. Arch Otolaryngol Head Neck Surg 32: 38-53, 1940.

Ruben RJ, Thaler SU, Holzer N: Radiation induced carcinoma of the temporal bone. Laryngoscope 87: 1613-1621, 1977.

Sasaki CT, Leder SB, Petcu L, Freidman CD: Longitudinal voice quality changes following Isshiki thyroplasty Type I: The Yale experience. Laryngoscope 100: 849-852, 1990.

Sataloff RT, Myers DL, Lowry LD, Spiegel JR: Total temporal bone resection for squamous cell carcinoma. Otolaryngol Head Neck Surg 96: 4-14, 1987.

Sataloff RT, Roberts BR, Myers DL, Spiegel JR: Total temporal bone resection. A radical but life-saving procedure. AORN J 48(5): 932-948, 1988.

Scholl LA: Neoplasms involving the middle ear. Arch Otolaryngol Head Neck Surg 22: 548-553, 1935.

Schuknecht HE, Allam AF, Murakami Y: Pathology of secondary malignant tumors of the temporal bone. Ann Otol Rinol Laryngol 77: 5-22, 1968.

Schusterman MA, Kroll SS: Reconstruction strategy for temporal bone and lateral facial defects. Ann Plastic Surg 26: 233-294,1983.

Sekhar LN, Pomeranz S, Janecka JP et al: Temporal bone neoplasm: A report on 20 surgically treated cases. J Neurosurg 76:578-587, 1992.

Sinha PP, Aziz HI: Treatment of carcinoma of the middle ear. Ther Rad 126: 485-487,1978.

Sorenson H: Cancer of the middle ear and mastoid. Acta Radiol 54: 460-468, 1960.

Spector JC: Management of temporal bone carcinomas: A therapeutic analysis of two groups of patients and long term follow-up. Otolaryngol Head Neck Surg 104: 58-66, 1991.

Spencer FR: Malignant disease of the ear. Arch Otolaryngol Head Neck Surg 28: 916-940, 1938.

Stokes HB: Primary malignant tumors of the temporal bone. Arch Otolaryngol Head Neck Surg 32: 1023-1030, 1990.

Tabb HG, Komet H, McLaurin JW: Cancer of the external auditory canal: Treatment with radical mastoidectomy and radiation. Laryngoscope 74: 634-643, 1964.

Tucker WN: Cancer of the middle ear. Cancer 16: 642-650, 1965.

Vize C: Laryngeal metastasis to the temporal bone causing facial paralysis. J Laryngol Otol 88: 175-177, 1974.

Wagenfield DJH, Keane T, Norstrand AWP, Bryce DP: Primary carcinoma involving the temporal bone: Analysis of 25 cases. Laryngoscope 90: 912-919, 1980.

Wahl JW, Gromet MT: Carcinoma of the middle ear and mastoid. Arch Otolaryngol Head Neck Surg 58: 121-126, 1953.

Wang CC: Radiation therapy in the management of carcinoma of the external auditory canal, middle ear or mastoid. Ther Rad 116: 713-715, 1975.

Ward GE, Loch WE, Lawrence W: Radical operation for carcinoma of the external auditory canal and middle ear. Am J Surg 82: 169-178, 1951.

Wiatrak BJ, Pensak ML: Rhabdomyosarcoma of the ear and temporal bone. Laryngoscope 99(11): 1188-1192, 1989.

Wilson CE, Shofstall WH: Carcinoma of the ear. Arch Otolaryngol Head Neck Surg 51: 724-738, 1950.

Yamada S, Schuh FD, Marsrin JS, Perot PL: En bloc subtotal temporal bone resection for cancer of the external ear. J Neurosurg 39: 370-379, 1973.

11

Complications of otologic surgery

Judgment is the result of experience, experience is the result of bad judgment.

SHEEHY J.

FACIAL NERVE TRAUMA

Post-operatively, if the continuity of the facial nerve has been preserved, the following events may take place:

– Normal

I. Neuroapraxy

Everything seems to be in order, but the nerve does not conduct well and the reason is not known. Recovery begins within two weeks.

II. Axonotmesis

Some axons are altered and die, and they take time to regenerate. Recovery begins within two months.

III. Neurotmesis

The neural sheath has been altered. The sheath may grow inside the axons, so that synkinesis may later appear. Recovery begins within 6 months.

If we are certain that the facial nerve has been preserved intact, but paralysis is observed post-operatively, it is necessary to wait at least a year before performing a hypoglossal-facial anastomosis. In fact, in most cases, recovery occurs or at least begins during this time period.

At times there may be a complete post-operative paralysis, though the nerve is intact. In these cases recovery should be expected to leave relics of weakness in the facial musculature and synkinesis.

If no hypotony is seen in the facial musculature when the patient awakens, or if it is slight or slowed, an almost complete functional recovery may be expected (see chapters 12, 13, 14, 15) (Figs. 11-1, 11-2, 11-3, 11-4, 11-5, 11-6) (Table 11-1).

LABYRINTHINE TRAUMA

The labyrinthine lesion may cause trauma to the semicirculars canals or the oval window (Fig. 11-7). Semicircular canal trauma may be due to the inadvertent exposure of a fistula during middle ear cholesteatoma surgery or to a traumatic fenestration with the drill. The fistula must be covered with fascia and bone wax as quickly as possible. In surgical treatment for Mèniére disease, the posterior semicircular canal must not be blue-lined, since the labyrinth is very fragile.

VASCULAR INJURY

The sigmoid sinus, superior and inferior petrosal sinus, jugular bulb and internal carotid artery may be injured (Figs. 11-8, 11-9, 11-10). (see (chapter 28, on the treatment of surgical complications). Sometimes a misdiagnosed high jugular bulb is injured in middle ear surgery (Figs. 11-11, 11-12). The internal carotid artery may be injured when it takes an anomalous course through the temporal bone, through the inferior tympanic canaliculus (Figs. 11-13, 11-14, 11-15). In this case, an intraoperative repair may be needed. The first steps to follow are:

- Pack gently with Surgicel.
- Block the eustachian tube orifice.
- Pack the ear canal.
- Prevent hypotension.

CSF LEAK IN MIDDLE EAR SURGERY

A CSF leak may occur during a stapedectomy (gusher), for a rare (1/10.000) CSF hypertension. In this case a perilymph leak immediately fills the middle ear and the IAC.

Once the surgeon notes CSF leaking from the stapedotomy, the following maneuvers must be performed:

Table 11-1. The most common complications of otologic surgery.

- Facial nerve trauma (chapter 12-15)
- Labyrinthine trauma
- Vascular injury
- CSF leak

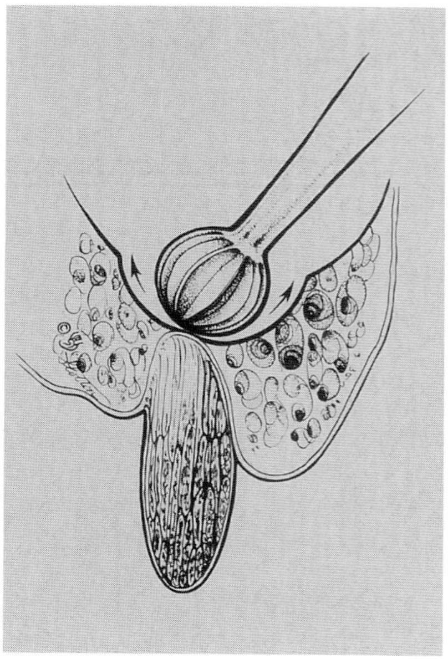

Fig. 11-1. The burr used for facial n. exposure should be larger then the underlying fallopian canal, to avoid slipping of the burr and lesioning of the nerve.

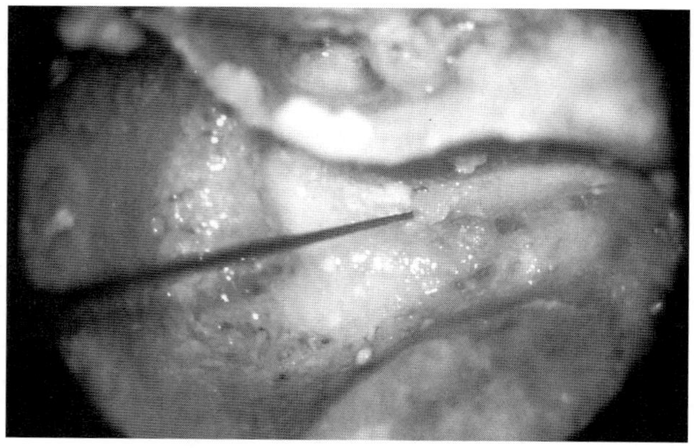

Fig. 11-2. Lesion of the facial n. (mastoid part).

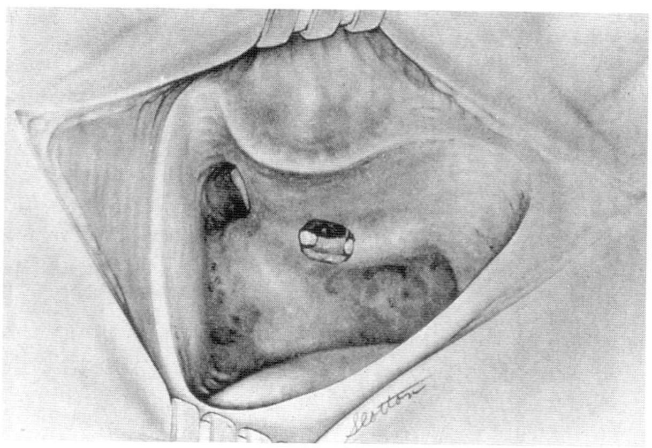

Fig. 11-3. Lesion of the facial n. (mastoid part).

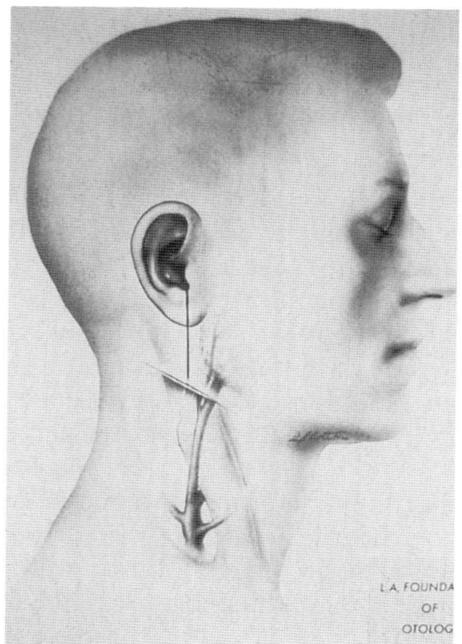

Fig. 11-4. Harvesting of the greater auricular n.

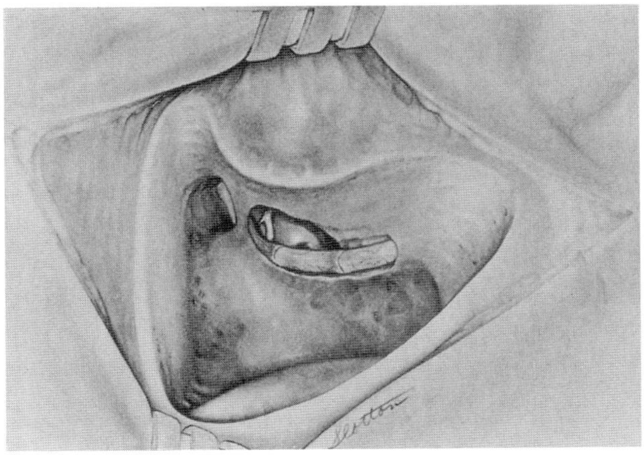

Fig. 11-5. The facial n. stumps are approximated, when possible.

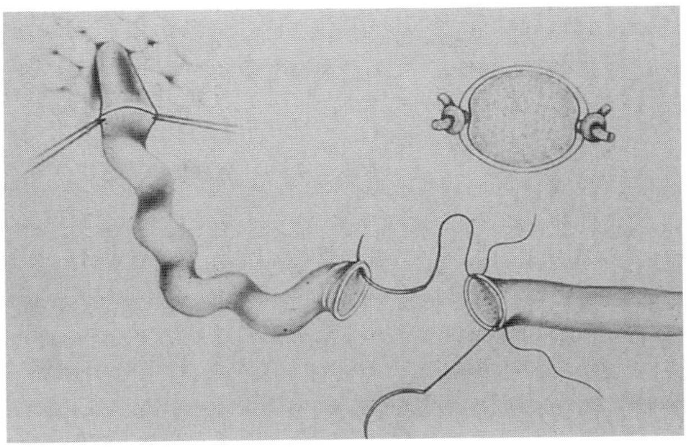

Fig. 11-6. Interposition graft: epineurial suture.

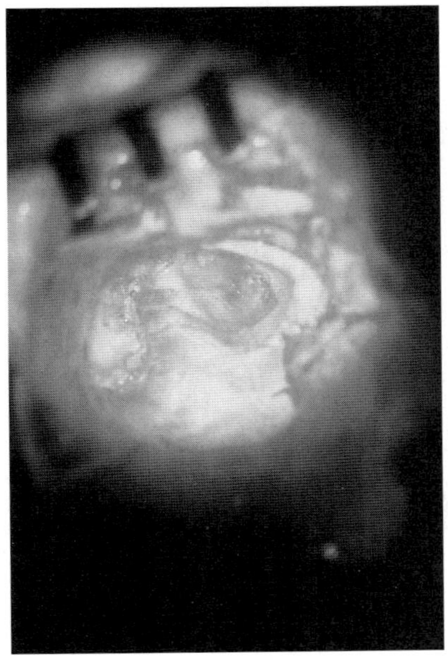

Fig. 11-7. Chronic otitis media with cholesteatoma: labyrinthine fistula. The most common location for labyrinthine fistulas to occur is in the lateral semicircular canal. The cholesteatoma matrix can be left in place and covered by temporalis fascia.

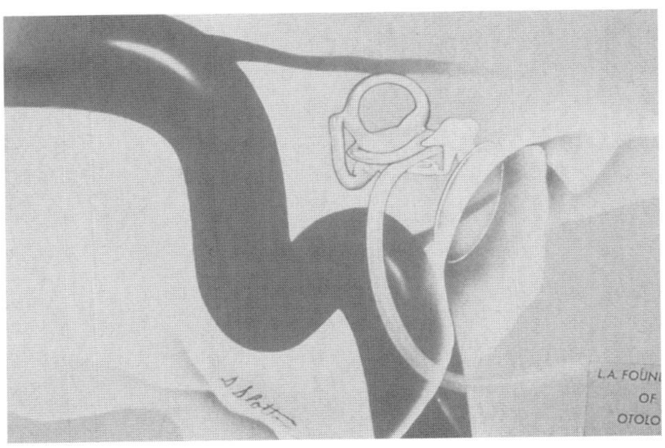

Fig. 11-8. Temporal bone and neurovascular structures.

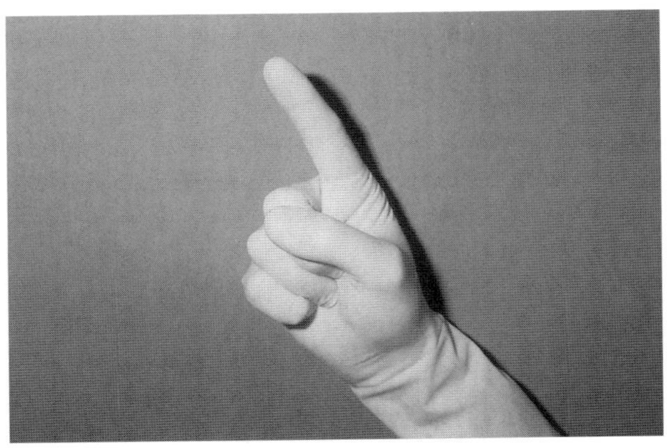

Fig. 11-9. When the sigmoid sinus is accidently opened, the bleeding can be quickly stopped with a finger, in order to reduce the blood loss, while preparing a large plug of Surgicel.

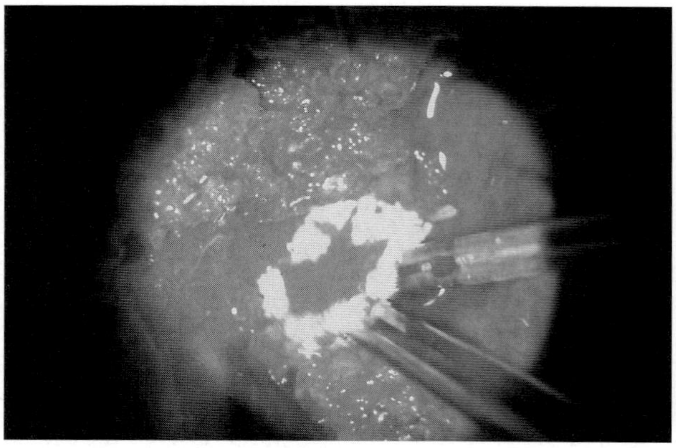

Fig. 11-10. A large plug of Surgicel is used to pack the injured vessel extraluminally: sigmoid sinus or jugular bulb. The bleeding is then controlled to continue the surgery (see Chapter 28, Management of surgical complications).

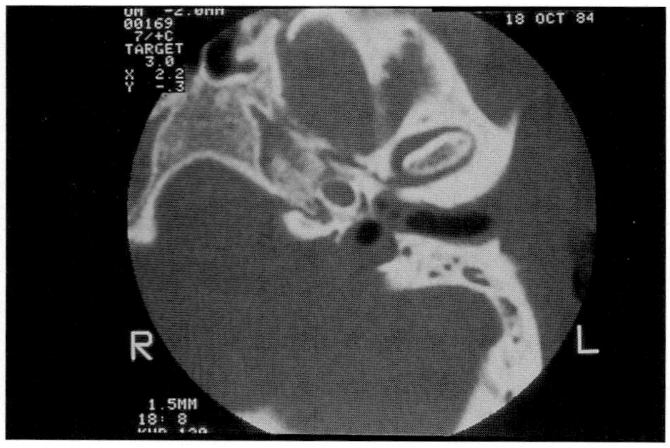

Fig. 11-11. CT. High jugular bulb: the jugular bulb occupies the middle ear.

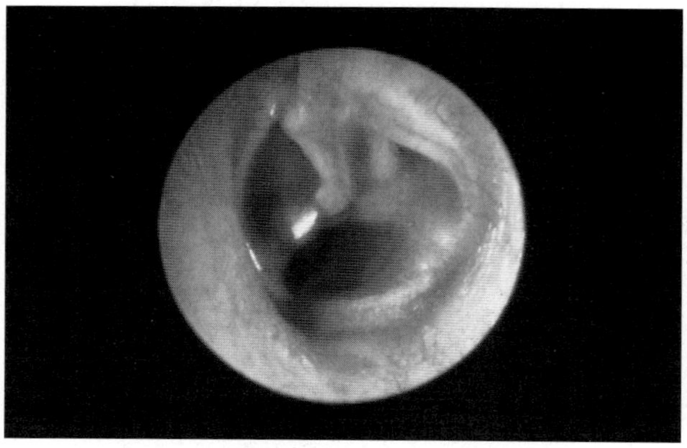

Fig. 11-12. High jugular bulb: otoscopic appearance of the right ear.

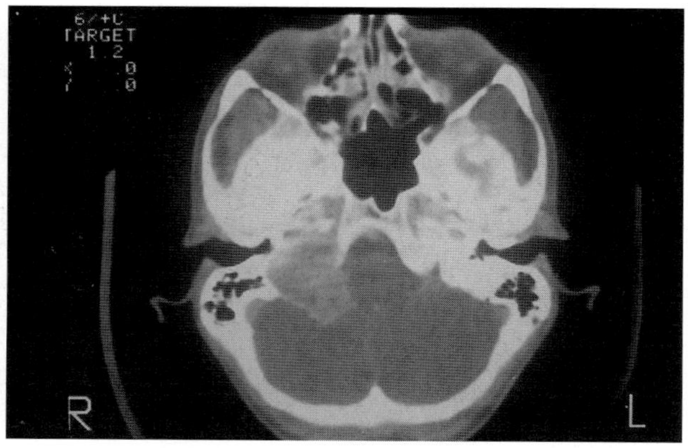

Fig. 11-14. CT. Exposed carotid in the right temporal bone.

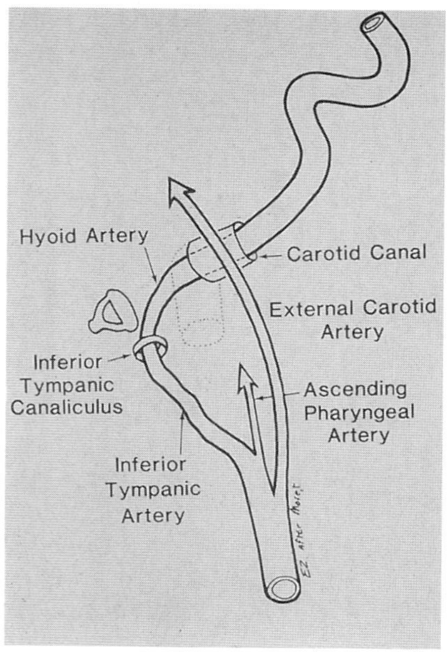

Fig. 11-13. Embryologic development of the carotid artery. The petrous carotid artery may take an anomalous course through the temporal bone, along the inferior tympanic artery and be exposed in the middle ear cavity.

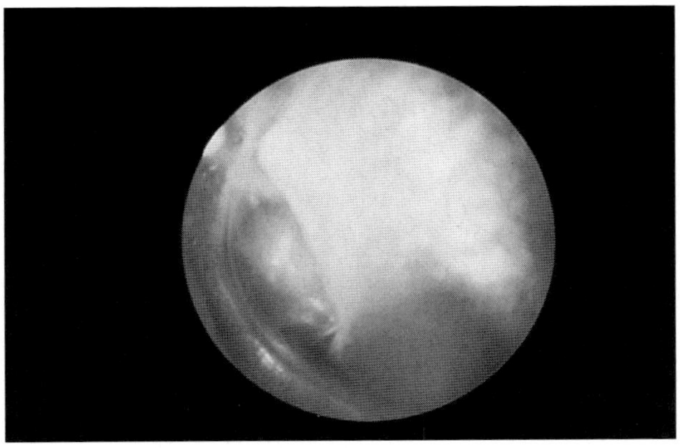

Fig. 11-15. Otoscopic appearance of an exposed carotid artery.

- Plug the oval window with Surgicel and then tamponade with Gelfoam. Tamponading with cotton is not suggested due to the risk of losing filaments in the labyrinth.
- Induce general anesthesia. Position a lumbar subarachnoid drain, to decrease the pressure on the perilymph.
- Incise the skin over the linea temporalis. Harvest temporalis muscle fascia. Create a 0.8 mm. or greater stapedotomy. Close the stapedotomy with temporalis fascia and insert the prosthesis.
- Elevate the patient's head 30° and limit ambulation in the postoperative period.
- Prescribe oral acetazolamide, 250 mg, four times a day, for 2 weeks.

A CSF leak may be a complication of neurootologic surgery (chapter 28).

REFERENCES

Effron MZ, Black FO, Burns D: Tension pneumocephalus complicating the treatment of postoperative CSF otorrhea. Arch Otolaryngol Head Neck Surg 107: 579-580, 1981.

Epstein GH, Weisman RA, Zwillenberg S, Schreiber A: A new autologous fibrinogen-based adhesive for otologic surgery. Ann Otol Rhinol Laryngol 95: 40-45, 1986.

Graf CJ, Gross CE, Beck DW: Complication of spinal drainage in the management of cerebrospinal fluid fistula: Report of three cases. J Neurosurg 54: 392-395, 1981.

Hoffman RA: Cerebrospinal fluid leak following acoustic neuroma removal. Laryngoscope 104:40-58, 1994.

House JL, Hitselberger WE, House WF: Wound closure and cerebrospinal fluid leak after translabyrinthine surgery. Am J Otol 4: 126-128, 1982.

Rodgers GK, Luxford WM: Factors affecting the development of cerebrospinal fluid leak after translabyrinthine acoustic tumor surgery. Laryngoscope 103: 959-962, 1993.

Sierra DH, Nissen AJ, Welch J: The use of fibrin glue in intracranial procedures: Preliminary results. Laryngoscope 100: 360-363, 1990.

Snow RB, Kuhel W, Martin SB: Prolonged spinal drainage after the resection of tumors of the skull base: A cautionary note. Neurosurgery 28: 880-883, 1991.

Swanson SE, Chandler WF, Kocan MJ: Flow-regulated continuous spinal drainage in the management of cerebrospinal fluid fistulas. Laryngoscope 95: 104-106, 1985.

Swanson SE, Kocan MJ, Chandler WF: Flow-regulated continuous spinal drainage: Technical note with case report. Neurosurgery 9: 163-165, 1981.

12

Facial nerve alterations

FACIAL NERVE ALTERATIONS

The facial nerve is the cranial nerve most frequently subject to paralysis. Peripheral paralysis is the most frequent due to the nerve's path in most of the inflexible canal (the fallopian canal) and to its contiguity with areas at risk for infections or tumors, such as the middle ear, the parotid, and the soft tissues. The causes and degree of facial paralysis are expressed in the Tables 12-1, 12-2.

ETIOLOGY

LESIONS OF THE SUPERIOR MOTOR NEURON

- These are lesions of the body of the superior motor neuron in the cortex, or of its axons projecting to the facial nucleus.
- Incomplete paralysis is seen, involving mainly the muscles of the lower half of the face, since the muscles of the upper half are innervated by homolateral and contralateral (decussated) fibers.
- Neither muscular atrophy nor loss of facial expression is seen, whereas voluntary movement is altered. The involuntary movements are preserved because the extrapyramidal system, which is responsible for involuntary facial movements, is spared.

NUCLEAR LESIONS

- These are lesions of the inferior motor neuron; the term "nuclear lesions" includes lesions both of the facial nucleus and its axons, in all parts of its nerve path. These lesions have in common the loss of both voluntary and involuntary movements, ipsilateral to the lesion.
- Among the pontine lesions that may provoke an involvement of the motor nuclei of nerve VII are glioma (neurogliocytoma), poliomyelitis, multiple sclerosis, brainstem infarction, and hemorrhage.

LESIONS OF THE INTRACRANIAL TRACT

- Lesions of the intracranial tract involve the part of the nerve between the cerebellopontine angle and the internal auditory canal.
- The most frequent alteration of the cerebellopontine angle is acoustic neuroma, which generally originates in the vestibular nerve, inside the internal auditory meatus. There may be various other reasons for endocranial extension, at times without other neurological signs. Other pathologies to consider are meningiomas, schwannomas of nerves V and VII, epidermoid tumors, cerebellar or pontine gliomas, local or metastatic carcinomas, lymphomas, sarcoidosis, fungal infections, and aneurisms.
- The nerve may be damaged in the internal auditory canal due to fractures irradiating from the petrous ridge.

Symptomatology

In clinical practice, the Otorhynolaryngologist most often observes peripheral facial paralysis. Paralysis involving the central nervous system is also frequent.

- When the corticobulbar structures are involved, complete paralysis of the lower half of the face may be seen, with the forehead spared due to the double innervation that the upper half of the face receives from direct or crossed fibers.
- We may classify the paralysis according to the degree of corticobulbar involvement. When the lesion is at the level of the cortex or just subcortical, the paralysis is observed when attempting to contract the face. Thus the patient is asked to open his eyelids, close his eyes, wrinkle his nose, and smile, looking for possible asymmetric facial contractions. Having the patient perform repetitive movements (e.g. batting his eyelids) may help to distinguish a subtle paralysis, demonstrating a slowed contraction time or fatigue.
- In deeper lesions involving corticobulbar elements, the patient can voluntarily activate facial

Table 12-1. Causes of facial paralysis.

- **Congenital**
  Bell's Paralysis, myotonic distrophy, Moebius syndrome, Melkersson's disease, familiar.
- **Contagious**
  Meningitis (acute and tubercular), malaria, leprosy, contagious mononucleosis, viral diseases (Coxsackie, Chickenpox, Measles, Herpes Zoster, Flu), otitis media, mastoiditis, malignant external otitis, encephalitis, sarcoidosis.
- **Traumatic**
  Skull base fracture, facial lesions, lesions penetrating the middle ear, height paralysis, forceps injuries at birth.
- **Metabolic**
  Diabetes, hypothyroidism, pregnancy.
- **Toxic**
  Thalidomide, tetanus, diphtheria.
- **Neurogical**
  Guillan Barre syndrome, Multiple Sclerosis, Serious Myasthenia, Opercular syndrome, Millard-Gubler syndrome.
- **Iatrogenic**
  Reactions to lockjaw shot, rabies vaccine, polio vaccine, mandibular block anesthesia.
- **Vascular**
  Wegener's granulomatosis, nodular periarteritis, sarcoidosis.
- **Tumors**
  Leukemia, cholesteatoma, jugular glomus, neurofibroma of VII and VIII CNs, meningioma, metastatic tumor, tympanic hemangioma, blastocytoma, sarcoma, osteopetrosis, facial nerve tumor (cylindroma), teratoma, Hand-Schuller-Christian's disease.

muscles, whereas spontaneous involuntary acts are associated with asymmetry of facial contractility (e.g. in laughing or smiling).

- Supranuclear lesions may be associated with deficit of the corticobulbar tract or other cranial nerves, and are manifested in movements of the throat or the tongue, or with a paralysis of the contralateral hemiface.
- In lesions underlying the facial nucleus, these motor deficits are on the same side as the alteration, given that the corticobulbar and corticospinal tracts are not yet decussated.
- If the corticobulbar lesion is near the facial nucleus (after decussation), homolateral flaccidity is seen in the contralateral limbs, indicating a pontine lesion.

PERIPHERAL NERVE LESIONS

- Peripheral nerve lesions involve the part of the nerve which goes from the acoustic foramen to the last branches.
- One of the most frequent causes of peripheral facial paralysis is Bell's paralysis. Its onset frequently follows exposure to cold, or is seen in diabetics. It is most frequent in middle-aged females. Viral causes are hypothesized (parotitis, measles, polio, parainfluenza) as are vascular causes (spasms of the arterioles supplying the nerve). Thus an edema is seen under the epineural sheath, which enlarges and crushes the nerve against the inflexible bone canal, causing nerve suffering.
- In herpes zoster oticus, or in the Ramsay-Hunt Syndrome, the virus, which may insinuate

Table 12-2. Degree of facial paralysis.

Alteration	Degree	Definition
1. Normal	I	Normal function
1-2.Slight disfunction, barely visible	II	Slight alteration visible only in a careful inspection. Complete closure of the eye with minimal effort, slight asymmetria of the glance with maximum effort; synkinesis barely visible, contractions or spasms absent.
2-3.Moderate dysfunction, easily seen.	III	Obvious but not disfiguring alteration. Inability to arch eyebrows may be seen. Complete closure of eyes. Mouth movement strong but asymmetrical with maximum effort. Synkinesis, spasms, contractions present but not disfiguring.
3.Moderately serious dysfunction	IV	Disfiguring alteration, inability to arch eyebrows. Eyes do not completely close, mouth asymmetric with maximum effort. Serious synkinesis, spasms, contractions.
3-4.Serious dysfunction	V	Barely perceptible movement. Incomplete closure of the eyes, slight movement in the corner of the mouth. Synkinesis, contractions, spasms generally absent
Complete paralysis	VI	No movement. Loss of tone. Absence of synkinesis, contractions, spasms.

On the left the old classification. On the right the new classification, proposed by House and Brackman and adopted by the Facial Nerve Disorders Committee of the American Academy of Otolaryngology-Head and Neck Surgery, 16 Sept. 1984.

silently into the geniculate ganglion after an infection, becomes active, causing geniculitis. Vesicles (blisters) are seen inside and around the ear, since the virus travels through the axons to afferent cutaneous neurons. The associated facial paralysis is a result both of the inflammation and of a direct viral invasion. The vesicles may spread to territory innervated by the trigeminal nerve. The geniculate ganglion is not always involved. Diphtheria and Guillan Barre Syndrome may cause facial paralysis, more frequently bilateral. Chronic purulent otitis media, both cholesteatomatous and hyperplastic, may injure the nerve with neurotoxins or by eroding the fallopian canal. One frequent cause is cranial trauma or the aftermath of an operation. The nerve is susceptible to stretching or injury at the level of the stylomastoid foramen. Tumors of the parotid gland may infiltrate the nerve, causing paralysis and local swelling.

Symptomatology
In complete monolateral peripheral facial nerve paralysis, facial asymmetry is seen, with lowering of the labial commissure, flattening of the nasolabial sulcus and the forehead wrinkles, enlarging of the palpebral slit, lid-lag, epiphora (stillicidium), deviation towards the healthy side of the buccal slit in the attempt to show teeth, rotation of the eyeball upward and outward (sign of Bell's paralysis). The corneal reflex is absent and the orbicular reflex of the eyelids is hypotonic to palpation.

FACIAL PARALYSIS IN CHILDREN

Among the causes of facial nerve paralysis in children is their high susceptibility to infection, the elevated incidence of temporal bone neoplasm, and the frequency of trauma (especially in boys)(Table 12-3).

CONGENITAL ABNORMALITIES

- Often anatomical deformities of the temporal bone can cause facial paralysis, which is manifested soon after birth. Among the causes are the absence of the fallopian canal in the middle ear, or its compression due to congenital abnormalities (e.g. craniofacial disostosis).
- X-rays exams will show the congenital anomaly since the bony part of the inner ear is clearly visible in newborns. What appears to be congenital facial paralysis may in reality be due to the development of a mass compressing the nerve, such as a congenital cholesteatoma or a meningioma. When X-rays do not indicate bone abnormalities causing facial paralysis in a newborn, a neoplasm of the central nervous system must be suspected.

Table 12-3. Causes of facial paralysis in in children.

- Congenital abnormalities.
- Inflammatory processes.
- Neoplasm
- Trauma.
- Hypertension.
- Idiopathic facial paralysis.

Birth trauma
At times a hypothetical congenital facial paralysis of a child or newborn is, in reality, due to a trauma to the peripheral trunk of the facial nerve caused by forceps during delivery. On the other hand, an apparent cause of forceps trauma during delivery may in reality have been caused by the pressure of the face of the fetus against the sacral bone of the mother during the last stages of pregnancy. Generally speaking, facial paralysis due to forceps or pressure against the sacral bone will regress spontaneously. Medical or surgical treatment in congenital alterations of VII is not effective.

INFLAMMATORY PROCESS

Paralysis of the facial nerve may be complicated by an otitis media with mastoiditis.
Generally, the paralysis will regress spontaneously if the infection is treated appropriately with medical procedures. Surgery must be performed when the indications for a mastoidectomy are present (e.g. no response to antibiotic therapy; postauricular edema; subperiosteal abscess). In cases of cholesteatoma, even if the nerve function returns to normal after antibiotic therapy, a relapse in the paralysis is almost certain, given the cholesteatoma's progression. The X-ray shows erosion of the aditus ad antrum and the ossicles. Surgery is necessary.

Herpes zoster
Rare in children. It manifests in paralysis of nerve VII, papular eruption in the external auditory canal and in other locations in the ear and the postauricular zone, hearing loss, and vertigo.

Guillan Barré Syndrome
This pathology is the result of a viral infection or non-specific polineuritis. Diagnosis is performed by the process of elimination. A high protein level in the spinal fluid is indicative.

Petrositis
Rare in children but may appear as a metastatic pathology due to osteomyelitis of the long bones.

Poliomyelitis

Though rare in this age group, it may cause an isolated paralysis, including that of nerve VII.

NEOPLASM

The facial nerve may be involved due to the expansion of a mass in the central nervous system. These neoformations may compress the facial nerve at the posterior fossa or along its course in the brainstem.

TRAUMA

Fractures of the temporal bone are a common cause of paralysis in children, especially males.

- If paralysis appears immediately after the accident, the nerve should be explored with decompression or suture, according to the lesion's extension.
- If paralysis appears after 7-8 days from the trauma, it usually will disappear spontaneously. If recovery does not take place within two weeks, however, decompression is indicated.
- In some traumas it may be difficult to evaluate if the paralysis was immediate or delayed: this is true in patients who are comatose for several days, or have a facial edema to the extent that an adequate evaluation of movement is not possible.
- A history of bleeding from the acoustic meatus or cerebrospinal otorrhea must lead us to suspect an immediate onset of facial paralysis. Thus we must proceed with nerve exploration when the patient's general conditions make general anesthesia and surgery possible.

HYPERTENSION

A facial paralysis reputed to be idiopathic may in reality be a symptom of a hypertensive child. The cause may be hemorrhage or edema of the fallopian canal.

IDIOPATHIC FACIAL PARALYSIS

- Idiopathic facial paralysis (Bell's palsy) is less common in children than in adults. When in the presence of a unilateral paralysis of nerve VII, X-rays and a hematological examination are necessary.
- Other rare causes of facial paralysis which may appear to be idiopathic are autoimmune diseases, such as granulomatosis of Wegener and periarteritis.

TOPOGRAPHIC DIAGNOSIS OF LESIONS OF NERVE VII

To correctly evaluate the site of a lesion of nerve VII, the following must be examined: auditory, lacrimal, stapedial functions; taste sensitivity, salivation, and motor activity.

SYMPTOMS IN FACIAL NERVE LESIONS

Distally to the chorda tympani

- Paralysis of facial muscles only.

Between the branch of the stapedial tendon and the chorda tympani

- Paralysis of the facial muscles.
- Loss of taste sensation on the anterior 2/3 of the tongue.
- Hearing loss.

Between the geniculate ganglion and the branch of the stapedial tendon

- Paralysis of the facial muscles.
- Loss of taste sensation of the anterior 2/3 of the tongue.
- Hearing loss (associated with a lesion of nerve VIII).
- Hyperacusia (from stapedial muscle dysfunction).

Between the internal auditory canal and the geniculate ganglion

- Facial muscle paralysis.
- Asymmetric salivation and lacrimation.
- Loss of taste sensation on the anterior 2/3 of the tongue.
- Hearing loss (associated with nerve VIII).
- Hyperacusia (from stapedial muscle dysfunction).

Posterior cranial fossa

- Paralysis of the facial muscles.
- Asymmetric salivation and lacrimation.
- Hearing loss (associated with a lesion of nerve VII).
- Hyperacusia (due to a stapedial muscle dysfunction).
- Signs of lesions intrinsic to the brainstem or other cranial nerves.

INSTRUMENTAL INVESTIGATION OF FACIAL PARALYSIS

For the etiological picture, it is important to distinguish between central and peripheral nerve lesions. This information is of great interest in tumors or traumas, but less so in neuropathies. This includes Bell's palsy, which tends to cause more extensive lesions. It is interesting to note that in Bell's palsy, the more proximal paralysis has a less favorable path.

The main objective in all the tests is to determine whether the nerve has degenerated or will degenerate, and to establish the degree.

If it has not degenerated, the paralysis may be considered the result of a focal point of neuroapraxia and demyelinization. These lesions tend towards to complete *restitutio ad integrum*, as long as there is no massive neural degeneration.

Neuropathies tend to progress in time, rather than causing sudden and total damage.

It is very important to define the pace of the advancement, for prognostic and therapeutic purposes. The sooner the therapy begins, the better the results.
The slower the initial pace, the more difficult a massive degeneration of the lesion will be.
The following are various functional tests. As a reminder, when based on tests of tears, taste and saliva flow, the topodiagnosis of lesions to nerve VII has a limited value when the lesion is acute, and is practically worthless after the passage of a significant period of time. This is because there are frequently collateral means of innervation, since the lesion may involve diverse segments of the nerve, because the recovery of the various parts may regress in time.
Some of these tests are only cited in the interests of thoroughness.

TEST OF THE CORNEAL REFLEX
The cornea has a motor innervation (facial nerve) and a sensory innervation (trigeminal nerve). The test will demonstrate any lesions to nerves V or VII.
In this test, the patient is asked to look to one side. A cotton-tip is brought towards the patient, out of the line of vision. The test is performed on both eyes.

- Normal response. The sclera is touched to check, without revealing a blinking reflex. The cornea is touched and a blinking reflex is seen.
- Pathological response. The cornea is touched, the patient has normal sensitivity but the blinking occurs only in the contralateral eye. This indicates motor deficit due to facial nerve involvement.
- Pathological response. The cornea is touched. Diminished sensitivity is seen. No blinking reflex is found. This is an indicator of sensory deficit (trigeminal nerve involvement).

SCHIRMER TEST
Parasympathetic fibers stimulate the lacrimal gland through the intermediate branch of Wrisberg, which separates from the facial nerve at the geniculate ganglion. A reduction or abolition of lacrimal secretion is an indicator of a lesion on or near the geniculate ganglion.
The test is performed by inserting a 0.5 cm strip of filter paper in each inferior fornix and comparing the imbibition of each eye after 5 min. It will be lesser or lacking in the injured eye.
Some variables that may influence the test:

- If the test is not performed in the days immediately following nerve involvement, the paralysis of the orbicular with subsequent xerophthalmia may indicate positivity even in the absence of geniculate ganglion involvement.
- Lacrimation may be excessive due to inadequate clearance of the conjunctive sac, even if total lacrimation is diminished.

STAPEDIAL MUSCLE REFLEX
Presenting a sound stimulus approx. 85 dB over the audiometric threshold, in the frequency from 250 to 4000 Hz, in each ear, a contraction reflex of the stapedial muscle is seen, recognizable with the impedenzometry.
This test is specific for the diagnosis of lesions located on the emergence of the stapedial muscle. When the stapedial reflex is positive, the lesion is distal to this area. Further, a positive stapedial reflex indicates that paralysis of the facial nerve is incomplete, and that the total degeneration of the fibers has not yet taken place. Thus the prognosis for recovery is relatively good, though this is not true in cases of Bell's paralysis.

SALIVA FLOW TEST
The submandibular and sublingual glands receive a parasympathetic innervation through the nervus intermedius and the chorda tympani. This examination tests alterations in saliva secretion due to lesions situated on top of these structures.
The test is performed by bilaterally probing the duct of Wharton and collecting saliva stimulated by lemon juice for one minute.
When the response is lowered by 25% in the first day of the paralysis, an incomplete recovery of the function is usually seen.
The test is not easy to perform, however, and can frequently lead to infection when repeated .

ELECTROGUSTATOMETRY
The taste fibers run from the anterior 2/3 of the tongue through the chorda tympani, to the facial nerve.
This test is based on the fact that a small positive electric current, when applied to the tongue, has a metallic bitter taste. To measure the function of the chorda tympani, a current is applied to the tip of the tongue, and is quantitatively controlled so that the taste response threshold may be measured.
This examination evaluates any possible alterations in taste sensation. Their manifestation is an early sign which generally precedes a clinically visible pathology. The return of the taste sensation often precedes movement reacquisition by weeks.

PALPEBRAL REFLEX TEST
The supraorbital nerve is stimulated electrically at its foramen and the responses reflected by the orbicular muscle of the eye are recorded.
There are two components to the electrical response: the first is a pontine response, while the second is trigeminal.

Information about the facial nerve is also obtained: a positive reflex indicates an anatomical continuity of the nerve through the lesion zone, even if conduction appears altered. The recovery of the reflex indicates the reinstatement of the conduction through the segment involved.

Electrical tests are more reliable, and thus, more useful.

ELECTRICAL TESTS

Electrical examinations answer the most important question in facial paralysis: What to do? Is recovery more likely with surgery or medical therapy?

The maximal stimulation test and the evoked electromyography or electroneurography are useful in revealing the initial degenerations, and are thus predominantly utilized in the first week of the paralysis.

The electromyography is useful for the most part from the 10th to the 14th day.

MAXIMAL STIMULATION TEST

This test is based on the principle that a nerve, though injured, continues to conduct distally to the lesion.

The test is carried out with a small portable apparatus. The stimulator is placed on the lateral region of the patient's face in nerve VII's peripheral path, and covered with electrode paste. The stimulus is brought to 5 mA or the highest intensity tolerated without forcing by the patient. Thus the responses of the following structures are compared: neck, lower lip, mouth, nose, eye, both sides of the forehead. They are classified as equal, lowered, or absent.

- In the first 3-5 days the test has no value, since even a completely sectioned nerve will continue transmitting distally to the lesion.
- Once this period has passed, in a first-degree lesion (without distal alterations) the responses from the two sides are the same.
- In a second or third-degree lesion, with axon alteration, the intensity of the stimulus must be increased to provoke a muscle contraction.
- For a third-degree lesion or above, where there is myelin distal axonal degeneration, no response is found apart from the intensity of the stimulus.
- When the response to maximal stimulation is symmetrical, 88% of patients will have a complete functional recovery. When the response is diminished, the complete recovery is presented in 27%. When the response is absent, in all patients we will see an incomplete functional recovery (Hilger).

In cases of trauma or infection, the test must be repeated until the response proves abnormal or until a recovery in voluntary movements is obtained (May).

- *Advantages*: Easy to perform, inexpensive, reproducible.
- *Limits*: Useful after 5th day of paralysis. Useful as long as a response is obtained; when the nerve has degenerated, the test is no longer practicable. Necessity of comparing the two sides, though the "healthy" side may no longer be so, as in general forms, with alternating bilateral involvement.

EVOKED ELECTROMYOGRAPHY OR ELECTRONEUROGRAPHY

Similar to the maximal stimulation test, this test is more precise because it is not based on a visual evaluation of the responses but rather on an evaluation of potentials and electromyographic summation recorded with an electromyographic recorder (Fisch, Esslen).

According to May, in cases of facial paralysis after a fracture of the temporal bone, surgery must be performed in the following situations:

- Sudden and total appearance of paralysis.
- 10% reduction in summation potentials after the 5th day.
- CT showing fallopian damage or fallopian canal not damaged, but no recovery in facial function after 6 months.

According to Fisch, in cases of Bell's palsy, surgery must be performed when summation potentials are reduced to 10% or less of the norm within 2 weeks after the appearance of the paralysis.

- In cases of Herpes zoster oticus, when symptoms of inner ear suffering are seen.
- In cases of acute otitis media, when summation potentials are reduced to 10% or less of the norm, even after medical treatment and/or paracentesis.

ELECTROMYOGRAPHY

- Electromyography studies the electrical activity of the muscular skeletal fibers. Needle electrodes are used, inserted into the belly of the facial muscles. First the spontaneous muscular activity subsequent to the needle's introduction is evaluated. The patient is then asked to contract the muscles, and the size and shape of the motor response is evaluated. The needle is moved in various directions, so as to examine a vast range of units. The patient is then asked to perform a maximal contraction, to detect any loss in motor units. Finally the needle is moved again in various directions, while having the patient relax and evaluating the spontaneous activity.

- Electrical potentials can be measured 10-20 days after the degeneration of a denervated muscle. Their presence during the patient's voluntary movements can exclude a total section of the nerve. Their reappearance, after nerve degeneration, is the first sign of regeneration, and frequently seen before the reappearance of voluntary motility (House, Brackmann).
- Poliphasic waves of small size and duration are characteristic of myopathic states, whereas large and longer waves suggest a neurogenic atrophy as well as a collateral innervation.
- An increase in polyphasic potentials may also be noted in various myopathies and neurogenic alterations.

All the tests described above, including the minimum excitability test and the maximum stimulation test (MST) and the electroneurography (ENOG) are based on a percutaneous stimulation of the facial nerve distally to the stylomastoid foramen. In any case, these tests prove normal up to 48-72 hours after the beginning of degeneration. Their main drawback is that they may indicate an axon degeneration only after two or three days from their manifestation. In this way the potential benefits of surgery are theoretically reduced. On the other hand, the MST has proved to be a reliable indicator in the prognosis of Bell's paralysis, with 94% accuracy.

TEST OF MAXIMUM STIMULATION

We use a Hilger 2-R and an H-3 (TM) facial nerve stimulator for this test (WR Medical Electronics Co., Stillwater Michigan).

REFERENCES

Andrews JC, Canalis RF: Otogenic pneumocephalus. Laryngoscope 96: 521-528,1986.

Arriaga MA, Brackmann DE: Facial nerve repair techniques in cerebellopontine angle tumor surgery. Am J Otol 13: 356-359, 1992.

Bailey CM, Graham MD: Intratemporal facial nerve neuroma: A discussion of five cases. J Laryngol Otol 97(1): 65-72, 1983.

Balkany T, Fradis M, Jafek BW, Rucker NC: Hemangioma of the facial nerve: Role of the geniculate capillary plexus. Skull Base Surg 1: 59-63, 1991.

Balliet R, Shinn JB, Gach Y, Rita P: Facial paralysis rehabilitation: Retraining selective muscle control. Int Rehabil Med 4: 67-74, 1982.

Barrs DM, Brackmann DE, Hitselberger WE: Facial nerve anastomosis in the cerebellopontine angle: A review of 24 cases. Am J Otol 5: 269-272, 1984.

Barrs DM: Facial nerve trauma: Optimal timing for repair. Laryngoscope 101: 835-848, 1991.

Belal A Jr: Structure of human muscle in facial paralysis: Role of muscle biopsy. In May M (ed): The Facial Nerve. New York, Thieme, 1986, pp 99-106.

Belluci RJ: Traumatic injuries of the middle ear. Otolaryngol Clin North Am 16: 633-650, 1983.

Broniatowski M, Grundfest-Broniatowski S, Davies CR, et al: Dynamic rehabilitation of the paralyzed face: III. Balanced coupling of oral and ocular musculature from the intact side in the canine. Otolaryngol Head Neck Surg 105: 727-733, 1991.

Brudny J, Hammerschlag PE, Cohen NL, Ransohoff J: Electromyographic rehabilitation of facial function and introduction of a facial paralysis grading scale for hypoglossal-facial nerve anastomosis. Laryngoscope 98: 405-410, 1988.

Burres S, Fisch U: The comparison of facial grading systems. Arch Otolaryngol Head Neck Surg 112, July 1986.

Caniff JP: Otorrhea in head injuries. Br J Oral Surg 8: 203-210, 1971.

Cannon C, Jahrsdoerfer R: Temporal bone fractures. Arch Otolaryngol Head Neck Surg 109: 285-288, 1983.

Chang CGS, Shen AL: Hypoglossofacial anastomosis for facial palsy after resection of acoustic neuroma. Surg Neurol (21): 282-286, 1984.

Chobaut JC: Intra-temporal facial nerve tumors. In Facial nerve. Portmann M Edit, Masson, New-York 417-423, 1985.

Chuang DCC, Wei FC, Noordhoff, MS: "Smile" reconstruction in facial paralysis. Ann Plast Surg 23: 56-65, 1989.

Coker NJ, Fordice JO, Moore S: Correlation of the nerve excitability test and electroneurography in acute facial paralysis. Am J Otol 13: 127-133, 1992.

Coker NJ, Jenkins HA, Psifidis A: Electrophysiological prognostication of acute facial nerve trauma. In Fisch U, Valavanis A, Yasargil MG (eds): Neurological Surgery of the Ear and the Skull Base. Amsterdam, Kugler & Ghedini, 1989, pp 355-362.

Coker NJ, Kendall KA, Jenkins HA, Alford BR: Traumatic intratemporal facial nerve injury: Management rationale for preservation of function. Otolaryngol Head Neck Surg 97: 262-269, 1987.

Coker NJ: Management of traumatic injuries to the facial nerve. Otolaryngol Clin North Am 24: 215-227, 1991.

Coker NJ, Fisch U: Disorders of the facial nerve. In English, G.M: Otolaryngology. Harper & Row, Philadelphia 1984 pp. 1-43.

Conley J, Baker DC: Hypoglossal-facial nerve anastomosis for reinnervation of the paralyzed face. Plast Reconstr Surg 63: 63-72, 1979.

Dort JC, Fisch U: Facial nerve schwannomas. Skull Base Surg 1: 51-55, 1991.

Dressler D, Schonle PW: Hyperkinesias after hypoglossofacial nerve anastomosis-treatment with botulinum toxin. Eur Neurol 31: 44-46, 1991.

Duncan NO, Coker NJ, Jenkins HA, Canalis RF: Gunshot injuries of the temporal bone. Otolaryngol Head Neck Surg 94: 47-55, 1986.

Esslen E: The Acute facial palsies: Investigations on the Localization and Pathogenesis of Meato-Labyrinthine Facial Palsies. Berlin, Springer-Verlag, 1977.

Farrior JB: Anterior facial nerve decompression. Otolaryngol Head Neck Surg 93;765-68, 1985.

Fisch U, Ruttner L: Pathology of intratemporal tumors involving the facial nerve. *In* Fisch U (ed): Facial Nerve Surgery. Birmingham, AL, Aesculapius, 1977, pp 448-456.

Fisch U: Facial paralysis in fractures of the petrous bone. Laryngoscope 84: 2141-2154, 1974.

Fisch U: Prognostic value of electrical tests in acute facial paralysis. Am J Otol 5: 494-498, 1984.

Gantz BJ, Gmuer AA, Holiday M, Fisch U: Electroneurographic evaluation of the facial nerve: Method and technical problems. Ann Otol Rhinol Laryngol 93: 394-398, 1984.

Gavron JP, Clemis JD: Hypoglossal-facial nerve anastomosis: A review of forty cases caused by facial nerve injuries in the posterior fossa. Laryngoscope 94: 1447-1450, 1984.

Ghorayeb BY, Yeakley JW: Temporal bone fractures: Longitudinal or oblique? The case for oblique temporal bone fractures. Laryngoscope 102: 129-134, 1992.

Glasscock ME, Smith PG, Schwaber MK, Nissen AJ: Clinical aspects of osseous hemangiomas of the skull base. Laryngoscope 94: 869-873, 1984.

Harrison DH: The pectoralis minor vascularized muscle graft for the treatment of unilateral facial palsy. Plast Reconstr Surg 75: 206-216, 1985.

Hitselberger WE: Hypoglossal-facial anastomosis. In House WF, Luetje CM (eds): Acoustic Tumors, Vol 2: Management. Baltimore/ University Park Press, 1979, pp 97-103.

Hough J, Stuart W: Middle ear injuries in skull trauma. Laryngoscope 78: 899-937, 1968.

House JW: Facial nerve grading systems, in M Portmann Edit Facial nerve, Masson Publi, NewYork Paris 34-41, 1985.

House JW: Facial nerve tumors and grafting. *In* Brackmann DE (ed:) Neurological Surgery of the Ear and Skull Base. New York, Raven Press, 1982, pp 77-80.

House JW, Brackmann DE: Facial nerve grading system. Laryngoscope 93: n.2, 146-147, 1985.

House WF, Shelton C: Middle fossa approach for acoustic tumor removal. Otolaryngol Clin North Am 25: 347-359, 1992.

Jackson CG, Glasscock ME III, Hughes G, Sismanis A: Facial paralysis of neoplastic origin: Diagnosis and management. Laryngoscope 90(10Ptl): 1581-1595, 1980.

King TT, Morrison AW: Primary facial nerve tumors within the skull. J Neurosurg 72(1): 1-8, 1990.

Lambert PR, Brackman DE: Facial paralysis in temporal bone fractures: A review of 26 cases. Laryngoscope 94: 1022-1026, 1984.

Lang J: Anatomy of the brainstem and lower cranial nerves, vessels, and surrounding structures. Am J Otol 6(Suppl): 1-19, 1985.

Lee KS, Britton BH, Kelly DL Jr: Schwannoma of the facial nerve in the cerebellopontine angle presenting with hearing loss. Surg Neurol 32(3): 231-234, 1989.

Leech PJ, Paterson A: Conservative and operative management for cerebrospinal fluid leakage after closed head injury. Lancet 1: 1013-1016, 1973.

Liliequist B: Neurinomas of the labyrinthine portion of the facial nerve canal. A report of two cases. Adv Otorhinolaryng 24: 58-67, 1978.

Lipkin AF, Coker NJ, Jenkins HA, Alford BR: Intracranial and intratemporal facial neuroma. Otolaryngol Head Neck Surg 96 (1): 71-79, 1987.

Litton W, Krause C, Anson B, Cohen W: Relationship of facial canal to the annular sulcus. Laryngoscope 79: 1584-604, 1969;

Lo WW, Brackmann DE, Shelton C: Facial nerve hemangioma. Ann Otol Rhinol Laryngol 98(2): 160-161, 1989.

Lore JM Jr: The parotid salivary gland. In Lore JM Jr. (ed): An Atlas of Head and Neck Surgery. Philadelphia, WB Saunders, 1988, pp 708-713.

Luxford WM, Brackmann DE: Facial nerve substitution: A review of sixty-six cases. Am J Otol (Suppl): 55-57, 1985.

Mangham CA, Carberry JN, Brackmann DE: Management of intratemporal vascular tumors. Laryngoscope 91: 867-876, 1981.

Marentette LJ, Valentino J: Traumatic anterior fossa cerebrospinal fluid fistulae and craniofacial considerations. Otolaryngol Clin North Am 24: 151-164, 1991.

Martin CH, Prades JM: Removal of selected infralabyrinthine lesions without facial nerve mobilization. Skull Base Surg 2:220-226, 1992.

May M, Sobol SM, Mester SJ: Hypoglossal-facial nerve interpositional jump graft for facial reanimation without tongue atrophy. Otolaryngol Head Neck Surg 104: 818-825, 1991.

May M: Total facial nerve exploration: transmastoid, extralabyrinthine, and subtemporal indications and results. Laryngoscope 89:906-917, 1979.

May M: Management of cranial nerves I through VII following skull base surgery. Otolaryngol Head Neck Surg 88: 560-575, 1980.

May M: Surgical rehabilitation of facial palsy. In May M (ed): The Facial Nerve. New York, Thieme, 1986, pp 695-777.

McCabe BF: Injuries to the facial nerve. Laryngoscope 82: 1891-1896, 1973.

Mincy JE: Post-traumatic cerebrospinal fluid fistula of the frontal fossa. Trauma 6: 618-622, 1966.

Murata T, Hakuba A, Okumura T, Mori K: Intrapetrous neurinomas of the facial nerve. Report of three cases. Surg Neurol 23(5): 507-512, 1985.

Neely JG, Alford BR: Facial nerve neuromas. Arch Otolaryngol Head Neck Surg 100(4): 298-301, 1974.

Nelson RA, House WF: Facial nerve neuroma in the posterior fossa: Surgical considerations. In Graham MD, House WF (eds): Disorders of the Facial Nerve. New York, Raven Press, 1982, pp 403-406.

O'Brien BM, Pederson WC, Khazanchi RK, et al: Results of management of facial palsy with microvascular free-muscle transfer. Plast Reconstr Surg 86: 12-22, 1990.

O'Donoghue GM, Brackmann DE, House JW, Jackler RK: Neuromas of the facial nerve. Am J Otol 10(1): 49-54, 1989.

Oberascher G: Cerebrospinal fluid otorrhea—new trends in diagnosis. Am J Otol 9: 102-108, 1988.

Orgel MG, Terzis JK: Epineural vs. perineurial repair. Plast Reconstr Surg 60: 80-91, 1977.

Pappas DG, Schneiderman TS, Brackmann DE, et al: Cavernous hemangiomas of the internal auditory canal. Otolaryngol Head Neck Surg 101: 27-32, 1989.

Pearman K, Welch AR: Schwannoma of the intratemporal facial nerve. Case report. J Laryngol Otol 94(7): 779-784, 1980.

Pensak ML, Jackson CG, Glasscock ME III, Gulya AJ: Facial reanimation with the VII-XII anastomosis: Analysis of the functional and psychologic results. Otolaryngol Head Neck Surg 94: 305-310, 1986.

Pillsbury HC, Price HC, Gardner LJ: Primary tumors of the facial nerve: Diagnosis and management. Laryngoscope 93(8): 1045-1048, 1983.

Pitty LF, Tator CH: Hypoglossal-facial nerve anastomosis for facial nerve palsy following surgery for cerebellopontine angle tumors. J Neurosurg 77: 724-731,1992.

Pulec JL: Facial nerve tumors. Ann Otol Rhinol Laryngol 78: 962-983, 1969.

Pulec JL: Facial nerve tumors. Ann Otol Rhinol Laryngol 78: 962-982, 1969.

Pulec JL: Facial nerve grafting. Laryngoscope 79: 1562-1583, 1969.

Pulec JL: Facial nerve neuroma. Laryngoscope 82(7): 1160-1176, 1972.

Rosenblum B, Davis R, Camins M: Middle fossa facial schwannoma removed via the intracranial extradural approach: Case report and review of the literature. Neurosurgery 21(5): 739-741, 1987.

Sabin HI, Bordi LT, Symon L, Compton JS: Facio-hypoglossal anastomosis for the treatment of facial palsy after acoustic neuroma resection. Br J Neurosurg 4: 313-318, 1990.

Samii M: Rehabilitation of the face by facial nerve substitution: Panel discussion. In Fisch U (Ved): Facial Nerve Surgery. Birmingham, AL, Aesculapius, 1977, pp 244-245.

Sanna M, Zini C, Gamoletti R, Pasanisi E: Primary intratemporal tumours of the facial nerve: Diagnosis and treatment. J Laryngol Otol 104(10): 765-771, 1990.

Shambaugh GE, Arenberg IK, Barney PL, Valvassori GE. Facial Neurilemmomas. Arch Otolaryng 90: 742-755, 1969.

Shelton C, Brackmann DE, Lo WW, Carberry JN: Intratemporal facial nerve hemangiomas. Otolaryngol Head Neck Surg 104(1): 116-121, 1991.

Stennert E: I. Hypoglossal facial anastomosis: Its significance for modern facial surgery. II. Combined approach in extratemporal facial nerve reconstruction. Clin Plast Surg 6: 471-486, 1979.

Tew JM Jr, Yeh HS, Miller GW, Shahbabian S: Intratemporal schwannoma of the facial nerve. Neurosurgery 13(2): 186-188, 1983.

Tran Ba Huy P, Monteil JP, Rey A: Results of twenty cases of transfacio-facial anastomosis as compared with those of XII-VII anastomosis. In Portmann M (ed): Facial Nerve. New York, Masson, 1985, pp 85-87.

Tucker HM: Restoration of selective facial nerve function by the nerve-muscle pedicle technique. Clin Plast Surg 6: 293-300, 1979.

Valvassori GE: Neuromas of the facial nerve. Adv Otorhinolaryngol 24: 68-70, 1978.

Westmore GA, Whittam DE: Cerebrospinal fluid rhinorrhea and its management. Br J Surg 69:489 492, 1982.

Wiet RJ, Pyle GM, Schramm DR: Middle fossa and intratemporal facial nerve neuromas. Otolaryngol Head Neck Surg 104(1): 141-142, 1991.

Wiet RS, Lohau AN, Brackmann DE: Neurilemmoma of the chorda tympani nerve. Otolaryngol Head Neck Surg 93: 119-121, 1985.

Xian-Xi G, Spector GJ: Labyrinthine segment and geniculate ganglion of facial nerve in fetal and adult human temporal bones. Ann Otol Rhinol Laryngol 90(Suppl 85): 1-12, 1981.

Ylikoski J, Brackmann DE, Savolainen S: Pressure neuropathy of the facial nerve: A case report with light and electron microscopic findings. J Laryngol Otol 98: 909-914, 1984.

Ylikoski J, Hitselberger WE, House WF, et al: Degenerative changes in the distal stump of the severed human facial nerve. Acta Otolaryngol (Stockh) 92: 239-248,1981.

Zini C, Sanna M, Gandolfi A: Hypoglosso-facial anastomosis in the rehabilitation of irreversible facial nerve palsies. In Portmann M (ed): Facial Nerve. New York, Masson, 1985, pp 519-522.

13

Facial nerve repair

When the continuity of the facial nerve has been preserved, the following events may take place post-operatively (Table 13-1).

If we are certain that the facial nerve has been preserved intact, but complete paralysis is observed after surgery, it is preferable to wait at least a year before performing a hypoglossal-facial anastomosis. In fact, in most cases, recovery occurs or at least begins during this time period.
At times there may be a complete post-operative paralysis, though the nerves are intact. In these cases recovery should be expected to leave relics of weakness in the facial musculature and synkinesis.
If no hypotony is seen in the facial musculature when the patient awakens, or if it is slight or slowed, an almost complete functional recovery may be expected.

INTRAOPERATIVE FACIAL NERVE TRAUMA

When an intraoperative facial nerve trauma has occurred, the surgeon has to perform a simultaneous intraoperative recognition.

- The neural sheath is exposed.
- When the nerve is intact, it is recorded in the operative note.
- When the sheath is opened, in case of a transection <33%, no maneuver is performed: the nerve will heal spontaneously.
- In case of a transection >33%, the nerve is completely transected and an end to end repair is performed.
- In case of a complete transection, an end-to-end repair is performed whenever possible, otherwise a nerve graft is used.

When there is a postoperative facial nerve paralysis, there may be an immediate or a delayed postoperative paralysis.
In case of an immediate postoperative paralysis:

- Wait 2 hours. If the paralysis recovers within two hours, it is due to local anesthetic.
- Loosen the packing. The nerve may suffer from an overly heavy packing.

When the paralysis does not recede, the following steps must be taken:

- Inform the patient and the family: There has been injury to the facial nerve.
- Re-explore within 24 hours.

When there is a delayed postoperative paralysis:

- Remove packing.
- Treat as Bell's palsy.

WHEN TO REPAIR THE NERVE

The facial nerve must be repaired following damaging events such as fracture of the temporal bone, iatrogenic lesions of the nerve, infratemporal facial trauma, nerve lesions following neuroma operations, glomus tumors, and meningiomas; or due to malignant tumors of the temporal bone and/or the parotid gland.

According to Pillsbury and Fisch, post-operative radiation therapy has a negative effect on the recovery of facial function, whereas according to Conley, the effect of radiation on nerve regrowth is slight.
We agree with Terris and Free's belief that immediate nerve reconstruction is preferable in cases of total parotidectomy, even when post-operative radiation therapy is planned:

- The proliferation of fibrous tissue is seen beginning on the fifth day. Afterwards, the operation becomes more complicated, especially in the horizontal and labyrinthine parts of the nerve.
- Another point in favor of early grafting is the need for adequate resection of the stumps of fibrotic and devitalized nerves when surgery is delayed. It is difficult to determine how much tissue should be removed to reach the fascicles in good condition (Barrs).

In conclusion, the sooner the injured nerve is repaired, the better the prospects of recovery will

Table 13-1. Integrity of the facial nerve. What to expect.

I. Neuroapraxy
Everything seems to be in order, but the nerve does not conduct well and the reason it is not known. Recovery begins within two weeks.

II. Axonotmesis
Some axons are altered and die, and they take time to regenerate. Recovery begins within two months.

III. Neurotmesis
The neural sheath has been altered. The sheath may grow inside the axons, so that synkinesis may later appear. Recovery begins within 6 months.

In all cases, a virtually complete recovery is likely to be had within 2 years.

be. For an intraoperative nerve section, the treatment indicated is immediate neurorrhaphy (Millesi, Mackinnon).
When necessary, the graft may nevertheless be performed with good chances of success even months after the trauma. This is demonstrated by the clinical data showing good axon regrowth even after years. Further, in delayed reconstructions, the positioning of epineural sutures is facilitated by a fibrotic epinevrium, which makes the nerve more resistant.

REPAIR TECHNIQUE

An ideal nerve repair matches each proximal fascicle with its distal partner (Sunderland; Lundborg; Millesi). Some AA maintain that a precise pairing of the fascicles leads to a precise approximation of the fascicles, creating an improved axon realignment, and providing the possibility of repairing only the damaged fascicles (Salvi, Bora).
In any case, the fascicular organization of the nerve changes progressively along its path. In particular, the proximal part of the facial nerve from the IAC to the horizontal tract is compact, with fascicles clinging to one another. The distal part of the nerve, in the mastoid and the parotid, is composed of highly diffused multiple fascicles.
The more substance lost, the less precise will be the juxtaposition of the bundles, when a termino-terminal suture is performed on the two stumps. The alteration is greater when a graft is utilized, since this has its own bundle organization (Barrs).
In the AA's opinion, the differing structures of the bundles make perineural or interfascicular sutures useless. Besides a more complex operating technique, they also require more time in surgery.
There are other disadvantages:

- A trauma to the nerve is unavoidable due to the repeated insertion of the needle.
- There is greater damage to the vascularization.
- The suture material in the anastomotic zone represents a *locus minoris resistentiae* for the formation of scars and neuromas, which may impede axon growth regenerating from the proximal to the distal segments.
- Small voids are created, allowing fibroblasts to enter. These may lead regenerating axons to occupy extraneural space inappropriately (M. Korff).

The epineural suture has fewer inconveniences and remains our chosen technique (Fig. 13-1).
Thread with greater tolerability should be used for suturing. Some examples are: silk, hair, stainless steel wire, tantalium. Repair with poliglycolic acid is also better tolerated than catgut, which provokes an intense reaction as a foreign body.
One of the better tolerated materials and one of the most readily available for clinical use is nylon. Single thread nylon 9-0 appears to be the most indicated, since 10-0 is too thin and 8-0 has a tendency to exit the nerve tissue (Giddens).

It is important to observe the following guidelines, no matter which repair technique is eventually chosen:

- The two extremities of the nerve must be juxtaposed without tension.
- The extremities must be completely cut for a better regeneration. For the cut, approx. 3 mm of the two extremities of the epineurium must be liberated, and only the perineurium and endoneurium must be cut. Trauma to the nerve is reduced. The following metaphor may be kept in mind: trauma to a banana (the nerve) is reduced if the peel (the epineurium) is removed before cutting (M. May).
- Anastomosis must be as trauma-free as possible, and must be adequately resistant.
- If a termino-terminal suture is used, the two stumps should be brought together without being twisted.
- If a nerve substitution technique is performed (e.g. VII-XII) for an older paralysis, it is important to check with a pre-operative histological exam that the distal extremity of the nerve has not undergone complete fibrosis. If it has, the nerve must be incised again until the healthy tissue is exposed.

USE OF FIBRIN

According to Moy, the use of fibrin, though technically facilitating the operation, has unsatisfactory clinical, electrophysiological and histological results compared to the epineural suture.
According to Boedts, the use of fibrin glue, alone or with tubes of fenestrated collagen, increases

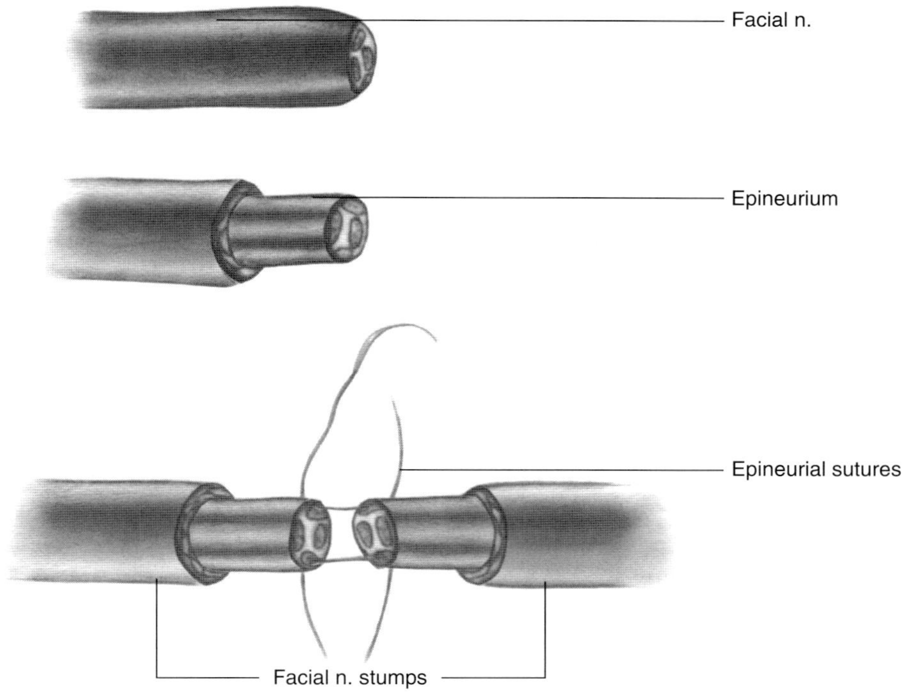

Fig. 13-1. End-to-end repair of the facial nerve. Epineural sutures.

the growth of connective tissue and the risk of neuroma formation. Becker and Smahel report just the opposite, demonstrating that in Schwann cell metabolism, the electrophysiological and histological parameters are comparable to epineural sutures.

The possible *advantages* of fibrin glue sutures are the following: better approximation of the nerve endings, reduced trauma to the nerve, the absence of a permanent foreign body (the suture), and the easy technique, applicable even in situations where positioning of the suture is problematic (Nishihara).

The possible *disadvantages* are related to the chances of a hitherto unknown fibrin glue toxicity, potential local inflammatory reaction and inadequate nerve stabilization during the repair period. The adhesive action of the fibrin glue lasts for 3-4 days (Nishihara).

Most AA's are convinced that a fibrin glue suture gives less satisfactory results than an epineural repair. To this, the risks of hepatitis or acquired immunodeficiency syndrome must be added. In any case, the possibility of deriving fibrinogen pre-operatively from the patient's own blood overcomes these inconveniences and permits its use even in the USA. The only problem is its elevated cost.

We use epineural repair whenever possible, but we use fibrin glue in the IAC and CPA, where the nerve's position makes interrupted suturing difficult. In these cases, the proximal stump fluctuates with the impulses transmitted to the liquor of the endocranial vascular structures, and the graft may be positioned only with a silk epineural stitch. Several stitches would be more stable but are difficult to position. Fibrin glue permits non-traumatic repair in an area where an epineural suture would necessitate a technical compromise.

In studies on cadavers, we have found that a nerve repaired with fibrin glue under traction, will be more likely to break elsewhere. This demonstrates the resistence of the suture.

Silicone tubes are prepared to wrap the nerve and the graft, to direct nerve regeneration. One proposal has been to wrap the nerve stumps in the silicone, attaching the ends of the tube but not the mixed nerves with fibrin glue (Matras, Kuderna, Wigand). The idea is persuasive, since it seems to exploit the advantages of fibrin glue, without entailing the disadvantages of its contact with the mixed nerves.

The use of a polypropylene tube with micropores has made for quicker sensory recovery in experimental models, compared to sutures alone (Edwards).

LASER NEURORRHAPHY

The aforementioned limits of the mechanical suture have led to research on new repair mechanisms, such as the laser.

The laser's repair mechanism involves protein denaturation and collagen fusion in the two segments (Eppley). Thus the collagen's suprastructure is modified with the interdigitation of altered fibrils (Schober). Laser repair involves the entire circumference, blocking the entrance of fibroblasts or the exit of regenerating axons and neurotrophic hormones.

Currently, the laser suture has not replaced the epineural suture.

The epineural suture with 10-0 nylon is superior to laser repair CO2 (200 μm, 90 mW, 2 msec burst) for its tensile force, and the compound action potential (Maragh).

To obviate the inadequate tensile force of laser anastomosis, a suturing technique with subcutaneous tissue (S-Q weld) has been proposed. A piece of subcutaneous tissue is drawn and stretched over a 2 cm aluminum plate. A suture thread container may be used, cutting it as needed (ethicon). The plate is placed under the two nerve stumps. The stumps are pulled closer together, and the subcutaneous tissue is rolled around the nerve and photocoagulated with the laser at the epineurium. The energy needed to fuse the subcutaneous tissue at the epineurium is 1.00 watts, with single impulses every 0.05 seconds and 0.36 diameter spots. Multiple photocoagulations are performed halfway around the subcutaneous tissue, several mm from the area to anastomose, to leave space for nerve expansion.

This technique was proposed to increase tensile force in the critical first week, before the elements of the connective tissue can provide the necessary stability.

Thus a greater tensile force is obtained for the suture compared to that of the laser alone, but it is still lower of that of an epineural suture. The CAP behavior in the sutures that stay intact seems greater compared to a nylon suture, but the percentage of dehiscences after 2 months is discouraging (Korff).

The YAG laser may not be utilized because it provokes significant damage to the endoneurium.

TROPHIC FACTORS

- When alfa-MSH is administered with a polypropylene tube, a faster recovery has been seen in experimental models compared to both tubulization alone and/or epineural sutures (P.M. Edwards).
- The systemic administration of ORG.2766, similar to ACTH, has reduced the time required for sensory recovery of a caudal nerve in rats undergoing lesions caused by crushing (Van der Hoop).
- The systemic administration of leupeptin in rats (after sciatic nerve division) has shown greater myelin growth, more axons, and faster nerve conductivity (Hurst).
- Cortisone has provided better axon regeneration and functional recovery in experimental models (Lipton). The steroids could work by decreasing scar formation and promoting axon regeneration with their antifibroblastic activity. Its effects on man and the best method of administration are still unknown.
- The administration of NGF in guide tubes for the nerve does not increase the number nor the diameter of the axons regenerating in the canal, but does distally increase Schwann cell activity in the distal stump, the myelin diameter, and the number of fascicles (Chen, Rich, Santos). In experimental studies, this has not led to significant clinical improvements. Thus we can conclude that the regenerating nerve and the Schwann cells associated with it find sufficient NGF already present in the organism for regeneration (Santos).

REFERENCES

Aldskogius H, Molander C, Persson J, Thomander L: Specific and nonspecific regeneration of motor axons after sciatic nerve injury and repair in the rat. J Neurol Sci 80:249-257, 1987.

Babcock WW: Nerve disassociation: a new method for the surgical relief of certain painful or paralytic affections of nerve trunks. Ann Surg 46:686-693, 1907.

Badalamente MA, Hurst LC, Paul SB, Stracher A: Enhancement of neuromuscular recovery after nerve repair in primates. J Hand Surg 12B :211-217, 1987.

Badalamente MA, Hurst LC, Stracher A: Neuromuscular recovery using calcium protease inhibition after median nerve repair in primates. Proc Natl Acad Sci USA 86:5983-5987, 1989.

Bailff JE, Cozzens JW, Hudson AR, et al: Laser-assisted nerve repair in primates. J Neurosurg 71:266-272, 1989.

Bansberg SF, McCaffrey TV: The effect of systemic triamcinolone acetonide on nerve repair. Otolaryngol Head Neck Surg 96:158-164, 1987.

Barrs DM: Facial nerve trauma: optimal timing for repair. Laryngoscope 101: 835-848, 1991.

Becker C, Gueuning C, Gilbert A, Graff GL: Increased muscle regeneration after repair of divided motor nerve with neuronotrophic factors containing glue. Arch Int Physiol Biochem 97:521-529, 1989.

Becker CM, Gueuning CO, Graff GL: Sutures or fibrin glue for divided rat nerves: Schwann cell and muscle metabolism. J Reconstr Microsurg 1:139-145, 1984.

Boedts D: A comparative experimental study on nerve repair. Arch Otorhinolaryngol 244:1-6, 1987.

Bolesta MJ, Garrett WE, Ribbeck BM, Glisson RR, Seaber AV, Goldner JL: Immediate and delayed neurorrhaphy in a rabbit model: a functional, histologic, and biochemical comparison. J Hand Surg 13A, 364-369, 1988.

Bora FW: Peripheral nerve repair in cats. J Bone Joint Surg Am 49:659-666, 1967.

Boyles IK, Zoellner CD, Anderson LJ, et al: A role for apolipoprotein E apolipoprotein a-1, and low density lipoprotein receptors in cholesterol transport during regeneration and remyelination of the rat sciatic nerve. J Clin Invest 83:1015-1031, 1989.

Bratton BR, Kline DG, Hudson AR, Coleman WT: Use of monofilament polyglycolic acid suture for experimental peripheral nerve repair. J Surg Res 31:482-483, 1981.

Braun RM: Comparative studies of neurorrhaphy and sutureless peripheral nerve repair. Surg Gynecol Obstetr 122:15-18. 1966.

Braun RM: Experimental peripheral nerve repair tubulation. Surg Forum. 15:452-454, 1964.

Brunetti O, Carretta M, Magni F, Pazzaglia U: Role of the interval between axotomy and nerve suture on the success of muscle reinnervation: an experimental study in the rabbit. Exp Neurol 90:308-321, 1985.

Campbell JB, Bassett CA, Husby I, Thulin CA, Feringa ER: Microfilter sheaths in peripheral nerve surgery. J Trauma 1:139-157, 1961.

Chen Y, Wang-Bennett LT, Coker NJ: Facial nerve regeneration in the silicone chamber: the influence of nerve growth factor. Exp Neurol 103:52-60, 1989.

Chiu DT, Janecka P, Krizek TJ, Wolff M, Lovelace RE: Autogenous vein graft as a conduit for nerve regeneration. Surgery 91:226 233, 1982.

Coker NJ: Management of traumatic injuries to the facial nerve. Otolaryngol Clin North Am 24:215-227, 1991.

Conley JJ: Facial nerve grafting. Arch Otolaryngol 73:322-327, 1961.

Crumley RL: Interfascicular nerve repair. Arch Otolaryngol 106:313-316, 1980.

De la Torre JC, Karaca M, Merali Z, Fortin T, Richard M: Laser or razor? a novel experimental peripheral nerve repair technique. Neurosurgery 22:531-538, 1988.

De Medinacelli L, Church AC: Peripheral nerve reconnection: inhibition of early degenerative processes through the use of a novel fluid medium. Exp Neurol 84:396-408, 1984.

De Medinacelli L, Freed WJ, Wyatt RJ: Peripheral nerve reconnection: improvement of long-term functional effects under simulated clinical conditions in the rat. Exp Neurol 81:488-496, 1983.

De Medinacelli L, Freed WJ: Peripheral nerve reconnection: immediate histologic consequences of distributed mechanical support. Exp Neurol 81:459-468, 1983.

De Medinacelli L, Seaber AV: Experimental nerve reconnection. Importance of initial repair. Microsurgery 10:56-70, 1989.

De Medinacelli L, Wyan RJ, Freed WJ: Peripheral nerve reconnection: mechanical, thermal, and ionic conditions that promote the return of function. Exp Neurol 81:469-487, 1983.

Denny-Brown D, Doherty MM: Effects of transient stretching of peripheral nerve. Arch Neurol Psichiatry 54:116-129, 1945.

Ducker TB, Hayes GL: Experimental improvements in the use of Silastic cuff for peripheral nerve repair. J Neurosurg 28:582-587, 1968.

Ducker TB, Kauffman FC: Metabolic factors in surgery of peripheral nerves. Clin Neurosurg 24:406-424, 1976.

Ducker TB, Kempe LG, Hayes GJ: The metabolic background for peripheral nerve surgery. J Neurosurg 30:270-280, 1969.

Edshage S: Peripheral nerve suture. Acta Chir Scand 331: 2-104, 1964.

Ellis JC, McCaffrey TV: Nerve grafting: functional results after primary vs delayed repair. Arch Otolaryngol 111:781 - 785, 1985.

Gabrielson Gl, Stenstrom SJ: A contribution to peripheral nerve suture technique. Plast Reconstr Surg 38:68-72, 1966.

Giddens GE, Wade PJ, Amis M: Primary nerve repair: strength of repair with different gauges of nylon suture material. J Hand Surg 14B 301-302, 1989.

Grabb WC. Median and ulnar nerve suture: J Bone Joint Surg Am 50:964-972, 1968.

Grafstein B: The nerve cell body response to axotomy. Exp Neurol 48(11):32-51, 1975.

Hentz VR, Rosen JM, Xiao SJ, McGill KC, Abraham G: A comparison of suture and tubulization nerve repair techniques in a primate. J Hand Surg 16A:251-261, 1991.

Highet WB, Sanders FK: The effects of stretching nerves after suture. Br J Surg 30: 355-369, 1943.

Hudson AR, Bilbao JM, Hunter D: Polyglycolic acid suture in peripheral nerve: an electron microscopic study. Can J Neurosci 2:17-21, 1975.

Hudson AR, Hunter D: Polyglycolic acid suture in peripheral nerve, Il: sutured sciatic nerve. Can J Neurosci, 3:69-72, 1976.

Humphrey MF, Levy WJ, Dietrich WD, Rumpf R, Mora J: Peripheral nerve repair across a gap studied by repeated observation through a new window implant chamber. Brain Res 497:132-137, 1989.

Hurst LC, Badalamente MA, Ellstein J, Stracher A: Inhibition of neural and muscle degeneration after epineurial neurorrhaphy. J Hand Surg 9:564-571. Abstract, 1984.

Iwagana M, Yamamoto E, Yamauchi M, Fukumoto M, Uchno R, Sawada S: Facial nerve neurinoma. Two cases located in the horizontal portion. Laryngoscope 94: 938-941, 1984.

Johns ME, Crumley RL: Facial nerve injury, repair and rehabilitation. Am Acad Otolaryngol 8:63, 1979.

Jung TT, Jun BH, Shea D, Paparella MM: Primary and secondary tumors of the facial nerve. A temporal bone study. Arch Otolaryng Head Neck Surg 112: 1269-1273, 1986.

Khodadad G: Microsurgical techniques in repair of peripheral nerves. Surg Clin North Am 52: 1157-1166, 1972.

Kline DG, Hayes GJ: The use of a resorbable wrapper for peripheral nerve repair. J Neurosurg 21:737-750, 1964.

Kline DG: Comment. Neurosurgery 22:538-539, 1988.

Korff M, Bent SW, Havig MT, Schwaber MK, Ossoff RH, Zealer DL: An investigation of the potential for laser nerve welding. Otolaryngol Head Neck Surg 106:345-350, 1992.

Labelle JJ, Allen DE: The peripheral nerve repair. J Maine Med Assoc. 63:164-166, 1972.

Langley JN, Hashimoto M: On the suture of separate nerve bundles in a nerve trunk and on internal nerve plexuses. J Physiol 51:318-346, 1917.

Lathrop FD: Management of the facial nerve during operations on the parotid gland. Ann Otol Rhinol Laryngol 72:780-801, 1963.

Levinthal R: Comparison of fascicular, interfascicular, and epineural suture techniques in the repair of simple nerve lacerations. J Neurosurg 47:744-750, 1977.

Lipton R, McCaffrey TV, Ellis J: The beneficial effect of triamcinolone acetonide on nerve repair with autogenous grafts. Otolaryngol Head Neck Surg 94:310-315, 1986.

Mackinnon SE: New directions in peripheral nerve surgery. Ann Plast Surg 22:257-272, 1989.

Madison RD, da Silva CF, Dikkes P: Entubulation repair with protein additives increases the maximum nerve gap distance successfully bridged with tubular prostheses. Brain Res 325-334, 1988.

Maragh H, Hawn R, Gould JD, Terzis JK: Is laser nerve repair comparable to microsuture coaptation? J Reconstr Microsurg 4 :189-195, 1988.

Marshall DM, Grosser M, Stephanides MC, Keeley RD, Rosen JM: Sutureless nerve repair at the fascicular level using a nerve coupler. J Rehab Res 26:63-76, 1989.

McCabe BF: Facial nerve grafting. Plast Reconstr Surg 45:70-75, 1970.

McGuirt WF, McCabe BF: Effect of radiation therapy on facial nerve cable autografts. Laryngoscope 87:415-428, 1977.

Medders G, Mattox DE, Lyles A: Effects of fibrin glue on rat facial nerve regeneration. Otolaryngol Head Neck Surg 100:106-109, 1989.

Merle M, Dellon AL, Campbell JN, Chang PS: Complications from silicon-polymer intubation of nerves. Microsurgery 10:130-133, 1989.

Midgley RD, Woolhouse FM: Silastic sheathing technique for the anastomoses of nerves and tendons. Can Med Assoc J 98:550-551, 1968.

Millesi H, Meissl G, Berger A: The interfascicular nerve-grafting of the median and ulnar nerves. J Bone Joint Surg Am 54:727-750, 1972.

Millesi H: Progress in peripheral nerve reconstruction. World J Surg 14:733-747, 1990.

Moy LJ, Peimer CA, Koniuch MP, Howard C, Zielezny M, Katikaneni PR: Fibrin seal adhesive vs nonabsorbable microsuture in peripheral nerve repair. J Hand Surg. 13A:273-278, 1988.

Muller HW, Ignatius MI, Hangen DH, Shooter EM: Expression of specific sheath cell proteins during peripheral nerve growth and regeneration in mammals. J Cell Biol. 12:393-402, 1986.

Nishihira S, McCaffrey TV: Repair of motor nerve defects: comparison of suture and fibrin adhesive techniques. Otolaryngol Head Neck Surg 100:17-21, 1989.

Pham HN, Padilla JA, Nguyen KD, Rosen JM: Comparison of nerve repair techniques: suture vs avitene-polyglycolic acid tube. J Reconstr Microsurg 7:31-36, 1991.

Pillsbury HC, Fisch U: Extratemporal facial nerve grafting and radiotherapy. Arch Otolaryngol 105:441-446, 1979.

Rice DH, Berstein FD: The use of autogenous vein for nerve grafting. Otolaryngol Head Neck Surg 92:410-412, 1984.

Rich KM, Alexander TD, Pryor JC, Hollowell JP: Nerve growth factor enhances regeneration through silicone chambers. Exp Neurol 105: 162-176, 1989.

Rosen JM, Hentz VR, Kaplan EN: Fascicular sutureless and suture repair of the peripheral nerves: a comparison study in laboratory animals. Orthop Rev 8:85-92, 1979.

Rosen JM, Pham HN, Hentz VR: Fascicular tubulization: a comparison of experimental nerve repair techniques in the cat. Ann Plast Surg 22:467-478, 1989.

Santos PM, Winterowd JG, Graham GA, Bothwell MA, Rubel EW: Nerve growth factor: increased angiogenesis without improved nerve regeneration. Otolaryngol Head Neck Surg 105:12-25, 1991.

Seddon HJ: The use of autogenous grafts for the repair of large gaps in peripheral nerves. Br J Surg 35:151-167, 1947.

Seifert V, Stolke D: Laser-assisted reconstruction of the oculomotor nerve: experimental study on the feasibility of cranial nerve repair. Neurosurgery 25:579-582, 1989.

Smahel J, Meyer VE, Bachem U: Glueing of peripheral nerves with fibrin: experimental studies. J Reconstr Microsurg 3 :211 -218, 1987.

Smith JW: Microsurgery of peripheral nerves. Plast Reconstr Surg 33 :317-329, 1964.

Snyder CG, Webster HF, Pickens JE, Hinff WA, Warden G: Intraneural neurorrhaphy: a preliminary clinical and histological evaluation. Ann Surg. 167:691-696, 1968.

Spector JG, Lee P, Derby A, Roufa DG: Early stages of facial nerve regeneration through silicone chambers in the rabbit. Laryngoscope 101:1109-1123, 1991.

Spreyer P, Schaal H, Kuhn G, et al: Regeneration-associated high level expression of apolipoprotein D mRNA in endoneurial fibroblasts of peripheral nerve. EMBOJ. 9:2479-2484, 1990.

Stensaas L, Bloch LM, Garcia R, Sotelo J: Snug tubular enclosures reduce extrafascicular axonal escape at peripheral nerve repair sites. Exp Neurol: 103:135-145, 1989.

Strange FG: An operation for nerve pedicle grafting. Br J Surg 34: 423-425, 1947.

Sunderland S: Factors influencing the course of regeneration and the quality of the recovery after nerve suture. Brain 75:19-54, 1952.

Sunderland S: Nerves and Nerve Injuries. 2nd ed. New York, NY: Churchill Livingstone Inc; 1978.

Sunderland S: The intraneural topography of the radial, median and ulnar nerves. Brain 68: 243-298, 1945.

Szal GJ, Miller T: Surgical repair of facial nerve branches: an analysis of different sheathing and suturing techniques. Arch Otolaryngol 101:160-165, 1975.

Tupper JW, Crick JC, Matteck LR: Fascicular nerve repairs: a comparative study of epineurial and fascicular (perineurial) techniques. Orthop Clin North Am. 19:57-69, 1988.

Van der Hoop RG, Brakkee JH, Kapelle A, Samson M, DeKoning P, Gispen WH: A new approach for the evaluation of recovery after peripheral nerve damage. J Neurosci Meth 26:111-116, 1988.

Waiton RL, Brown RE, Matory E, Borah GL, Dolph JL: Autogenous vein graft repair of digital nerve defects in the finger: a retrospective clinical study. Plast Reconstr Surg 84:944-949, 1989.

Waller A: Experiments on the section of the glossopharyngeal and hypoglossal nerves of the frog and observations of the alterations produced thereby in the structure of their primitive fibres. Phil Trans 140:423-429, 1850.

Weiss P: The technology of nerve regeneration: Sutureless tubulation and related methods of nerve repair. Neurosurgery l:400-450, 1944.

Wilkolm RP, Swett JE, Torigoe Y, Blanks R: Repair of severed peripheral nerve: a superior anatomic and functional recovery with a new reconnection technique. Otolaryngol Head Neck Surg 99:353-361, 1988.

Wise AJ, Topuzlu C, Davis P, Kaye IS: A comparative analysis of macro and microsurgical neurorrhaphy technics. Am J Surg 117: 566-572, 1969.

Young JZ, Medawar BB: Fibrin suture of peripheral nerves: measurement of the rate of regeneration. Lancet 239:126-128, 1940.

Zini C, Sanna M, Jemmi G, Gandolfi A: Transmastoid extralabyrinthine approach in traumatic facial palsy. Am J Otol 6:216-221, 1985.

14

Facial reinnervation techniques

The facial nerve lesion may be seen in otologic, otoneurological and skull base surgery. Often the nerve must be transposed in surgery of the skull base (e.g. in the infratemporal approach).

In oncological surgery of the skull base, a malignant tumor may invade the nerve. The tumor must be partially removed, so that it does not impede the most propitious access. In the latter case, the microscopic section of the nerve significantly increases operating space, and paves the way for reconstruction. This will give better results compared to a nerve which has undergone intraoperative retraction and stretching.

After a voluntary or iatrogenic neurotmesis, the nerve must be repaired.

- Whenever possible, the direct reconstruction of the nerve is always the best choice. Better functional recovery is obtained, as well as fewer involuntary expression movements compared to VII-XII anastomosis.
- When the substance loss is such that it does not permit the two stumps to rejoin, it is preferential to graft a segment of another nerve, such as the greater auricular nerve, the ileo-inguinal nerve, the lateral cutaneous femoral nerve, the sural nerve, or the transverse nerve of the neck. The stumps of the graft, inserted into the fallopian canal, are sutured at the ends of the nerve according to the aforementioned technique (Figs. 14-1, 14-2, 14-3).

In some cases, neither of these two options is possible. One example is when there is the certainty after surgery that the facial nerve has been preserved intact, but it shows no signs of functional recovery post-operatively, even a year after surgery. Another example is when, during neuroma removal surgery, the facial nerve breaks at the brainstem and there is no proximal stump to be grafted.
In these situations, other reparatory techniques must be used.

The objectives in every facial reinnervation procedure are those indicated by Conley:

- Normal resting facial aspect.
- Symmetry of voluntary movements.
- Controlled equilibrium in expressing emotions.
- Restitution of control of oral, nasal, and ocular sphincters.
- No loss of other important functions.

It is impossible to completely reach these goals, even with an immediate suture. Research has been developed on techniques that approximate these goals as much as possible, when neither termino-terminal suturing nor grafting is possible (Figs. 14-4, 14-5, 14-6).

NERVE SUBSTITUTION PROCEDURE

- The procedure of facial anastomosis with the accessory spinal nerve has been almost abandoned due to its side effects: postoperative atrophy of the trapezius muscle and the sternocleidomastoid muscle, with pain and lowering of the shoulder.
- The utilization of the glossopharyngeal nerve or the phrenic nerve have been abandoned because these lead to excessive involuntary facial spasms. Further, the injured phrenic nerve may further compromise the pulmonary systems protection capacity.
- The nerve substitution procedures have the advantages of providing an adequate number of axons to the musculature and require a single microneural anastomosis. The disadvantages include the necessity of distally intact endoneural tubules and a non-atrophied musculature. There is also the deficit due to the sacrifice of the donor nerve, and recruitment movements are frequent. Hyperkinesis is a sign when a cranial motor nerve is substituted because the neural input may be superior to the normal stimulus required.

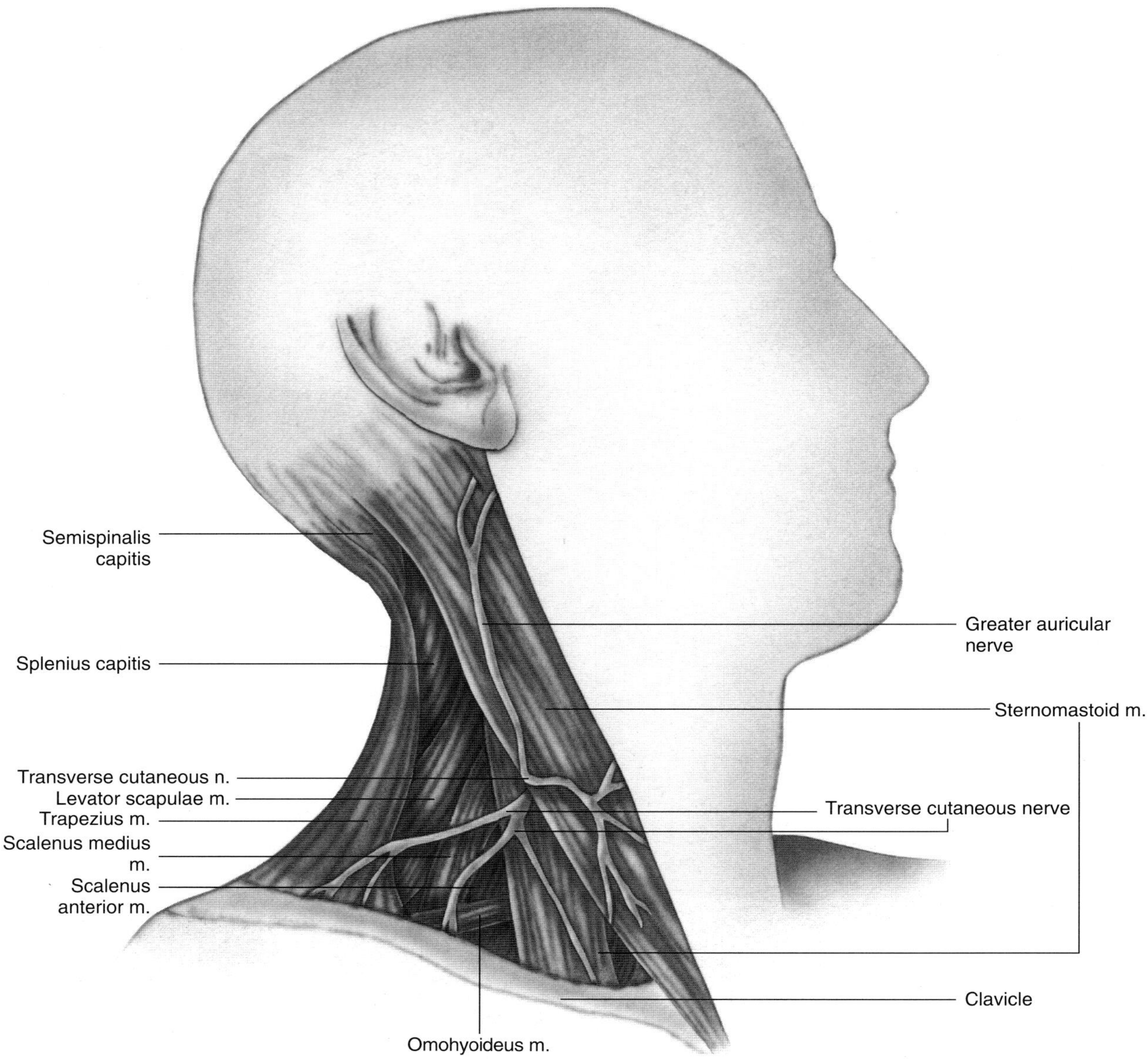

Fig. 14-1. Posterior triangle of the neck (behind the sternocleidomastoid muscle). The muscles and the greater auricular nerve.

HYPOGLOSSAL-FACIAL ANASTOMOSIS

When direct repair or grafting are not possible, a nerve substitution procedure is followed. The most effective is currently the hypoglossal-facial anastomosis. This technique was made popular by Conley and Baker, who cite the numerous points in its favor:

- The tongue and the facial movements originate in areas adjacent to the motor cortex.
- In the brainstem, the centers of the hypoglossal and the facial nerves have a pattern similar to motor nuclei.
- Most of the facial movements are associated with a certain degree of voluntary and involuntary lingual movements.
- Nerves VII and XII have a similar diameter (2-3 mm), though the hypoglossal nerve is slightly larger.

The prerequisites for surgery are:

- Intact extracranial facial nerve. Intact hypoglossal nerve.
- Facial expression muscles intact.
- Patient prepared to accept deficits caused by hypoglossal nerve sacrifice.
- Patient's life expectancy adequate (time needed for recovery may not justify the approach).
- Patient not at risk for other neurological deficits, such as alterations of nerves IX and X, since these may present serious alterations in language and swallowing.

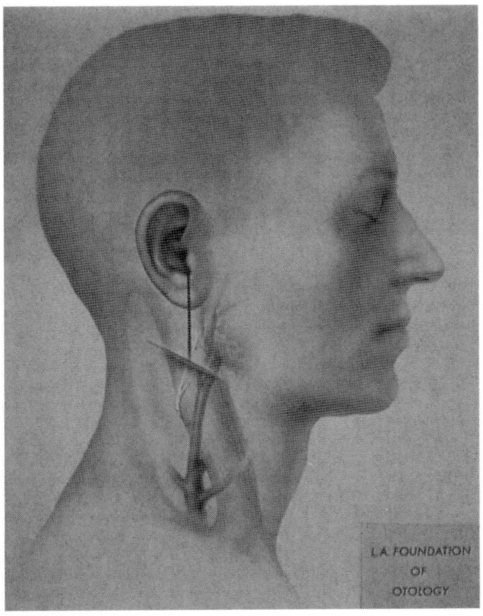

Fig. 14-2. The course and the harvesting of the greater auricular nerve.

Good results can be guaranteed with a homolateral hemilingual paralysis, which is generally well tolerated in any case.

Hypoglossal-facial anastomosis may not be utilized in the following instances:

- The hypoglossal nerve is intact on only one side.
- Reanimation of both sides of the face in patients with bilateral facial paralysis. In patients with Type 2 Neurofibromatosis in which there is the risk of a contralateral extension of the paralysis and/or a lesion of the mixed nerves.
- Patients who refuse the consequences of the hypoglossal nerve sacrifice, especially patients whose profession requires them to speak in public.
- When there is also a deficit of the mixed nerves or nerve X.

The disadvantages of hypoglossal-facial anastomosis are the following:

- Hypertony of facial musculature in 2/3 of patients. In general this is in the medial third of the face and most frequently seen during chewing.
- Loss of emotional facial mobility.
- Slight alteration in chewing, swallowing, and language capacity. Patients need their food cut into small pieces and must frequently extract food manually from the buccal and lingual sulci on the affected side.

SURGICAL TECHNIQUE

- Incision: (Fig. 14-7). The incision begins one cm above the tragus, descends, passes horizontally under the lobe for approx. 1/2 cm, then curves

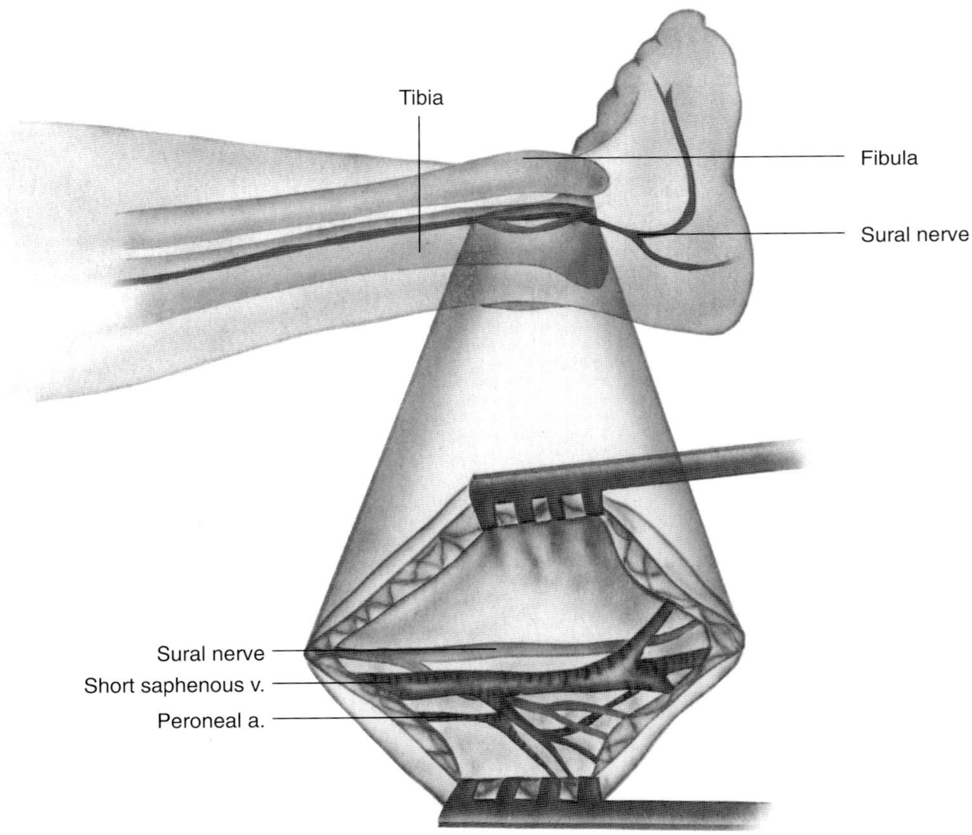

Fig. 14-3. Harvesting of the sural nerve (Adapted from Sekhar LN).

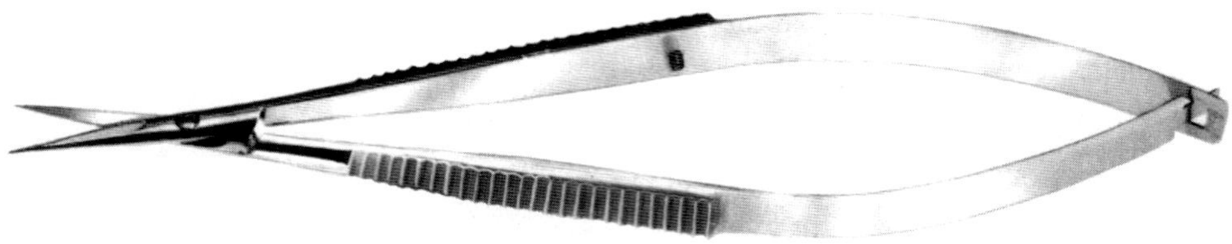

Fig. 14-4. Microscissors.

skirting the sternocleidomastoid muscle, and reaches the great horn of the hyoid passing approx. 2 cm from the mandibular angle.

- Elevation of the skin flaps.
- Separation of the posterior face of the gland from the sternocleidomastoid muscle posteriorly, from the mastoid apex superiorly and from the external auditory canal above.
- With the tip of the forceps or with a knife (n. 15 blade), the superficial aponeurosis of the sternocleidomastoid muscle is cut, and the parotid gland is placed on its superficial face. Thus the great auricular nerve is identified, running over the sternocleidomastoid muscle and approx. 2 cm under the mastoid tip. It has an oblique and superior course, towards the vertical branch of the mandible.
- Section of the temporoparotid fascia which is the only thing attaching the gland posteriorly. Forward traction of the gland. Thus cartilage of the external auditory canal is exposed.
- With the rounded point of scissors or forceps, the cartilage is separated from the external auditory canal of the parotid. After a few mm, a cleavage plane is reached which leads to the end of the cartilage, where a finger shaped projection is found called the "tragal pointer".
- Thus the "tragal pointer" has been identified above and the mastoid process and the insertion of the posterior belly of the digastric muscle posteriorly.
- The dissection proceeds medially and posteriorly to the "tragal pointer", until reaching the stylomastoid foramen, where the facial nerve exits.
- With curved blunt forceps or with scissors the dissection of the nerve is continued anteriorly into the parotid, until the main trunk is freed and the *pes anserinus* has been exposed.
- Retraction of the sternocleidomastoid muscle posteriorly and exposure of the large vessels of the neck.
- Superior retraction of the posterior belly of the digastric muscle, and identification of the hypoglossal nerve descending between the jugular vein and the internal carotid.
- At the level of the bifurcation of the common carotid, superior to the great horn of the hyoid bone, a loop is formed. The branch going in an anterior direction is the true hypoglossal nerve. The descending branch "descends" and then unites with the inferior root of the cervical loop and forms a loop, called the cervical or hypoglossal loop (see chapter 6).
- The nerve in contact with the facial artery superiorly and the lingual artery inferiorly runs on the surface of the hyoglossal muscle, enters in contact with the lingual nerve, the submandibular gland and its duct, passes above the mylohyoid margin, and proceeds to innervate the lingual muscles.
- The hypoglossal nerve is followed and isolated from its fascial adherences in the neck with blunt scissors to its entrance into the lingual musculature.
- Section of the facial nerve at the level of the stylomastoid foramen.
- Section of the hypoglossal nerve as anteriorly as possible, to acquire greater length (Fig. 14-8).

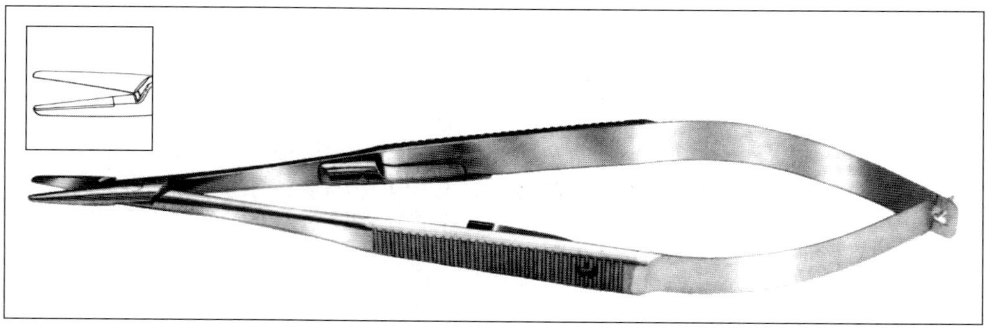

Fig. 14-5. Nerve anastomosis equipment. Needle holder.

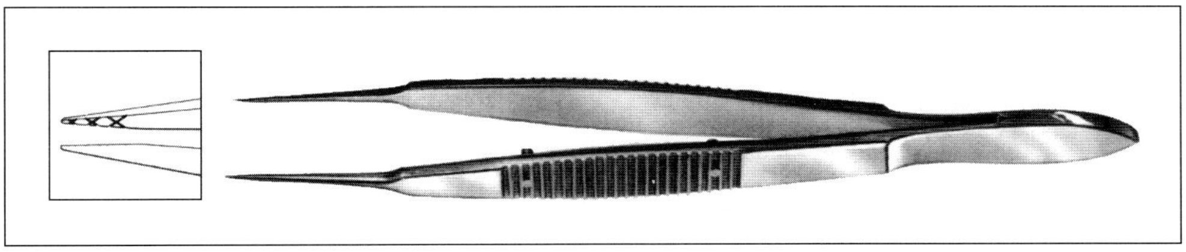

Fig. 14-6. Nerve anastomosis equipment. Forceps.

- The hypoglossal nerve is rotated superiorly and anastomosed to the facial nerve.
- Anastomosis is performed according to the common techniques (Fig. 14-9).

RESULTS

The facial nerve innervates 16 complex muscles on each side of the face, and contains components of the sensory and autonomous nervous system.
The normal organization of the innervation is altered after a neurotmesis.
After even the most careful nerve suture, an inappropriate connection is seen between neurons (Crumley). The neurons go to innervate agonistic and antagonistic facial muscular groups, haphazardly, causing a cancellation effect.
It is not known to what extent the supraspinal system of the central nervous system can compensate the altered connection between neurons (R. Leffert), but it is impossible to obtain a normal facial function.
Due to the altered direction of the axons, synkinesis and mass movement are always observed, which are very bothersome to the patients.

Management of Hyperkinesis

To reduce synkinesis, exercise or biofeedback may be useful during recovery. In serious cases the selective section of facial nerve branches has been proposed, as well as the use of botulin toxin injections. Botulin toxin is injected into hyperkinetic muscles. When its effects vanish after 2-7 months, the injections can be repeated.

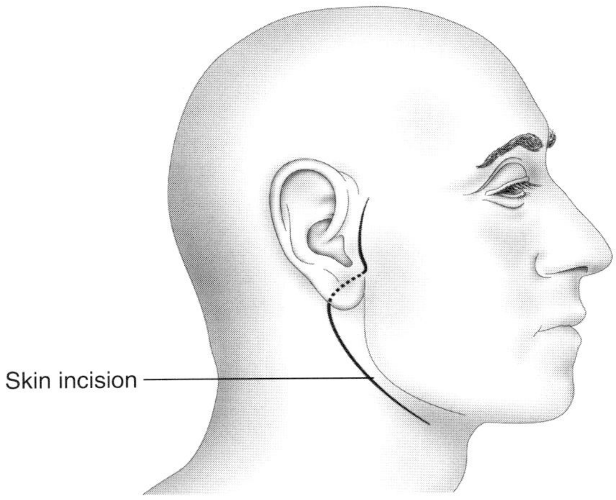

Fig. 14-7. Skin incision for hypoglossal facial anastomosis.

- Selective neurolysis can be used in the management of hyperkinesis, in order to weaken or paralyze the innervation of the muscles involved.
- The most lasting results, however, are obtained with regional myectomy. A portion of the involved muscle is selectively excised.
- Hyperkinesis of muscles around the eye: excision of the orbicularis oculi muscle. Chin spasm: mentalis myectomy. Hyperkinesis of the oral levator muscles: resection of the zygomaticus and levator labii superioris muscles.
- After anastomosis of VII and XII, the blinking reflex cannot be obtained even in the best of cases. Thus xerophthalmia and cheratitis from exposure can be seen, necessitating a palpebral reanimation procedure (see chapter 15).
- The first signs of functional recovery are obtained after 4 to 6 months.
- The functional interaction between the facial nerve and the hypoglossal nerve for chewing, swallowing and phonation facilitate the functional recovery compared to the use of the phrenic nerve or the spinal accessory nerve. The patient may also become accustomed to provoking facial movements by attempting to move the tongue.
- The rehabilitative procedure may be strengthened with an electromyographic feedback-enhanced rehabilitation.
- In time, with recovery of the facial muscular tension and the atrophy of the hemilingua, chewing capacity is improved. Food is mantained in the buccal vestibule, and the bothersome accumulation of food in the lingual sulcus is reduced.

The classification of the results obtained with rehabilitation may not be done with the House-Brackmann grading system, which was conceived to evaluated the function of the facial nerve, without undergoing a reinnervation process. To examine the results of the hypoglossal-facial anastomosis, we use the Luxford and Brackmann classification (Table 14-1).

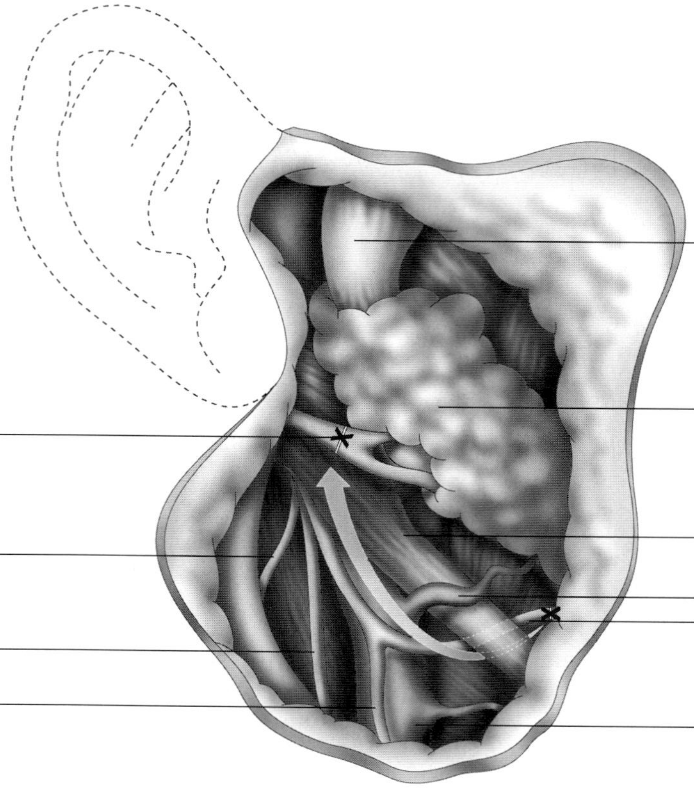

Fig. 14-8. The hypoglossal nerve is exposed and cut as far anteriorly as is possible. The distal end of the facial nerve is cut and sutured to the proximal end of the hypoglossal nerve. (Adapted from Luxford WM and House JR).

The sooner the anastomosis is performed, the better the functional results and the surpassing of the hypoglossal deficit will be.

In conclusion, the hypoglossal-facial anastomosis attains the following objectives:

- Normal facial symmetry at rest.
- Good voluntary mobility of the hemiface.

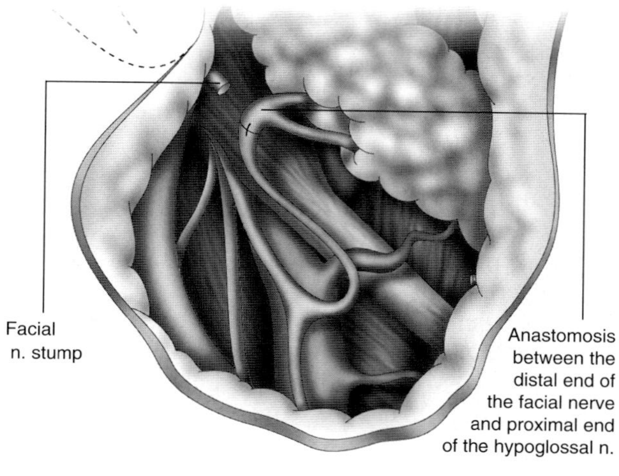

Fig. 14-9. The distal end of the facial nerve is sutured to the proximal end of the hypoglossal nerve. (Adapted from Luxford WM and House JR).

- Absence of reflexes or emotional facial movements.
- A certain degree of synkinesis in facial movements.
- Slight functional deficit of the hemilingua for hypoglossal paralysis.

The results obtained by the Otologic Medical Group revealed an excellent functional recovery in 25% of cases, good in 35%, fair in 32%, and poor in 8%.

INTERPOSITIONAL JUMP GRAFT

The technique of hypoglossal-facial jump grafting was proposed by May, as a facial reanimation

Table 14-1. Facial nerve function after VII-XII Anastomosis: Qualitative Recovery Criteria.

Poor muscular tone with no symmetry or mobility (motility)
Fair muscular tone, symmetry, reduced mobility
Good muscular tone, symmetry, fair mobility, moderate synkinesis
Excellent muscular tone, symmetry, fair mobility, slight synkinesis

From Luxford WM, Brackmann DE: Facial nerve substitution. A review of 66 cases. Am J Otol (Suppl): 55-57, 1985.

technique for those patients who cannot tolerate an alteration of the lingual functionality.
This is an interposition of a nerve graft between the partially sectioned hypoglossal nerve and the main trunk, or a few distal branches of the injured facial nerve.
It may provide a significant improvement in facial function, if associated with other facial reanimation techniques, without sacrificing lingual function.

Surgical Technique.

- Skin incision: typical incision for parotid surgery.
- Mobilization of the parotid, identification of the facial nerve to its bifurcation.
- Isolation of the hypoglossal nerve between the internal jugular vein and the internal and external carotid arteries, under the digastric muscle.
- Identification of the main trunk of the hypoglossal nerve and the descending branch with umbilical threads of different colors. The hypoglossal nerve is sectioned from 1/3 to halfway, and the proximal axons are exposed. The hypoglossal nerve is stimulated electrically near the partial section: a sudden contraction of the hemilingua indicates that a sufficient number of axons have been spared. This data enables the prediction of the degree of preservation of lingual function.
- Harvesting of graft to position: greater auricular, cutaneous cervical or sural, approx. 5-7 cm in length. The graft must be twice as long as needed, to guarantee the absence of traction (Fig. 14-10).
- Suture of the graft, according to the usual technique: one part to the sectioned half of the hypoglossal nerve, and the other to the distal extremity of the facial nerve. The extremities of the nerves must demonstrate vital tissue, swollen and white. The epineurium is sutured with a no. 9-0 or 10-0 monofilament nylon suture (Fig. 14-11).
- The hypoglossal nerve is not a polifascicular nerve; thus it is not possible to identify the fascicles. It is, however, possible to use a splitting technique with the hypoglossal nerve, since its diameter is greater than that of the facial nerve.

Advantages.

- Good recovery of facial tone, symmetry and fair facial musculature movement.
- Absence of mass movement and fewer problems in swallowing, mastication and phonation compared to the classical VII-VII anastomosis.

Disadvantages.

- Facial muscles contractions of lower intensity and longer recovery time compared to classical VII-XII anastomosis.

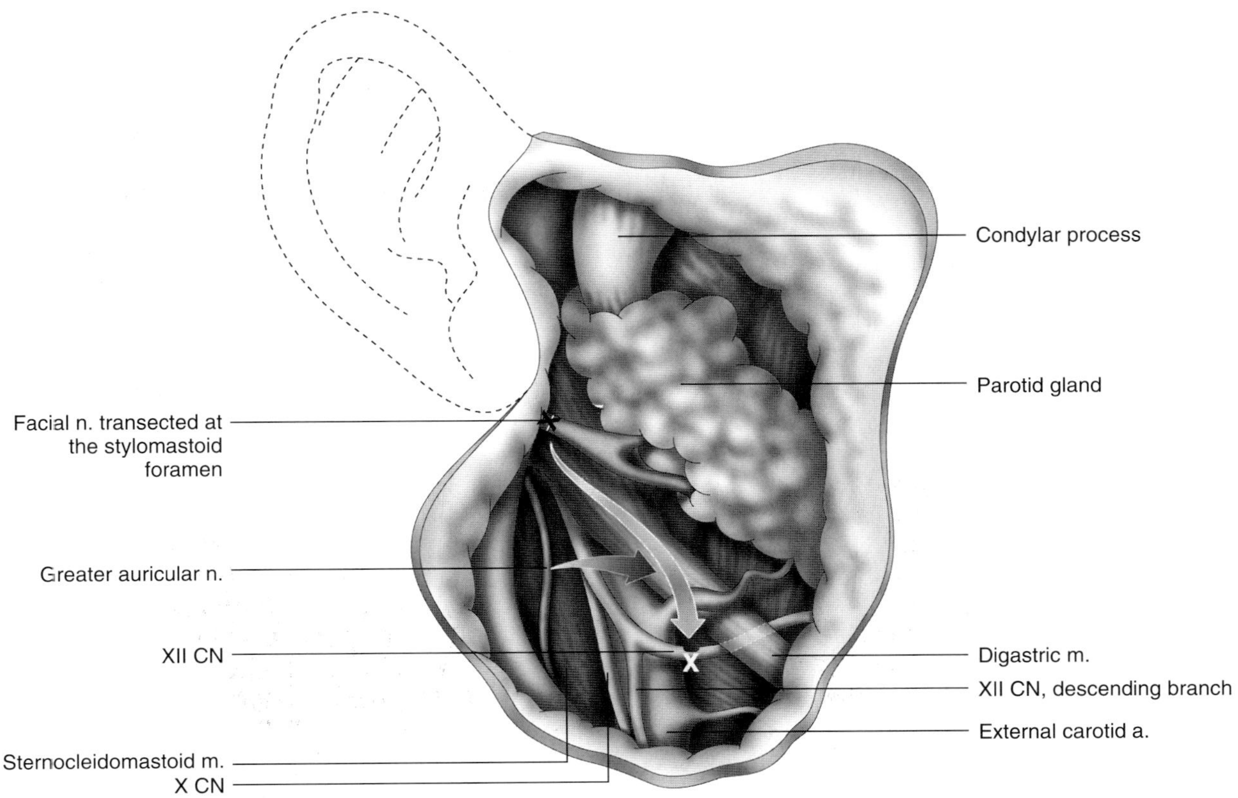

Fig. 14-10. VII-XII jump graft (May M.). The greater auricular nerve is harvested.

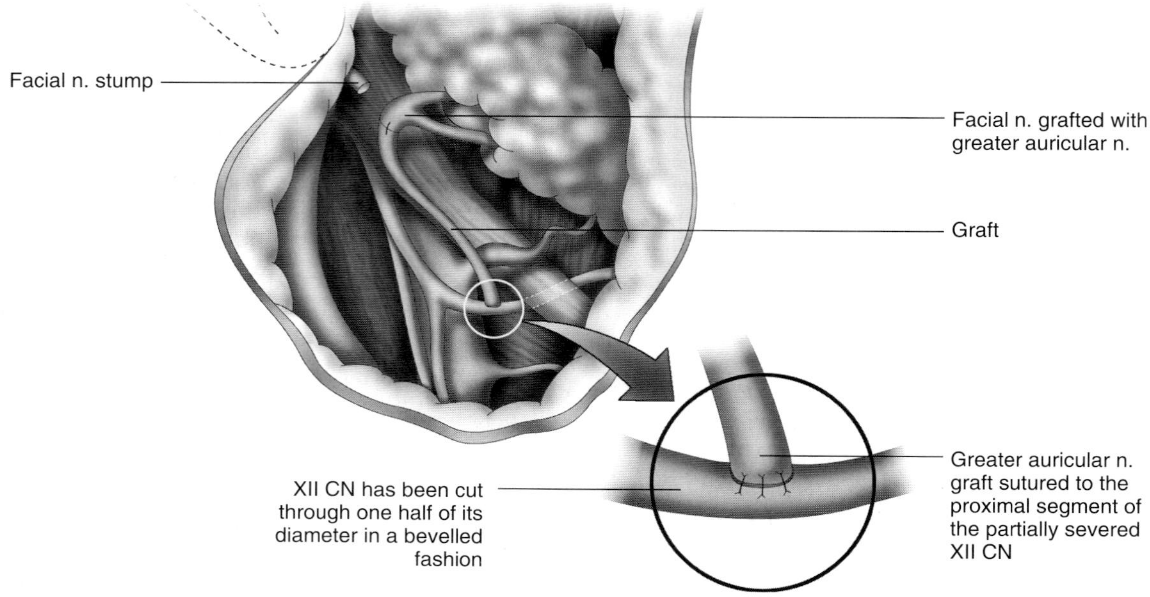

Fig. 14-11. The distal end of the facial nerve is severed, the hypoglossal nerve is partially severed. The greater auricular nerve graft is sutured to the facial nerve and to the partially severed hypoglossal nerve (May M).

- Better results are obtained when the technique is performed within a year of the lesion, whereas VII-XII anastomosis can be done up to two years later.
- An error to be avoided: if a branch of the cervical loop of the hypoglossal nerve is mistakenly used instead of the hypoglossal nerve itself, the results are less promising.

PARTIAL ANASTOMOSIS OF THE HYPOGLOSSAL NERVE WITH THE FACIAL NERVE

A procedure similar to May's has been proposed by Cusimano and Sekhar, but is differentiated by the facial nerve being sutured to the partially sectioned hypoglossal nerve, without the interposition of other nerves.

Surgical Technique

- Exposure of the hypoglossal nerve and the facial nerve by means of a cervical incision, from the skull base to the mylohyoid muscle.
- Section of the facial nerve as near as possible to the stylomastoid foramen.
- Section of the hypoglossal nerve to verify its capacity to conduct the stimulus to the tongue. If the nerve does not transmit adequately, the descending branch of the hypoglossal nerve may be anastomosed with the main trunk, following the usual procedure (see following section) .
- It is very important to perform a suture without tension. Thanks to a section as proximal as possible to the two nerves, this objective is almost always reached. In other cases the great auricular nerve or the sural nerve is interposed.
- In Cusimano and Sekhar's experience, on a single patient, the facial function recovery is comparable to that of VII-XII anastomosis. A sufficient lingual functionality is also obtained, due probably to hypertrophy of the non-paralyzed muscles.

CROSS FACIAL GRAFTING

This technique, proposed by H. Anderl, is based on the connection of some fibers of the contralateral facial nerve (intact) with the paralyzed facial musculature.
It has the advantage of permitting symmetrical voluntary and emotional movements and not provoking motor deficit. It does, however, partially alter the normal nerve, and furnishes the muscles with a scarce supply of neural elements. These disadvantages have made this technique less widely-used.

TIPS AND PITFALLS

- When a facial nerve synthesis is performed at the level of or distal to the geniculate ganglion, it is helpful to section the greater superficial petrosal nerve, to avoid axon regeneration through this nerve (U. Fisch).
- The nerve is like a banana (May) (see chapter 13).

To avoid damage to the facial nerve:

- Never touch the nerve with the tip of the aspirator.
- Preserve the arteries going to the nerve.
- In case of a nerve reroute, dissect it with a knife or sharp (not blunt) instruments.
- In case of a CPA tumor, it is important not to stretch the nerve; for the tumor dissection, a medial to lateral direction is preferable.
- It is well to use high powered enlargements (25x) when working with the nerve, since once the cleavage plane is lost, it becomes very difficult to find it once again.
- When removing a tumor from the CPA, part of the facial nerve must be devascularized, which causes its suffering.
- In neuromas of nerve VII with normal facial function, we believe the best route is to remove the neuroma and perform a graft. Thus a response is obtained equal to grade III on the House-Brackmann scale. If too much time has elapsed and the facial nerve is already paralyzed, grade III can no longer be obtained.
- Most of nerve VII's vascularization is along the greater superficial petrosal nerve, which is cut to perform a posterior rerouting of the facial nerve (transcochlear surgery). The interruption of this arterial supply is the primary cause of reduced post-operative function in nerve VII (House-Brackmann III).
- In choosing the reparatory technique, the duration of the paralysis should be considered. The facial nerve remains in good conditions and does not degenerate even 10 years after the lesion, though it may form a fibrosis. On the other hand, the facial muscles, consequent to the denervation, proceed rapidly towards atrophy and irreversible degeneration. This degenerative process becomes evident at around 12-14 months. Thus, within a year of the onset of paralysis due to a lesion of nerve VII, VII-XII neurorrhaphy or grafting is preferable, since this has a greater effect on the nerve. After a year, VII-XII anastomosis is preferable, since only 4 months are required for regeneration, whereas 12 months are necessary for grafting. This latency provokes an increase in the muscular degeneration which compromises rehabilitative results.

One factor to consider in the choice of a reparatory technique. If grafting is considered, it is essential to keep the length of the reparatory graft in mind. The longer it is, the less favorable the results will be.

REFERENCES

Anderl H: Cross-face nerve grafting: up to 12 months of seventh nerve disruption. In: LR Rubin, ed. Reanimation of the paralyzed face. St. Louis: CV Mosby Co, 1977: 241-277.

Balliet R, Shinn JB, Gach-Y-Rita P: Facial paralysis rehabilitation: Retraining selective muscle control. Int Rehabil Med 4: 67-74, 1982.

Belal A Jr: Structure of human muscle in facial paralysis: Role of muscle biopsy. In May M (ed): The Facial Nerve. New York, Thieme, 1986, pp 99-106.

Broniatowski M, Grundfest-Broniatowski S, Davies CR, et al: Dynamic rehabilitation of the paralyzed face: III. Balanced coupling of oral and ocular musculature from the intact side in the canine. Otolaryngol Head Neck Surg 105: 727-733, 1991.

Brudny J, Hammerschlag PE, Cohen NL, Ransohoff J: Electromyographic rehabilitation of facial function and introduction of a facial paralysis grading scale for hypoglossal-facial nerve anastomosis. Laryngoscope 98: 405-410, 1988.

Cannoni M, Pech A, Zanaret M, Thomassin JM, Goubert JL: Notre experience de l'anastomose hypoglosso-faciale. Ann Oto-Laryng (Paris) 99: 299-302, 1982.

Chang CGS, Shen AL: Hypoglossofacial anastomosis for facial palsy after resection of acoustic neuroma. Surg Neurol (21): 282-286, 1984.

Chuang DCC, Wei FC, Noordhoff MS: "Smile" reconstruction in facial paralysis. Ann Plast Surg 23: 56-65, 1989.

Conley J, Baker DC: Hypoglossal-facial nerve anastomosis for reinnervation of the paralyzed face. Plast Reconstr Surg 63: 63-72, 1979.

Dressler D, Schonle PW: Hyperkinesias after hypoglossofacial nerve anastomosis-treatment with botulinum toxin. Eur Neurol 31: 44-46, 1991.

Fisch U: Reconstruction intra-cranienne du nerf facial apres exerese du neurinome de l'acoustique. Communication colloque "Neurinomes de l'acoustique acquisitions et controverses." Toulouse 7 et 8.11. 1986 (a paraitre), 1986.

Gavron JP, Clemis JD: Hypoglossal-facial nerve anastomosis: A review of forty cases caused by facial nerve injuries in the posterior fossa. Laryngoscope 94: 1447-1450, 1984.

Harrison DH: The pectoralis minor vascularized muscle graft for the treatment of unilateral facial palsy. Plast Reconstr Surg 75: 206-216, 1985.

Hitselberger WE: Hypoglossal-facial anastomosis. In House WF, Luetje CM (eds): Acoustic Tumors, Vol 2: Management. Baltimore, University Park Press, 1979, pp 97-103.

Janecka IP, Sekhar LN, Sen CN: Facial nerve management in cranial base surgery. Laryngoscope 103: 291-298, 1993.

Janecka IP, Sen CN, Sekhar LN: Facial Translocation. A new approach to the cranial base. Otolaryngol Head Neck Surg, 25: 931-941, 1989.

Sekhar LN, Janecka IP, Jones NF: Subtemporal-infratemporal basal subfrontal approach to extensive cranial base tumors. Acta Neurochir (Wien) 92: 1, 1988.

Janecka IP: Integrity of Facial Function: Its Preservation and Repair. Critical Reviews in Neurosurgery: 1:60-71, 1991.

Luxford WM, Brackmann DE: Facial nerve substitution: A review of sixty-six cases. Am J Otol (Suppl): 55-57, 1985.

May M: Management of cranial nerves I through VII following skull base surgery. Otolaryngol Head Neck Surg 88: 560-575, 1980.

May M, Sobol SM, Mester SJ: Hypoglossal-facial nerve interpositional jump graft for facial reanimation without tongue atrophy. Otolaryngol Head Neck Surg 104: 818-825, 1991.

O'Brien BM, Pederson WC, Khazanchi RK, et al: Results of management of facial palsy with microvascular free-muscle transfer. Plast Reconstr Surg 86: 12-22, 1990.

Pensak ML, Jackson CG, Glasscock ME III, Gulya AJ: Facial reanimation with the VII-XII anastomosis: Analysis of the functional and psychologic results. Otolaryngol Head Neck Surg 94: 305-310, 1986.

Pitty LF, Tator CH: Hypoglossal-facial nerve anastomosis for facial nerve palsy following surgery for cerebellopontine angle tumors. J Neurosurg 77: 724-731, 1992.

Qay M: Surgical rehabilitation of facial palsy. In May M (ed): The Facial Nerve. New York, Thieme, 1986, pp 695-777.

Sabin HI, Bordi LT, Symon L, Compton JS: Facio-hypoglossal anastomosis for the treatment of facial palsy after acoustic neuroma resection. Br J Neurosurg 4: 313-318, 1990.

Samii M: Rehabilitation of the face by facial nerve substitution: Panel discussion. Fisch U (ed): Facial Nerve Surgery. Birmingham, AL, Aesculapius, 1977, pp 244-245.

Stennert E: 1. Hypoglossal facial anastomosis: Its significance for modern facial surgery. II. Combined approach in extratemporal facial nerve reconstruction. Clin Plast Surg 6: 471-486, 1979.

Tran Ba Huy P, Monteil JP, Rey A: Results of twenty cases of transfacio-facial anastomosis as compared with those of XII-VII anastomosis. *In* Portmann M (ed): Facial Nerve. New York, Masson, 1985, pp 85-87.

Tucker HM: Restoration of selective facial nerve function by the nerve-muscle pedicle technique. Clin Plast Surg 6: 293-300, 1979.

Ylikoski I, Hitselberger WE, House WF, et al: Degenerative changes in the distal stump of the severed human facial nerve. Acta Otolaryngol (Stockh) 92: 239-248, 1981.

Zini C, Sanna M, Gandolfi A: Hypoglosso-facial anastomosis in the rehabilitation of irreversible facial nerve palsies. *In* Portmann M (ed): Facial Nerve. New York, Masson, 1985, pp 519-522.

15

Facial reanimation techniques

The facial reanimation procedures, as well as the reinnervation techniques, are classified as either static or dynamic.

STATIC PROCEDURES
Brow lift
Static slings
Lower Lip Rehabilitation
Canthoplasty
Treatment of Hyperkinesis

DYNAMIC PROCEDURES
Reanimation of the eye
Gold weight implantation
Eyespring implantation
Silastic prosthesis implantation

Temporary sutures
Taped suture of the upper lid to cheek
Temporary tarsorrhaphy

Transposition of the temporalis muscle
Free muscle flaps

- If a facial paralysis is left untreated, the following consequences on the paralyzed eye become evident in a few days: Lagophthalmus (lid-lag), ectropion, epiphora, exposure keratitis, blurred vision, and corneal ulceration.
- Appropriate eye care must be adopted for the duration of the paralysis. A suitable eye reanimation procedure must be chosen within a few days of onset.
- Facial reinnervation procedures are valuable, but a few months are needed for them to become effective. During this period, regional techniques are useful to protect the eye and correct deformities of the mouth, while the potential for recovery from nerve grafts or substitution is left unaffected.

STATIC PROCEDURES

In each of the following procedures, the eye is protected with a scleral shell.

Brow Lift

A paralyzed eyebrow may be seen as the result of a Bell's paralysis or herpes zoster oticus. The main symptomps are visual field reduction and feeling of heaviness in the upper eyelid.
Treatment:
- In cases of dermatochalasis of the eyebrow, blepharoplasty is the treatment of choice.
- If there is a contemporary diminishing in the orbicularis oculi muscle function, an eyelid reanimation procedure is performed.
- In other cases, a brow lift is done.

This operation is performed with the patient under local anesthesia, in order to control the results of surgical manipulation.

Static Slings

- In cases of facial paresis, static slings are used to correct the ptosis of lower facial tissues, to improve at rest facial symmetry.
- Preparation of a tunnel in the superficial musculoaponeurotic system. The palmaris longus muscle or the fascia lata graft are sutured to the levator angularis muscles of the mouth and then suspended from the zygomatic arch with a miniplate. This results in an elevation of the corner of the mouth and a collapsed nasal ala, slightly more than necessary.

Lower Lip Rehabilitation

This technique can be used to depress the paralyzed lower lip.
The tendon of the anterior belly of the digastric muscle is transposed and sutured to the lower lip of the depressor muscles, after having prepared a tunnel. The digastric muscle thus counteracts the action of the muscles elevating the lips.

Canthoplasty

Canthoplasty can be medial or lateral.
Medial canthoplasty
The globe is protected with a scleral shell. Probes are inserted into the canaliculi to protect them.

An incision is made at the mucocutaneous junction. The two medial canthal tendons are exposed, and sutured together with 5.0 polyester. The skin is closed.
This technique is useful as a temporary or permanent measure for correcting mild degrees of lower lip droop and eversion of the lower lacrimal punctum.

Lateral Canthoplasty

This is helpful in reducing lateral lid opening. The inferior canthal tendon is sectioned; traction is placed on the tendon until it reaches the desired position, and it is sutured with 5-0 polyester. The excess tissue surrounding the tendon is cut, leaving a tarsal tongue. The tarsal tongue is pulled under the superior tendon and sutured to the periosteum of the rim. The skin is closed.

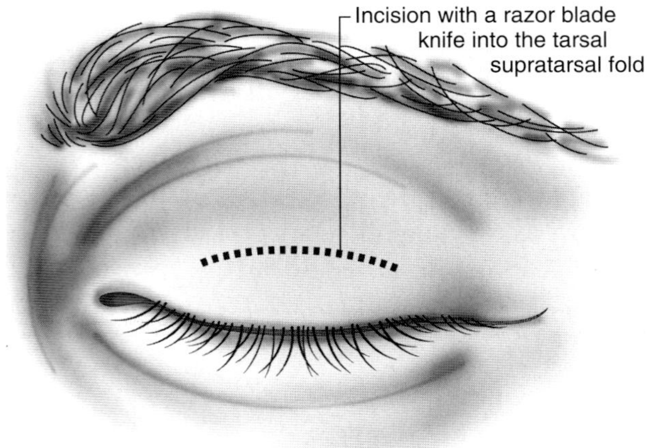

Fig. 15-1. Incision in the lid fold, for gold weight implantation.

DYNAMIC PROCEDURES

Gold Weight Implantation

A gold weight of an adequate size is selected and attached to the patient's upper eyelid with cyanoacrilate glue. The patient opens and closes his eyes to permit the surgeon to select the correct weight. Through an incision in the fold of the eyelid (Fig. 15-1), the orbital septum is exposed and the gold weight is sutured onto the levator aponeurosis with 5.0 polyester (Fig. 15-2). The patient opens and closes his eyes once more to ensure that the adequate weight has been chosen. The incision is closed with 7.0 catgut (Fig. 15-3). The implant works better when the patient is upright. The patient is counseled to sleep with his

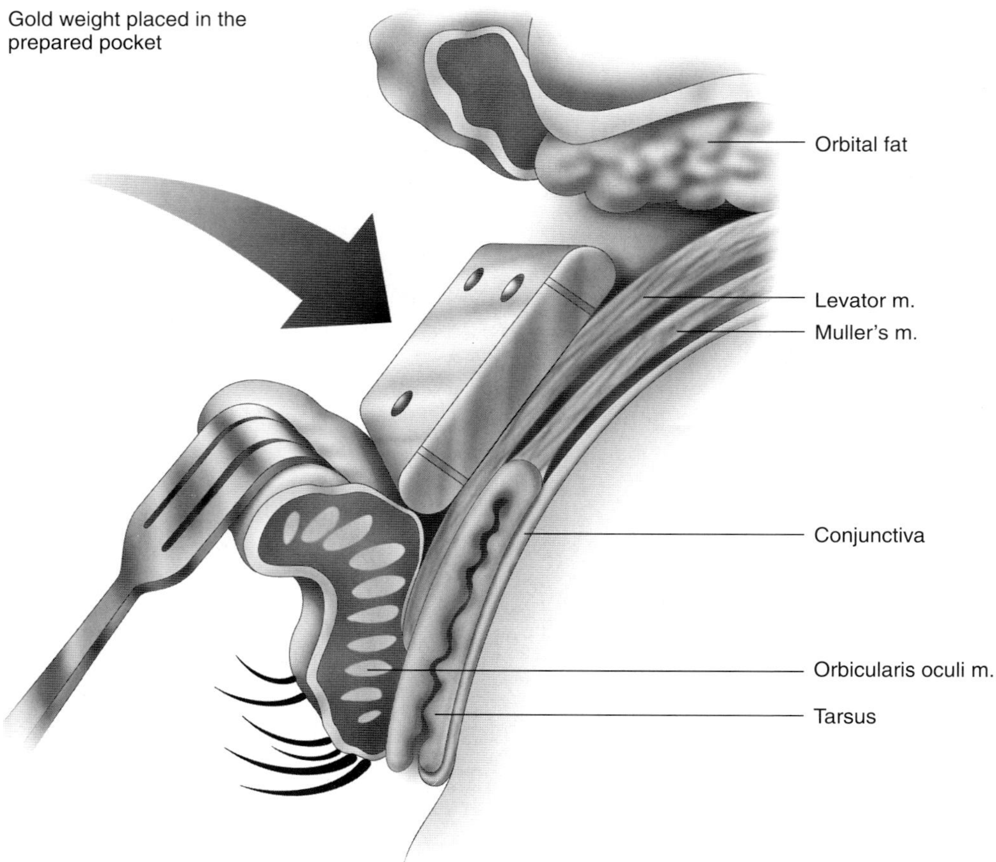

Fig. 15-2. The orbital septum is exposed (Adapted from May M. and from Levine RE).

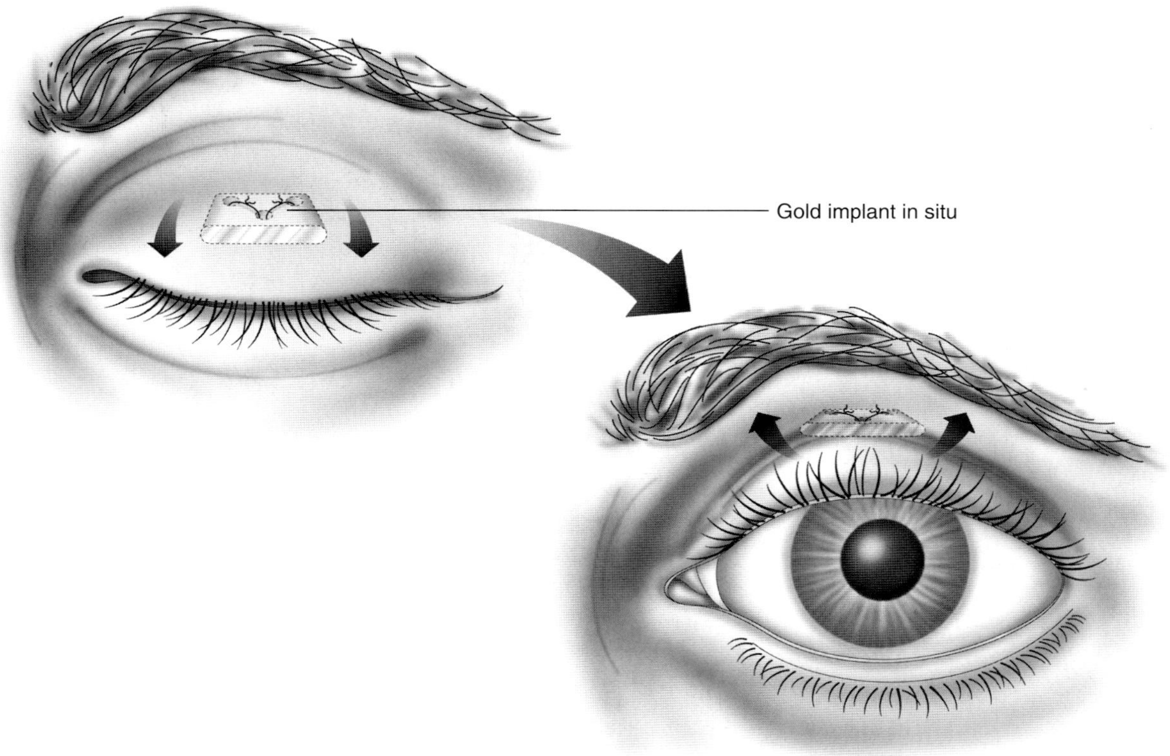

Fig. 15-3. The weight is fixated supratarsally to the levator m., with a 5.0 polyester suture. The gold weight is suitable for the degree of lagophtalmos (Adapted from May M. and from Levine RE).

head elevated with one or two pillows, to allow the force of gravity to act.

Eyespring implantation

The implantation of a wire spring into the upper eyelid is helpful for patients with powerful lid retraction or a weak Bell's phenomenon in the treatment of lagophthalmos (Figs. 15-4, 15-5, 15-6, 15-7, 15-8).

The spring acts mechanically and tends to counteract the action of the levator palpebrae superioris. The tension of the wire is adjusted to permit

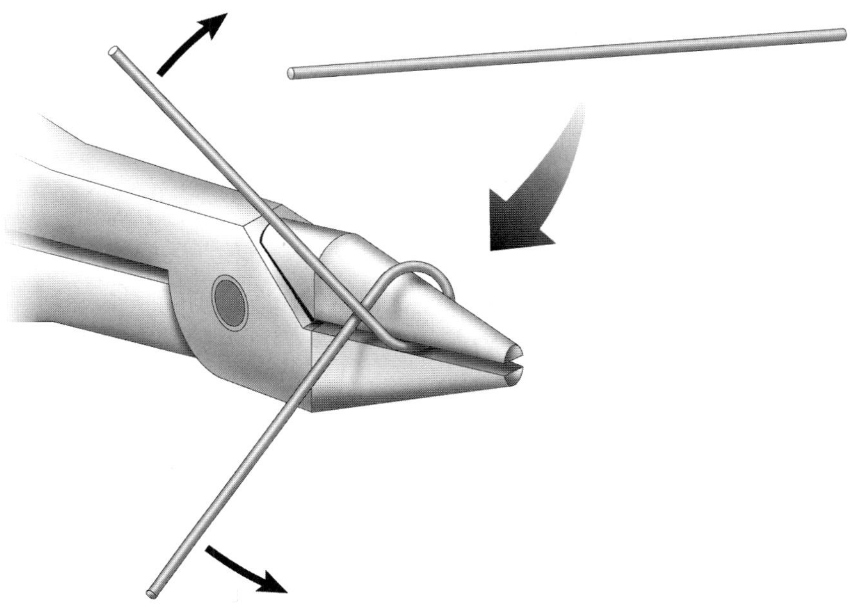

Fig. 15-4. The palpebral spring is prepared preoperatively

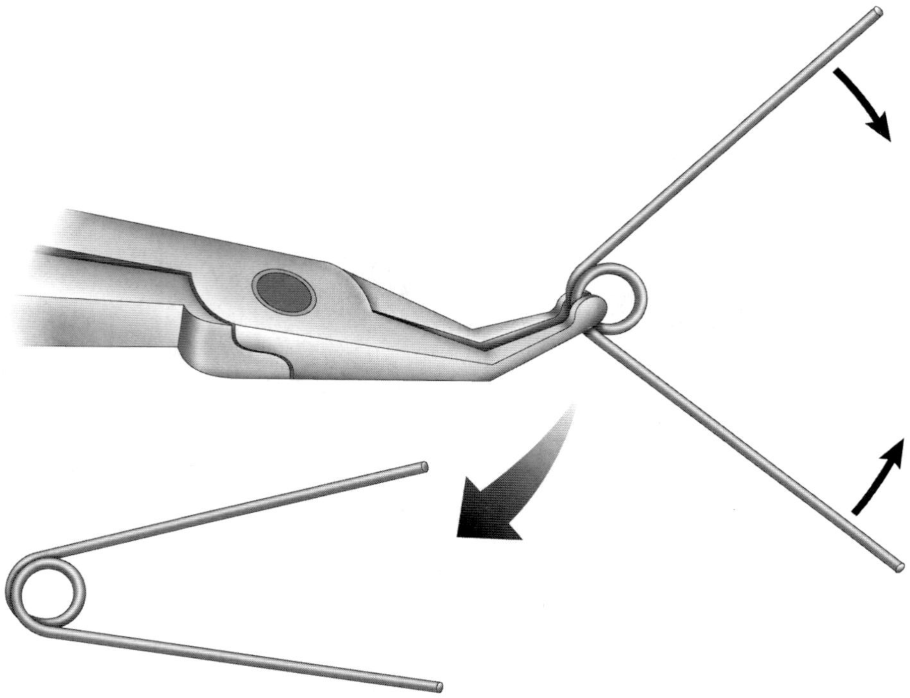

Fig. 15-5. In surgery, the spring is modeled to conform to the curvature of the patient's orbit, and proper tension is adjusted.

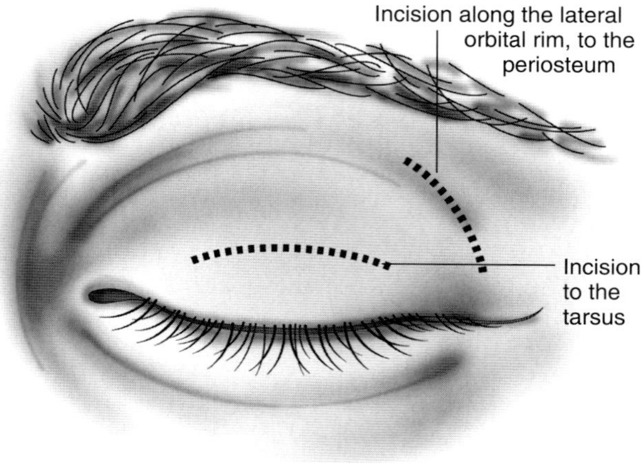

Fig. 15-6. Two incisions are made.

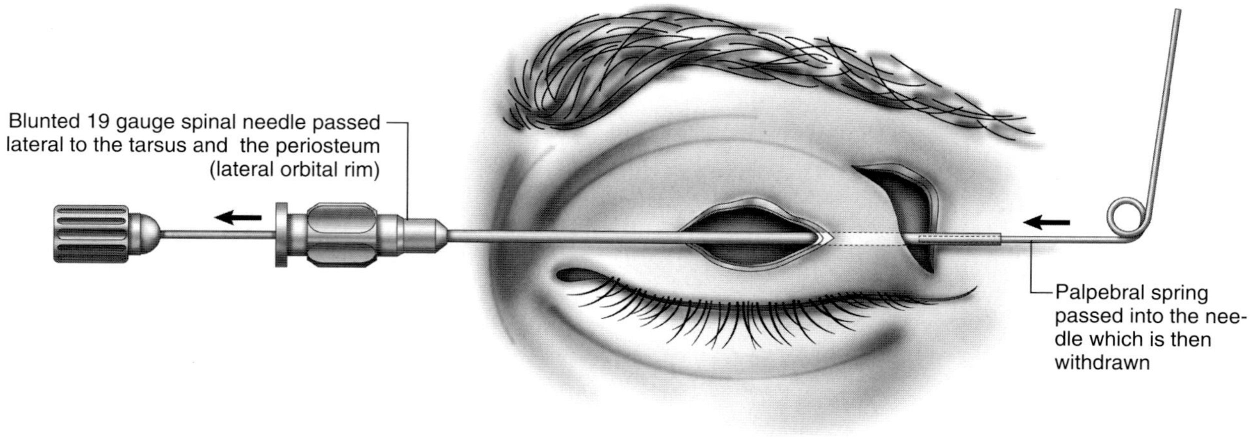

Fig. 15-7. A blunted 19 gauge spinal needle is passed lateral to the tarsus and the periosteum (lateral orbital rim). The obturator is then removed, and the wire spring is passed through the needle, which is then withdrawn (Adapted from May M. and from Levine RE).

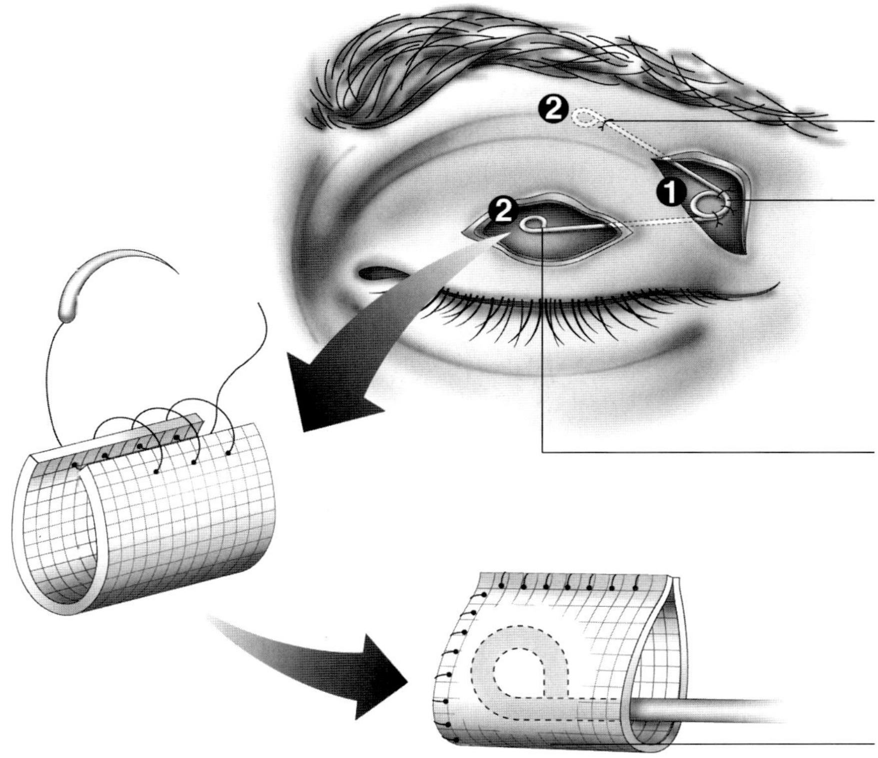

Fig. 15-8. The fulcrum of the spring is brought into the desired position and sutured to the periosteum with 4-0 mersilene sutures. The tension of the spring is adapted to the degree of lagophtalmos, by changing the angulation of the upper end of the wire. The upper limb of the spring is sutured to the periosteum. The lower limb is enveloped in Dacron and sutured (Adapted from May M. and from Levine RE).

the levator to elevate the eyelid, opening the spring (Fig. 15-9).

The enhanced palpebral spring implantation consists of a simultaneous tightening of the levator, to strengthen it. Thus greater tension can be placed on the spring, resulting in a faster blink (Figs. 15-10, 15-11).

Silastic elastic prosthesis

A silicone prosthesis is available as a 1.0 mm diameter rod. The implant of this prosthesis is useful in selective cases: marked lower lid droop, and mild or moderate lagophthalmos.

Temporary Procedures

These procedures are useful in buying time before utilizing a facial nerve restoration procedure or a facial reanimation technique.

Taped suture of the upper lid to the cheek

- A 5.0 silk suture is passed through skin and orbicularis muscle. The extremity is knotted and anchored by a strip of tape (TM Mefix), and reinforced by another one.
- The elevation of the entire blocking system permits inspection and medication of the eye. The suture may be left in place no more than 3 weeks, or scarring complications of the upper lid may ensue.

Temporary Tarsorrhaphy Suture

- This temporary suture protects the eye for several weeks, without causing scarring of the upper lid.
- A double-armed 5-0 silk suture is passed through the center of the upper and lower lids, through skin and orbicularis muscle. Cotton is placed under the area of suture tension. The suture is closed with a temporary knot so that the eye can be opened and medicated.

TRANSPOSITION OF THE TEMPORALIS MUSCLE

Transposition of the temporalis muscle is a technique useful in establishing a certain level of facial function in patients whose problem cannot be treated with the restoration of the neuromuscular system (Fig. 15-12).

Indications

- Patients with inadequate facial function, 2 years after an operation which has left the facial nerve intact, or 2 years after repair surgery on the nerve.

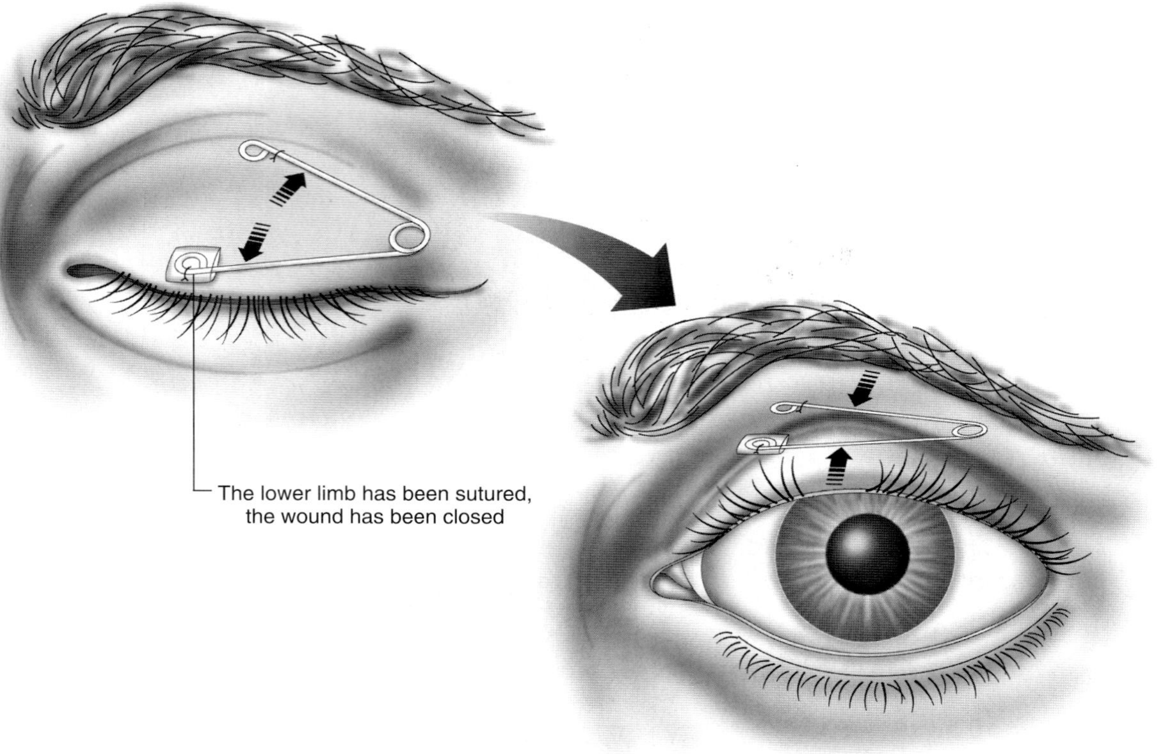

Fig. 15-9. Eyelid spring implanted. The wound has been closed.

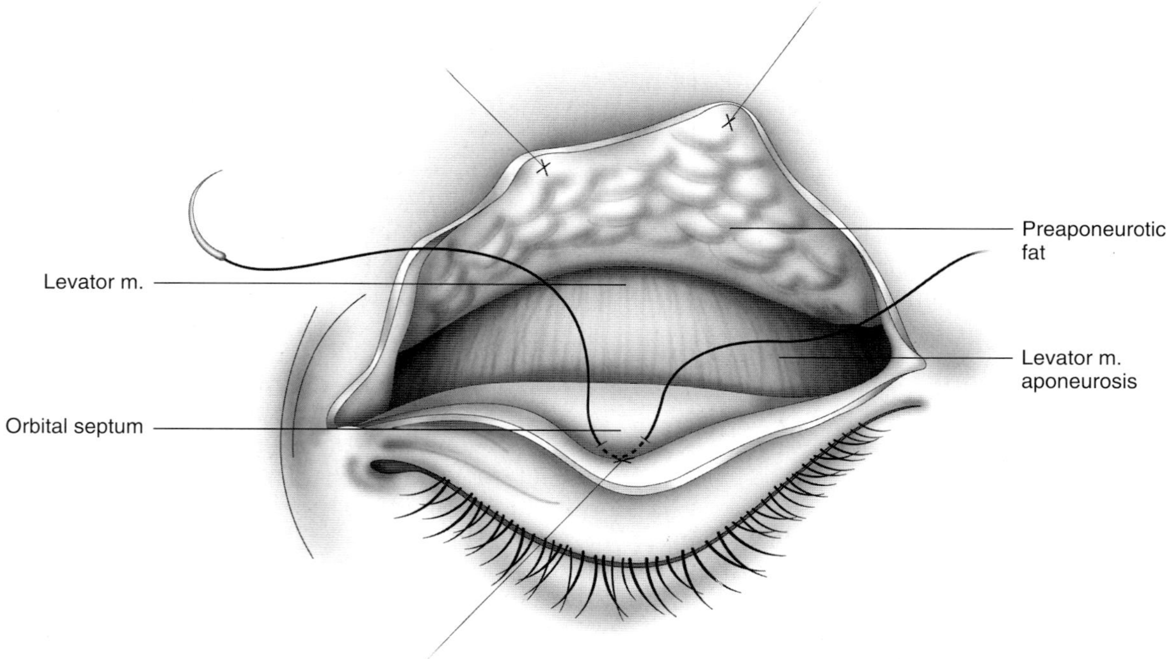

Fig. 15-10. Preaponeurotic fat is seen, the septum is opened. The tarsus is exposed and transfixed by a 5-0 mersilene suture (Adapted from May M. and from Levine RE).

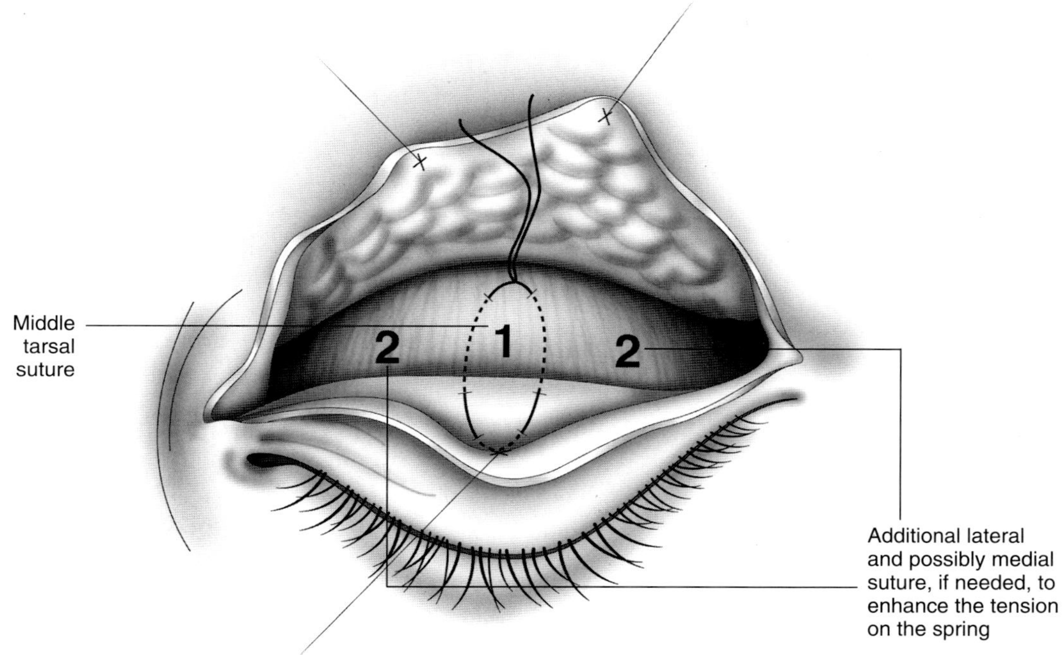

Fig. 15-11. A temporary knot is put in place and the result evaluated. To reduce lid strengthening, the knot is loosened; to enhance, additional lateral and medial suture may be placed (Adapted from May M. and from Levine RE).

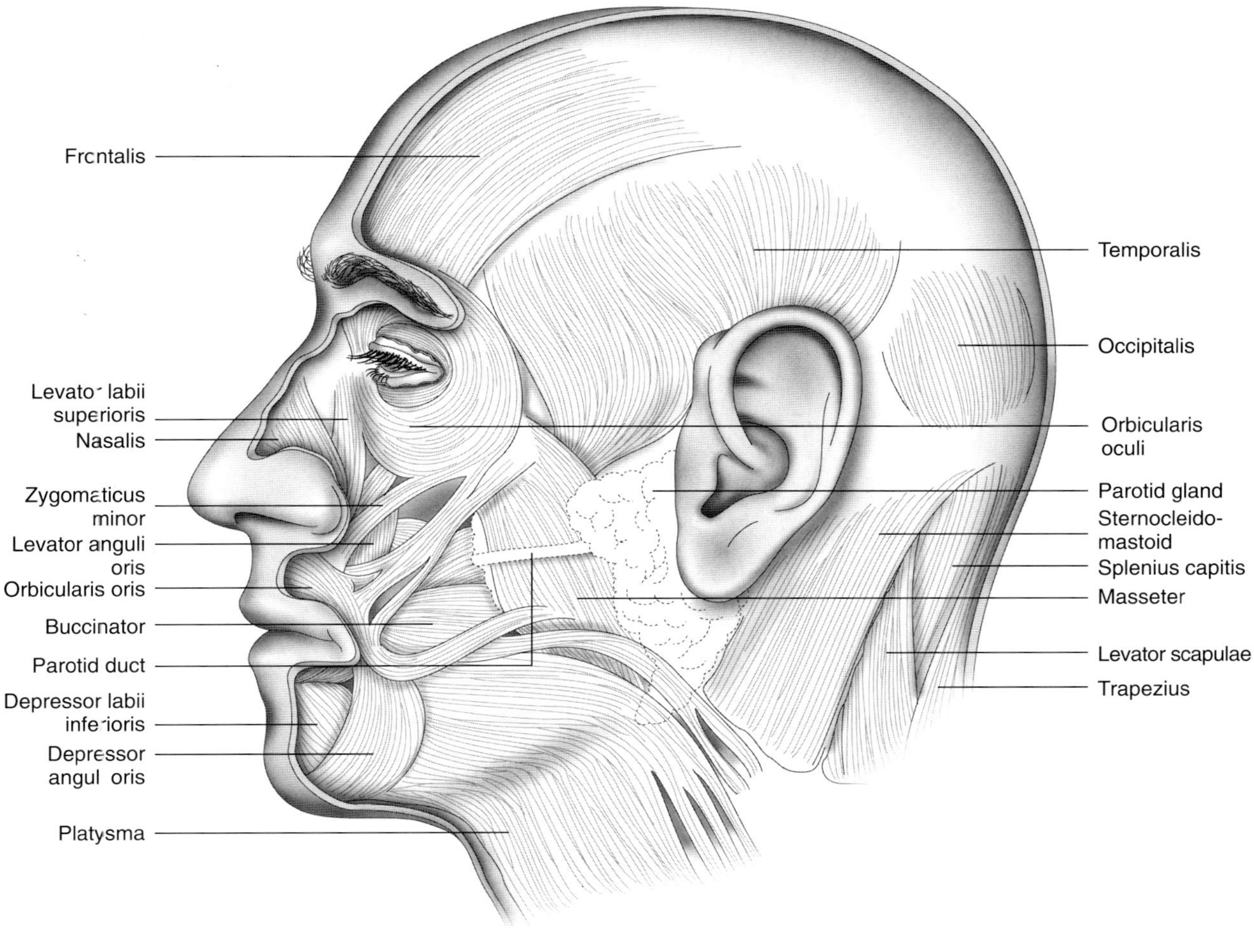

Fig. 15-12. Muscles of the face.

- Paralysis following operation in which the stump proximal to the facial nerve cannot be located or used for grafting.
- Patients who refuse other neuromuscular restoration techniques.
- Paralysis following oncological surgery in which the long-term prognosis is poor.
- Patients with other neurological deficits, such as alterations of nerves IX and X, and thus cannot undergo hypoglossal-facial grafting, due to the risk of serious alterations in language and swallowing.
- Patients with hypodevelopment of the facial nerves and facial musculature, such as that found in the syndrome of Mobius.
- Paralysis following an operation where the facial nerve is preserved but full recovery still has not been attained after one year.
- Temporalis muscle transposition may also be utilized along with a hypoglossal-facial anastomosis. Thus an immediate restoration of facial function, without compromising neuromuscular recovery, occurs within 4-6 months.

Surgical Technique (May modification of Rubin and Conley technique)
- The operative site is shaved.
- Disinfection with povidone-iodine.
- A tarsorrhaphy is performed to protect the affected eyelid during the procedure
- Intubation.
- Positioning of a sticky drape to hold the tube at the patient's chin, without modifying the motility of the lips.
- Lidocaine (Xilocaine) infiltration with 1:100:000 adrenalin.
- Incision of the skin and the subcutaneous tissue with a cutting cautery.
- Exposure of the temporalis fascia.
- Temporalis muscle outline of 2 × 5 cm with a needle tip cautery (Fig. 15-13).
- Subperiosteal dissection of temporalis muscle (Fig. 15-14).
- Tunnelization lateral to the superficial musculo-aponeurotic system (SMAS). If a medial direction is pursued, there is the risk of injury to the facial nerve or the parotid duct (Fig. 15-15).
- Incision of the vermilion-cutaneous border and tunnelization lateral to the superficial system, until connecting with the superior tunnel (Fig. 15-16).
- Splitting of the temporalis muscle for 1 cm. A bit of prolene is placed at each extremity. The threads serve as guides for the inferior eversion of the muscle, the heads of which are then sutured to the facial musculature, above and below the oral commissure (Fig. 15-17). Other points (bits) are positioned in the angle between the two peduncles, so as to attract the corner of the mouth until the first molar is

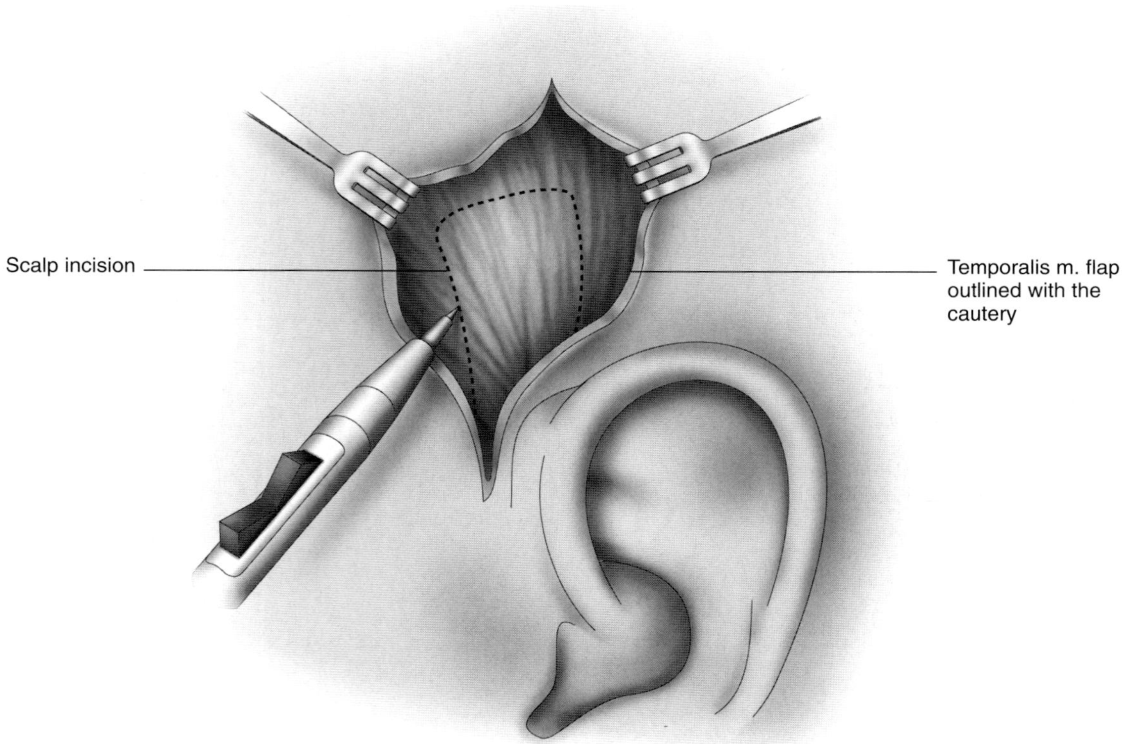

Fig. 15-13. The scalp is incised. A temporalis muscle flap, inferiorly based, is outlined (Adapted from May M).

Fig. 15-14. The muscle flap is elevated from the temporal bone, with a Lempert elevator (Adapted from May M).

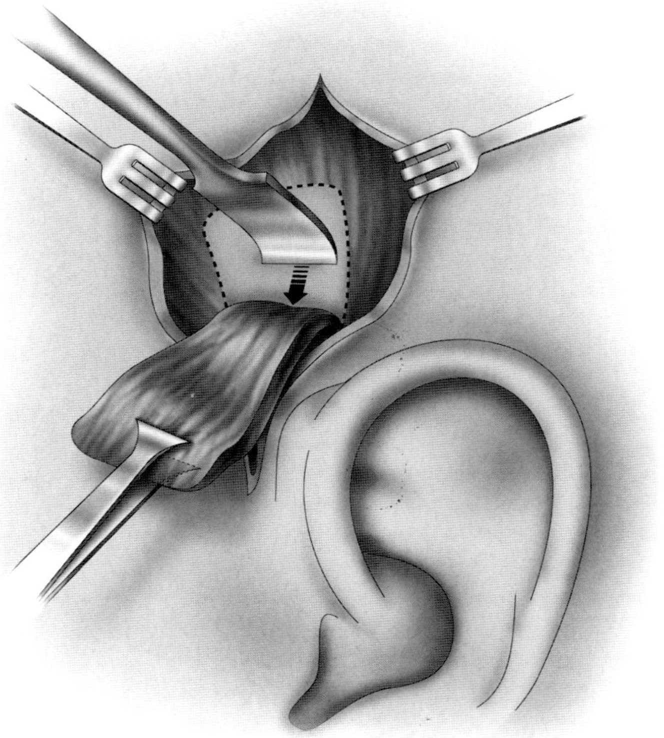

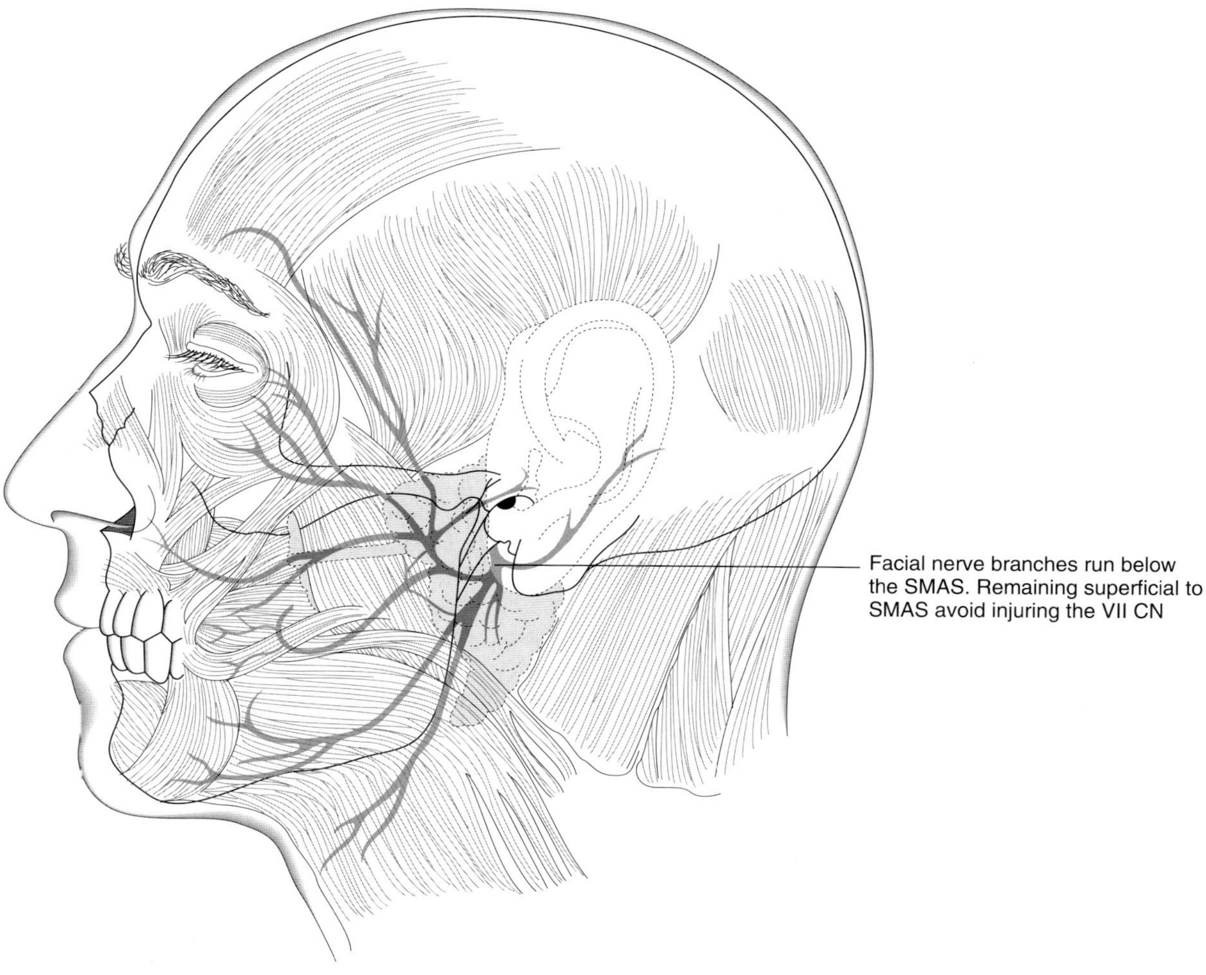

Fig. 15-15. The facial nerve branches run under the superficial musculoaponeurotic system (SMAS).

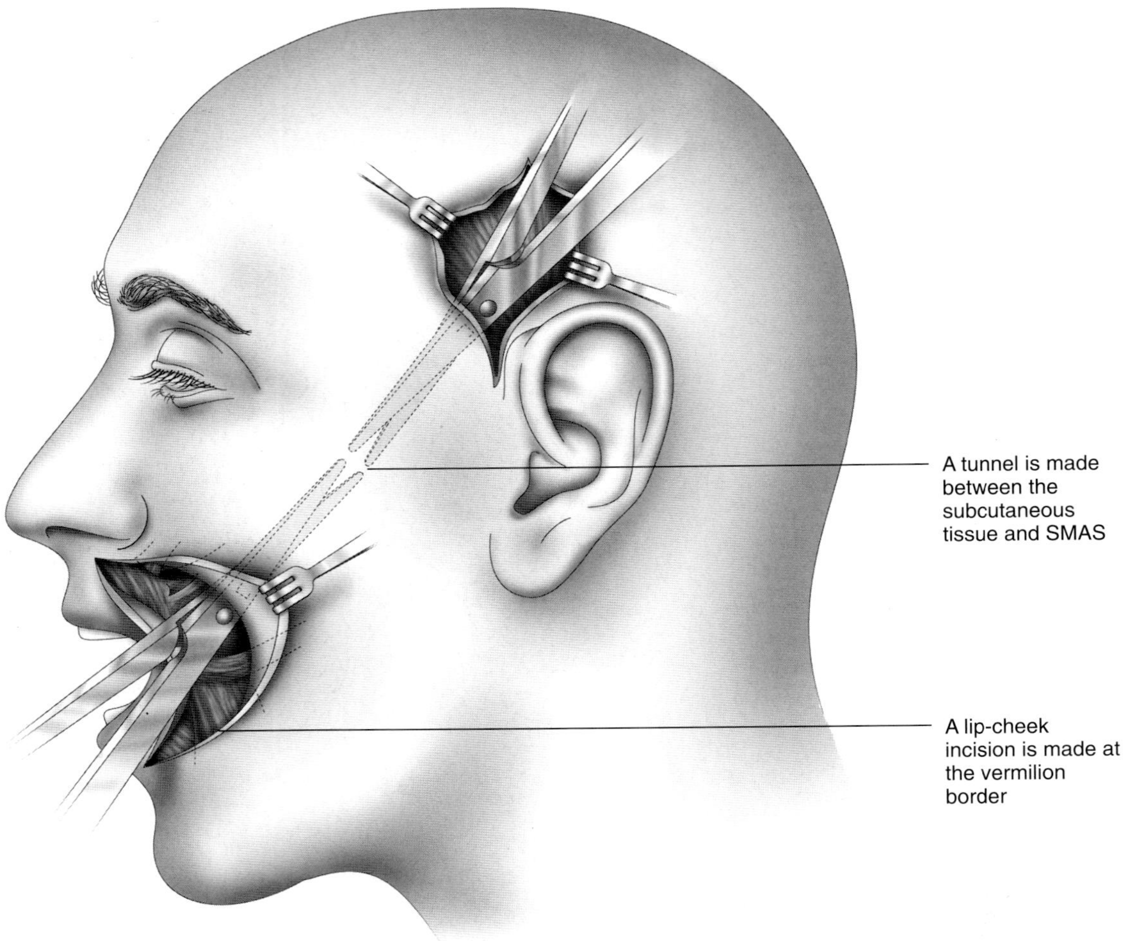

Fig. 15-16. A lip-cheek incision is made in the vermilion. A tunnel is made, superficial to the SMAS, to avoid injuring the underlying facial nerve branches (Adapted from May M).

seen (overcorrection of the lateral smile) (Figs. 15-18, 15-19). After the operation, the smile generally flattens. If it remains hypercorrected, the incision must be reopened and the sutures repositioned at the corner of the mouth.

- To close the defect of the temporalis muscle, a flap of the superficial fascia of the pedunculized muscle may be used (Cheney).
- Positioning of two drains, one at the corner of the mouth and one posterior to the scalp incision. They are removed after three days.
- Antibiotic treatment, begun perioperatively, is interrupted the third day after surgery.

Complications

Rare: 2-5%.

- Hematoma: if precocious, it must be drained in the operating room.
- Seroma: This can be needle aspirated and its reformation prevented with pressure dressings.
- Infections: Abscess is drained. Wide spectrum i.v. antibiotics are admistered.

FREE MUSCLE FLAPS

- The donor muscle must be able to be removed from the donor site with minimal residual functional disability.
- The muscle must have a long neurovascular pedicle -gracilis, latissimus dorsi, serratus anterior, pectoralis minor, rectus abdominis-. The pedicled artery and vein are anastomosed to the superficial temporal artery and vein end to end, with 9-0 monofilament nylon sutures. The donor and recipient nerves are joined with epineural sutures.
- The free muscle flap must be larger than deemed necessary, since a decrease in postoperative volume is normal, due to atrophy.

Good results have been reported using this technique. In the future, if the results are backed by significant statistics, this technique may be a valid alternative to muscle transposition.

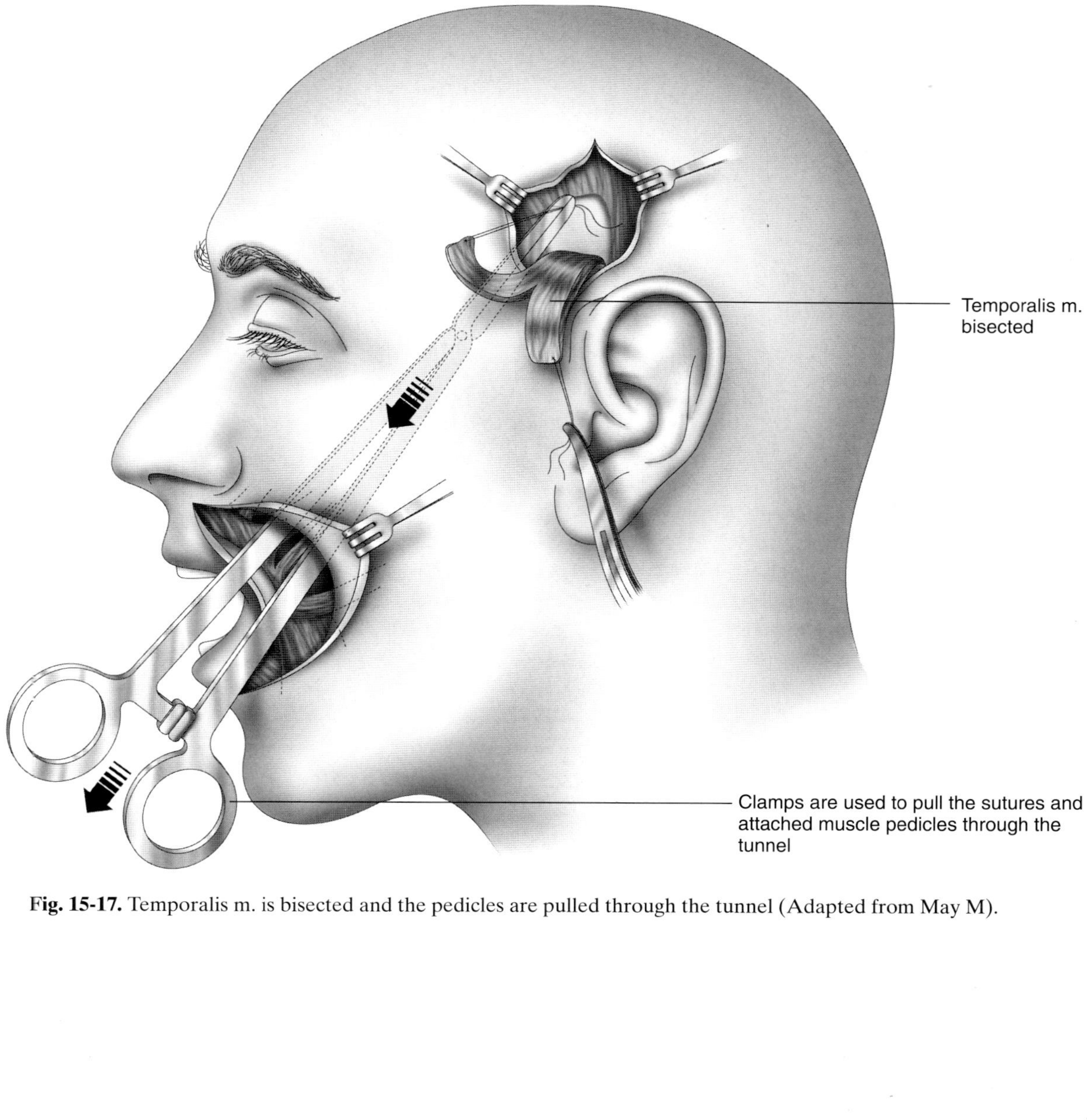

Fig. 15-17. Temporalis m. is bisected and the pedicles are pulled through the tunnel (Adapted from May M).

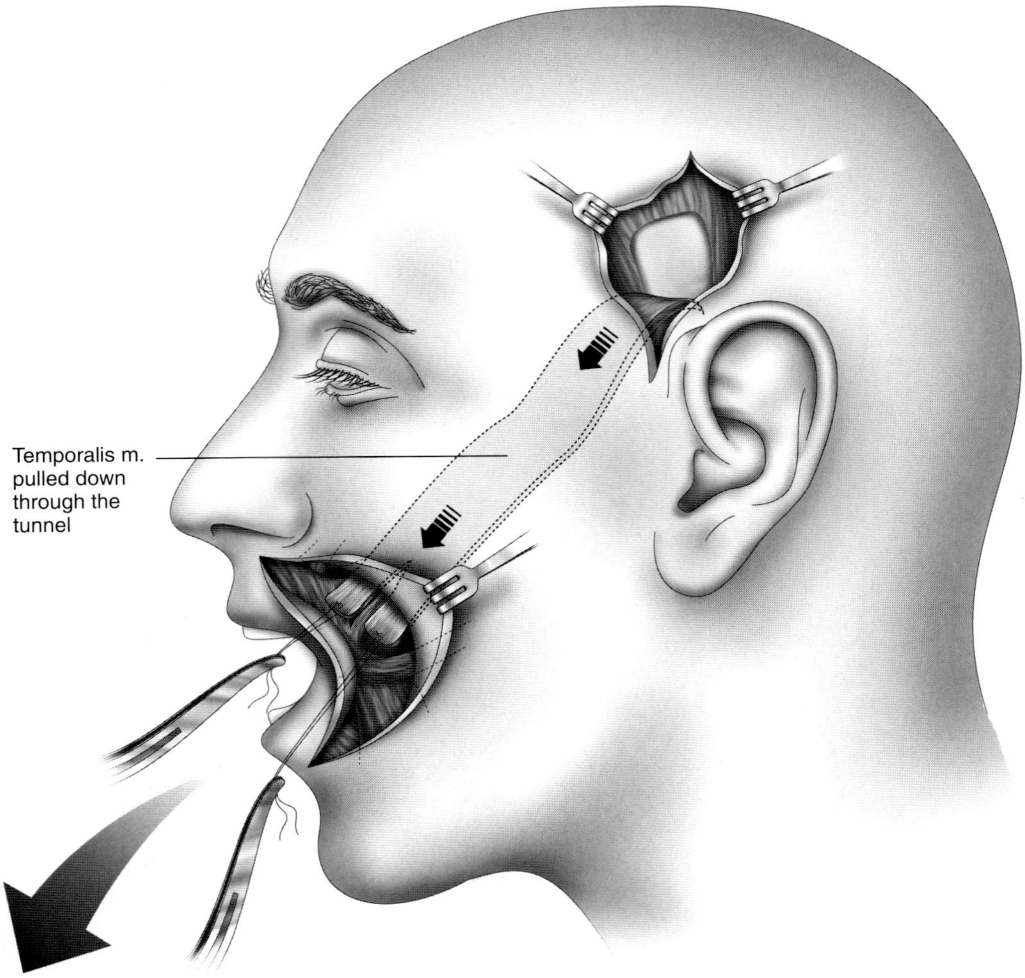

Fig. 15-18. Temporalis m. transposed (Adapted from May M).

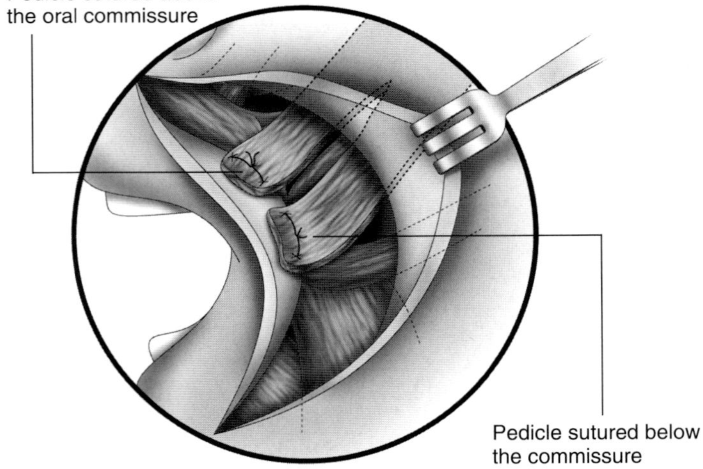

Fig. 15-19. The superior pedicle is sutured above the commissure, the inferior pedicle below the commissure (Adapted from May M).

REFERENCES

Arion HG: Dynamic closure of the lids in paralysis of the orbicularis muscle. Int Surg 57: 48,1972.

Baker D, Conley J: Regional muscle transposition for rehabilitation of the paralyzed face. Clin Plast Surg 6: 317-31, 1979.

Beard C: Canthoplasty and brow elevation for facial palsy. Arch Ophthalmol 71: 386-388, 1964.

Bridger GP: Surgery and facial nerve grafting and malignant parotid disease. Aust N Z J Surg 39: 232-238, 1970.

Chiu D, Janecka IP, Krizek TJ, Wolff M, Lovelace RD: Autogenous vein graft as a conduit for nerve regeneration. Surgery 91:226, 1982.

Chiu D, Lovelace R, Yu L, Wolff M, Stergel S, Middeltown L, Janecka IP, Krizek T: Comparative electrophysiologic evaluation of the nerve grafts and vein grafts as nerve conduits—an experimental study. Surg Forum 34:601, 1983.

Conley J, Baker DC, Seife TW: Paralysis of the mandibular branch of the facial nerve. Plast Reconstr Surg 70: 569-576, 1982.

Conley JJ: Facial rehabilitation following radical parotid gland surgery. Arch Otolaryngol 66: 58-66, 1957.

Cosman B, Janecka IP: Facial palsy. Plastic surgery of the head and neck. New York: Churchill Livingstone, 839-873, 1987.

Freed WJ, Medinacelli L, Wyatt RJ: Promoting functional plasticity in the damaged nervous system. Science 227:1544-1552, 1985.

Frielinger G: A new technique to correct facial paralysis. Plast Reconstr Surg 56: 44-48, 1975.

Gullane PJ, Havas TJ: Facial nerve grafts: effects of postoperative radiation therapy. J Otolaryngol 16: 112-5, 1987.

Harii K, Ohmori K, Torii S: Free gracilis muscle transplantation with microneurovascular anastomoses for the treatment of facial paralysis. Plast Reconstr Surg 57: 133-143, 1976.

Harii K: Microneurovascular free muscle transplantation for reanimation of facial paralysis. Clin Plast Surg 6: 361-375, 1979.

Hugo NE, Stone E: Anatomy for a blepharoplasty. Plast Reconstr Surg 53:381-383, 1974.

Janecka IP: Integrity of facial function: its preservation and repair. Crit Rev Neurosurg 1, 1991.

Jelks GW, Smith B, Bosniak S: The evaluation and management of the eye in facial palsy. Clin Plast Surg 6(3): 397-419, 1979.

Jobe RP: A technique for lid-loading in the management of lagophthalmos in facial paralysis. Plast Reconstr Surg 53: 29-31,1974.

Johnson JB, Hadley RC: The aging face. In: Converse JM, ed. Reconstructive plastic surgery. Philadelphia: Saunders, 1964.

Laage Hellman JE: Facial nerve in parotidectomies. Arch Otolaryngol 81: 527-33, 1965.

Levine RE, House WF, Hitselberger WE: Ocular complications of seventh nerve paralysis and management with the palpebral spring. Am J Ophthalmol 73: 219, 1972.

Levine RE: Eyelid reanimation surgery. In May M (ed): The Facial Nerve. New York, Thieme-Stratton, 1985, pp 681-694.

Levine RE: Lid reanimation with the palpebral spring. In Wright K, Tse D (eds): Color Atlas of Ophthalmic Surgery. Philadelphia, JB Lippincott, 1992, pp 231-238.

Levine RE: Management of lagophthalmos with palpebral spring and silastic elastic prosthesis. In Homblass A (ed): Ophthalmic and orbital plastic reconstructive surgery, Vol 1. Baltimore, Williams & Wilkins, 1989, pp 384-392.

Levine RE: Management of the eye after acoustic tumor surgery. In House WF, Luetje CM (eds): Acoustic Tumors, Vol 2. Baltimore, University Park Press, 1979, pp 105-149.

Levine RE: Management of the ophthalmologic complications of facial paralysis. Trans Pac Coast Ophthalmol Otolaryngol Soc 61: 85-93, 1980.

Levine RE: Palpebral spring for lagophthalmos due to facial nerve palsy. In Wesley RE (ed): Techniques in Ophthalmic Plastic Surgery. New York, John Wiley & Sons, 1986, pp 424-427.

Levine RE: Protection of the exposed eye in facial paralysis. In Graham MD, House WF (eds): Disorders of the Facial Nerve. New York, Raven Press, 1982, pp 336-375.

Levine RE: Protection of the exposed eye. In Brackmann DE (ed): Neurological Surgery of the Ear and Skull Base. New York, Raven Press, 1982, pp 81-87.

Maar M, Croxson GR, Klein SR: Bell's palsy: Management of sequelae using EMG rehabilitation, botulinum toxin, and surgery. Am J Otol 10: 220-229, 1981.

Marrone AC, Soll D: Modification of the Arion encircling silicone spring. Thesis for membership in the American Society of Ophthalmic Plastic and Reconstructive Surgery, 1977.

May M (ed): The Facial Nerve. New York, Thieme Medical Publishers, 1986.

May M: Facial reanimation and skull base trauma. Am J Otol suppl 62-7, 1985.

May M: Reanimation of the paralyzed eyelid following cancer surgery. J Head Neck Cancer 1: 481-91, 1985.

May M: Surgical rehabilitation of facial palsy. In: May M, ed. The facial nerve. New York: Thieme 695-780, 1986.

May M: Muscle transposition for facial reanimation. Arch Otolaryngol Head Neck Surg 110: 184-189, 1984.

May M: Muscle transposition for facial reanimation. Arch Otolaryngol Head Neck Surg 110: 184-189, 1984.

McGuirt WF, Welling DB, McCabe BF: Facial nerve function following irradiated cable grafts. Laryngoscope 99: 27-34, 1989.

Morel-Fatio D, Lalardrie JP: Le ressort palpebral: Contribution a l'etude de la chirurgie plastique de la paralysie faciale. Neurochirurgie 11: 303,1965.

Morel-Fatio D, Lalardrie JP: Palliative surgical treatment of facial paralysis: The palpebral spring. Plast Reconstr Surg 33: 446, 1964.

O'Brien BM, Pederson WC, Khazanchi RK, et al: Results of management of facial palsy with microvascular free-muscle transfer. Plast Reconstr Surg 86: 12-22, 1990.

Rosenstock TG, Hurwitz JJ, Nedzelski JMJ, Tator CH: Ocular complications following excision of cerebellopontine angle tumours. Can Opthalmol 21(4): 134-139, 1986.

Rubin L: Reanimation of the paralyzed face. St. Louis, CV Mosby, 1977.

Samii M, Jannetta PJ, eds. The cranial nerves. New York: Springer Verlag, 649, 1981.

Seiff SR, Chang J: Management of ophthalmic complications of facial nerve palsy. Otolaryngol Clin North Am 25(3): 669-690, 1992.

Sobol S, Alward P: Early gold weight implantation for reanimation of the paralyzed eye. Head and Neck 149-53, 1990.

Sobol SM, May M, Mester S: Early facial reanimation following radical parotid and temporal bone tumor resections. Am J Surg 160: 382-386, 1990.

Tenzel RR, Buffam FV, Miller GR: The use of the lateral canthal sling in ectropion repair. Can J Ophthalmol 12: 199-202, 1977.

Tenzel RR: Treatment of lagophthalmos of the lower lid. Arch Ophthalmol 81: 366-368, 1969.

Wells MD, Manktelow RI: Surgical management of facial palsy. Clin Plast Surg 17: 645-653, 1990.

Wells MD, Manktelow RT: Surgical management of facial palsy. Clin Plast Surg 17: 645-653, 1990.

Wood-Smith D: Experience with the Arion prosthesis. In Tessier P (ed): Symposium on Plastic Surgery in the Orbital Region. St. Louis, CV Mosby, 1976.

Zlotnik El, Smeyanovitch AF, Tyappo EP: Method of eyelid closure in facial nerve paralysis. Technical note. J Neurosurg 57: 722-723, 1982.

16

Glomus tumors

To become a master temporal bone surgeon is a real challenge – like graduating from medical school or parenting a child – and as gratifying. And no one can do it for you.

HOUSE W.F.

Glomus tumors are neoplasms originating in the paragangliar system of the temporal bone. They are generally found in the dome of the jugular bulb, but may also be seen in the tympanic plexus on the promontory of the middle ear.

These paraganglia are part of the non-chromaffin system and consist of highly vascularized residual epithelial cells derived from neural crest tissue.

They are found in various perivascular locations and it is believed that they function as chemoreceptors. These lesions may be confined to the promontory or may involve the mastoid, the jugular bulb, the internal carotid artery, the dura, the endocranium (see classification).

SYMPTOMATOLOGY

The most common symptoms of glomus tumors limited to the middle ear are the following:

- Pulsating tinnitus.
- Conductive hearing loss.
- Bleeding.
- Retromandibular swelling.

As the tumor progresses, the following symptoms may be seen:

- Deafness.
- Vertigo.
- Hydrocephalus.
- Otorrhagy.
- Paresis of the cranial nerves VII-IX-X-XI-XII with the related problems (facial paresis, facial spasms, difficulty in swallowing, voice changes).
- Pain is rare.

DIAGNOSIS

- Otoscopy with a 25X microscope shows the tumor's pulsations through the tympanic membrane. This is confirmed by a tympanometry. The tumor is bluish in color.
- The caloric tests are not reliable because of the vascular shunt around the external auditory canal, which alters response to caloric stimulation.
- Normal audiometric tests (air, bone, and vocal) are useful in evaluating the degree of hearing impairment.
- Auditory evoked potentials are useful if an intracranial invasion is suspected. A high resolution CT is the best choice because of its capacity to define the degree of bone involvement. It demonstrates the tumor's extension in the temporal bone, the neck and the intracranial space. With it we can diagnose possible jugular bulb involvement and any medial extension into the internal carotid artery.
- The MRI is particularly useful in evaluating the intradural extension of the tumor, its relationship with the cerebral parenchyma, and the degree of endocranial involvement. It is helpful in defining jugular bulb involvement, since the flow signal is altered when the lumen has been invaded. The MRI may overestimate the degree of petrous apex involvement. In this zone the bone marrow is hyperintense, and indistinguishable from the tumor in the T1 images.
- The arteriography confirms the hypothesis of a vascular tumor and evidentiates the tributary vessels. It is an essential preoperative test, to define any ICA involvement and to diagnose any paragangliomas in other locations. If narrowing or irregularity is noted in the arterial wall, the collateral flow and the patient's tolerance to a possible carotid resection must be checked. The suspicion of carotid involvement must be very well-founded, since complication rates in occlusion tests go from 3-7% (R.W. Tarr 1991) to 9% (U. Fisch). Among the possible complications are cerebrovascular ischemia and embolization. When the balloon occlusion test is performed, a neurological monitor is used along with an electroencephalogram, a xenon CT map of the cerebral flow, and a positron emission tomography.

DIFFERENTIAL DIAGNOSIS

Glomus tumors with tympanic expansion are clinically diverse from an aberrant carotid artery which is more anterior and more reddish in color, or from the jugular bulb, which is a darker blue in color. The CT is recommended for a differential diagnosis.

Laboratory tests

Laboratory tests evaluate the production of catecholamines and serotonin. Vanilmandelic acid is sought in the urine, as well as methanefrin, idrossindolacetic acid, catecholamines metabolites and serotonin production. This data may identify an endocrine tumor in its active phase, which may provoke serious pressure bounces during surgical manipulation. The clinical history of a patient with a secernent tumor may show hypertension, hydrocephalus, diarrhea, hot flashes in the head and tachyarrhythmia.

BRAIN PERFUSION AND FLOW STUDIES

The clinical-radiological data is sufficient to make a diagnosis. A diagnostic biopsy of the tumor should be avoided, since profuse bleeding results and there is the risk of injuring an aberrant carotid artery or a high jugular bulb.
When a vessel restriction is shown by the angiography, the collateral flow and the patient's tolerance to a carotid resection must be evaluated.

Evaluation of the collateral flow

- *Compression of the ipsilateral ICA and angiography of the contralateral ICA.* A frontal projection will show whether or not there is a rapid filling of the ipsilateral medial cerebral artery and its branches, through the anterior communicating artery.
- *Compression of the ipsilateral ICA and angiography in a lateral projection of the dominant vertebral artery.* The test is positive if the ipsilateral medial cerebral artery fills rapidly and completely through the communicating posterior artery.

Temporary Balloon Occlusion

A temporary ballon occlusion or a tolerance test is performed on the ipsilateral ICA with the patient sedated but awake. This state ensures early identification of negative neurological consequences.
A balloon catheter (5 French catheter with a non-detachable double lumen: Meditech, Watertown, Massachusetts) is inserted with a transfemoral approach into the ipsilateral internal carotid artery. A second catheter, 5 French, of the type used for angiographies, is inserted through the contralateral femoral artery into the ipsilateral carotid, up to 5 cm from the previous catheter.
The response to the test is monitored with continuous neurologic monitoring and EEG. Radioisotope or Xenon studies or positron-emission tomography are used to assess cerebral perfusion during occlusion studies. If necessary, the balloon can be deflated immediately to restore cerebral perfusion.
During the test, the part above the occlusion is heparinized with an injection through the two-way catheter and the underlying part is heparinized with the conventional catheter. A contrast agent is injected through the conventional catheter. If a complete occlusion is present, the contrast agent will pool, and will not surpass the balloon in the angiographic evaluation.

Permanent Balloon Occlusion

When the ICA wall is involved with part of the tumor, or an extended tumor receives blood from branches of the ICA, a permanent balloon occlusion must be considered.
This is indicated in glomus tumors for the following:

- Tumors that englobe the ICA in its horizontal segment, without reaching the foramen lacerum (Fisch's C3) or for tumors that involve the foramen lacerum and englobe the ICA up to the cavernous sinus (Fisch's C4). Thus removal is easier and safer since the tumor is less vascularized and the risk of a mortal hemorrhage caused by an ICA laceration is surpassed. E.g.:
- Spheno-petro-clival meningiomas or carcinomas of the rhynopharynx involving the cavernous sinus.
- Glomi with intracranial extension into the cerebello-pontine angle and rhynopharynx angiofibromas with parasellar extension, since these receive blood from the carotico-tympanic and cavernous branches of the ICA.

A 7 French catheter is used to introduce the balloon into the ICA. It is continuously bathed in heparine. Through it a balloon attached to a microcatheter is introduced into the ICA and advanced to the cavernous tract, before the emergence of the ophthalmic artery. An angiography with the introduced catheter evaluates complete ICA occlusion and the permeability of the ophthalmic artery.
The internal catheter is removed under fluoroscopic control and the balloon is left in place.
The patient is moved to intensive care for 24 hours.

COMPLICATIONS

If ischemic deficit or a significant lowering of pressure is seen (less than 100 mm Hg), plasma

expanders or vasopressor drugs are administered. Even in the presence of a good collateral flow, during the phase of hypotension there is a very high risk of ischemic deficit.
One rare complication is blindness from emboli that reach the ophtalmic circulation through branches of the internal maxillary artery anastomised with the ophtalmic artery.

Bleeding
Profuse bleeding may take place during surgery, especially in glomi of the jugular bulb and when carotid artery or transdural arteries are involved.

- Preoperative embolization is performed.
- All patients are advised to use autotransfusion, to reduce the risks inherent in intraoperative transfusion. This is done several weeks before surgery is scheduled.
- During surgery we use a Cell Saver whenever possible (Hemonics, Braintree, MA) which intraoperatively retransfuses the lost blood. The apparatus may only be used if no coagulant substances are present in the surgical field, such as oxidized cellulose (Surgicel), gelatine sponge (Gelfoam), and bovine collagen (Avitene). We begin the operation with this apparatus, and interrupt its use only when the conditions of the surgical field no longer support it.

Angiofibromas
Angiofibromas receive blood from the ipsilateral maxillary artery and from the superior pharyngeal branch of the ascending pharyngeal artery. Tumors with intracranial intradural extensions receive blood from the cerebral arteries.
Glomi
Preoperative embolization, in comparison with patients not undergoing embolization, significantly reduces hematic loss and time in the operating room; it does not reduce the risk of lesions to nerves IX-X-XI. Both balloon occlusion of the carotid artery and selective embolization are performed at least 1 day before the neurotologic surgery.
Tributary arteries are embolized with Ivalon, usually during angiography.
Embolization is usually begun at the distal branches of the external carotid and proceeds towards the proximal branches.
Embolization has a particular morbidity. The most serious complications are heart attack and death. Other neurological deficits may be seen, such as paralysis of the cranial nerves. There is some risk of vascular lesions, especially in arteriosclerotic vessels.

EMBOLIZING MATERIALS

IVALON in microparticles from 250-500 micron (IVALON, Unipoint Laboratories, High Point, North Carolina). This is an alcohol and polivinyl foam. It is often used since it is both effective and long-lasting due to its resistance to absorption. It is a foam suspended in a saline contrast agent, and is injected into the angiographic catheter through a well-lubricated syringe.

IBCA: Isobutil-2-cyanoacrilate (Unipoint Industries Inc., High Point, NC). This is a fluid substance with rapid polymerization, which occurs at its first contact with saline solution, blood and vessel interiors... To slow the polymerization, a mixture of 0.5 cc of IBCA and 0.5 cc of Pantopaque (an oily contrast agent) is used. 1 gr. of Tantalium powder is added to make the substance opaque.
To avoid polymerization, the catheter must be rinsed with a 5% glucose solution and it must be rapidly removed after the injection.

Risks of embolization
The risks of embolization are relative to the diffusion of the embolizing material along collateral branches of the external carotid artery (ECA) with damage to the corresponding districts involuntarily ischaemized:

- Anastomosis between the ECA and the internal carotid (IC) or the vertebral artery (AV).
- Cerebral arteries that may originate in meningeal branches of the ECA.
- Branches of the ECA which may supply the peripheral cranial nerves.

The presence of a tumor may often provoke an inversion of the flow.
For example, anastomosis of the terminal branches of the occipital artery with the terminal branches of the muscular branches of the vertebral artery is frequent. If the ECA loses blood to the AV, the risk of embolization becomes concrete.

CAROTID ARTERY INVOLVEMENT

In most tumors it is possible to cleave the tumor from the adventitia of the carotid.
The part of the ICA most frequently involved by tumors is the petrosal vertical part.
When the tumor involves the ICA, the surgical procedure depends on the preoperative ICA occlusion test. The ICA, when possible, is sacrificed intraoperatively by clipping it before the exit of the ophthalmic branch. When the risk is moderate, the ICA may be sacrificed and reconstructed with a saphenous vein bypass graft. Sometimes a partial removal of the artery wall with reconstruction is possible, though this is acceptable only in benign tumors.
After a partial transection, the artery wall may be reconstructed. After a total transection, the ICA

is reconstructed with a bypass graft of the saphenous vein. The risks inherent to this procedure are related to temporary blood flow interruption. During this phase, the cerebral metabolic rate is reduced with barbiturates or etomidate while the systolic blood pressure is elevated 30 mm Hg above the normotensive state, to maintain adequate blood flow in the contralateral ICA.
There are postoperative risks of thrombosis, which may interfere with the collateral haematic flow of embolisms, and hemorrhage.
In patients who cannot tolerate the balloon occlusion test (20%) the preservation of the ICA segment is advised and the residual tumor is treated with radiation therapy.

ROLE OF RADIATION THERAPY

Radiation therapy is not, in our experience, definitive. The response is typical of highly vascularized neoplasms. Sclerosis and fibrosis are present, due to the microvascular damage, but the low mitotic index reduces the number of cells killed by radiation (Spector; Brackmann).
Radiation therapy acts partially on the vascularization, but the number of tumor cells remains unchanged.
The pathology tends to progress in time, despite the radiation, so that the best therapeutic approach calls for precocious diagnosis and surgery. The best possibilities for surgical radicality and the preservation of neurological functions are obtained when the tumor is still small.

The role of radiation therapy, in agreement with Anand, is limited to the following:

- Tumors with ICA involvement where the performance of a balloon occlusion test is impossible.
- Bilateral glomus tumors where a deficit of the mixed nerves is seen on the opposite side from where the operation is to take place.
- Patients in poor health.
- Patients who refuse surgery.
- Patients with contralateral sensorineural hearing loss.

Side effects

The most common side effects are a temporary cutaneous reaction, nasal crust, dry mouth, mucositis and tearing.
The most serious consequence is post-radiation necrotization of the brain or the temporal bone, seen in 2-4% of cases with doses of 50 GY.
The most widely-used dose with the fewest side effects is between 40 and 50 GY, using a conventional fractioning (Boyle; Dawes; Tildwell).

CLASSIFICATION

Various classifications have been proposed (Tables 16-1, 16-2, 16-3).

Table 16-1. Classification of glomus tumors (Fisch).

Type A	Limited to the middle ear
Type B	Limited to the tympanomastoid area with no infralabyrinthine involvement
Type C	Infralabyrinthine involvement and extension into the petrosal apex
Type D1	Intracranial extension less than 2 cm in diameter
Type D2	Intracranial extension greater than 2 cm in diameter

TYMPANIC GLOMUS TUMOR

This tumor originates in the glomus bodies of the tympanic plexus, along Jacobson's nerve, in the submucosa of the promontory.
A tympanic glomus tumor limited to the mesotympanum may be symptomatically silent, or may manifest itself in a pulsating tinnitus and a conductive hearing loss. The typical symptoms of larger tumors are not seen, such as total sensorineural hearing loss, vertigo, and cranial nerve deficit. The otoscopic exam shows a reddish neoformation within the limits of the annulus tympanicum.

TRANSCANAL APPROACH

A tympano-meatal flap is prepared with an endoaural approach, wider than that used for the stapedectomy. The superior transversal incision is at approx. 10 mm from the fibrous annulus, whereas the superior vertical incision reaches 12 o'clock and the inferior vertical incision goes to 6 o'clock of the annular sulcus.

Table 16-2. Classification of Glomus Tumors (Jackson/Glasscock).

Tympanic Glomus	
Type I	Small mass of the cavum tympani, the jugular bulb and the mastoid
Type II	Complete involvement of the cavum tympani
Type III	Involvement of the cavum tympani and the mastoid
Type IV	As above, with extension through the tympanic membrane or the carotic canal.
Jugular Glomus	
Type I	Small mass of the cavum tympani, the jugular bulb and the mastoid
Type II	Extension under the internal auditory canal with or without intracranial extension
Type III	Extension to the petrosal apex with or without intracranial extension
Type IV	Extension beyond the petrosal apex to the clivus or the infratemporal fossa with or without intracranial extension.

We use the De la Cruz classification for the stadiation of the lesion. Various surgical approaches are related to this classification.

Table 16-3. Classification of glomus tumors and surgical approach (De La Cruz).

Classification	Surgical approach
Tympanic	Transcanal
Tympanomastoid	Mastoid-extended facial recess
Jugular bulb	Mastoid-neck (possible limited facial nerve rerouting)
Carotid artery	Infratemporal fossa
Transdural	Infratemporal fossa/intracranial

The entire tumor is visible with this approach, including its edges.
The vascular peduncle of the tumor is formed by the inferior tympanic ramus of the ascending pharyngeal artery. Hemostasis of this vessel may be performed using bipolar coagulation or Surgicel to occlude the osseous canaliculus where the artery originates. Monopolar coagulation must never be used on the promontory, since the passage of electrical energy may irreparably damage the cochlear nervous structures. The tumor is dissected from the promontory with a dissector and a flap of Surgicel and is then removed with cupped forceps. Anterior bleeding generally occurs, proximal to the pyramidal eminence, from the tributary artery; this can be halted with Surgicel. Bovine collagen is used (Avitene) and left in situ. The tympano-meatal flap is replaced and the external auditory canal is packed (Fig. 16-1).

ANTERIOR HYPOTYMPANIC APPROACH

(JB Farrior)
This is indicated for tumors with limited hypotympanic involvement.

These tumors are seen by means of otoscopy: a bluish mass occupies the hypotympanic zone, and can be seen through the inferior quadrants.

- A postauricular incision is made sliding from under the periosteal plane and the external auditory canal is sectioned, at the osteo-cartilaginous junction.
- The skin is removed from the lower two-thirds of the external auditory canal, from approx. 2 mm from the fibrous annulus, inferiorly, up to 8 mm superiorly. The exposed bone is then drilled until is reached the vertical tract of the facial nerve and the hypotympanum. Drilling of the anterior wall of the bony auditory canal makes it possible to retract the mandible for-

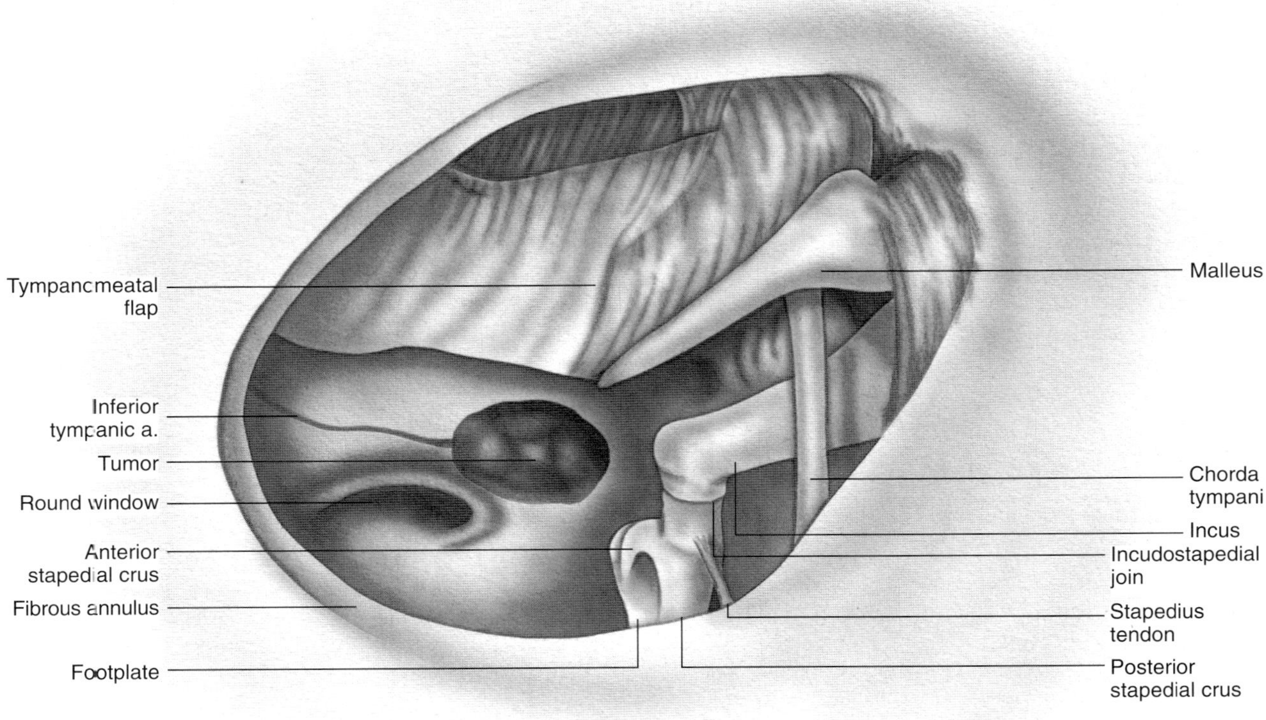

Fig. 16-1. Small tympanic glomus tumor.

ward and to obtain a better exposure of the carotid artery and the eustachian tube (see chapter 9).
- The tympanic membrane is elevated from the annular sulcus of the exposed bony area and is folded upward on the malleus handle.
- Bone removal from the hypotympanum is completed with a burr, until the bony annulus is reached, which should not be damaged.
- Using a cottonoid and beginning anteriorly, the tumor is cleaved from the eustachian tube, the carotid artery and from the promontory. It is then displaced from the ossicular chain and cleaved inferiorly. Then it is removed from the jugular bulb and from the hypotympanum.
- Small flaps of Surgicel are left in place in the tympanic cavity. A flap of temporalis fascia is placed on the hypotympanic bone deficit and superiorly the tympanum is replaced. A skin-free flap covers the bone of the exposed external auditory canal, and stabilizes the fascia graft.

At the operation's conclusion, hearing and facial function have been preserved.

Tumors treated with this approach are small, with hypotympanic involvement. They may reach the ICA and the jugular bulb, but the contact zone must be very limited and there must not be deep infiltration of these vessels. There is no proximal or distal control of the ICA, which is necessary in the presence of larger lesions. If an extended laceration of the jugular bulb is provoked, bleeding must be quickly controlled with a large flap of Surgicel. Due to the horizontal position of the patient, there is no risk of air embolization. When continuing surgery, small flaps of Surgicel may not safely be used, due to the risk that they may transverse the breach into the bulb and from there, go reach the right heart and on to the lungs, causing an infarction. It is then necessary to ligate the jugular vein in the neck (chapter 28: Treatment of surgical complications).

TYMPANIC MASTOID GLOMUS TUMOR

This tumor originates in the glomus bodies of the tympanic plexus. Besides the cavum tympani, the tumor also occupies the mastoid but does not involve the jugular bulb.
Thus a mastoidectomy must be performed by opening the facial recess. The facial recess is a collection of cells situated just lateral to the facial nerve, at the second genu.

ENLARGED FACIAL RECESS MASTOIDECTOMY

- Mastoidectomy.
- Under continuous irrigation, with a cutting burr, the lateral semicircular canal and the body of the incus are identified. The bony posterior wall of the external auditory canal (EAC) is thinned in the area indicated by the extremity of the short process of the incus. This surgical step may be performed with a cutting burr, which has the advantage of not creating bone paste typical of the diamond burr, which obscures the view of the underlying field. The cutting burr is also more penetrating: to avoid injuring the underlying structures, a wide diameter burr (3-3.5 mm) must be used in this first step, cutting with the side and never the tip. The tip masks the underlying view and has a slower rotation, making the burr's action more similar to lacerating than cutting. The oscillation of the burr must be tangent to the facial nerve, and never transversal, due to the risk of injuring the facial nerve. This is more easily achieved with the side than the tip of the burr.
- *Opening of the facial recess.* The facial recess may be opened without having to expose the facial nerve or the chorda tympani, as for example in the case of closed tympanoplasty. In this situation the identification of these structures provides the maximum opening of the recess and the best underlying visibility. The third tract of the facial nerve is identified. It is anterior and just below the dome of the horizontal semicircular canal. It describes an anterior concavity and passes underneath the tympanic membrane anterior and medial to the annulus. The chorda tympani detaches from the third tract of nerve VII proximally to the digastric crest and lies with anterior concavity. The facial recess has a mean maximum size of 2-4 mm. Even in two-year old children, it is generally no smaller than 2 mm. The recess is opened with small diamond burrs (1-2 mm). With the facial recess completely open, the horizontal part of the facial nerve may be seen, as well as the lenticular process of the incus, the incudostapedial articulation, the head of the stapes, the tendon of the stapes, and, by inclining the microscope forward, the cochleariform process. The bony spur dividing the short process from the incus of the facial recess must be preserved. If this spur is drilled, the ligaments of the short process from the incus may be torn, and the incus dislodged. Through the thinned bone canal, the chorda tympani may be seen, and inferiorly, the facial nerve (Fig. 16-2).
- *Enlarged opening of the facial recess.* In general the enlarged facial recess approach is used in

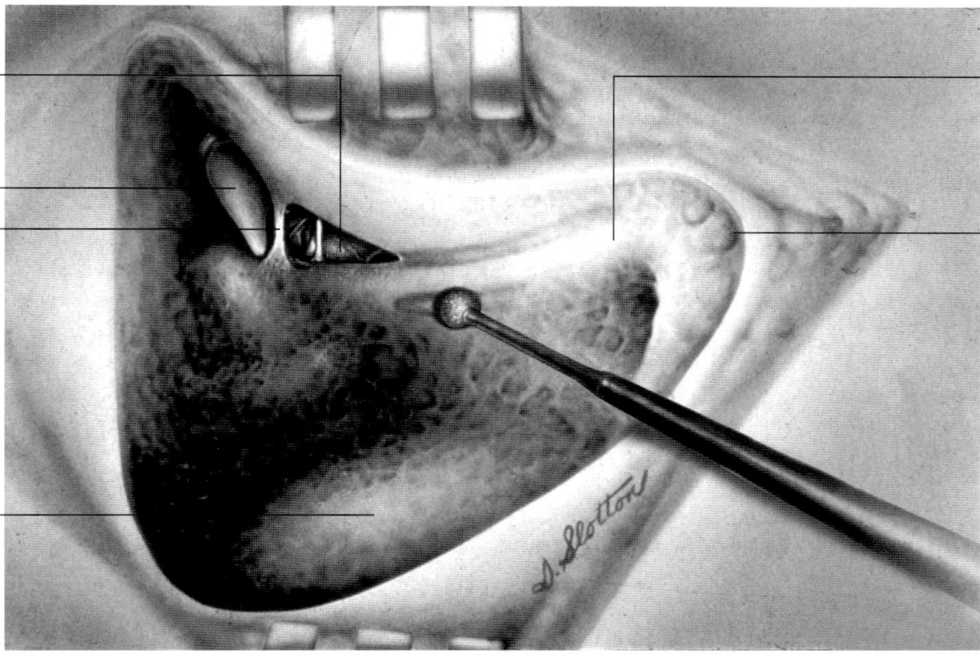

Fig. 16-2. Facial recess. Skeletonization of the facial nerve.

glomus tumors extending to the hypotympanic area. The chorda tympani is sacrificed and the lateral limit of the dissection thus proves to be the annular ligament of the tympanic membrane. The medial limit is the facial nerve and the inferior limit is the jugular bulb. Thus a view of the so-called crotch is obtained, where the jugular bulb unites with the carotid artery.

- In glomus tumors extending to include the hypotympanic region and the retrofacial region, the latter must be opened in the inferior part of the mastoid cavity. The superior limits of this dissection are the posterior semicircular canal and the cochlea. The posterior limit is the bone layer of the middle fossa, and the inferior and anterior limit is the jugular bulb. The facial nerve is suspended from a thin bone sheath and complete access is available to the hypotympanum, passing over and under the facial nerve (Figs. 16-3, 16-4).
- The approach described above is limited to tumors not involving the jugular bulb. At the end of the bone removal phase, all the vital structures have been identified. This occurs before tumor removal, which leads to profuse bleeding and makes removal more difficult (Fig. 16-5).
- The tumor is reduced by means of electrocoagulation with a bipolar cautery, acting on the vascularization. Monopolar coagulation must never be used due to the risk of electrical transmission through the cochlea to the ganglion of Corti. Flaps of Surgicel complete the haemostatic effect (Fig. 16-6). The tumor is freed superiorly, inferiorly, and posteriorly. Laterally it is liberated from the tympanic membrane with blunt instruments. In the presence of a significant infiltration of the tympanic membrane, it may be necessary to section the membrane or one of its parts and then perform a miringoplasty.
- The last part of the tumor to be removed is the anterior part, which involves the ICA. The tumor is cleaved from the arterial wall. If the tumor adheres to the wall, it is dangerous to proceed since there is no proximal or distal control in cases of lacerations to the ICA. Thus, in these cases, the approach must be modified to an infratemporal one.
- In glomus tumors with mastoid and neck involvement, this approach may be combined with a transcochlear or translabyrinthine approach and associated with a facial nerve rerouting (see chapter 28, 37, 38).

For tumors involving the jugular bulb, but not extending to the ICA or the neck or the posterior fossa, a mastoid and neck approach is used.

APPROACH THROUGH MASTOID AND NECK

As above, a complete mastoidectomy is performed, and the aperture of the facial recess is enlarged (Figs. 16-7, 16-8, 16-9).

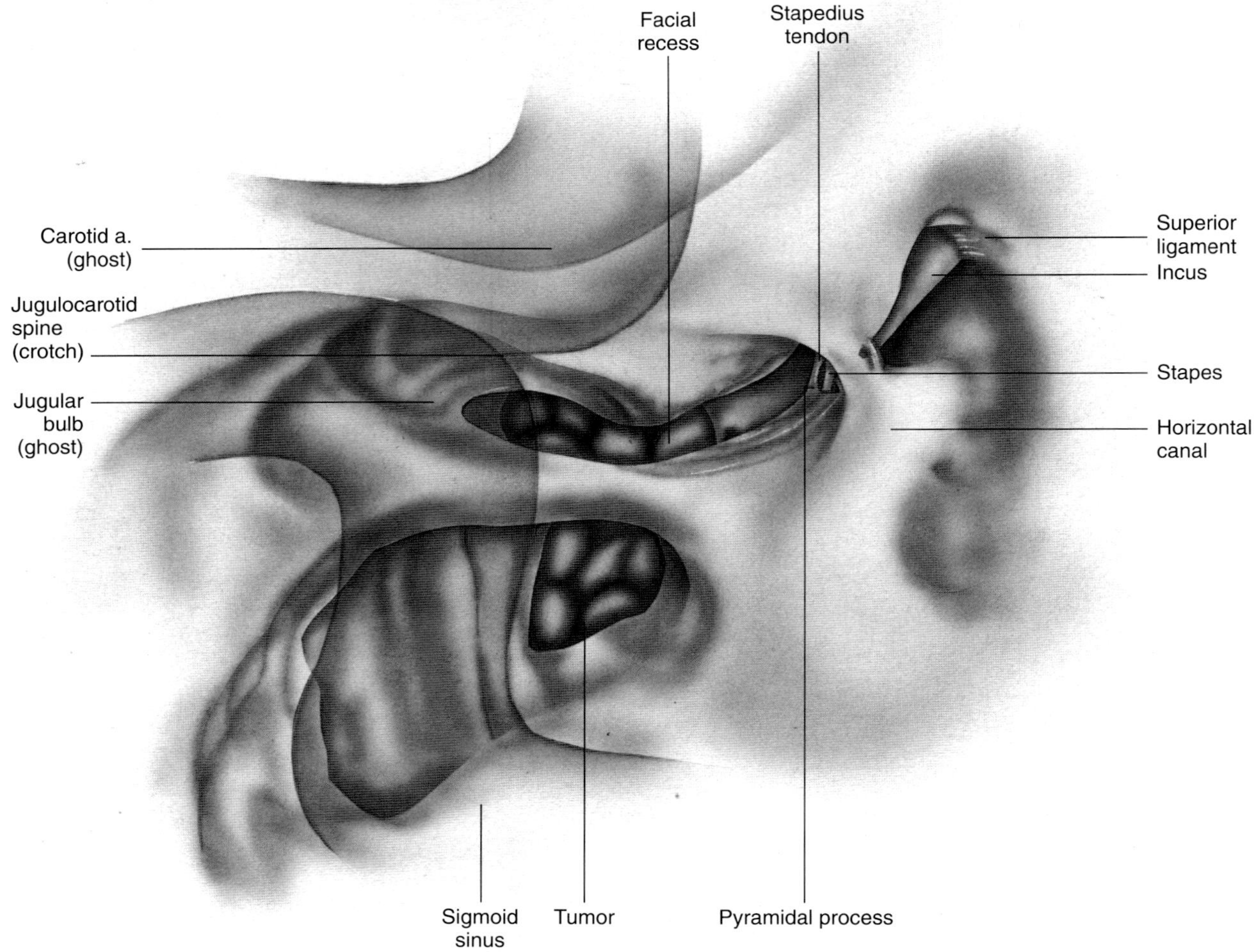

Fig. 16-3. Extended facial recess. Removal of retrofacial cells allows the surgeon to enter from the mastoid in the middle ear cavity, below the facial nerve, to expose tumor in the hypotympanum.

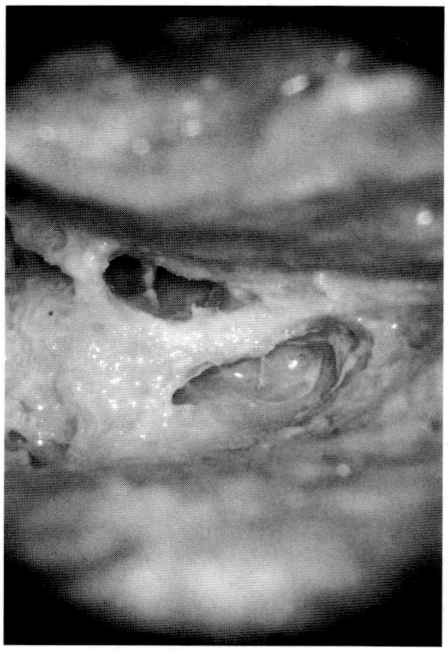

Fig. 16-4. The facial recess is opened and the facial n. is skeletonized. Tumor extension beneath the facial n. may be reached by removing the retrofacial air cells.

- The mastoidectomy is enlarged towards the tip, until reaching the digastric crest. It is better to use a large cutting burr and the tip may be used until reaching tissue of a hard but elastic consistency: this is the digastric crest. We continue along the crest until the mastoid tip has been completely liberated. There are no structures at risk during this phase, if we keep in mind that anteriorly and medially the digastric crest joins with the periosteum of the stylomastoid foramen, at the emergence of nerve VII.

The mastoid tip is drilled or removed with rongeurs while inferiorly the transition surface between bone and digastric is incised with Mayo scissors.

- The sigmoid sinus and the jugular bulb are skeletonized with diamond burrs. It is better to perform this step now, after having tied the jugular, since there is no possibility of embolization in the packing, in cases of laceration.

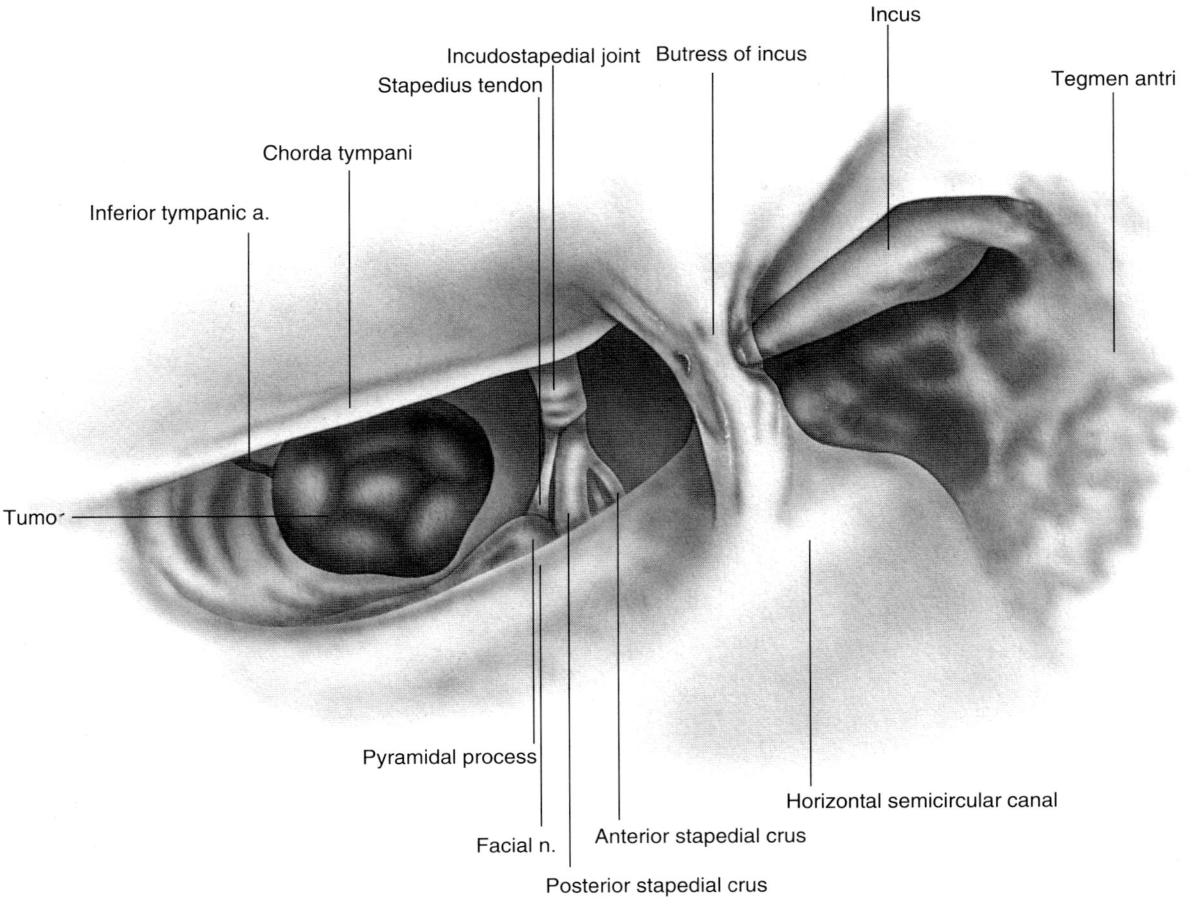

Fig. 16-5. Tympanic glomus tumor with hypotympanic extension.

Some bone is left on the medial part of the sinus. Between bone and sinus wall, an extraluminal pressurized packing is positioned.

A flap of Surgicel is placed just distal to the packed area. The sinus is incised and the Surgicel is advanced into the lumen of the bulb, to arrest bleeding coming from the inferior petrosal sinus and the condylar vein. The packing must be neither too pressurized nor too abundant (the Surgicel expands) so that nerves IX-X-XI are not injured. The tumor is then removed together with the jugular bulb.

Post-operatively, the patient is kept in intensive care due to the risk of hemorrhage or paralysis of the mixed nerves.

TUMORS INVOLVING THE VERTICAL TRACT OF THE FACIAL NERVE AND THE INFRALABYRINTHINE RETROFACIAL CELLS

In these glomus tumors, which must not involve the internal carotid artery, or in neuromas of the jugular foramen, the approach to the mastoid and neck may be amplified with a limited rerouting of the facial nerve. The facial nerve is exposed from the second genu on for the entire vertical tract. (See facial nerve exposure).

APPROACH THROUGH MASTOID AND NECK WITH PARTIAL FACIAL NERVE REROUTING

The facial nerve is exposed.

- The perineurium must be preserved to reduce trauma to the facial nerve. The periosteum of the stylomastoid foramen is incised underneath the facial nerve. The nerve is elevated from the stylomastoid foramen along with the periosteum and at the posterior belly of the digastric muscle.
- The limited rerouting of the nerve provides good control of the jugular bulb. The approach is not appropriate, however, for tumors involving the carotid artery, since the vertical view is

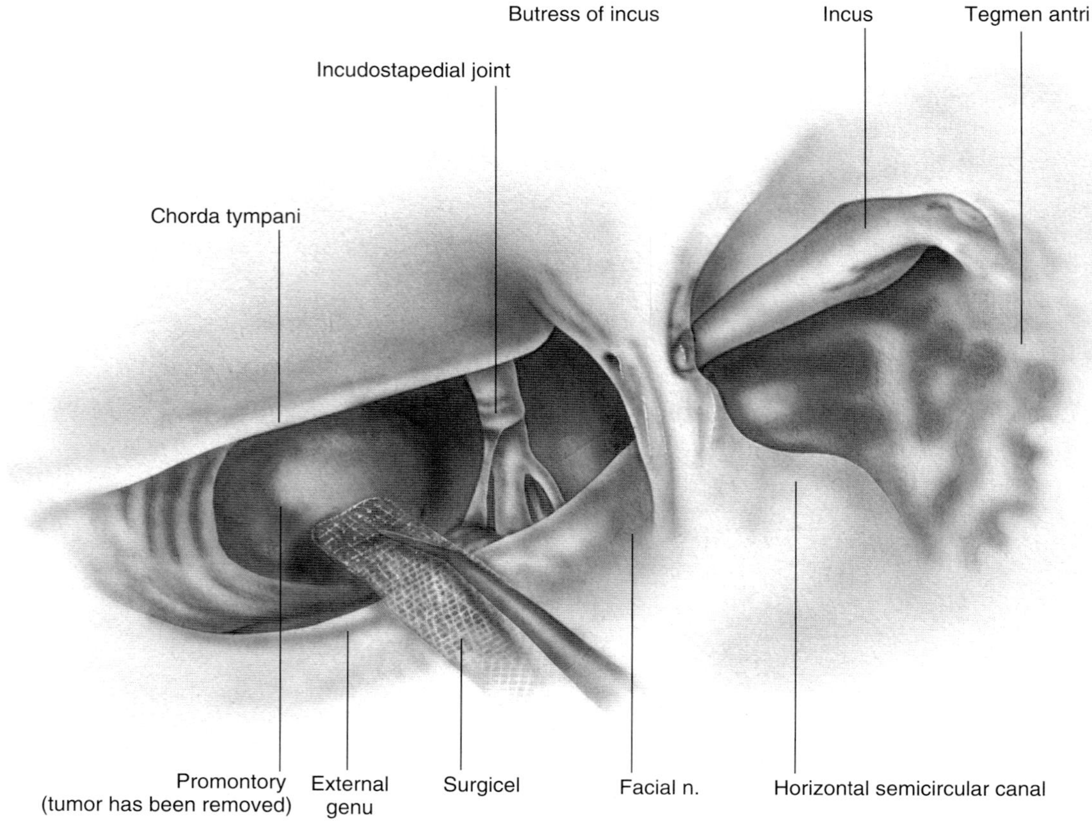

Fig. 16-6. Mastoid extended facial recess allows complete exposure of the middle ear and the hypotympanum, for tympanomastoid glomus tumors. The tumor has been removed. Surgicel is used to coagulate.

limited by the annulus tympanicum and the posterior bony canal wall.

FACIAL NERVE DECOMPRESSION

An enlarged mastoidectomy is performed with the largest cutting burr possible. The lateral semicircular canal (LSC) is identified as well as the body of the incus in the epitympanum. The posterior semicircular canal (PSC) is seen. The mastoid tip is opened wide until the digastric crest is reached. The posterior bony wall of the external auditory canal is thinned, working with the side of the burr.

Now, with the main landmarks identified, it is important to note that:

- The second genu of VII is just anterior and 2-3 mm medial to the dome of the LSC.
- The extremity of the PSC projects and almost reaches the third tract of the nerve.
- Near the stylomastoid foramen, the periosteum of the digastric muscle joins the facial nerve sheath. The entrance of the nerve into the sty-

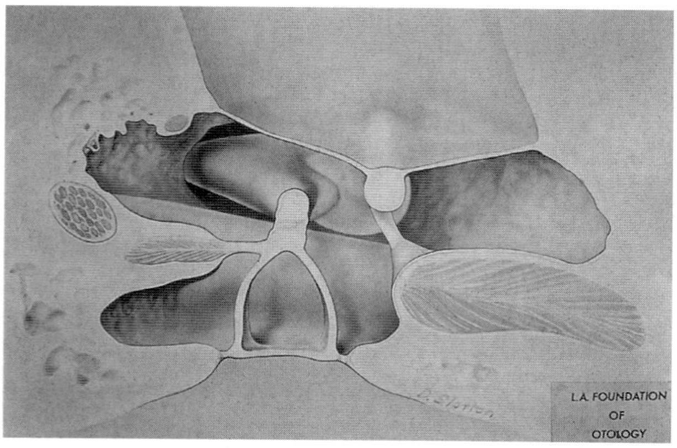

Fig. 16-7. Progressive saucerization of the facial recess.

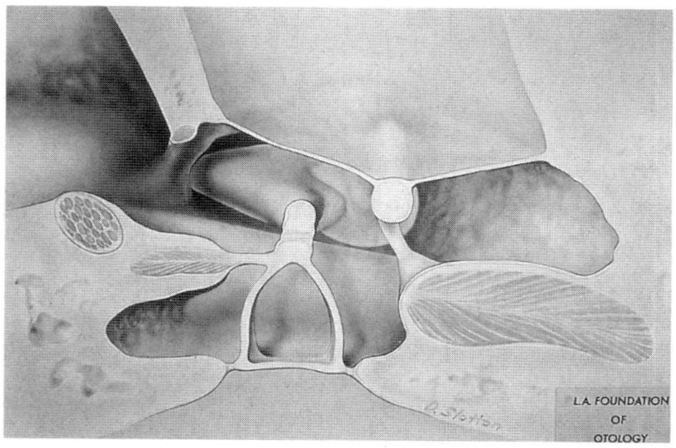

Fig. 16-8. Opening of the facial recess.

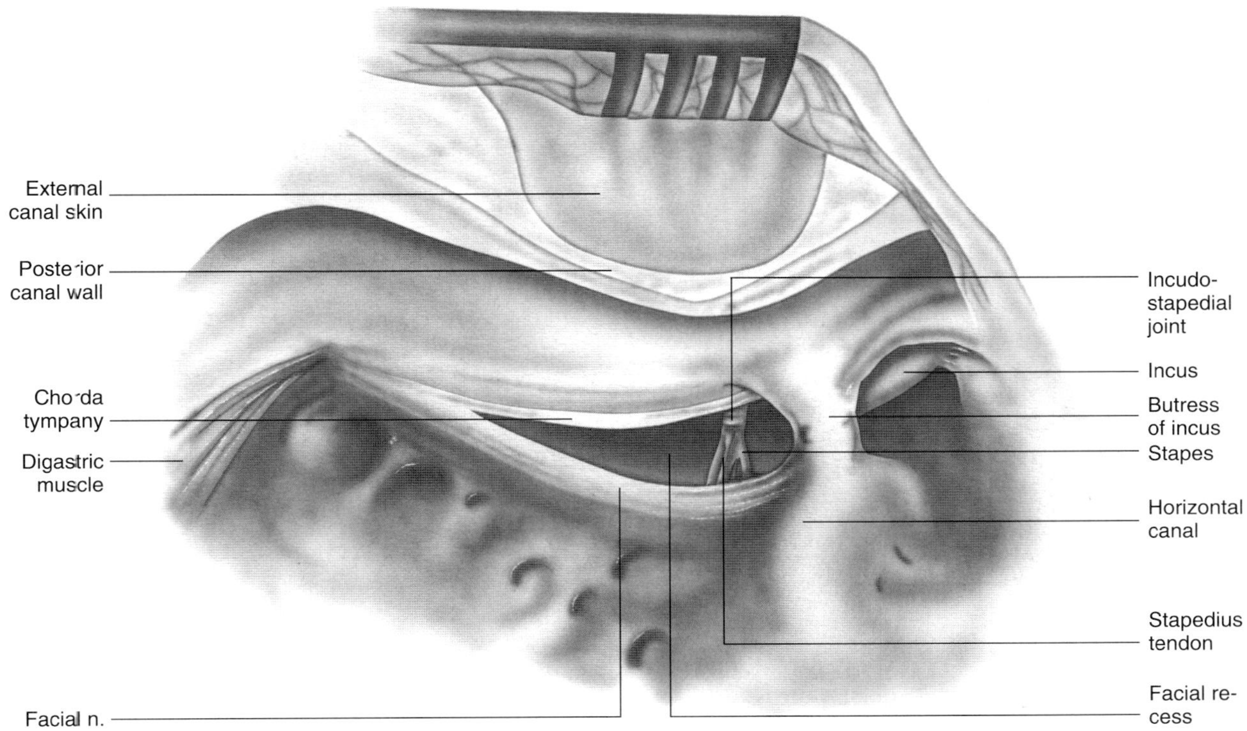

Fig. 16-9. Facial recess and related structures.

lomastoid foramen is approx. 2/3 mm lateral to the second genu of VII and is aligned at the level of the chorda tympani. The third tract of nerve VII describes an anterior concavity.

- With the side of the burr, the bony wall of the external auditory canal is thinned. With continuous irrigation the intersinuso-facial cells are drilled. The facial nerve is neared and a compact osseous sheath is seen, through which nerve VII may be viewed at its genu and its vertical tract. The nerve is distinguished by its yellowish-pinkish color, contrasting with the white of the bone. The bone is removed with a large diamond burr and profuse irrigation, to avoid damaging the nerve by overheating.
- The removal of the bone overlying the nerve is begun posteriorly to the vertical tract near the stylomastoid foramen and followed to the posterior semicircular canal. Thus injury to the chorda tympani is avoided. In the third tract, from the posterior semicircular canal to the II genu, the burr must act centrally, to avoid injuring the canal. On the second genu, the burr goes anteriorly, to avoid injuring the lateral semicircular canal. In the second tract, the burr acts centrally, following the nerve to the cochleariform process and then to the geniculate ganglion. Anteriorly there is the tendon of the stapes muscle and the posterior branch of the stapes. The lateral canal is posterior. The size of the diamond burr is reduced for this phase because of the necessity of passing through a restricted space among the stapes and the cochleariform process anteriorly, the lateral semicircular canal posteriorly and the body of the incus superiorly (Figs. 16-10, 16-11, 16-12, 16-13, 16-14, 16-15).

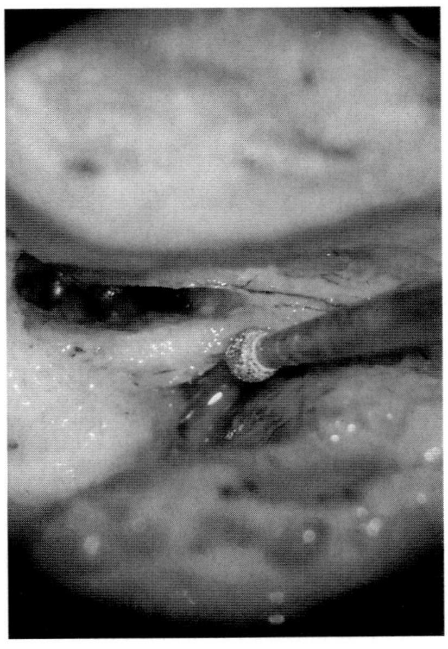

Fig. 16-10. Exposure of the second and third part of the facial nerve is performed moving the diamond burr from posterior to lateral to anterior, to avoid injury to the surrounding structures (chorda tympani and horizontal canal).

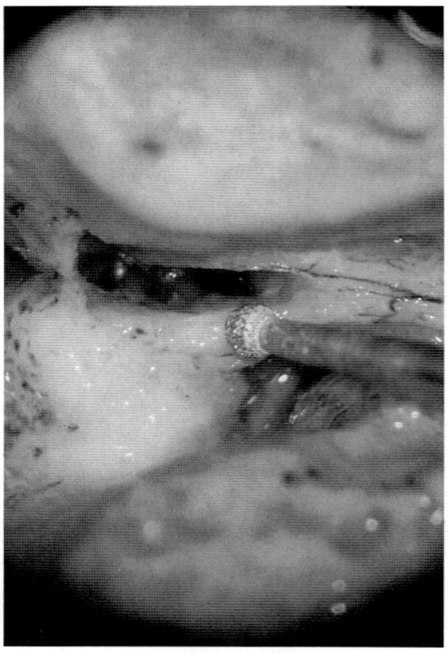

Figs. 16-11. Exposure of the second and third part of the facial nerve is performed moving the diamond burr from posterior to lateral to anterior, to avoid injury to the surrounding structures (chorda tympani and horizontal canal).

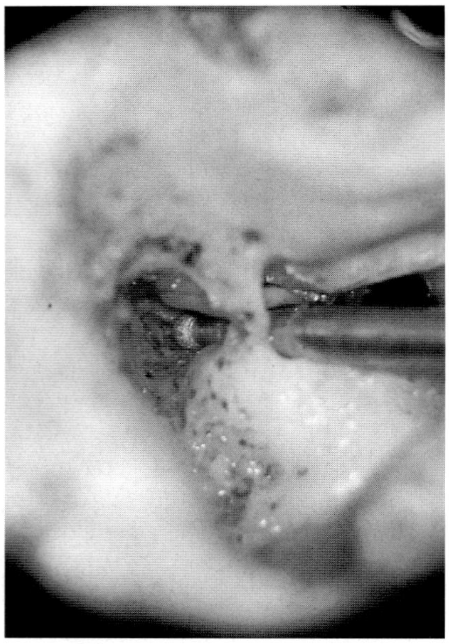

Fig. 16-13. The facial nerve can be exposed up to the geniculate ganglion, through the facial recess. In the infratemporal approach, the canal wall down technique allows a wider exposure of the facial nerve.

- When working with the nerve with a 10x or 16x enlargement, slight bleeding may take place at the vasa nervorum. Heavier bleeding is due to the lesion of one or both arterial vessels exiting the nerve in its vertical path. One artery reaches the fallopian canal in its medial part, the other is a branch of the stylomastoid artery.

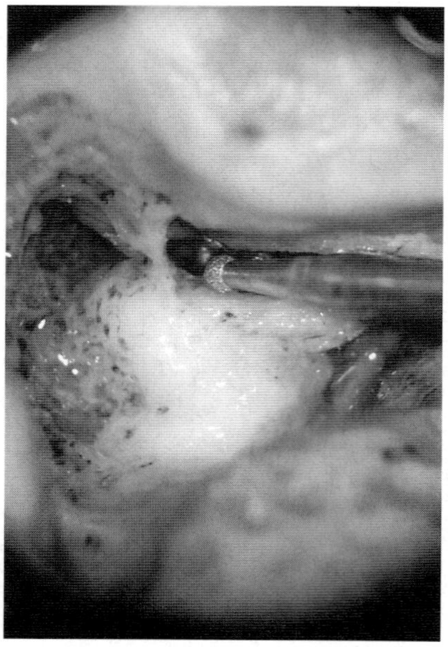

Figs. 16-12. Exposure of the second and third part of the facial nerve is performed moving the diamond burr from posterior to lateral to anterior, to avoid injury to the surrounding structures (chorda tympani and horizontal canal).

- The last layers of bone covering the nerve are removed. We prefer a modified dental dissector, similar to the whirlybird in middle ear surgery (Fisch). It has the advantage of acting both as a curette and as a dissector, and is fairly sturdy. For the right ear a curvature to the right is used; vice versa for the left. A Rosen needle may also be used, especially in the second tract, where the space is narrower. The tip must be checked, keeping in mind not to use the fulcrum above the nerve.

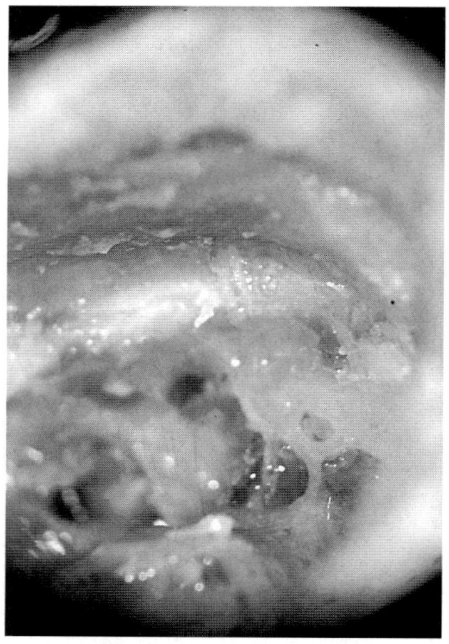

Fig. 16-14. At the stylomastoid foramen, the periosteum of the digastric muscle blends with the sheath of the facial nerve.

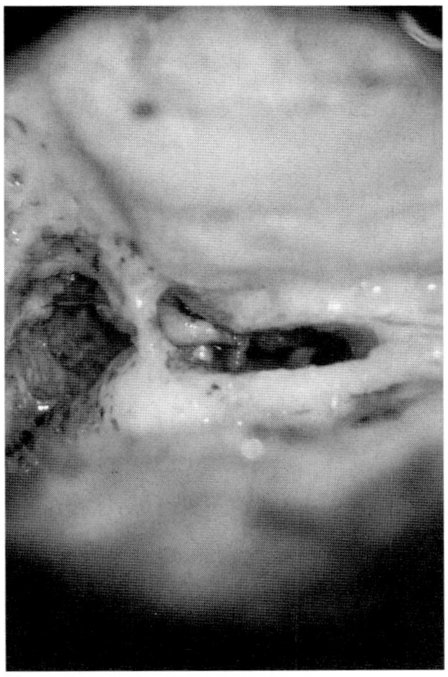

Fig. 16-15. Right ear. The facial recess.

TUMORS INVOLVING THE JUGULAR BULB AND THE INTERNAL CAROTID ARTERY

The infratemporal approach, developed by Fisch has greatly improved the possibilities of operating on tumors previously considered inoperable (Fig. 16-16).
Fisch names three separate infratemporal approaches: Type A, Type B, and Type C.

TYPE A APPROACH TO THE INFRATEMPORAL FOSSA
This approach is specific to glomus tumors involving the jugular bulb and the internal carotid artery, in its horizontal and/or vertical part. It enables us to treat tumors reaching the cavernous sinus and/or those with an intracranial extension. It may be utilized for cholesteatomas and cholesterinic cysts of the petrosal apex, and for neuromas of nerves IX-X-XI-XII in the jugular foramen.

- C shaped postauricular incision. The incision is extended to the neck tissue (Fig. 16-17).
- Cul-de-sac closure of the external auditory canal. The canal skin is transected at the bony-cartilaginous junction and is undermined laterally. Extra cartilage is removed, and the skin is closed with interrupted 5-0 nylon sutures in a dimple-like fashion at the external auditory meatus. A periosteal flap is used to oversew the undersurface of the canal skin (Figs. 16-18, 16-19, 16-20, 16-21, 16-22, 16-23).

The original description by Fisch foresees:

- Exposure of the intraparotid facial nerve and partial exposure of the temporo-zygomatic and cervico-facial branches.
- Extension of the skin incision to the neck.
- Identification of the large vessels and the nerves of the neck.
- Ligation of the branches of the external carotid.
- Subtotal petrosectomy.
- Preparation of a new fallopian canal in the anterior epitympanum, from the geniculate ganglion to the anterior parotid, and anterior transposition of the nerve into the new canal (Fig. 16-24).
- Sigmoid sinus ligation.

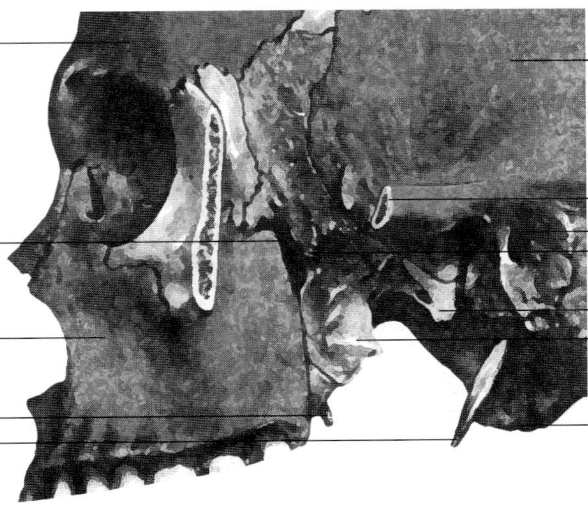

Fig. 16-16. The infratemporal fossa.

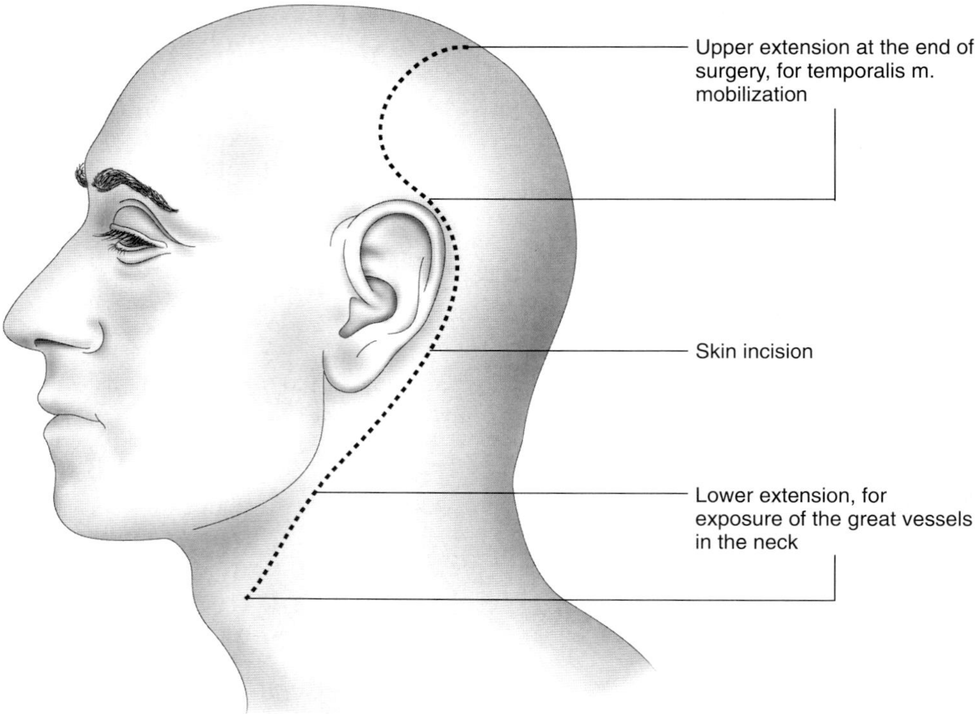

Fig. 16-17. Incision for infratemporal fossa approach type A.

- Separation of the parotid gland from the tympanic bone.
- Fracture of the styloid process.
- Anterior dislocation of the mandible with the introduction of a retractor through the infratemporal fossa (Fischer and Storz, Germany).
- Tumor removal.

The technique proposed by Brackmann, which we use, has made some technical modifications to the technique proposed and codified by Fisch:

- Cul-de-sac closure of the external auditory canal, in the same chronology as Fisch.
- Mastoidectomy with facial nerve exposure.

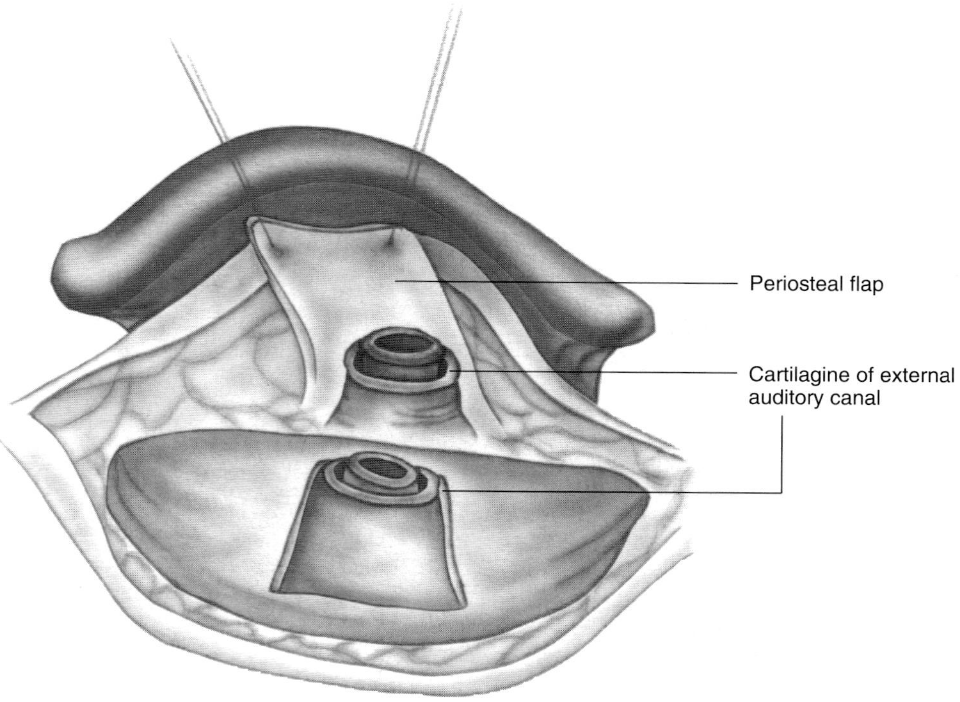

Fig. 16-18. Transection of the external auditory canal (Adapted from Fisch U).

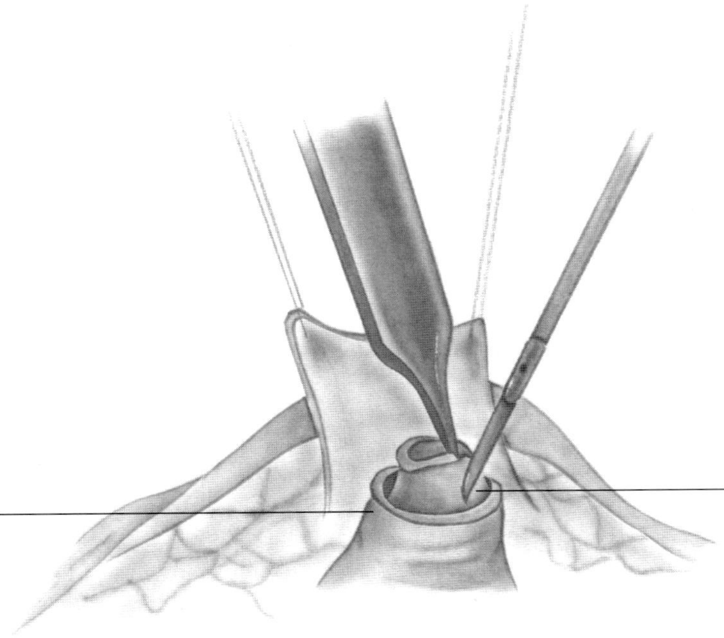

Fig. 16-19. The cartilage is dissected from the canal skin.

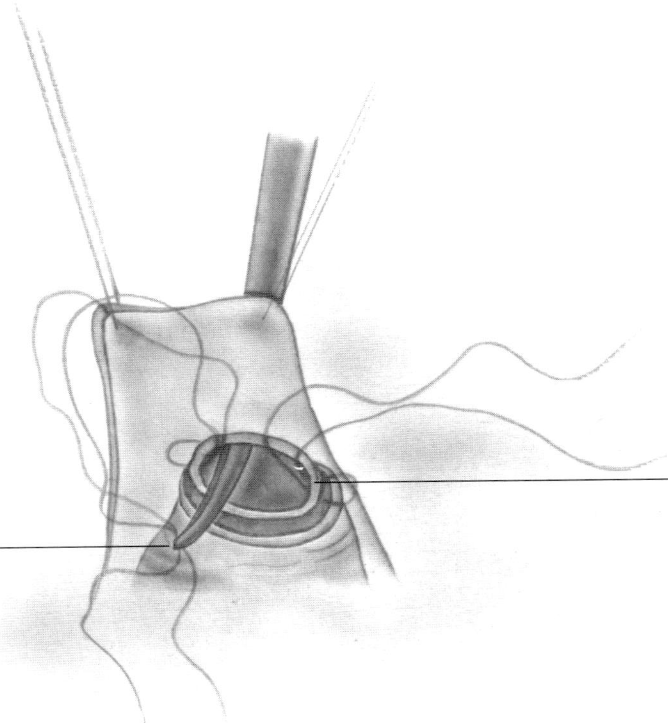

Fig. 16-20. Two catgut sutures are passed through the canal skin and then through the meatus. The stay sutures are pulled, thus everting the canal skin (Adapted from Fisch U).

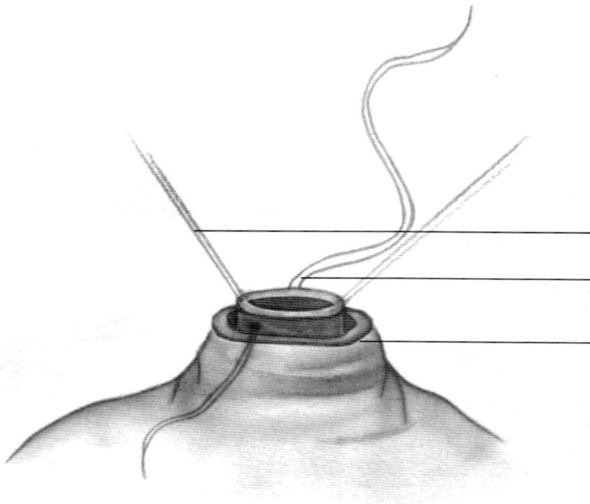

Fig. 16-21. The everted canal skin is closed with 4-0 nylon sutures.

- Preparation of the jugular vein and the internal carotid artery, and neck exposure.
- Transposition of the facial nerve.
- Identification of nerves IX-X-XI-XII.
- Tumor removal.

SURGICAL TECHNIQUE

SUBTOTAL PETROSECTOMY AND INTRAMASTOID FACIAL NERVE EXPOSURE

- The skin of the IAC is removed with a suction aspirator and an elevator, according to the technique used in the tympanoplasty. The fibrous annulus is also removed along with the tympanic membrane.
- Mastoidectomy.
- Opening of the facial recess and separation of the incudo-stapedial articulation. Once the facial recess has been identified, the posterior bony wall of the external auditory canal covering the recess and the facial nerve may be safely removed. This is done with a burr or rongeurs.
- A complete mastoidectomy is performed (see approach through mastoid and neck), with the additional exposure of the sigmoid sinus.

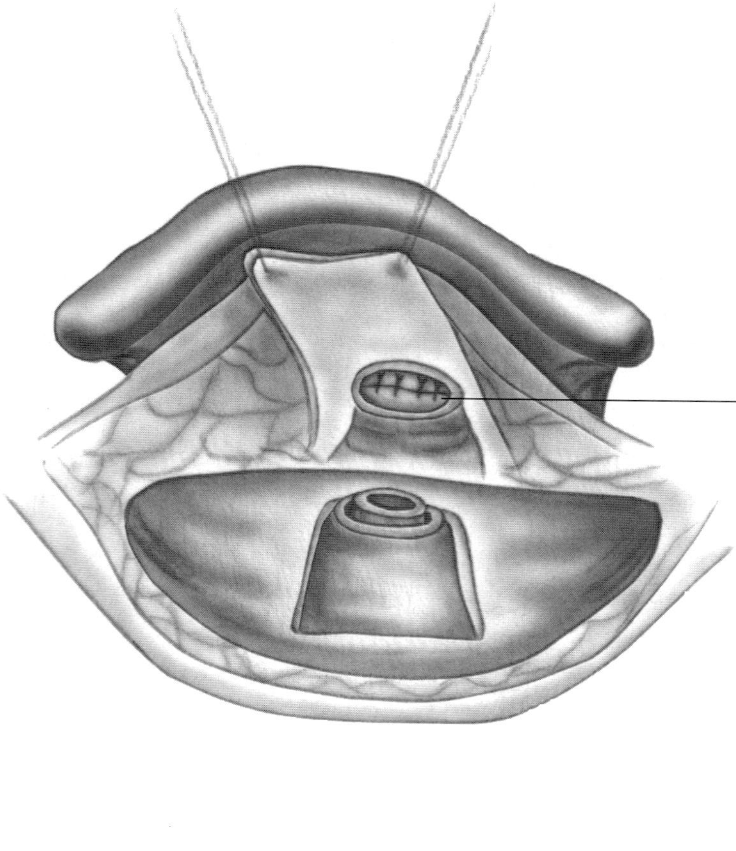

Fig. 16-22. A periosteal flap, for a second layer of closure, is pedicled.

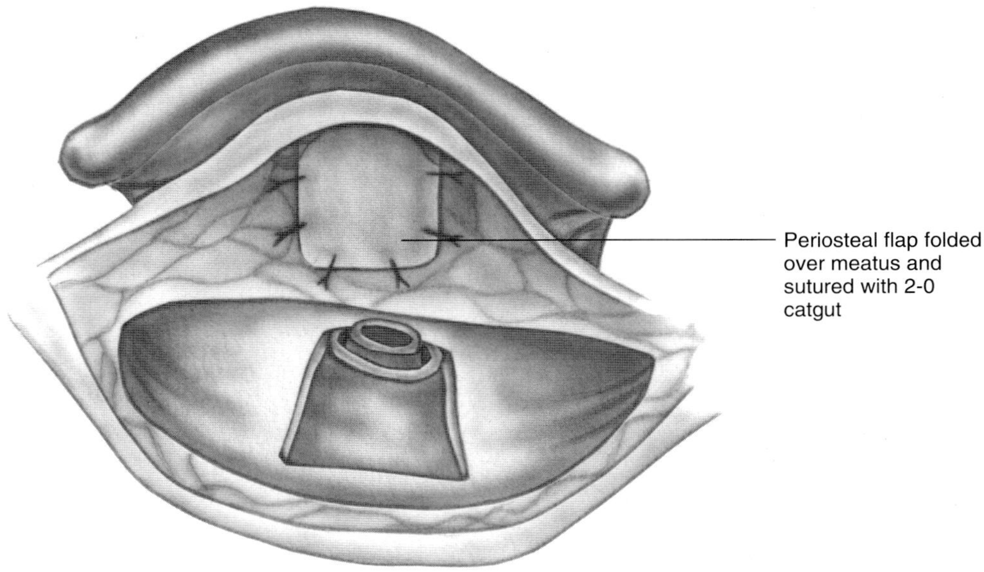

Fig. 16-23. The periosteal flap is rotated anteriorly and sutured with absorbable sutures (Adapted from Fisch U).

- The jugular bulb is identified. Anteriorly to the "crotch", the internal carotid artery is identified. The bone of the anterior external auditory canal is removed until the periosteum of the temporomandibular articulation is reached. In this area there may be bleeding which can be easily halted with a dissector placed on the periosteum, upon which electrocoagulation is performed.

THE NECK

- The incision is extended along the anterior border of the sternocleidomastoid muscle. The mastoid tip is safely removed with a burr or rongeurs, since the stylomastoid foramen has already been identified.
- The internal jugular vein is identified, as is the trunk of the internal carotid artery and the external carotid artery. Silk threads are used but not tied (Fig. 16-25).

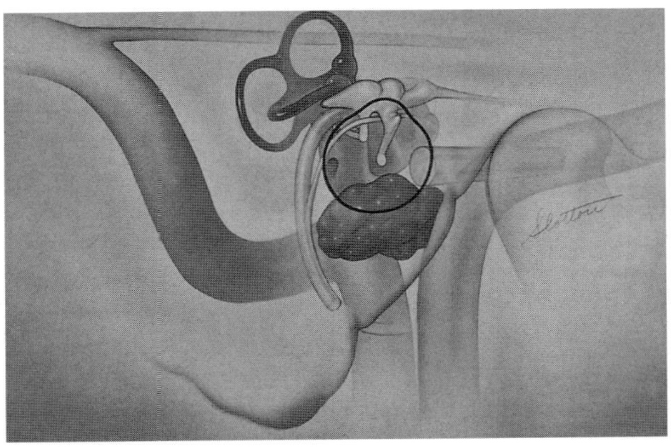

Fig. 16-24. The facial nerve is an obstacle for the successful removal of glomus tumors with jugular bulb and/or carotid artery and/or transdural extension, therefore facial nerve rerouting is necessary.

- Exposure of the facial nerve from the geniculate ganglion to the stylomastoid foramen and its transposition.
- To improve the possibilities of working on the tympanic segment of nerve VII, which runs from the lateral canal to the stapes, the suprastructure is cut with crurotomy scissors. This also helps to avoid leaving residual tumor in situ. The incision goes from the anterior crus to the posterior crus, finally reaching the tendon of the stapedial muscle. The footplate remains intact and in place.
- The thin bony sheaths are removed. The nerve is exposed for 270° in the mastoid and 180° in the tympanic tract. The nerve is elevated from the fallopian canal, moving it with the side of the suction-irrigator. A cottonoid is positioned below the suction-irrigator to avoid aspiration trauma and the fibrous adherences are sectioned with a sickle knife. The stapedial muscle is separated medially at the level of the stapes in the third segment of the nerve.
- Fisch's technique calls for the identification of the nerve at the exit of the stylomastoid foramen. The nerve is then exposed, including the two branches, the temporo-zygomatic branch and the cervico-facial branch (Fig. 16-26).
- The landmarks for finding the extratemporal facial nerve at its exit from the stylomastoid foramen are the tympanomastoid suture, the external ear canal cartilage, called the "pointer", and the digastric muscle (Fig. 16-27).

Brackmann's Technique

- Brackmann's technique does not call for the exposure of the facial nerve in the parotid. The

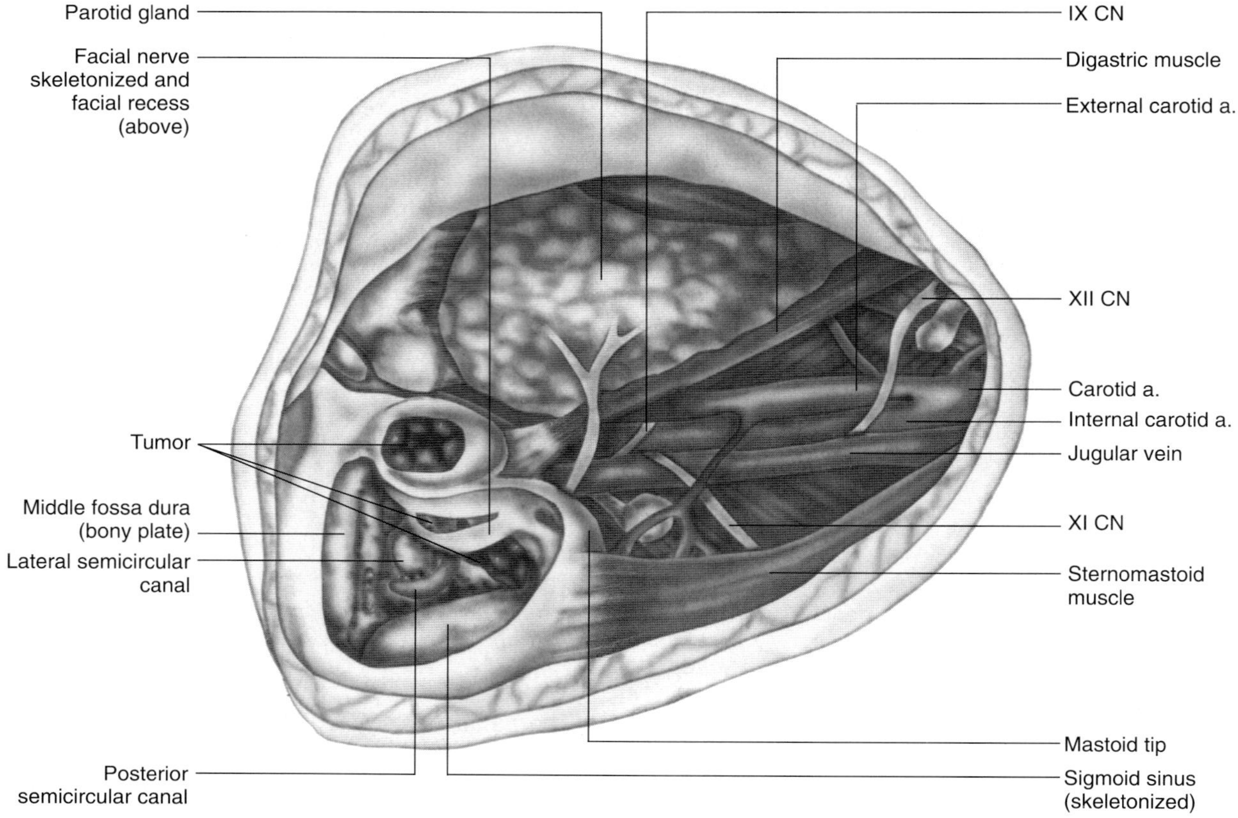

Fig. 16-25. Mastoidectomy and facial recess. The facial n. is exposed up to the parotid gland. The great vessels in the neck are exposed. (Adapted from Glasscock ME.).

nerve is rather transposed along with the periosteum of the stylomastoid foramen and moved with the tail of the gland. This variation makes it possible to maintain the vascularization of the facial nerve to the stylomastoid foramen and reduce intraparotid trauma, (since it does not call for the exposure of the nerve in the parotid). In our experience, the incidence and intensity of postoperative paresis is reduced (Brackmann 1987).

- Once the second and third segments of the facial nerve have been exposed, the incision is ex-

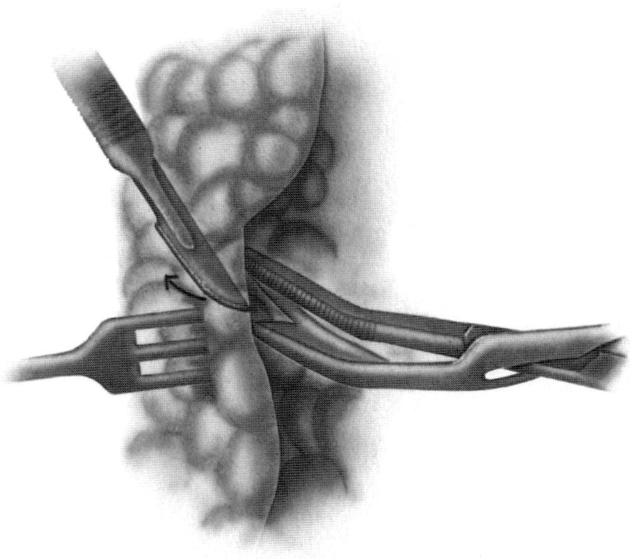

Fig. 16-26. Exposure of the facial nerve up to temporo-zygomatic and cervico-facial branches. A curved clamp is opened over the nerve and the overlying parotid is cut.

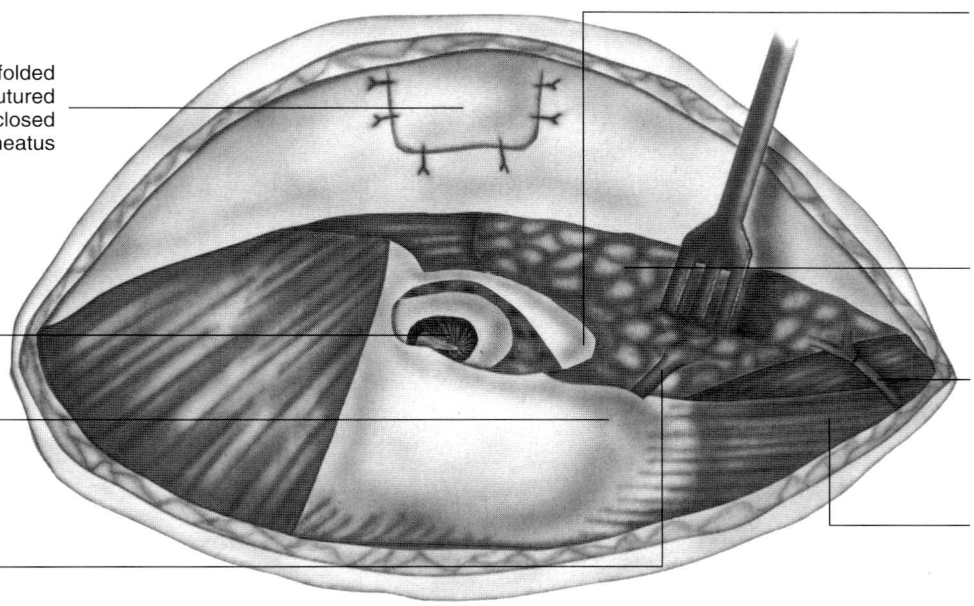

Fig. 16-27. Exposure of the facial and greater auricular nerves.

tended to the neck. The digastric crest is laterally exposed in the mastoid tip, lateral to the facial nerve.

- The sternocleidomastoid muscle is detached from the bone of the mastoid tip and retracted posteriorly. The posterior belly of the digastric muscle is dissected and retracted anteriorly.
- The facial nerve is not exposed in the stylomastoid foramen. Rather, the soft tissues and the periosteum of the stylomastoid foramen are incised to reduce trauma, and are elevated along with the facial nerve (Figs. 16-28, 16-29, 16-30). The contents of the stylomastoid foramen are reflected forward along with the tail and the

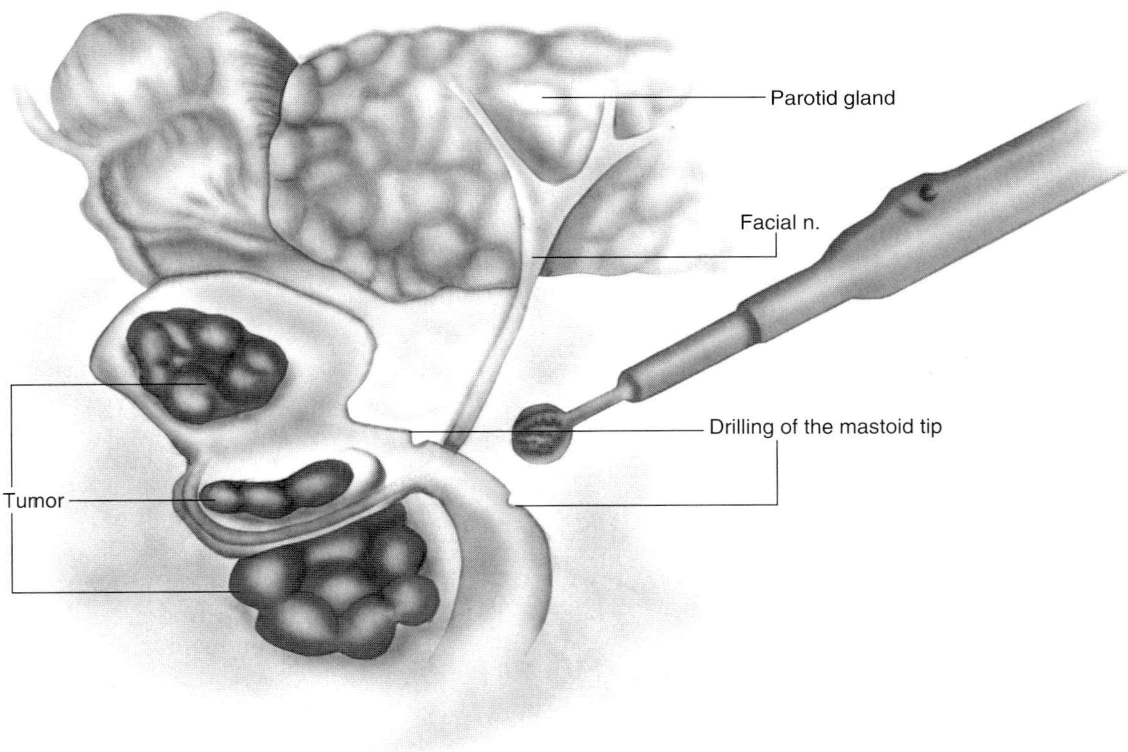

Fig. 16-28. The mastoid tip is drilled

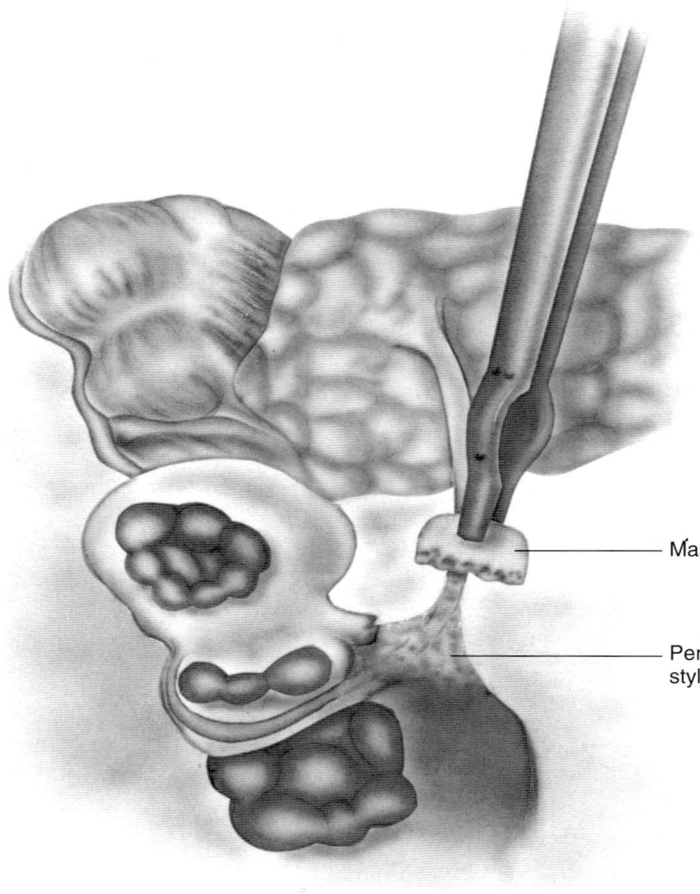

Fig. 16-29. The mastoid tip is removed.

deep lobe of the parotid, while the parotid gland is dislodged lateral to the mandible branch. The periosteum of the stylomastoid foramen is anchored with 2-0 silk thread at the fibrous tissue of the glenoid fossa. Thus the nerve is temporarily transposed anteriorly and access to the sigmoid sinus is freed, at the jugular bulb and the carotid artery (Fig. 16-31). At the end of the operation the skin suture is removed and the nerve is repositioned in the original site. Abdominal fat is used to fill the void and to keep the nerve in place.

- To expose the internal carotid artery at the cranial base during the operation, we place a large Perkins retractor (V. Mueller, Chicago) with a wide blade behind the blade of the mandible, with the teeth in the soft tissue of the neck. The mandible is thus anteriorly dislodged and this avoids having to section the mandibular condyle.

THE NECK AGAIN

- The course of the ICA is followed from the neck into the cranial base and into the petrosal tract. Nerves IX-X-XI are identified into the jugular foramen and nerve XII is identified at its foramen.
- Double ligation and section between the two ligations of the jugular vein.
- Ligation of the external carotid artery, to reduce the hematic supply which is the principle task of the ascending pharyngeal artery. Silk threads are kept in situ for a possible ligation of the ICA, in case of non repairable lacerations.
- Opening of the sigmoid sinus and occlusion of the sigmoid sinus with Surgicel.
- If the tumor is intradural, the sinus is ligated. The dura of the posterior fossa is exposed pre and retrosigmoid. The retrosigmoid dura is incised approx. 3 mm from the sinus. An aneurism needle is passed under the sinus, the presigmoid dura is incised in relation to the salience of the needle, a double silk thread is passed in the eye, the needle is removed, the thread is divided in two and tied.
- The jugular vein is elevated from bottom to top, including the bulb. The tumor is cleaved from the nervous part of the jugular foramen.
- The tumor is separated anteriorly from the ICA. Tumors may invade the periosteum of the carotic canal, necessitating the separation of the periosteum from the adventitia of the ICA with a Kelly forceps and curved scissors. Hemostasis

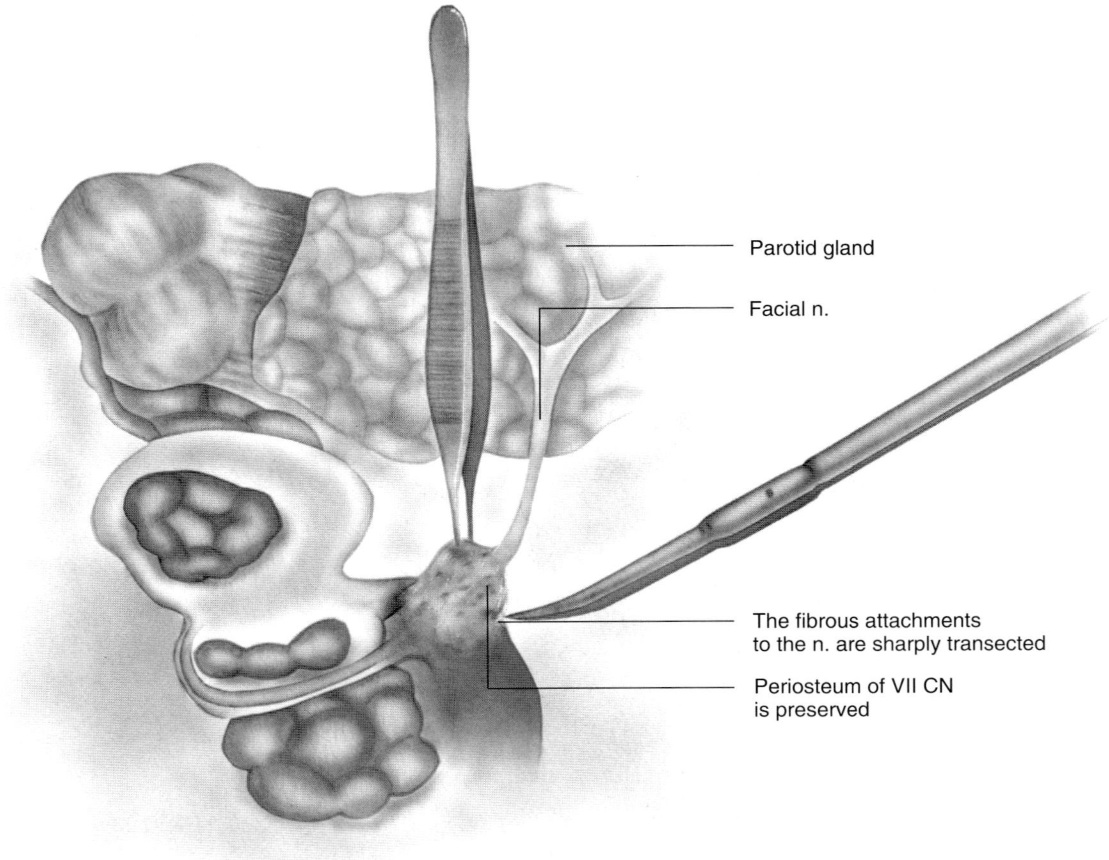

Fig. 16-30. Dissection of the periosteum of the stylomastoid foramen, around the facial nerve.

sis is performed of the tympanic-carotic vessels of the ICA and of the tumor with a bipolar cautery, reducing the tumor's dimensions. Bleeding of the inferior petrosal sinus is halted with Surgicel.

- The tumor is removed from bottom to top, including the jugular vein, the bulb and part of the sigmoid sinus.
- The mixed nerves must be preserved whenever possible. The point in which they are most easily injured is the jugular foramen, where they run in the pars nervosa.
- When the tumor removal phase is terminated, the inferior bone is drilled at the labyrinthine capsule, to remove any residual tumor in the cavity. Then the bleeding spots are occluded with a diamond burr without irrigation.

Closure

The ostium of the eustachian tube is closed with muscle fragments. The operating cavity is closed with abdominal fat. If a CSF leak has occurred, the fat may be anchored to the dura with silk threads. The fat thus takes the path of least resistance and occludes the fistule. More fat may be placed in the cavity, to prevent the CSF leakage; an important rule to follow is that too much fat is better than too little. Closure of the skin must leave salience due to the underlying fat. If residual fat is left between the lips of the wound, it is removed by rubbing with a gauze strip.

To cover the cavity before skin closure, a flap may be created with the temporalis muscle, with the bottom up.

TUMORS WITH INTRACRANIAL EXTENSION

- While working with the jugular bulb, the tumor may penetrate into the intracranial spaces. The glomus generally follows two paths of least resistance, i.e. the jugular bulb and the inferior petrosal sinus lumen. Small tumor extensions are removed.
- *Large Endocranial Tumor Extensions.* Before beginning the endocranial phase, the possibility of staging should be considered. One deciding factor is blood loss. Generally, in an average subject (average age, weight, general health conditions), the cut-off is 3000 ml. Beyond this limit, despite transfusions, bleeding problems may occur, due to the depletion of coagulating factors.

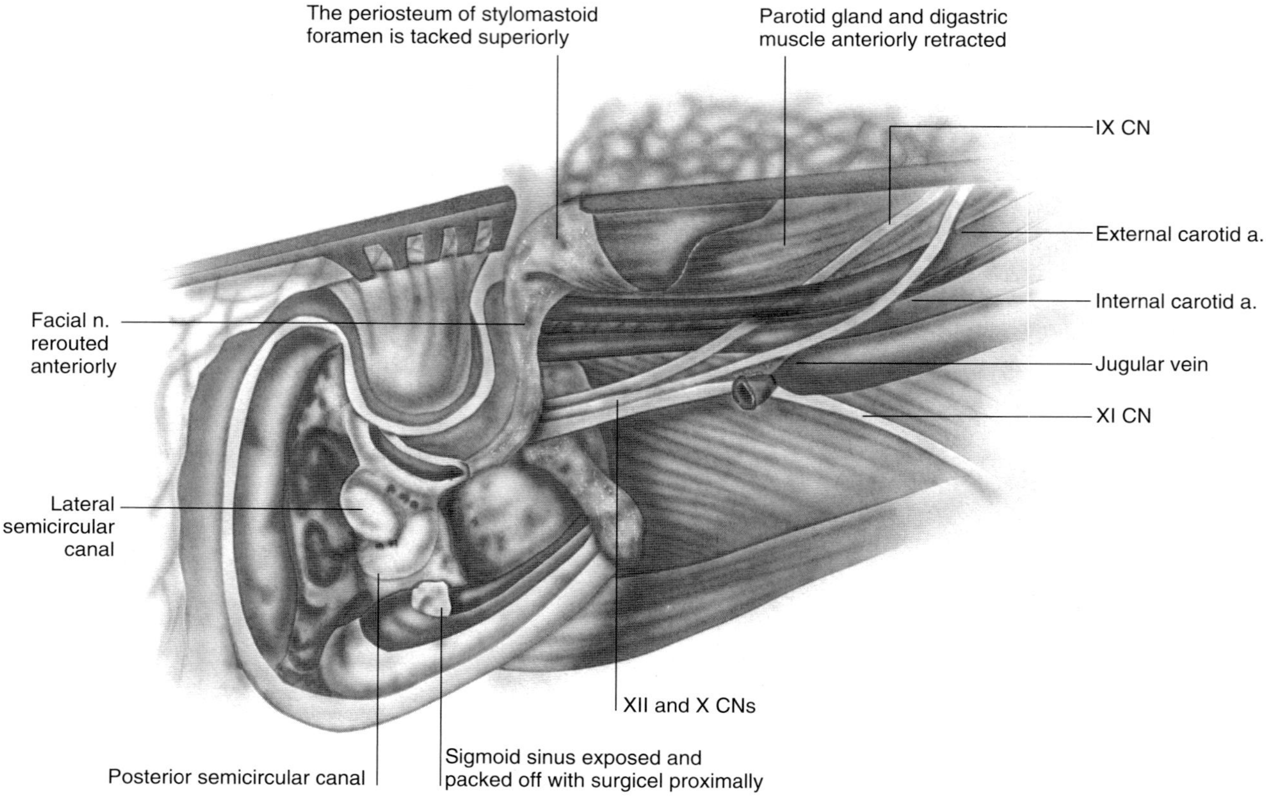

Fig. 16-31. The facial nerve, with the periosteum of the stylomastoid foramen, is transposed anteriorly along with the tail of the parotid. The periosteum of the stylomastoid foramen is sutured to the soft tissues of the root of the zygoma (Adapted from Brackmann DE).

- We generally tend to remove the tumor in one single step, since once the extracranial part is finished, the worst of the trauma has already been faced. The possibility of postoperative contamination should be noted, due to the risks of communication between the endocranial and extracranial spaces. This can be prevented by means of careful closure.
- Removal of the intracranial part provokes less bleeding, since its vascularization is lesser and since much of the hemostasis has already been accomplished in the previous phase. Hemostasis is then achieved with bipolar coagulation.
- In these instances, the tumor goes through the dura and enters the endocranium. Thus, if the radicality is to be pursued, the dura must be contextually removed.
- Once it has been decided not to stage the operation, the extracranial phase may be eliminated in order to go directly to the intracranial phase: part of the tumor is left above the dura of the posterior cranial fossa and the jugular bulb, and is later removed along with the dura and the intracranial part. This saves time and thus reduces bleeding.
- Closure of the dural breach is performed with a fascia lata flap closed with a watertight suture.

The phases following closure are those already described.

RESULTS

Glomus tympanycum tumors

The experience of the House Ear Clinic includes 73 tympanic glomus tumors treated from 1957-1990 (O'Leary) 20% treated with a transcanal approach, and 80% with a mastoid, facial recess approach.
Hearing stayed within the preoperative levels.
The morbidity was minimum: 3 tympanic perforations treated with tympanoplasty, one paresis of VII resolved after a decompressive surgery, one postoperative cholesteatoma. In 3 cases an incomplete removal of the tumor was performed and a relapse followed.
Average blood loss was over 500 ml.

Glomus Jugularis Tumors, from the Carotid and Transdural Arteries.

The experience of the House Ear Clinic includes 52 cases treated in the period from 1980 to 1991 (Green), 83% with an infratemporal fossa approach, 10% with a mastoid-neck approach and a limited reroute of the facial nerve, 7% with a mastoid-neck approach. Complete removal was obtained in 85% of cases. 95% of the patients showed good post-operative facial function: I and II degree. In 85% of cases it was possible to achieve the same physical efficiency as before the operation.

Eight patients underwent facial nerve sections for radical surgery, followed by grafting. In ten patients it was necessary to increase the thickness of the vocal cords. In percentages under 4%, a tracheotomy or a gastrostomy was necessary.

The risk of lesions to the internal carotid artery and the repair possibilities are evaluated with preoperative examinations (deVries).

Risk factors in recurring glomus tumors, with intracranial extension

- In patients with tumors that recur after surgery or after radiotherapy, it is harder to distinguish the tumor from normal tissues. Thus preservation of the cranial nerves is more difficult, as is cleavage of the neoplasm from the ICA and complete tumor removal. The risk of lesion to the ICA is increased. Dural repair is complicated, due to weakening of the dura from the previous treatment.
- In these situations, protracted time in surgery and the prolonged use of blades for cerebral retraction may provoke an ischemic lesion of the cerebellar, occipital or temporal lobes. We have never witnessed these particular complications, since the only retraction has been exerted by the suction-irrigator. Thus the pressure exerted is only fleeting, and does not have the ischemic effect of continuous pressure exerted by a spatula.

TYPE B INFRATEMPORAL APPROACH (FISCH)

This is recommended for lesions to the petrosal apex, such as cholesteatomas and cholesterinic cysts and for chordomas to the clivus.

- Skin incision (Fig. 16-32).
- Closure of the external auditory canal.
- Identification of the facial nerve in the parotid.
- The emergence of the nerve is identified at the stylomastoid foramen and followed to the bifurcation. The frontal branch of the bifurcation is followed to the zone overlying the zygomatic arch and to the entrance of the facial musculature. Identification of the superior ramus prevents future lesions. The periosteum of the zygomatic arch is dissected and reflected downwards along with the frontal ramus of nerve VII.
- The temporalis muscle is dissected from the medial surface of the zygomatic arch.

Section of the zygomatic arch

The zygomatic arch is divided as proximally and distally as possible with a 1 mm cutting burr. The zygomatic arch is reflected inferiorly, attached to the masseter muscle.

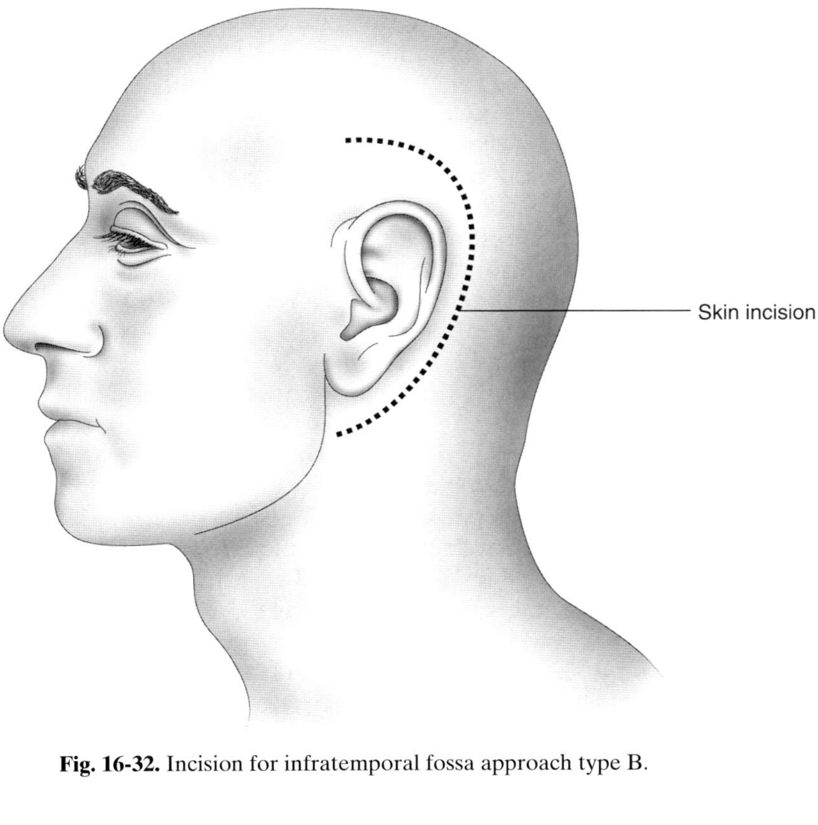

Fig. 16-32. Incision for infratemporal fossa approach type B.

Dissection of the temporalis muscle

The temporalis muscle is dissected from the squamous portion of the temporal bone and reflected downwards, pedicled at the coronal process of the mandible.

Subtotal petrosectomy

- The skin of the external auditory canal is removed, as well as the tympanum, the malleus, and the incus.
- All the tympano-mastoid cells are drilled.
- The second segment of the facial nerve is identified and followed along the third (mastoid) tract, while removing the overlying bone. A sheath of bone is left on the nerve.
- The jugular bulb and the internal carotid artery are identified in the tympanic cavity with diamond burrs. A thin sheath of bone is left on these structures.

Exposure of the Mandibular Condyle

- The entire anterior and posterior tympanic annulus is removed. The bone is removed anteriorly from the floor of the middle cranial fossa and the glenoid fossa. The articulated disc is removed and the condyle exposed.
- The retractor of the infratemporal fossa is inserted with the two blades between the wound superiorly and the mandibular condyle inferiorly. It is important to take care that the blade does not slip from the condyle and injure the frontal ramus of nerve VII.
- The medial meningeal artery and V3 are incised and coagulated to widen access to the infratemporal fossa.
- The bone and cartilaginous part of the eustachian tube are removed. The horizontal tract of the internal carotid is identified medial to the tube.
- The tensor tympani muscle is removed from the tympanum and the carotid artery is followed to the foramen lacerum.
- The bone around the carotid artery is removed anteriorly and posteriorly. The artery may thus be elevated with an umbilical thread, which permits the removal of the lesion at 360° around the ICA.
- If a rerouting of nerve VII is performed and the ICA is elevated, the path is opened to the entire petrosal apex. In cases of congenital cholesteatomas, it may be necessary to remove the cochlea with a diamond burr. The ICA is found just 1 mm from the anterior margin of the basal turn of the cochlea. Once the cochlea has been opened, there will be a CSF fistula both from the cochlear duct and particularly from the internal auditory canal. These areas are closed with bone wax.

Clivus Exposure

Fisch's Type B infratemporal approach is appropriate for the removal of the petrosal apex and of the posterior clivus. The steps are those already described above.

- To reach the clivus, it is necessary to expose the petrosal tract of the ICA and the artery is anteriorly penetrated in the soft tissues and the periosteum above the clivus. The petro-occipital fissure is identified. Bleeding of the inferior petrosal sinus is stopped with Surgicel. The tumor is removed with large curettes and the bone is drilled to follow its branchings. With a curved dissector the tumor may be followed medially to the horizontal part of the internal carotid, which may be only partially moved.
- The dura of the posterior fossa must be spared as far as possible. If proceeding with the exposure anteriorly, the contralateral internal carotid artery is reached, inferior to the hypoglossal canal and superior to the hypophyseal gland.
- The combination of a Type B approach with a Type A approach makes it possible to treat chordomas with a cervical extension.
- The exposure of chordomas or lesions with a more anterior extension, towards the infratemporal fossa, the sella and the rhynopharynx calls for a Type C (Fisch) infratemporal approach.

Closure

The membranous part of the eustachian tube is closed with Vicryl 4-0 thread. To be safe, a muscle fragment is also passed through the tip, to fill any gaps. The zygomatic arch is replaced anteriorly with metallic thread (wire). The cavity is closed with abdominal fat. A flap of temporalis muscle with an anterior opening may be rolled over it.

The cavity is filled with fat.

TYPE C INFRATEMPORAL APPROACH

This is an approach enabling us to treat lesions involving the infratemporal fossa and/or the pterygopalatine and/or the parasellar region and/or the rhynopharynx (Fig. 16-33).

The surgical steps are analogous to those described in the Type B approach.

- The exposure is wider anteriorly because once the ICA has been exposed, the ligaments of the petro-occipital fissure are cut. Then the periosteum and the soft tissue are elevated and the base of the greater wing of the sphenoid is exposed, along with the lateral pterygoid lamina and the clivus.

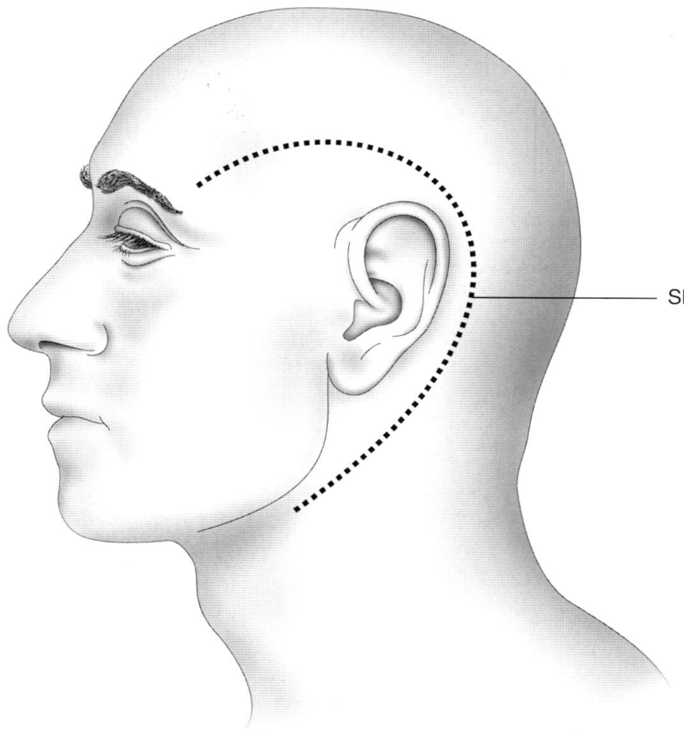

Fig. 16-33. Incision for infratemporal fossa approach type C.

- To expose the lateral wall of the rhynopharynx, the base of the lateral and medial plates of the pterygoid process are drilled. The external pterygoid muscle is separated from the condyle process and removed along with the residual pterygoid process.
- The lateral wall of the nasal cavity, consisting of mucosa, is incised at the inferior limit of the base of the pterygoid process, from the superior to the posterior parts. Thus the rhynopharynx is penetrated, and the vomer and the tail of the inferior turbinates can be seen bilaterally, as well as the eustachian tube contralaterally.

Excision Boundaries

- The entire peritubaric area may be removed en bloc.
- *Upper limit*: The anterior extension may reach the cavernous sinus, the parasellar extradural region, the lateral wall of the sphenoid sinus, the posterior ethmoidal cells, and the maxillary sinus.
- *Inferior limit*: The inferior extension may reach the superior surface of the palate.

Closure

The ample communication between the operating field and the rhynopharynx calls for a careful closure. A mobilization of the temporalis muscle is performed. The latter is reflected into the wound. The muscle is sutured around the rhynopharyngeal deficit. If this does not suffice, a free flap may be used with the abdominal rectus, since its removal has minimal consequences.

REFERENCES

Anand V, Leonetti JP, Al-Mefty O: Neurovascular consideration in surgery of glomus tumors with intracranial extensions. Laryngoscope 103: 722-727, 1993.

Andrews JC, Valavanis A, Fisch U: Management of the internal carotid artery in skull base surgery. Laryngoscope 99: 1224-1229, 1989.

Arriaga MA, Brackmann DE: Differential diagnosis of primary petrous apex lesions. Am J Otol 12(6): 470-474, 1991.

Arriaga MA, Janecka IP: Facial translocation approach to the cranial base: The anatomic basis. Skull Base Surg 1: 26-33, 1991.

Arriaga MA, Lo WWM, Brackmann DE: Imaging case study of the month. Magnetic resonance angiography of synchronous bilateral carotid body paragangliomas and bilateral vagal paragangliomas. Ann Otol Rhinol Laryngol 101: 955-957, 1992.

Bickerstaff ER, Howell JS: The neurological importance of tumors of the glomus Jugulare. Brain 76: 576-593, 1953.

Boyle JO, Shimm DS, Coulthard W: Radiation therapy for paragangliomas of the temporal bone. Laryngoscope 100:896-901, 1990.

Brackman DE: The facial nerve in the infratemporal fossa approach. Otolaryngol Head Neck Surg 97:15-17, 1987.

Brackmann DE, House WF, Terry R, et al: Glomus jugulare tumors: Effect of irradiation. Trans Am Acad Ophthalmol Otolaryngol 76:1423-1431, 1972.

Brackmann DE: The facial nerve in the infratemporal approach. Otolaryngol Head Neck Surg 97: 15-17, 1987.

Brown JS: Glomus jugulare tumors revisited: A ten-year statistical follow-up of 231 cases. Laryngoscope 95: 284-285, 1985.

Buckingham RA, Kenji Amii Perrelli SL: Multicentric origin of glomus jugulare tumors. Arch Otolaryng 70: 104-107, 1959.

Cantrell RW, Kaplan MJ, Atukn O, Winn HR, Jahrsdoerferr A: Cathecolamine secreting infra temporal fossa paraganglioma. Ann Otol Rhinol Laryngol 93: 583-588, 1984.

Coker NJ, Jenkins HA, Fisch U: Obliteration of the middle ear and mastoid cleft in subtotal petrosectomy: indications, technique and results. Ann. ORL 95: 5-11, 1986.

De Vries EJ, Sekhar LN, Horton JA, et al: A new method to predict safe resection of the internal carotid artery. Laryngoscope 100: 85-88, 1990.

Djindjian R, Merland JJ: Superselective arteriography of the external carotid artery. Springer, Berlin 1978.

Donald PJ: Skull base surgery: Combined results of treatment of malignant disease. Skull Base Surg 2: 76-79, 1992.

Farrior JB: Glomus tumors -Postauricular hypotympanotomy. Arch Otolaryngol Head Neck Surg 86: 367-373, 1967.

Felix H, Fisch U: Uncommon causes of facial paralysis. In Portmann M: Facial Nerve. Masson, Paris 1985 (pp.286-290).

Fisch U, Dobie RA, Gmur A, Felix H: Intracranial facial nerve anastomosis. Amer J Otol 8: 23-29, 1987.

Fisch U, Esslen E: Total intratemporal exposure of the facial nerve. Pathologic findings in Bell's palsy. Arch Otolaryngol 95: 335-34, 1972.

Fisch U, Fagan P, Valvanis A: The infratemporal fossa approach for the lateral skull base. Otolaryngol Clin North Am 17(3): 513-552, 1984.

Fisch U, Felix H: On the pathogenesis of Bell's palsy. Acta Otolaryngol 95: 532-538, 1983.

Fisch U, Mattox DE: Petrosectomy and facial rehabilitation in malignant tumors of the retromandibular fossa. In Bull TR, Myers E: Plastic Reconstruction in the Head and Neck. Butterworth London 1986(pp.79-97).

Fisch U, Mattox DE: Microsurgery of the Skull Base. New York, Georg Thieme, 1988.

Fisch U, Nedzelski J, Wellauer J: Diagnostic value of meatocisternography. Arch Otolaryngol 101: 339-343, 1975.

Fisch U, Oldring DJ, Senning A: Surgical therapy of internal carotid artery lesions of the skull base and temporal bone. Otolaryngol Head Neck Surg.88: 548-554, 1980.

Fisch U, Pillsbury HC: Infratemporal fossa approach to lesions in the temporal bone and base of skull. Arch Otolaryngol 105: 99- 107, 1979.

Fisch U, Rouleau M: Facial nerve reconstruction. J Otolaryngol 9: 478-492, 1980.

Fisch U, Ruettner J: Pathology of intratemporal tumors involving the facial nerve. In Fisch U: Facial Nerve Surgery. Aesculapius, Birmingham 1977 (pp.448-456).

Fisch U, Wegmuller A: Early diagnosis of acoustic neuromas. J Oto Rhino-Laryngol 36: 129, 1974.

Fisch U, Yasargil MG: Der translabyrinthare Zugang fur die Akustikusneurinome. Pract Oto Rhino Laryngol 31: 111, 1969.

Fisch U: Carotid lesions at the skull base. In Brackmann DE: Neurological surgery of the ear and skull base. Raven Press, New York 1982 (pp.269-281).

Fisch U: Carotid lesions at the skull base. In Brackmann DE: Neurological Surgery of the Ear and Skull Base. Raven Press, New York 1982 (pp.269-281).

Fisch U: Cross-face grafting in facial paralysis. Arch Otolaryngol 102: 453-457, 1976.

Fisch U: Die mikrochirurgie des felsenbeines. H.N.O. 25: 193-197, 1977.

Fisch U: Facial nerve grafting. Otolaryngol Clin N Amer 7: 517-529, 1974.

Fisch U: Infratemporal approach for extensive tumors of the temporal bone and base of skull. In Silverstein, H, Norell, H: Neurological surgery of the ear. Aesculapius, Birmingham 1977 (pp.34-53).

Fisch U: Infratemporal fossa approach for extensive tumors of the temporal bone and base of the skull. In Silverstein H, Norell H: Neurological Surgery of the Ear. Aesculapius, Birmingham 1977 (pp. 34-53).

Fisch U: Infratemporal fossa approach for glomus tumors of the temporal bone. Ann Oto-Rhino-Laryngol 91: 474-479, 1982.

Fisch U: Infratemporal fossa approach to tumors of the temporal bone and base of the skull. J Laryngol Otol 92: 949-967, 1978.

Fisch U: Intracranial complications of cholesteatoma. In Sade J: Cholesteatoma and Mastoid Surgery. Kugler, Amsterdam 1982 (pp.336-379).

Fisch U: Lateral (infratemporal fossa) approach to the skull base. In Chretien PB, Decker BC: Head and Neck Cancer. Mosby, St. Louis 1985 (pp.251-262).

Fisch U: Management of intratemporal facial palsy. Advanc Tech Stand Neurosurg 7: 215-238, 1980.

Fisch U: Petrosektomie und gesichtsrehabilitation bei tumoren des retromandibularen Raumes. ORL 8. Huber Bern 137-144, 1985.

Fisch U: Subtotal petrosectomy with permanent anterior dislocation of the facial nerve and obliteration of the cavity. In Naumann, H.H: Head and Neck Surgery, vol. III. Thieme, Stuttgart 1982 (pp.544-551).

Fisch U: Subtotale Petrosektomie (mit permanenter vorderer Dislokation des N. facialis und Obliteration der Operationshohle). In Naumann, k. H: Kopf- und Halschirurgie, vol.III. Thieme, Stuttgart 1976 (pp.536-543).

Fisch U: The infratemporal fossa approach for nasopharyngeal tumors. Laryngoscope 93: 36-44, 1983.

Fisch U: Transmastoid translabyrinthine access to the internal meatus. Naumann, HH: Head and Neck Surgery, vol. III. Thieme, Stuttg. 1982 (pp.508-543).

Fisch U: Zur Diagnose und therapie der speicheldrusentumoren. Schweiz. med. Wschr: 108: 927-932, 1978.

Gantz BJ, Fisch U: Modified transotic approach to the cerebellopontine angle. Arch. Otolaryngol: 109: 252-256, 1983.

Gantz BJ, Gmur A, Fisch U: Intraoperative evoked electromyography in Bell's palsy. Amer J Otolaryngol 3: 273-278, 1982.

Gantz BJ, Gmur A, Holliday M, Fisch U: Electroneurographic evaluation of the facial nerve: Method and technical problems. Ann Oto Rhino Laryngol 93: 394-398, 1984.

Gates GA: The lateral facial approach to the nasopharynx and infratemporal fossa. Otolaryngol Head Neck Surg 99: 321-325, 1988.

Glasscock ME, Harris FH: Glomus tumors: diagnosis and treatment. Laryngoscope 84:2006-2032, 1974.

Gleeson M J, Fisch U, Felix H: A morphological study of the effect of CUSA near human peripheral nerves. Archives of Otolaryngology Head Neck Surgery 113: 530-532, 1987.

Gordon E: A basis and practice of neuroanaesthesia, 2nd ed. Excerpta.

Guild SR: The glomus jugulare, a nonchromaffin paraganglion, in man. Ann Otol Rhinol Laryngol, 62:1045-1071, 1953.

Hardesty RA, Jones NF, Swartz WM, et al: Microsurgery for macrodefects: Microvascular free-tissue transfer for massive defects of the head and neck. Am J Surg 154: 399-405, 1987.

Hawthorne MR, Makek MS, Harris JP, Fisch U: The histopathological and clinical features of irradiated and non-irradiated temporal paragangliomas. Laryngoscope 98: 325-331, 1988.

Hitselberger WE, Horn K, Hankinson H, Brackmann DE, House WF: The middle fossa transpetrous approach for petroclival meningioma. Skull Base Surg 3:130-5, 1993.

Holliday MJ, Nachlas N, Kennedy DW: Uses and modifications of the infratemporal fossa approach to skull base tumors. Ear Nose Throat J 65: 101-106, 1986.
House WF, Glasscock ME III: Glomus tympanicum tumors. Arch Otolaryngol 87: 124-128, 1968.
House WF: Middle cranial fossa approach to the petrous pyramid: report of 50 cases. Arch Otolaryngol 78:460-468, 1963.
House WF: Surgical exposure of the internal auditory canal and its contents through the middle cranial fossa. Laryngoscope 71:1363-1935, 1961.
Jackson CG: Skull base surgery. Am J Otol, 3: 161-171, 1981.
Jackson CG, Cueva RA, Thedinger BA, Glasscock ME: Conservation surgery for glomus jugulare tumors: the value of early diagnosis. Laryngoscope 100:10, 1990.
Jackson IT, Bailey MH, Marsh WR, Juhasz P: Results and prognosis following surgery for malignant tumors of the skull base. Head Neck 13: 89-96, 1991.
Jackson IT, Marsh WR, Bite U, Hide TA: Craniofacial osteotomies to facilitate skull base tumor resection. Br J Plast Surg 39: 153-160, 1986.
Jackson IT: Advances in craniofacial tumor surgery. World J Surg 13: 440-453, 1989.
Janecka SP, Sekhar LNS, Horton JA: General blood flow evaluation. In Cummings CW, et al. (eds): Otolaryngology Head and Neck Surgery Update II. St. Louis, Mosby Year Book, 1990, pp 54-63.
Jenkins HA, Fisch U: Glomus tumors of the temporal region: Technique of surgical resection. Arch Otolaryngol 107: 209-213, 1981.
Jenkins HA, Fisch U: The transotic approach to resection of difficult acoustic tumors of the cerebellopontine angle. Amer J Otol 2: 70-76, 1980.
Jenkins HA, Fisch U: Glomus tumors of the temporal region: technique of surgical resection. Arch Otolaryngol 107: 209-214, 1981.
Jenkins HA, Fisch U: The transotic approach to resection of difficult acoustic tumors of the cerebellopontine angle. Amer J Otol 2: 70-76, 1980.
Jones NF, Schramm VL, Sekhar LN: Reconstruction of the cranial base following tumor resection. Br J Plast Surg 40: 155-162, 1987.
Jones NF, Sekhar LN, Schramm VL: Free rectus abdominis flap reconstruction of the middle and posterior cranial base. Plast Reconstr Surg 78: 471-479, 1986.
Kumar A, Fisch U: The infratemporal fossa approach for lesions of the skull base. Adv Neurosurg 10: 187-220, 1983.
Lachard A, Hassoun J, Charpin C, Toga M: Les paragangliomes de la tete et du cou chemodectomes. Aspects anatomo-pathologiques, in Les chemodectomes cervicocephaliques, Leroux, Robert J, Pech A. Edit Masson Publ Paris 3-16, 1984.
Lasjaunias P, Berenstein A: Surgical Neuroangiography, vol. II: Endovascular treatment of craniofacial lesions. Springer, Berlin 1987.
Lasjaunias R, Berenstein A: Surgical neuroangiography, vol. 1: Functional anatomy of craniofacial arteries. Springer, Berlin 1987.
Leonetti JP, Brackmann DE: Glomus vagale tumors: The significance of early vocal cord paralysis. Otolaryngol Head Neck Surg 100: 533-537, 1989.
Leonetti TP, Brackmann DE, Prass RC: Improved preservation of facial function in the infratemporal fossa approach to the skull base. Otolaryngol Head Neck Surg 101: 74-78, 1989.
Mattox D, Felix H, Fisch U: Effect of ligating peripheral branches on facial nerve regeneration. Otolaryngol Head Neck Surg 98: 558-5 1988.
Mattox DE, Fisch U: Surgery of the skull base. In Johns ME: Complications in Otolaryngology-Head and Neck Surgery vol II: Head and Neck. Decker BC, Philadelphia, 1986 (pp.307-313.)
Mc Cabe BF, Fletcher J: Selection of therapy of glomus jugulare tumors. Arch Otolaryngol 89: 156-159, 1969.
Mc Neill KA, Milner GAW: Bilateral tumor of the glomus jugulare. J Laryngol Otol 69: 430-431, 1955.
Murphy TP, Brackmann DE: Effects of preoperative embolization on glomus jugulare tumors. Laryngoscope 99: 1244-1247, 1989.
Neterrville JD: Primary thyroplasty in glomus jugulare surgery. Oral presentation, American Neurotology Society Fall Meeting, Washington DC, September 13, 1992.
O'Leary MJ, Shelton C, Giddings N, et al: Glomus tympanicum tumors: A clinical perspective. Laryngoscope 101: 74-78, 1989.
Oldring D, Fisch U: Glomus tumors of the temporal region: surgical therapy. Amer J of Otology 1: 718, 1979.
Pech A, Cannoni M, Thomassin JM, Abdul S, Zanaret M: Le diagnostic d'extension des tumeurs du glomus jugulaire. Ann Otolaryng Paris 98: 215-222, 1981.
Pellet W, Cannoni M, Lavieille J, Lehmann G, Vacherat S, Mouren P: Volumineuse tumeur du glomus jugulaire: voie d'abord combinee oto-neuro-chirurgicale. Neurochirurgie Paris 19: 567-579, 1973.
Pillsbury HC, Fisch U: Extratemporal facial nerve grafting and radiotherapy. Arch Otolaryngol 105: 441-446, 1979.
Rogers GP, Brackmann DE, Lo WWM: Magnetic resonance angiography, a technique for evaluation of skull base lesions. Am J Otol 14 (1) 56-62, 1993.
Rosenwasser H: Carotid body-like tumor of the middle ear and mastoid bone. Arch Otolaryngol 41: 64-67, 1945.
Rossenwasser H: Glomus jugulare tumors. Arch Otolaryng 89: 186-192, 1969.
Schwaber MK, Glasscock ME, Nissen AJ, Jakson CG, Smith PG: Diagnosis and management of catecholamine secreting glomus tumors. Laryngoscope 94: 1008-1015, 1984.
Sekhar LN, Schramm VL Jr, Jones NF: Subtemporal-preauricular infratemporal fossa approach to large lateral and posterior cranial base neoplasms. J Neurosurg 67: 488-499, 1987.
Shapiro MJ, Neues DK: Technique for removal of glomus jugulare tumors. Arch Otolayngol 79: 219 224, 1964.
Spector JG, Compagno J, Perez CA, et al: Glomus jugulare tumors: effects of radiotherapy. Cancer, 35: 1316-1321, 1975.
Spector GJ, Fierstein J, Ogura JH: A comparison of therapeutic modalities of glomus tumors in the temporal bone. Laryngoscope 86: 690-696, 1976.
Spector GJ, Maisel R, Ogura JH: Glomus jugulare tumors. A clinicopathologic analysis of the effect of radiotherapy. Ann Oto-Laryngol 83: 26-32, 1974.
Steinkerg N, Holz WG: Glomus jugulare tumors. Arch Otolaryngol Head Neck Surg 82: 387-394, 1965.
Terracol J, Guerrier Y, Guibert HL: Le glomus jugulaire. Masson Edit Paris 1-119, 1956.
Thomassin JM, Zanaret M, Sarrat P, Cannoni M, Pech A: Les problemes diagnostiques et therapeutiques des chemodectomes tympanojugulaires. In les chemodectomes cervicocephaliques, Leroux Robert J, Pech A, Edit. Masson Publ Paris 140-148, 1984.
Valavanis A, Schubiger O, Naidich TP: Clinical imaging of the cerebellopontine angle. Springer, Berlin 1987.
Valavanis A: Preoperative embolization of the head and neck: Indications, patient selection, goals and precautions. Amer J Neuroradiol 7: 943-952, 1987.
Wang ZW, Kishimoto S, Felix H, Fisch U: Experimentell erzeug Dehnung des Nervus facialis bei Katzen. ORL: Aktuelle Probleme d' Otorhinolaryngologie 6. Huber, Bern 1983.
Wetmore SJ, Herrmann P, Fisch U: Spontaneous cerebrospinal fluid otorrhea. Amer J Otol 8, March 1987.
Williams IG: Radiotherapy of tumors of the glomus jugulare. J Fac Radiol 8: 325-338, 1957.

Wylder AR, Leech RW, Reynolds AF, Ojemann GA, Mead C: Cholesterol granuloma of the petrous apex: case report. J Neurosurg 41: 765-768, 1974.

Yamamoto E, Fisch U: Effect of electron irradiation on results of fast nerve grafting. In Graham MD, House WF: Disorders of the facial nerve. Raven Press, New York 1982 (pp.179-185).

Yamamoto E, Fisch U: Experimentally induced facial nerve compression in cats. Acta Oto-Laryngol 79: 390-395, 1975.

Yamamoto E, Fisch U: Experiments on facial nerve suturing. Oto Rhino Laryngol 36: 193-204, 1974.

Zack FG, Lawson W: The paragangliome chemoreceptor system. Physiology-pathology and clinical medicine. Springer Verlag Edit, New York Heidelberg Berlin 15-23, 1982.

17

Mèniére's disease and labyrinthine syndromes. Clinical aspects Surgical treatment of Mèniére's disease

The etiology of Mèniére's disease has not yet been determined, but an alteration in endolymph reabsorption mechanisms at the duct and the endolymphatic sac has been experimentally confirmed (Figs. 17-1, 17-2).

SYMPTOMS

- The disease manifests with vestibular symptoms, episodic vertigo, and cochlear symptoms, as well as progressive fluctuating sensorineural hearing loss, tinnitus, sound intolerance, and diplacusia.
- Vertigo is seen episodically, and may last from a few seconds to a few days, and is often part of a symptomatologic triad: tinnitus, feeling of "stopped up" ears and hearing loss, vertigo.
- The patient "senses" the crisis coming on. These generally occur with increasing frequency, only to diminish with the progressive degeneration of the inner ear. The crises are manifested with feelings of dizziness, pallor, nausea, and frequently vomiting. Even the smallest body movements exacerbate the symptoms. Spontaneous nystagmus accompanies the crises.
- In the intercritical periods, positional vertigo may be seen, generally brought on by rapid head movements, manifested as a rapid loss of equilibrium. The patient may in rare instances fall suddenly and violently to the floor, as if pushed from behind; these crises are called utricular crises.
- The hearing loss has a distinctive characteristic, i.e. it fluctuates, varying in degree. It is greater during the utricular crises. It tends to worsen in time with the degeneration of the inner ear. It is accompanied by a feeling of fullness in the ears, due to hydropsy and diplacusia, with perceived sounds distorted in the diseased ear. Intense sounds are bothersome and painful, due to the phenomenon of recruitment.
- Tinnitus accompanies the hypoacusia but may also precede it, even by years. Its frequency is correlated to the hypoacusia, e.g. low-frequency tinnitus, low-frequency hypoacusia. Tinnitus is not pulsating, nor modified by the carotid pressure (Table 17-1).

DIAGNOSIS

- History.
- Audiometric tests.
- Tonal audiometry demonstrates sensorineural hypoacusia for low tones, and fluctuates at subsequent checks.
- The reflex threshold shows recruitment.
- The Fowler test shows recruitment, when this is monolateral.
- The glycerol test may show an improvement in the symptoms and the hypoacusia. This may foresee a possible recovery, and thus favor a conservative surgical procedure rather than a destructive one (see endolymphatic shunt).
- ABR: generally normal.
- ELECTRONYSTAGMOGRAPHY. Vestibular hypofunction of the affected side. Spontaneous nystagmus or position nystagmus, more marked with closed eyes or eyes open in the dark.
- CT. Mastoid alterations may be seen, though not always, due to previous otitis mediae.

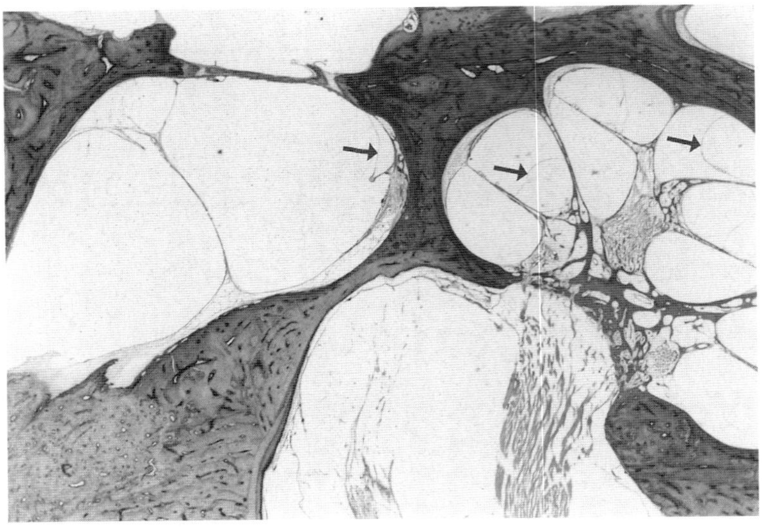

Fig. 17-1. Courtesy of Linthicum FH. Endolymphatic hydrops due to a blockage of the endolymphatic duct by abnormal bone (white arrow). The saccular and Reissner's membranes are distended (black arrows). ×15.

- MRI. Useful in cases of suspected intracranial pathology
- LABORATORY TEST. In at-risk patients, the treponemal test for syphilis is useful.

MEDICAL TREATMENT

- *Restriction* in the intake of sodium and administration of diuretics: Hydrochlorothiazide, 50 mg/day. These do not have a determining effect, but do reduce the frequency and the seriousness of the crises.
- *Antihystamines*. These have a sedative action on the vestibular system, all the more effective when their anticholinergic effect is greater. They have a blocking effect on the monoamines and the synaptic nerve endings.
- *Sedatives*. Diazepam has a sedative effect on the vestibular nuclei. Fenotiazine has a dopamine blocking action, besides an antihystaminic and anticholinergic action. Sedatives in general have a positive effect since they diminish the patient's level of anxiety, which can trigger the crises.
- *Vasoactive drugs*. These are administered to increase the vascularization of the labyrinth and endolymph reabsorption. Their clinical efficacy is controversial.
- *Vestibulotoxins*. If common medical therapy is unsuccessful, some AA suggest the use of streptomycin (see chapter 26). This treatment has a damaging action on the ampullar cells of the semicircular ducts. Treatment is continued until caloric tests show no response. Hearing is not affected.
- *Hyperbaric chamber*. Hyperbaric chamber treatment of patients with acute attacks leads to a fairly long symptom remission (Tjernstrom).
- *Psychological aspect*. Last but certainly not the least, the patient must know the cause of his

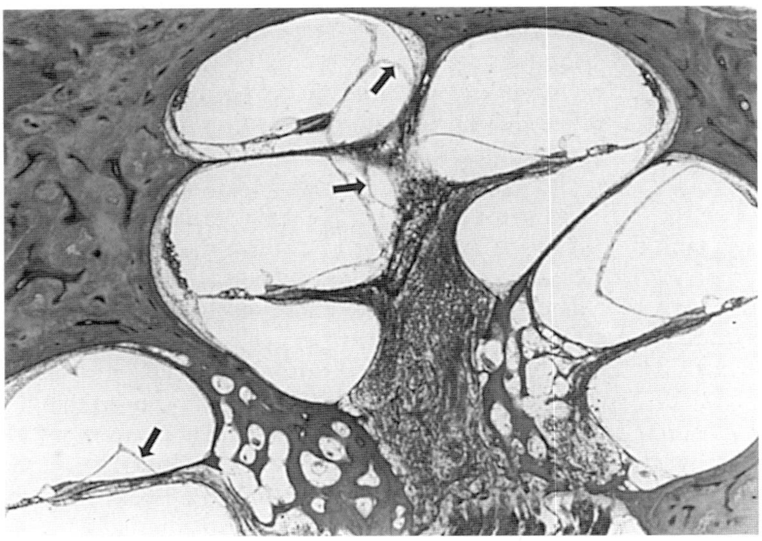

Fig. 17-2. Courtesy of Linthicum FH. Menièré's disease. Ruptures of the hydropic membrane are represented by redundancies in the membrane (arrows). ×35.

Table 17-1. Some predisposing causes for Mènière disease.

- Familiar.
- Genetic (20% of cases)(Paparella).
- Otitis Media.

Experimental evidence has shown a concomitance of chronic otitis and endolymphatic hydrops of 15% in the temporal bone. This can be explained by a labyrinthitis of the endolymphatic spaces, with the subsequent chemical alteration in the endolymph.

- Otosclerosis.
- Otosclerosis may involve the vestibular acqueduct, with the subsequent alteration of the duct and the endolymphatic sac (Paparella and Chasin, 1966, Ghorayeb and Linthicum 1978).
- Syphilis.
- Syphilis may involve the inner ear, provoking progressive endolymphatic hydropsy and a degeneration of the membranous labyrinth (Schuknecht).
- Leukemia.
- Leukemic infiltration may provoke a narrowing in the vestibular aqueduct and the endolymphatic sac, with subsequent hydropsy (Sando and Egami, 1977).
- Autoimmune Diseases.
- Autoimmune alterations may involve the labyrinth and cause Mènière's syndrome (McCabe, Yoo).
- Trauma.
- An acoustic or physical trauma may alter the cells of the saccule and the utricle, provoking an altered endolymph reabsorption with the subsequent hydropsy (Paparella, Mancini).

disease and its clinical progression, in order to live with the invalidating symptoms.

BENIGN PAROXYSMAL POSITIONAL VERTIGO

This manifests in brief vertiginous episodes, provoked by changes in position. One possible cause is cupololitiasis (Schuknecht), or carbonate crystals of the utricular and saccular otocones pressing on the cupola of the posterior semicircular canal. Moving the patient from a sitting to a lying-down position with his head hyperextended and turned to the side, a rotational (or horizontal) nystagmus is evoked, after a latency of approx. 5 seconds. This beats on the side of the underlying ear. The nystagmus builds to a crescendo and then disappears over a period of approx. 30 seconds but beats on the opposite side when the patient is made to resume the sitting position.

Therapy is based on position exercises. The patient is in a sitting position with his eyes closed. He is made to lie laterally on the bed on his side, with the lateral part of the head resting on the bed, so as to guarantee the stimulation of the posterior semicircular canal. The patient awaits the disappearance of the vertiginous symptomatology, and then returns swiftly to a sitting position for 30 seconds. The patient then repeats the maneuver on his other side, and the procedure is repeated until the positional vertigo is significantly reduced. The patient continues this rehabilitation every 4-5 hours. The maneuvers are interrupted after 3 consecutive days of symptomatologic quiet. The therapeutic effects seems to refer to the dispersion of the degenerated otoliths, with the subsequent functional resumption of the cupola of the posterior semicircular canal.

VESTIBULAR NEURONITIS

This manifests with sudden vertigo, frequently accompanied by nausea and vomiting. Instability may last for months. Generally, a complete resolution is had within 6 months. The disease may reappear even after a great deal of time has passed. The etiology is probably viral. Therapy is based on sedatives and cortisone.

LABYRINTHITIS

Among the causes, non-infective agents should be remembered, such as autoimmune diseases or intoxication and infective agents, such as bacteria, viruses, fungi, protozoas, and treponema pallidum. In cases of purulent chronic otitis, the germs that most frequently reach the labyrinth through the two windows are Streptococcus Haemoliticus, Diplococcus pneumoniae and Haemophilus influenzae. The disease manifests with vertigo, nausea, vomiting and vestibular alterations that show an irritative state, with nystagmus beating on the diseased side. The disease's progression may lead to a deficit form with Ny inversion. The limbs deviate in the direction of the slow Ny phase.

The therapy is directed to the causal agent.

POST-TRAUMATIC VERTIGO

Longitudinal or transverse fractures may follow a cranial trauma involving the temporal bone. Longitudinal fractures (the most frequent) run parallel to the greater axis of the petrous ridge. The line of fracture predominantly involves the middle ear, with subsequent conductive hypoacusia. The labyrinthine block is rarely involved. The transversal fractures have a perpendicular path to the greater axis of the petrous ridge. The inner ear is almost always involved, with the loss of vestibular and cochlear function. Vertigo, nausea, and vomiting are also seen.

In the absence of fractures, a positional vertigo is generally seen, due to cupololitiasis, which tends to disappear anywhere from six weeks to two years later.

A sudden hearing loss may occur, due most probably to the pressurizing wave after the trauma, which propagates through the bone to the cochlea. The hearing loss is usually reversible.

Post-traumatic syndrome. A slight sense of instability, headache, and insomnia may last for months. The causes are the traumatic action on the labyrinth, but also psychosomatic factors.

SURGICAL TRAUMA

Surgery with a mastoid approach may provoke a fistula of the lateral semicircular canal. If the membranous canal is also damaged, there is a loss of auditory and vestibular function.

After a stapedectomy operation, a perilymphatic fistula of the oval window may be seen, with unbalance, occasional vertigo, sensorineural hearing loss of fluctuating degrees, and nystagmus. Surgical revision is necessary.

OVAL AND ROUND WINDOW TRAUMA

A sudden variation in middle ear pressure, due to barotrauma or impact trauma, may provoke a rapid increase in cerebrospinal liquid pressure, forming a fistula in the round or oval window.

Thus sudden hearing loss, objective vertigo, and nystagmus are seen. The picture may however be variable, with fluctuating hearing loss, or with positional vertigo, or with symptoms analogous to Mèniére's Disease (tinnitus, feeling of fullness in the ears, diplacusia and sound intolerance). Therapy calls for rest and frequent audiometric checks. If there is no improvement, an exploratory tympanotomy is called for, and possible fistula repair (using connective tissue, fascia, perichondrium, and fat...).

OTOTOXIC DRUGS

The most common ototoxic drugs are aminoglycosides (gentamycin, neomycin, streptomycin, kanamycin). The patient shows a sense of instability and caloric tests demonstrate a progressive loss of vestibular response. A sensorineural hearing loss reveals a progressive onset. There are many other ototoxins to be investigated with a careful investigation on the patient's medical history.

CENTRAL ALTERATIONS

- *Vertebro-basilar deficit.* This manifests with decrease in the visus, headache, fainting, ataxia, and dysarthria. The angiography is rarely significant. CT is negative. Therapy is based on anti-aggregant platelet drugs (aspirin) and, in serious instances, anticoagulants with heparine.
- *Cerebellar infarction.* This manifests in sudden appearance of vertigo, nausea, and vomiting. Nystagmus, ataxia, dysrhythmia, and dysmetria. There are obvious alterations to the CT and the ENG. Therapy may call for surgical decompression, in serious cases.
- *Cerebellar hemorrhage.* This manifests with headache, vertigo, nausea, and vomiting. Nystagmus, nuchal rigidity, facial paralysis, dysmetria, and myotic pupils are seen. There are obvious alterations to the CT and the ENG. Therapy calls for surgical decompression.

LABYRINTHINE HEMORRHAGE

This manifests in sudden vertigo, nausea, vomiting, and hearing loss.

Hemorrhagic diathesis is also seen, e.g. leukemia. Therapy is based on the control of the hemorrhagic diathesis and on the symptomatic treatment of the vertigo.

MULTIPLE SCLEROSIS

This is a demyelinating disease of the central nervous system. The pathology may be seen in varying symptoms: decrease in visus, due to demyelinization of the optic nerve, weakness, diplopia, ataxia. At times vertigo and/or hearing loss may be seen. A definite diagnosis can be made with a MRI.

VERTEBROBASILAR INSUFFICIENCY

This disease is seen predominantly in the elderly. Vertigo (sudden or progressive), nystagmus (vertical or horizontal) are seen, as well as hemiparesis, headache, diplopia, and fainting spells. Diagnosis is based on arteriograms, CT, and MRI. Therapy ranges from simple anticoagulants to surgical removal of the obstruction.

VASCULAR COMPRESSION SYNDROME

This is a rare syndrome, due to a loop in the anterior inferior cerebellar artery exerting pressure on nerve VIII in the posterior cranial fossa. Tinnitus, diplacusia, vertigo, and hearing loss are among the symptoms. A definite diagnosis is problematic, and is based essentially on the clinical history of the patient. The onset is frequently seen in an intense and sudden vertigo, or more rarely a gradual vertigo. There is a constant sense of instability, which increases with the activity level of the patient and almost disappears when the patient is resting. The marching test demonstrates a lateral deviation. The evoked potentials demonstrate an elongation in the latency of peak II, a division in peak II and /or peak III, and a decreased size of peak III. Peak I is generated by the distal part of the acoustic nerve, while peak II is generated by the intracranial (proximal) part (M.B. Møller, A.R. Møller). The arteriography and the MRI are rarely helpful. Surgical therapy (Janetta) is based on a retrosigmoid approach, through which the loop compressing the vestibular nerve is identified. It is separated with a small piece of Gelfoam. This therapy allows disabilitated patients to resume work 70% of the time (See chapter 27).

Hearing loss, though rare, is among the possible complications of this type of therapy, and results from lesions of the acoustic nerve.

TUMORS

Many tumors involve the ear, the cerebellum, and the brainstem, and show vestibular symptoms.

Table 17-2. Treatment of Mèniére's Disease.

Conservative procedures
Extradural procedures (Chapter 18)
Endolymphatic mastoid shunt
Endolymphatic subarachnoid shunt

Intradural procedures (Chapter 19)
Retrolabyrinthine vestibular nerve section
Retrosigmoid vestibular nerve section
Retrolabyrinthine-retrosigmoid vestibular nerve section
Middle fossa vestibular nerve section

Destructive procedures
Transcanal labyrinthectomy (Chapter 20)
Transmastoid labyrinthectomy (Chapter 23)
Cochleosacculotomy (Chapter 25)

Chemical procedures
Administration of Aminoglycosides (Streptomycin, Gentamycin) (Chapter 26)

The therapeutic procedure for Mèniére's disease followed at the House Ear Institute is the following:

Medical treatment
When medical treatment fails
symptomatology with a true limiting or invalidating significance:
Usable hearing
• Endolymphatic mastoid shunt
Non-usable hearing
• Youth: Translabyrinthine vestibular nerve section (Chapter 24)
• Older individual: Transcanal labyrinthectomy (Chapter 20)

Failure of the mastoid endolymphatic shunt
If vertigo is controlled for at least 5 years: Revision of the endolymphatic shunt.
If failure occurs within 5 years:
Usable hearing
• Retrolabyrinthine section of the vestibular nerve
Non-usable hearing
Elderly individual with good vestibular function:
• Cochleosacculotomy
Elderly individual with poor vestibular function:
• Transcanal labyrinthectomy
Youth:
• Section of vestibular nerve with translabyrinthine approach

Among the tumors located in the cerebello-pontine angle and the posterior cranial fossa, are (in order of occurrence):
Benign tumors, such as acoustic neuromas, meningioma, primitive cholesteatoma, glomus tumor, facial neuroma, arachnoid cysts, hemangioma, osteoma and cholesterinic granuloma.
Malignant tumors, such as squamous cell carcinoma, condrosarcoma, cordoma, rabdomiosarcoma, medulloblastoma.
Metastasizing tumors of the breast, lung, prostate, kidneys, etc.

Surgical treatment of Mèniére's disease

Surgical treatment of Mèniére's disease is based on functional and destructive operations.
The functional operations tend to maintain as far as possible the auditory function, whereas the others destroy not only vestibular but also auditory function. The purpose of both is the abolition of vertigo.
Destructive surgery is reserved for cases in which the ear is non-hearing or in cases of non-usable hearing. The concept of non-usable hearing tends to be more and more limited, due to progressive improvements in prosthetics devices (Table 17-2).

Before each operation, audiometric, vestibular, metabolic and radiological exams are carried out in order to evaluate the origins of the vertigo. Thus, a complete picture of the pathology is obtained, assuring the surgeon that possible unknown etiological motives have not been ignored.

REFERENCES
See Chapter 18.

18

Endolymphatic sac shunt

The surgical approaches for an endolymphatic sac shunt are basically:
• Endolymphatic sac-mastoid shunt
• Endolymphatic sac-subarachnoid shunt

ENDOLYMPHATIC SAC-MASTOID SHUNT

The indications for surgery of the endolymphatic sac are essentially Mèniére's disease and Mondini's malformation, considered a variant of hydrops (Fig. 18-1).
Surgery is performed after medical treatment has failed to elicit a response: antihystamines, sedatives, vasoactive drugs, osmotic decompressors (macromolecules), for at least 12 months.
There are some symptoms which can predict a better therapeutic outcome to the surgery: recent fluctuations in threshold, sense of pressure in the ear in question, intense dizzy spells with periods of symptoms remission, positive response to diuretic dehydrating therapy: glycerol, urea, furosemide.
Effective therapeutic results are less probable when the vertigo is moderate but constant, and there are no variations in threshold. This is the phase in which irreversible changes in the membranous labyrinth take place. An endolymphatic shunt with introduction of Silastic would act by increasing the lumen of the sac, reducing the osseous pressure, improving vascularization and increasing the surface of sac absorption (Paparella).

• Surgery is usually carried out using general anesthesia.
• In the postauricular approach, an enlarged mastoidectomy is performed. A thin plate of bone is left on the dura of the middle fossa and the posterior fossa (Fig. 18-2). The cells of the mastoid tip are drilled up to the digastric crest. The sigmoid sinus is exposed. It is very important to fully expose the sino-dural angle. The more this angle is opened, the better the view of the underlying sac. Thus there is more room for the surgeon to operate. It is through this space that the instruments pass which serve for the subsequent procedure on the endolymphatic sac (Fig. 18-3).
• It is unnecessary to uncover the body of the incus or the facial nerve. The posterior semicircular canal is exposed first laterally, and then posteriorly (Fig. 18-4).
• A "blue line" of the posterior canal is not recommended. It presents a pointless risk, especially when we consider the greater fragility of the labyrinth shown in Mèniére's Disease.
• According to some AA, a line drawn from the lateral canal perpendicular to the posterior canal (Donaldson line), and prolonged posteriorly to the dura of the posterior cranial fossa should indicate the location of the endolymphatic sac. In reality it indicates where the sac is not: it is never above this line (Fig. 18-5).
• The sac is usually inferior and medial to the retrofacial cells and inferior to the posterior semicircular canal.
• The dura of the posterior cranial fossa is skeletonized, between the posterior semicircular canal, the sigmoid sinus and the jugular bulb. The bulb is not reached. The sigmoid sinus is not decompressed, except in cases where it is very prominent.
• The surgeon proceeds with a cutting burr until a thin bony layer is identified behind the posterior canal, which is then removed with a diamond burr (Fig. 18-6). The sac is almost never in this position. Thus we see where the sac is not. The surgeon proceeds by exposing the inferior dura, which appears thicker, and paler or pinkish compared to the surrounding dura: this is the endolymphatic sac (Figs. 18-7, 18-8, 18-9). The sac is completely exposed; the sac is decompressed anteriorly with a House elevator.
• The instrument is inserted flat between the sac and the concavity of the posterior canal and the

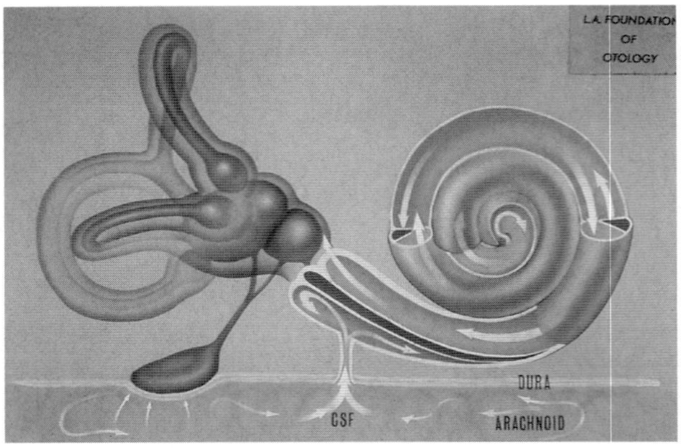

Fig. 18-1. The membranous labyrinth.

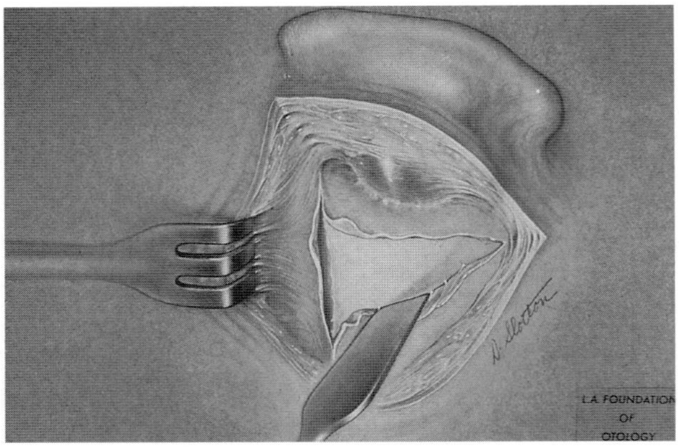

Fig. 18-2. The dural plate over the posterior fossa dura is thinned.

endolymphatic duct is identified. The residual bone fragments are removed with a diamond burr and a curette between the posterior canal, the external auditory canal wall and the sac. The sac is thus decompressed (Fig. 18-10).

- Before incision, the mastoid cavity is bathed in a physiological solution, to remove debris and bone dust. Thus the accumulation of residual bone is prevented in the lumen of the sac, and through the aditus of the middle ear, with possible conductive hearing loss. The contamination of the endolymphatic spaces is also prevented, which could otherwise lead to labyrinthitis and a consequent sensorineural damage.
- With a Gimmick elevator the dura below the mastoid bone and the posterior semicircular canal is decompressed. The elevation of the dura under the posterior semicircular canal fur-

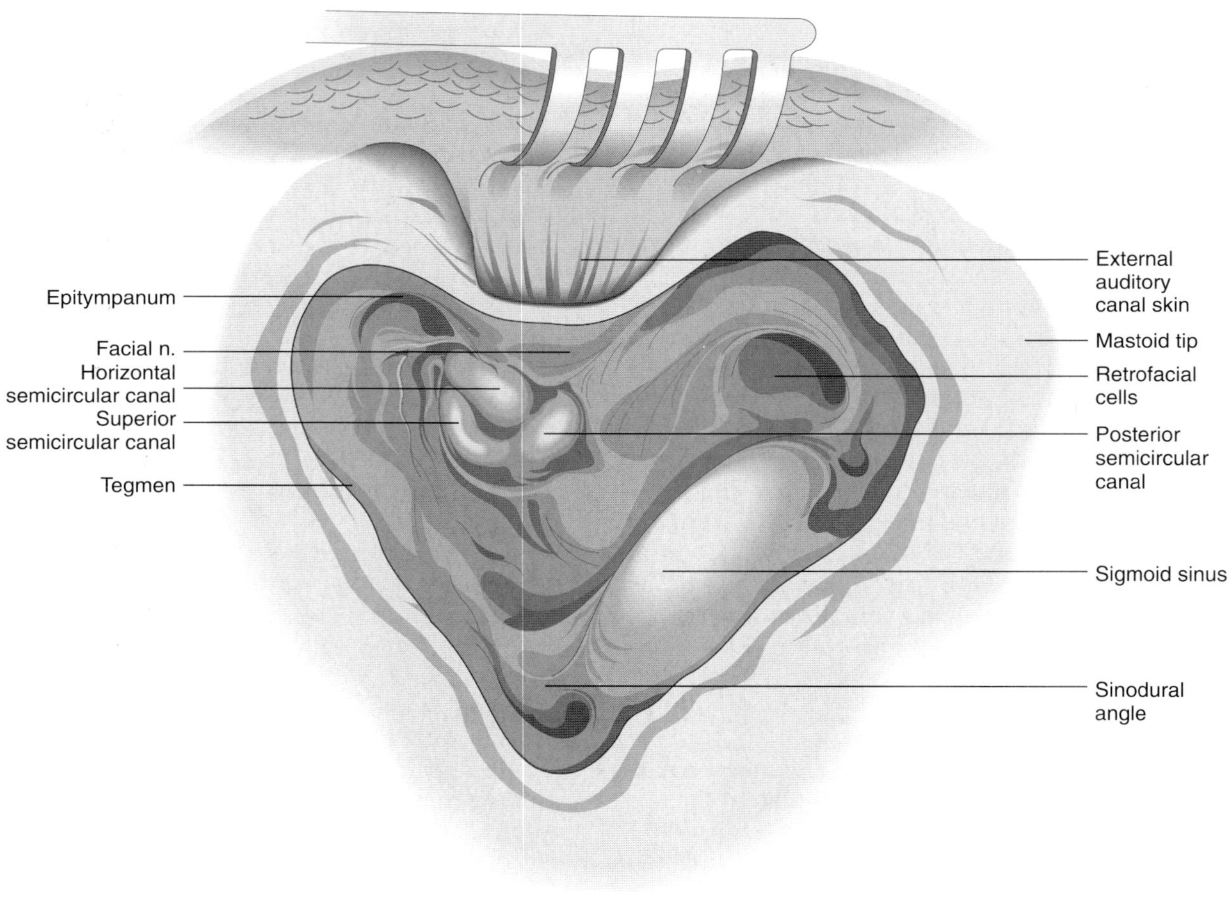

Fig. 18-3. Right ear. Complete mastoidectomy.

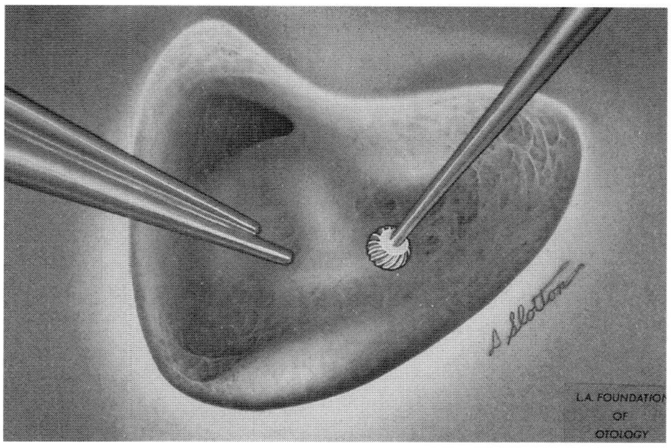

Fig. 18-4. The posterior semicircular canal is outlined.

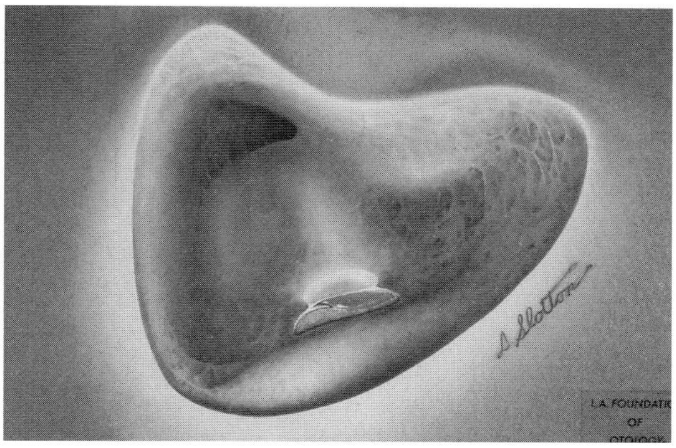

Fig. 18-6. Partial removal of bone posterior to the posterior semicircular canal.

ther allows us to follow the white trace of the endolymphatic duct, confirming the sac's correct identification.

In order to obtain the maximum decompression effect, Paparella uses strips of silastic positioned between dura and bone.

- The lateral wall of the sac is then incised with a straight n. 67 disposable Beaver blade for eye surgery. It is cut lengthwise, following the line of the sac fibers, for a lesser trauma. The cut is eccentric, in the upper two-thirds, to allow a greater endoluminal space at the introduction of the shunt, which occurs in a top-to-bottom direction (Fig. 18-11).
- The incision may also be done with a hook.
- The incision must enter the lumen of the sac, and not simply penetrate into the first layer of

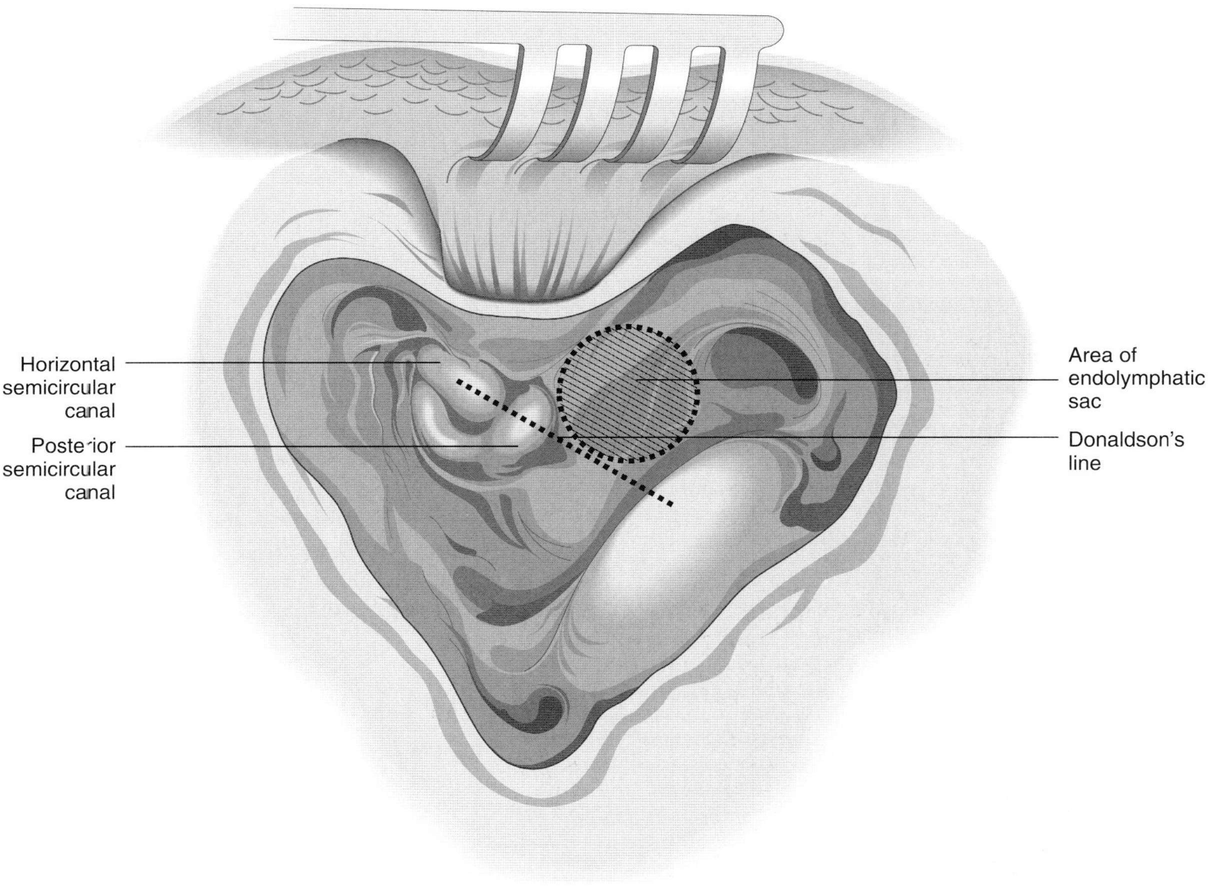

Fig. 18-5. The sac is located somewhere below Donaldson's line, an imaginary line along the lateral semicircular canal.

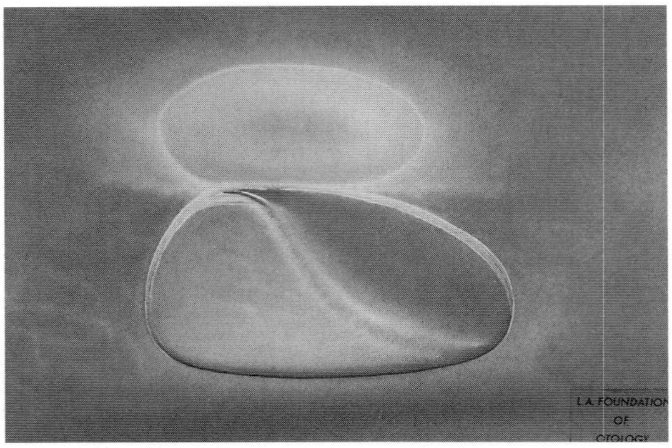

Fig. 18-7. The sac appears as thickened white dura, next to the darker and single-layered normal dura.

fibers of the lateral wall. On the other hand, it must not be deep enough to penetrate the medial wall of the sac. To this end, it is helpful to perform the incision while at the same time elevating the dural surface with the blade.

- The lumen is recognized for its smooth and lucid surface, luminous under the microscope light. A probe is inserted in the lumen to verify the correct position in the structure and also to separate the walls from the sac (Figs. 18-12, 18-13, 18-14).
- A T-shaped silastic prosthesis is inserted into the lumen. The arms of the T are bent over and under and inserted into the lumen, while the leg sticks out. The two arms divaricate inside, elevating the lateral wall of the sac and maintaining opened the lumen and preventing the shunt from exiting.

A silicon apron may be placed over the sac and in the surrounding areas, and kept in place with two large flaps of Gelfoam soaked in antibiotic solution. Its purpose is to impede fibroblast migration into the endolymphatic sac, causing mechanical obstruction (Paparella) (Figs. 18-15, 18-16).

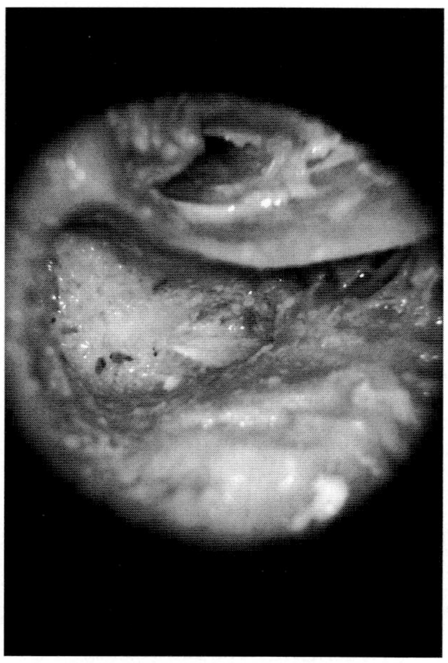

Fig. 18-8. The sac is outlined.

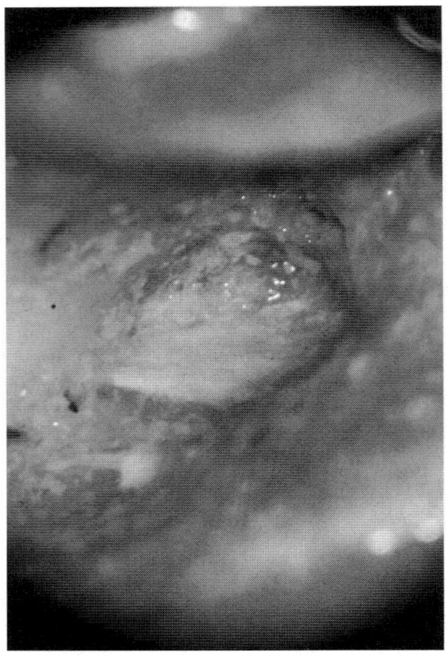

Fig. 18-9. Same as fig. 18-8.

The postauricular incision is closed in layers, with 3-0 Vycril subcutaneously and 4-0 silk on the skin, according to the usual procedure.

COMPLICATIONS

Iatrogenic lesions to the bony wall of the external auditory canal, to the incus, to the horizontal or posterior semicircular canal, to the facial nerve, to the sigmoid sinus, and to the jugular bulb are treated according to the techniques described on chapter 11 and 28 (treatment of surgical complications).

RESULTS

There is great controversy surrounding the physiological basis for endolymphatic sac surgery, but the fact remains that many patients have had satisfactory postoperative data (Brackmann). Because of the low incidence of morbidity of this nondestructive procedure, we consider endolymphatic sac mastoid shunt the procedure of choice for patients with disabling Mèniére's disease who have aidable hearing and who have showed no response to medical treatment.

ENDOLYMPHATIC SAC-SUBARACHNOID SHUNT

- This operation is similar to the previous one up to the opening of the sac. The lumen is tested with a probe. In this type of surgery it is unnecessary to

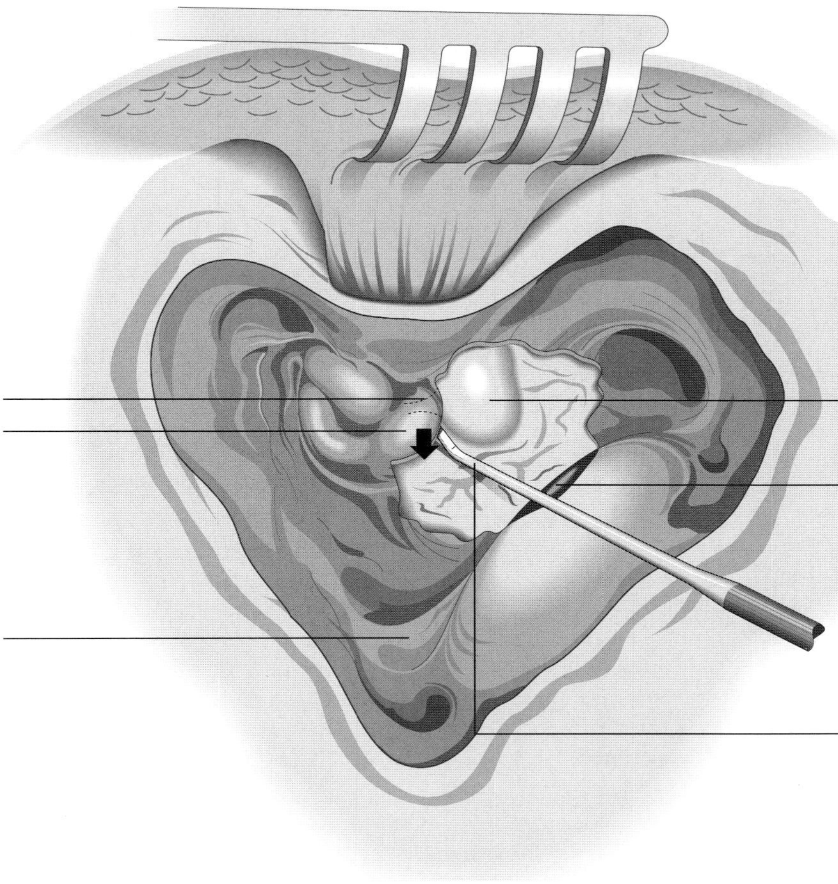

Fig. 18-10. Part of the sigmoid sinus has been exposed. The dural plate over the sac has been removed. Dura below the posterior semicircular canal is decompressed and the endolymphatic duct is seen.

completely decompress the sac, unlike in the endolymphatic mastoid shunt (Figs. 18-17, 18-18).

- The medial wall of the sac is cut using a straight disposable n. 59 Beaver blade. The remaining fibrous attachments are removed until the arachnoid appears, herniated across the incision. The arachnoid is enlarged to permit the introduction of a shunt tube (Fig. 18-19).
- Drainage (e.g. a De la Cruz valve) is close to the tip with an "alligator" clamp and pushed inside the arachnoid, in the subarachnoid space (Fig. 18-20). The shunt tube must be positioned with an anterior angle, to penetrate into the cerebellopontine cistern. It is important to avoid advancing posteriorly, where the cerebellum is located.
- Once in place, the valve can be seen draining the spinal fluid. If this does not occur, the permeability of the valve may be tested with a light suction of the valvular surface, keeping it still by means of pressure with a House elevator. The lateral extremity of the valve, with its orifice, is housed in the lumen of the sac. The sheet of silicone around the orifice protrudes from the two dural sheaths and contributes to keeping the sac opened.
- To close the dural defect, a small piece of muscle is positioned over the dural aperture and is kept in place with one silk suture. The wound is closed in layers.

COMPLICATIONS

Besides the complications already described for the mastoid endolymphatic shunt, this operation comports a specific risk-bleeding.

Bleeding

Light bleeding from small vessels in the external or internal surfaces of the dura may be controlled with bipolar coagulation. Following the introduction of the shunt valve, uncontrolled bleeding may occur, due to the trauma exerted by the valve on a subarachnoid or cerebellar vessel. Complications may be fatal, due to blood pooling in the posterior cranial fossa. The approach to the cerebellopontine angle, for hemostasis, may be a retrolabyrinthine or retrosigmoid approach.

No lesion to the AICA upon introduction of the valve has ever been mentioned in any literature.

The greater morbidity of the subarachnoid shunt compared to the mastoid shunt is not justified by the results. Brackmann and Nissen have found a percentage of vertigo control very similar in both

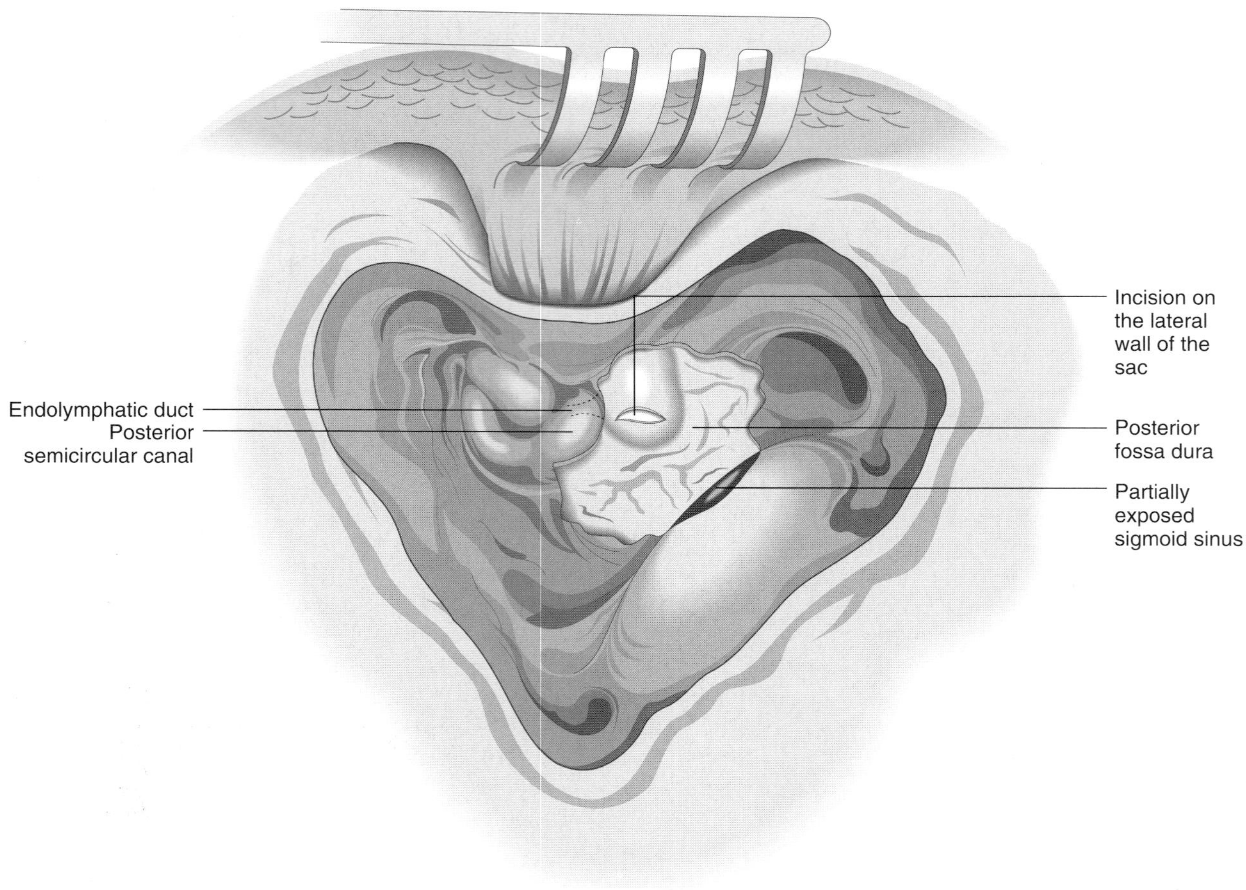

Fig. 18-11. The endolymphatic sac is opened with an incision on its lateral wall.

procedures (67%). Their experience therefore suggests an endolymphatic mastoid shunt, when a shunt is needed.

TIPS AND PITFALLS

- In Mèniére's disease, 30-50% of patients will develop the pathology in the other ear. This data must be considered before practicing destructive procedures.
- Surgery on the endolymphatic sac has a low morbidity since it is an extradural procedure,

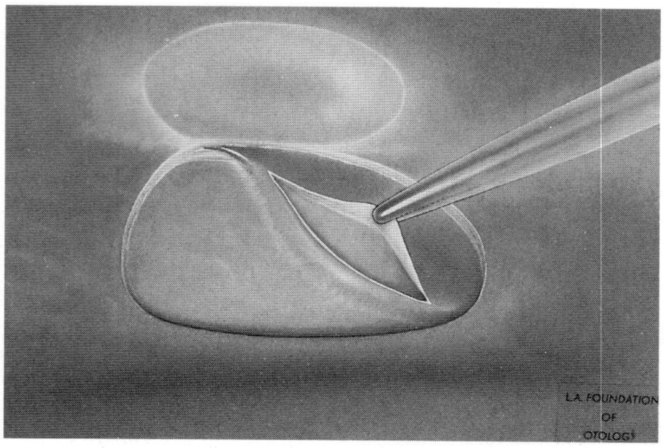

Fig. 18-12. The lateral dural wall of the sac is incised; the interior is exposed.

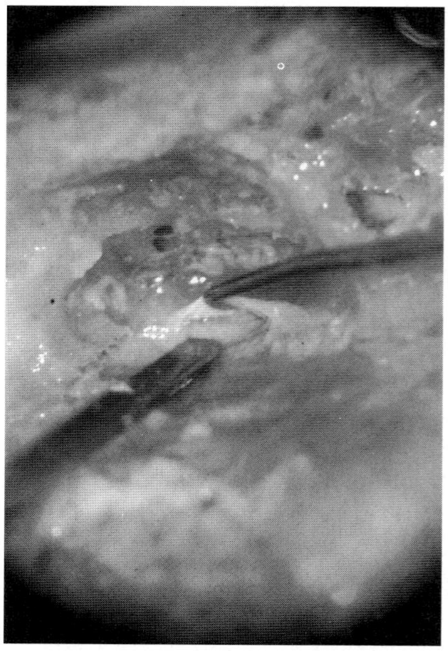

Fig. 18-13. The lumen of the sac is probed.

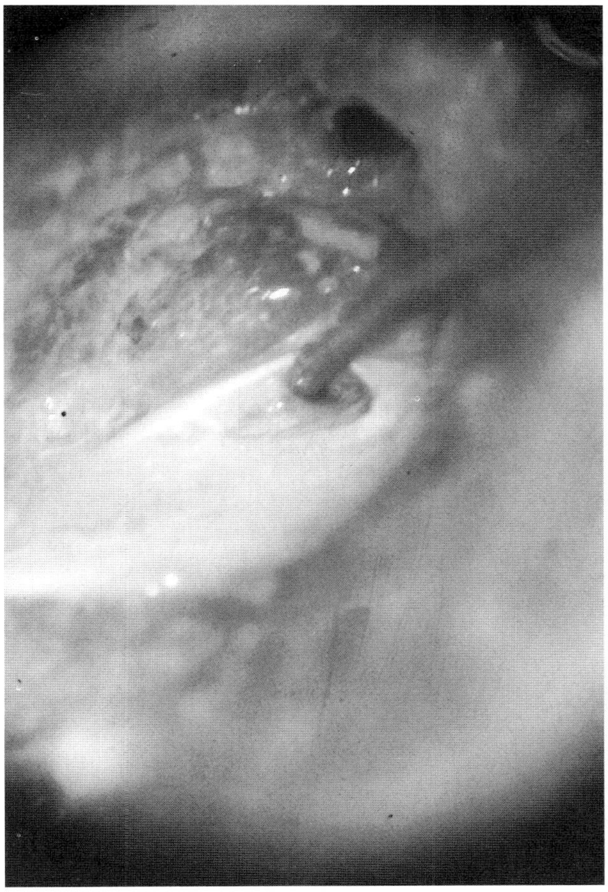

Fig. 18-14. Close-up view of Fig. 18-13.

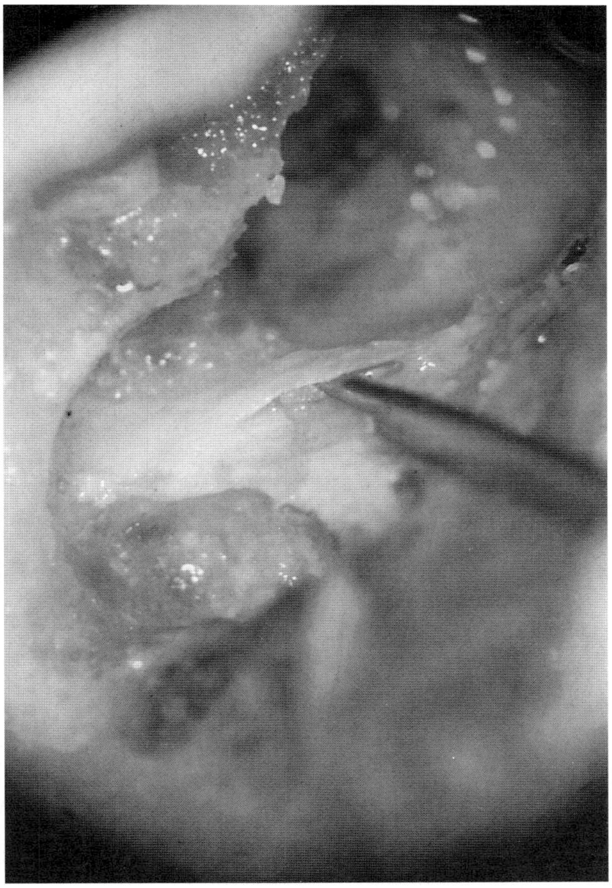

Fig. 18-15. A silicone sheeting T-strut is placed within the sac.

and treats all the symptoms of Mèniére's Disease, including the sense of pressure.

- In Mèniére's disease, hearing will theoretically decrease up to 50 dB, remaining fairly stable thereafter. This is because once all the internal hair cells are destroyed, 50% of hearing has already been lost, the external ciliated cells remain, transmitting sounds over 50 dB. In reality, there may be hearing loss much greater than 50 dB.

- A small translucent plate of bone may be left on the sac. The bone is later removed with a House elevator and the sac is exposed. This procedure prevents tiny lacerations on the lateral wall of the sac, which can occur even when using the diamond burr. The bone sheath must be paper-thin, so that very little force is required in its removal. If the bone is too thick, it forms adherences which lacerate the dura when the bone is lifted.

- To locate the sac, the sigmoid sinus and the dura medial to it are followed.
- The identification of the sac can be double-checked by dissecting the dura of the posterior cranial fossa from the labyrinthine block and identifying the endolymphatic duct passing under the posterior semicircular canal.

- Endolymphatic shunt failure is frequently caused by the difficulty in finding the lumen of the sac. It is then advisable to depress the sac with the fenestrated suction while a hook is used to elevate the external wall layer after layer (Brackmann).

- The sac may be very low and medial and may be almost completely beneath the posterior semicircular canal. In these cases (3% according to Paparella), the shunt is abandoned in favor of a simple decompression. The sac, following the increases in endolymph pressure, may then freely expand without being compressed by bone walls (Shambaugh).

- At times the sac is very anteriorized and there is little space between the posterior canal and the bony part of the canal. The third part of the facial nerve must then be identified. In this way all structures surrounding the sac are identified, including the dura.

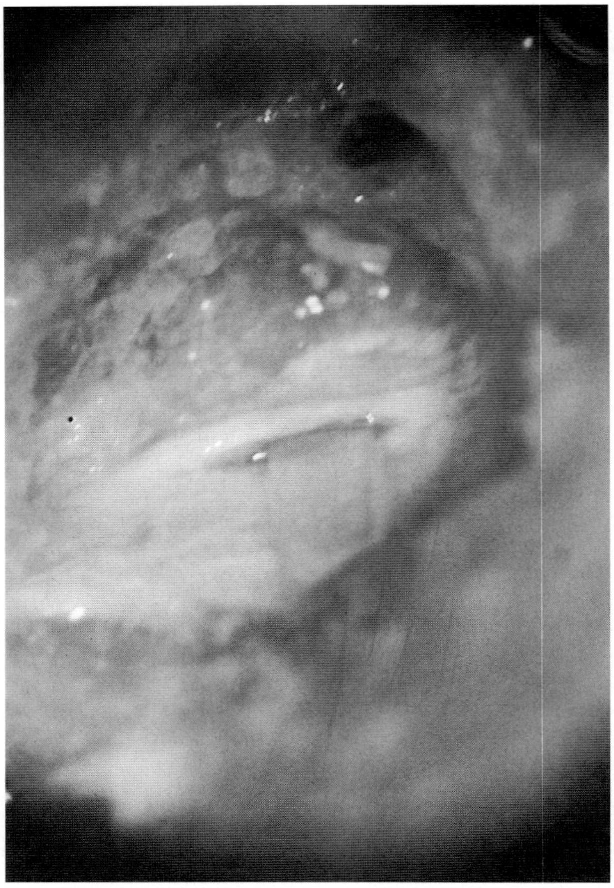

Fig. 18-16. Close-up view of Fig. 18-15.

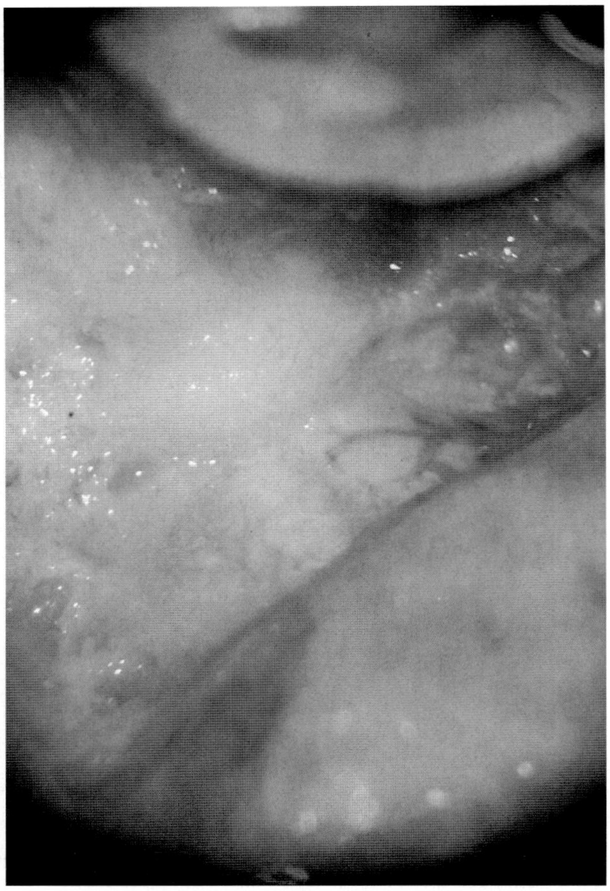

Fig. 18-17. Endolymphatic subarachnoid shunt. The lateral surface of the sac appears as thickened white dura, next to the darker and single-layered normal dura.

- At times bone removal from the dura of the posterior cranial fossa may provoke a laceration, especially in elderly patients where the meninges are particularly fragile. A CSF fistula is observed. The patient is placed in an anti-Trendelenburg position; the lacerated area is compressed with Gelfoam, an adrenaline-soaked gauze is placed on if the blood ooze; the operation is then terminated.

- The gauze and Gelfoam are removed. The small dural breach is repaired with a temporal fascia and fibrin glue (Tissucol). Otherwise a small piece of temporalis muscle (twice as large as the perforation, using 4-0 silk) may be used to cover the edges of the breach, stretching the pieces of muscle between the two edges. The closure of the point leads the muscle to move in the path of least resistance, closing the deficit completely. This method is very effective and we also recommend it in closure of approaches at the cerebellopontine angle, and in reconstruction when an incomplete dural closure is suspected.

- The incision of the superior surface of the sac is performed one-third posteriorly and two-thirds anteriorly to the sac. The incision is in an asymmetric position so that more anterior space is available for the prosthesis. It is generally not a good idea to cut further back. Although anterior space is increased, we risk losing the plane and entering the dura or under the sac.

- The incision is performed practically parallel to the direction of the fibers, to cause the least trauma possible. Thus the incision is less likely to injure the arterioles, which are located axially, whereas the venules are smaller and circumferential. The venules are closer to the epithelium of the sac while the arterioles, which receive blood from the external carotid artery, are deeper, in the perisaccular connective tissue (Gadre).

- At times Mèniére's disease may mimic otosclerosis. There is in fact a simultaneous conductive hearing loss greater than 40 dB, due to the sac's pushing under the oval window.

- To prepare the prosthesis for the shunt, a small piece of thin silastic rubber sheeting is fashioned into a T-shape and inserted into the lumen.

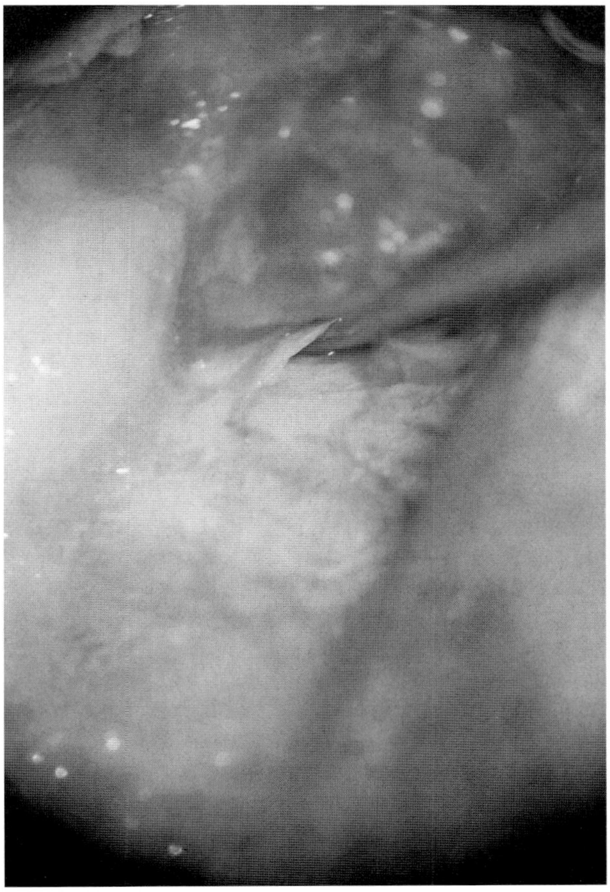

Fig. 18-18. The lateral wall of the sac is incised and the lumen is exposed.

- A toothless clamp is used (the same utilized in taking the prosthesis in stapedectomy). Using the clamp, the first arm is bent under the bit of the prosthesis, then the second arm is bent over the bit, using the index and the middle finger of the right hand, then the clamp is opened and closed, so that both extremities of the arms are bent under the tip of the prosthesis.

- The Donaldson line tells us that the sac is somewhere inferior. One useful method is thus to expose the dura of the posterior fossa along the Donaldson line: we know in this way that the sac is not there. The dura is then followed inferiorly and anteriorly, until the sac is identified. At times, in Mèniére's disease, the sac is very fragile and may be damaged. If the landmarks are recognized and followed, it is very difficult to go wrong. The internal surface of the sac is always slightly humid and shines under the light of the microscope.

- When a simple sac decompression is performed, the mastoid must be opened wide to the tip, otherwise there is insufficient access to the operculum of the sac. Ample access and decompression of the sac are necessary as well in the endoymphatic shunt. It is useful to associate the effects of decompression to that of the shunt.

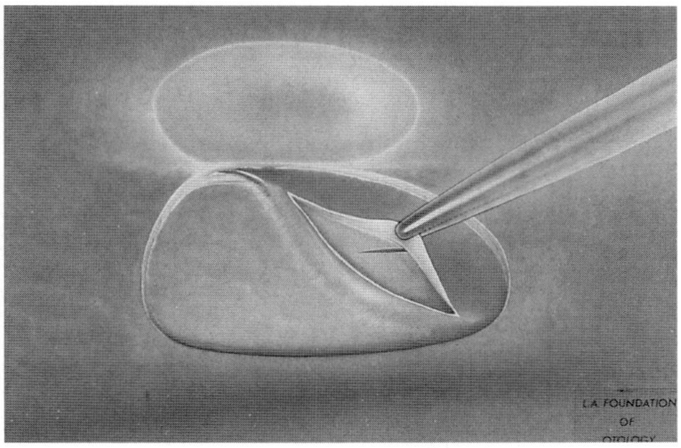

Fig. 18-19. Endolymphatic subarachnoid shunt. The medial wall of the sac is incised.

- The prosthesis is inserted into the sac by grasping it with a toothless clamp. When the clamp divaricates and one extracts, it is possible that the prosthesis will come back out. We thus advise that a hook be inserted between the jaws of the clamp while pushing down, while simultaneously retracting the clamp.

- The sac is thicker, whiter and more vascularized than the surrounding dura. Its walls are composed of radiated fibers, which become visible when pressing on the external wall of the sac.

COMPLICATIONS

- In approx. 1% of cases a profound sensorineural hearing loss may be demonstrated, as a result of the sac being opened. The accidental opening of the posterior semicircular canal should be avoided, since it provokes vertigo and postoperatively deafness syndrome.

- If there have been lesions to the facial nerve, signs of paresis or paralysis of the facial nerve may appear. This should not, however, occur in this operation.

- In rare instances a blood loss may occur in the tympanic cavity, with consequent conductive hearing loss, which generally can be cured within a few days.

- In the case of a subarachnoid shunt, a liquor fistula may appear, with subsequent rhynoliquorrea; in rare cases, meningitis may also appear.

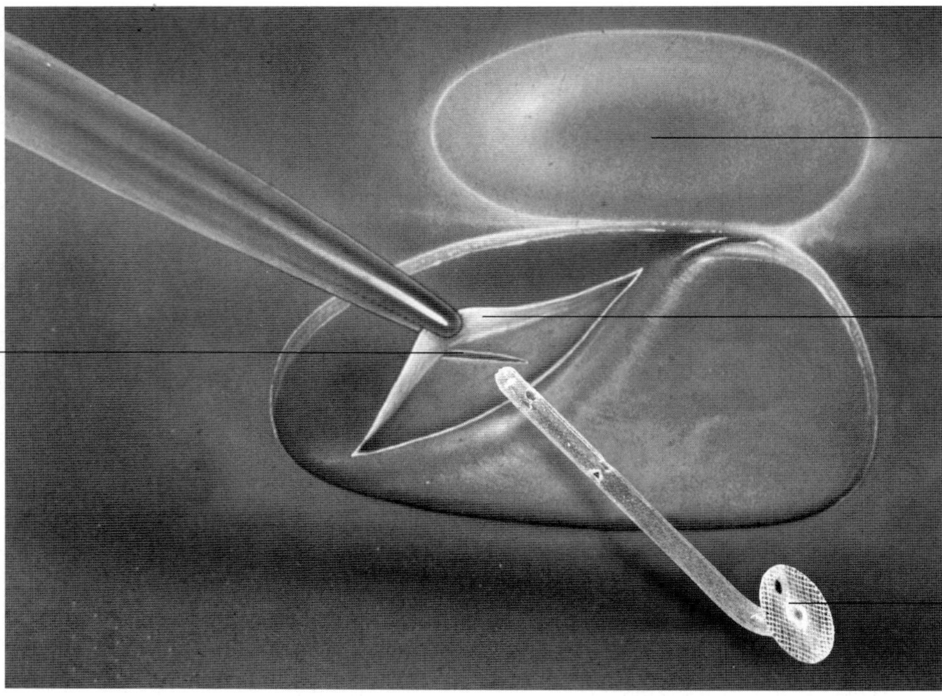

Fig. 18-20. Endolymphatic subarachnoid shunt. The medial wall of the sac is incised and a shunt tube is inserted in the subarachnoid space.

REFERENCES

Arenberg IK, Balkany TJ: Revision endolymphatic sac and duct surgery for recurrent Mèniére's disease and hydrops: Failure analysis and technical aspects. Laryngoscope 92: 1279-1284, 1982.

Arenberg IK, Stahle I, Wilbrand H, Newkirk JB: Unidirectional inner ear valve implant for endolymphatic sac surgery. Arch Otolaryngol Head Neck Surg 104(12): 694-704, 1978.

Arenberg IK: Results of endolymphatic sac to mastoid shunt surgery for Mèniére's disease refractory to medical therapy. Am J Otol 8(4): 335-344, 1987.

Arenberg IK: The fine points of valve implant surgery for hydrops: an update. Am J Otol 3:359-74, 1982.

Austin DF: Endolymphatic fistulization. Ann Otol Rhinol Laryngol 93(Pt 1): 534-539, 1984.

Belal A Jr: Pathology as it relates to ear surgery. IV. Surgery of Mèniére's disease. J Laryngol Otol 98(2): 127-138, 1984.

Brackmann DE, Anderson RG: Mèniére's disease: Results of treatment with the endolymphatic subarachnoid shunt. ORL J Otorhinolaryngol Relat Spec 42(1-2): 101-118, 1980.

Brackmann DE, Nissen RL: Mèniére's disease: Results of treatment with endolymphatic subarachnoid shunt compared with the endolymphatic mastoid shunt. Am J Otol 8(4): 275-282, 1987.

Bretlau P, Thomsen J, Tos M, Johnsen NJ: Placebo effect in surgery for Mèniére's disease: A three-year follow-up study of patients in a double blind placebo controlled study on endolymphatic sac shunt surgery. Am J Otol 5(6): 558-561, 1984.

Brown JS: A ten year statistical follow up of 245 consecutive cases of endolymphatic shunt decompression with 328 consecutive cases of labyrinthectomy. Laryngoscope 93(Pt 1): 1419-1424, 1983.

Chui RT, McCabe BF, Harker LA: Mèniére's disease at the University of Iowa: 1973-1980. Otolaryngol Head Neck Surg 90(4): 482-487, 1982.

Fisch U, Ruttner J: Pathology of intratemporal tumors involving the facial nerve. In facial nerve surgery. Fisch U Edit Aesculapius pub Co Birmingham, Alabama 448:456, 1977.

Ford CN: Results of endolymphatic sac surgery in advanced Mèniére's disease. Am J Otol 3(4): 339-342, 1982.

Futaki T, Nomura Y: The surgical procedures and evaluation of two modifications of endolymphatic sac surgery: The epidural shunt and vein graft drainage. Acta Otolaryngol (Stockh) 468(Suppl): 117-127, 189.

Gardner G: Shunt surgery in Mèniére's disease: A follow-up report. South Med J 81(2): 193-198,1988.

Goldenburg RA, Justus MA: Endolymphatic mastoid shunt for treatment of Mèniére's disease: A five year study. Laryngoscope 93(Pt 1): 1425-1429, 1983.

Graham VID, Kemink JL: Surgical management of Mèniére's disease with endolymphatic sac decompression by wide bony decompression of the posterior fossa dura: Technique and results. Laryngoscope 95: 680-683, 1984.

Gya K, Yangihara N: Endolymphatic-mastoid shunt operation: Results of the 24 cases and revision surgery with the Silastic sheet. Auris Nasus Larynx 9(2): 59-66, 1982.

Hallpike CS, Cairns H: Observations on the pathology of Mèniére's syndrome. J Laryngol 53: 625-655, 1938.

House WF, Fraysee B: Revision of the endolymphatic subarachnoid shunt for Mèniére's disease. Review of 59 cases. Arch Otolaryngol Head Neck Surg 105(10): 599-600, 1980.

House WF: Subarachnoid shunt for drainage of endolymphatic hydrops. Laryngoscope 72: 713-729, 1962.

Huang TS, Lin CC: Endolymphatic sac surgery for Mèniére's disease: A composite study of 339 cases. Laryngoscope 95 (Pt 1): 1082-1086, 1985.

Huang TS, Lin CC: Endolymphatic sac surgery for refractory luetic vertigo. Am J Otol 12(3): 184-187, 1991.

Huang TS, Lin CC: Surgical treatment of chronic otitis media and Mèniére's syndrome. Laryngoscope 101: 900-904, 1991.

Jackler RK, Luxford WM, Brackmann DE, Monsell EM: Endolymphatic sac surgery in congenital malformations of the inner ear. Laryngoscope 98(7): 698-704, 1988.

Kaye AH, Hahn JF, Kinney SE, Hardy RW, Bay JW: Jugular foramen schwannomas. J Neurosurg 60: 1045-1053, 1984.

Kimura R: Experimental blockage of the endolymphatic duct and sac and its effect on the inner ear of the guinea pig. Ann Otol Rhinol Laryngol 76: 664-669, 1976.

Kitahara M, Kitajima K, Yazawa Y, Uchida K: Endolymphatic sac surgery for Mèniére's disease: Eighteen years' experience with the Kitahara sac operation. Am J Otol 8(4): 283-286, 1987.

Kitahara M, Kitano H: Surgical treatment of Mèniére's disease. Am J Otol 6(1): 108-109, 1985.

Liston S, Nissen RL, Paparella MM, daCosta SS: Surgical treatment of vertigo. In Paparella MM, Shumrick DA (eds): Otolaryngology, 3rd ed, Vol II, Otology. Philadelphia, WB Saunders, 1990, pp 1715-1732.

Maddox HE: Surgery of the endolymphatic sac. Laryngoscope 91(7): 1058-1062, 1981.

Meyerhoff WL, Paparella MM, Shea D: Mèniére's disease in children. Laryngoscope 88(Pt 1): 1504-1511, 1978.

Miller GW, Welsh RL: Surgical management of vestibular Mèniére's disease with endolymphatic mastoid shunt. Laryngoscope 93(Pt 1): 1430-1440, 1983.

Morrison AW: Cochleostomy or endolymphatic sac surgery for advanced Mèniére's disease. Otolaryngol Clin North Am 16(1): 135-142, 1983.

Morrison AW: Management of sensorineural deafness. London, Butterworth's, 1975, pp 109-144.

Morrison AW: Sac surgery on the only or better hearing ear. Otolaryngol Clin North Am 16: 143-151, 1983.

Morrison GA, O'Reilly BJ, Chevreton EB, Kenyon GS: Longterm results of revision endolymphatic sac surgery. J Laryngol Otol 104: 612-616, 1990.

Nadol JB Jr, Weiss AD, Parker SW: Vertigo of delayed onset after sudden deafness. Ann Otol Rhinol Laryngol 84(6): 841-846, 1975.

Naito T: Notre experience de l'operation de G. Portmann (ouverture du sac endolymphatique dans la maladie de Mèniére). Rev Laryngol Otol Rhinol (Bord) 83: 643-645, 1962.

Paparella MM, daCosta SS, Fox R, Yoon TH: Mèniére's disease and other labyrinthine diseases. In Paparella MM, Shumrick DA (eds): Otolaryngology: Otology and Neurology. Philadelphia, WB Saunders, 1990.

Paparella MM, deSousa LC, Mancini F: Mèniére's syndrome and otitis media. Laryngoscope 93: 1408-1415, 1983.

Paparella MM, Goycoolea MV, Schachern PA: Multiple otological pathologies. Ann Otol Rhinol Laryngol 91(1): 14-18, 1988.

Paparella MM, Hanson DG: Endolymphatic sac drainage for intractable vertigo (methods and experience). Laryngoscope 86(5): 697-703, 1976.

Paparella MM, Kim CS, Shea DA: Sac decompression for refractory luetic vertigo. Acta Otolaryngol (Stockh) 89(5-6): 541-546, 1980.

Paparella MM, Mancini F, Liston SL: Otosclerosis and Mèniére's syndrome: Diagnosis and treatment. Laryngoscope 94(Pt 1): 623-629, 1984.

Paparella MM, Mancini F: Vestibular Mèniére's disease. Otolaryngol Head Neck Surg 93(2): 148-151, 1985.

Paparella MM, Morizono T, Matsunaga T: Kyoshiro Yamakawa and temporal bone histopathology of Mèniére's patients reported in 1938. Arch Otolaryngol Head Neck Surg 118: 660-662, 1992.

Paparella MM, Sajjadi H: Endolymphatic sac revision for recurrent Mèniére's disease. Am J Otol 9(6): 441-447, 1988.

Paparella MM: Pathogenesis of Mèniére's disease and Mèniére's syndrome. Acta Otolaryngol (Stockh) 406(Suppl): 10-25, 1984.

Pearson BW, Brackmann DE: Committee on Hearing and Equilibrium: Guidelines for reporting treatment results in Mèniére's disease. Otolaryngol Head Neck Surg 93: 579-581, 1985.

Pillsbury HC, Arenberg IK, Ferraro J, Ackley RS: Endolymphatic sac surgery: The Danish sham surgery study—an alternative analysis. Otolaryngol Clin North Am 92(Pt 1): 113-118, 1983.

Plester D: Surgery of endolymphatic hydrops. J Otolaryngol Soc Aust 3(3): 393-395, 1972.

Portmann G: The saccus endolymphaticus and an operation for draining the same for the relief of vertigo. Arch Otolaryngol 6: 309, 1927.

Portmann M: The Portmann procedure after sixty years. Am J Otol 8(4): 271-274, 1987.

Pulec IL: Endolymphatic subarachnoid shunt for Mèniére's disease in the only hearing ear. Laryngoscope 91(5): 772-783, 1981.

Shambaugh GE Jr: Effect of endolymphatic sac decompression on fluctuant hearing loss. Otolaryngol Clin North Am 8(2): 537-540, 1975.

Shambaugh GE Jr: Surgery of the endolymphatic sac. Arch Otolaryngol Head Neck Surg 83(Suppl): 305-315, 1966.

Shea DA, Chole RA, Paparella MM: The endolymphatic sac: Anatomical considerations. Laryngoscope 89: 88-94, 1979.

Shea JJ: Teflon film drainage of the endolymphatic sac. Arch Otolaryngol Head Neck Surg 83: 316-319, 1966.

Silverstein H: The effect of the endolymphatic subarachnoid shunt operation on vestibular function. Laryngoscope 88(10): 1603-1611, 1978.

Silverstein H: Vestibular neurectomy in the United States-1990. Trans Am Otol Soc 149-156, 1991.

Smith WC, Pillsbury HC: Surgical treatment of Mèniére's disease since Thomsen. Am J Otol 9: 39-43, 1988.

Spector GJ, Smith PG: Endolymphatic sac surgery for Mèniére's disease. Ann Otol Rhinol Laryngol 92(Pt 1): 113-118, 1983.

Stahle J, Stahle C, Med B, Arenberg IK: Incidence of Mèniére's disease. Arch Otolaryngol Head Neck Surg 104: 99-102, 1978.

Williams A, Horton B, Day L: Endolymphatic hydrops without vertigo. Trans Am Otol Soc 35: 116, 1947.

Yamakawa K: Uber die Pathologische Varanderung bei einem Mèniére-Kranken. Z Otol 44: 192-193, 1938.

19

Vestibular nerve section

The surgical approaches for vestibular nerve section are basically:

- Retrolabyrinthine approach
- Retrosigmoid approach
- Middle fossa approach.

RETROLABYRINTHINE VESTIBULAR NERVE SECTION

Pathways of CNs VII-VIII in the cerebellopontine angle.

- In the retrolabyrinthine or retrosigmoid approaches it is essential to know the surgical anatomy of CNs VII and VIII. At the fundus of the IAC and medial to the labyrinth, the cochlear nerve is hidden from view by the inferior vestibular nerve. The inferior vestibular nerve joins with the superior vestibular nerve in the superior or medial third of the IAC, forming one single nerve. The cochlear nerve unites with it almost immediately, rotating in a counterclockwise direction in the right ear and in a clockwise direction in the left ear. Most of the rotation occurs in the IAC and the rest occurs in the cerebellopontine angle. The cochlear nerve enters the pons in a caudal position, slightly lateral in regard to the vestibular nerve (Silverstein).
- The facial nerve is superior and slightly medial in its intralabyrinthine part to the superior vestibular nerve. Entering the IAC, it becomes medial to the vestibular nerve, which hides it from view. It then runs parallel to the vestibular-cochlear nerve to the brainstem, and enters the caudal part of the pons medially and the slightest bit caudally in relation to nerve VIII.
- In the cerebellopontine angle, between the trunk of the facial nerve and the cochlear nerve, the intermediate Wrisberg nerve is found. This is a branch of the facial nerve.
- The superior vestibular nerve originates in the superior and horizontal semicircular canals, the saccule and the utricle. The singular nerve (or posterior ampullary nerve) originates in the posterior semicircular canal while the saccular nerve originates in the saccule. These two nerves join medially to the labyrinth to form the inferior vestibular nerve. The size ratio of the singular and saccular nerves is approx. 1/4.
- **V**. The trigeminal nerve is the largest of the cranial nerves. It is located approx. 1.5 cm above CNs VII and VIII, from the pons to its exit through Meckel's cave. The motor root of the trigeminal nerve is smaller than the sensory root and is situated rostrally and medially. The fibers which conduct the pain stimuli are concentrated in the posterior part of the sensitive root, whereas the fibers responsible for fine sensitivity are situated in the opposite part of the nerve. This organization of the sensitive root of the nerve makes it possible to selectively section the pain-sensitive fibers while preserving the tactile-sensitive fibers (Brackmann DE, Hitselberger WE).
- **VI**. The abducens nerve is medial to CNs VII-VIII in the posterior fossa. It may in rare cases cross the medial surface of the trigeminal nerve.
- **VII**. The facial nerve originates in the pons, caudally to the trigeminal nerve and rostrally and medially to nerve VIII. This position is maintained for the entire pathway of the posterior fossa to the internal auditory canal.
- **VIII**. The acoustic nerve exits the pons in a single trunk, immediately lateral and caudally to the facial nerve. When the nerve enters the IAC, it divides into three main branches: the cochlear nerve situated anterior and medial to the facial nerve; and the two branches of the vestibular nerve, superior and inferior, in a posterior position. A smaller branch, the singular nerve, separates from the inferior vestibular nerve and reaches the ampulla of the posterior canal.

- **IX**. Nerve IX is the smallest of the nerves in the posterior cranial fossa. It is caudal and distant from CNs VII-VIII but close to the vagus nerve. Together these nerves transverse the jugular foramen, to exit from the endocranium.
- **X**. The vagus nerve is composed of 8-10 roots which emerge from the bulb and group together in one single nerve. They are located inferior to IX. IX and X exit the posterior cranial fossa together through the jugular foramen.
- **XI**. The accessory nerve exits with four or five roots from the side of the bulb. It runs alongside the jugular foramen, caudally to CNs IX and X.

DISADVANTAGES

- In cases of a contracted mastoid or protruding sigmoid sinus, the extension of the posterior cranial fossa dura is too small to obtain a good view of the cerebellopontine angle.
- In patients who have already undergone open tympanoplasty with a retrolabyrinthine approach, a bacterial contamination in the subarachnoid spaces is possible.

In both cases, the retrosigmoid approach must be used for the section of the vestibular nerve.

SURGICAL TECHNIQUE

- The patient is supine, positioned as for a mastoidectomy. The electrodes are placed in the usual way for intraoperative monitoring of VII and VIII CNs.
- The postauricular incision is brought back approx. 3 cm behind the postauricular fold, going from the mastoid line above to the tip of the mastoid below. The periosteum-muscle flap is elevated by following the usual procedure. The area of bone freed up is extensive enough to permit a complete check of the sigmoid sinus and the posterior cranial fossa dura in the steps to follow.
- An extensive mastoidectomy is performed and the sigmoid sinus is decompressed 1-2 cm posteriorly until the posterior cranial fossa dura is exposed (Figs. 19-1, 19-2, 19-3, 19-4, 19-5).
- The retrofacial cells are removed near the jugular bulb, so that a thorough view of the mixed nerves may be obtained. The endolymphatic sac is exposed as well as the lateral and posterior semicircular canals. The posterior canal is the anterior limiting structure of the dissection. It is important to remove all the bone between the labyrinth and the lateral sinus in order to obtain the best exposure possible in the cerebellopontine angle (Fig. 19-6).
- It is not necessary to blue line the posterior canal. The distance between the anterior surface of the lateral sinus and the posterior surface of the posterior canal varies 2-3 mm in smaller mastoids and more than 1 cm in larger ones.

DURAL INCISION

- The sinus is outlined as a bluish, venous structure, with the dura as its reflection limit. It is not easily seen anteriorly. It should be kept in mind that the sinus is developed as a duplication of the dura, which does not immediately assume a cylindric aspect. The dural sheath is

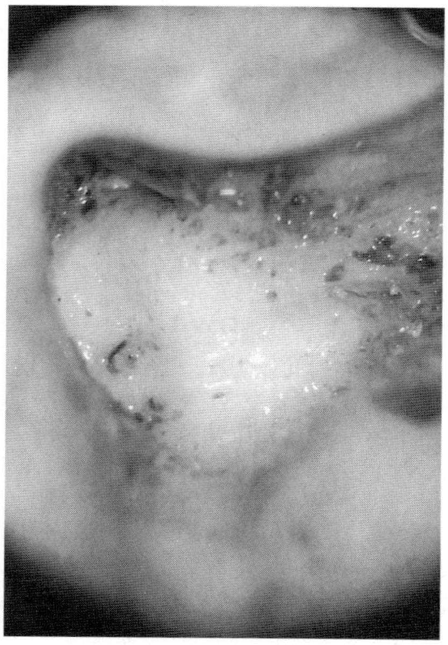

Fig. 19-1. Right ear. A mastoidectomy is performed. The horizontal and posterior semicircular canals are outlined.

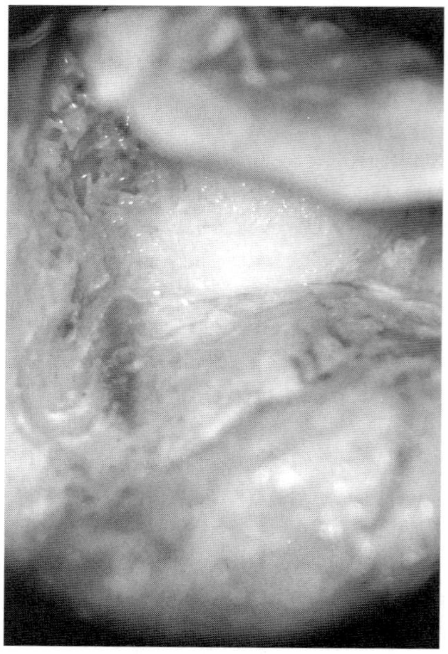

Fig. 19-2. The sigmoid sinus, the presigmoid dura and approximately 2 cm of dura posterior to the sigmoid sinus are exposed. The endolymphatic sac and the semicircular canals are preserved.

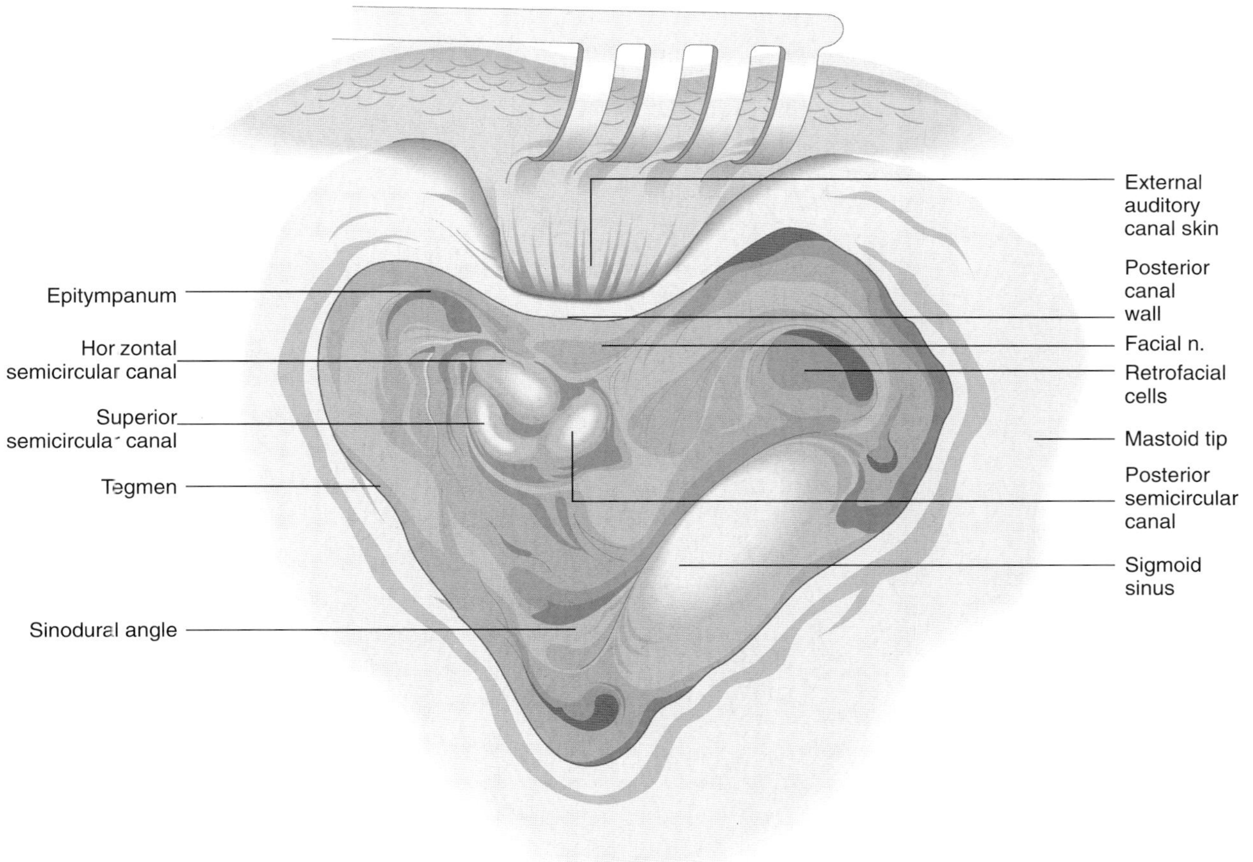

Fig. 19-3. Right ear. Complete mastoidectomy.

doubled at the sinus edges. Here the space between the two walls is less than 1 mm, then the two sheaths progressively enlarge, and the sinus reaches its largest size (1-1.5 cm).

- To avoid opening the sinus anteriorly, where the sheaths join, the incision must be parallel to the sinus and 1 cm away.
- The incision is in the shape of a C, with the concavity towards the labyrinth. The inferior incision is first, since the dura is thicker here. The endolymphatic sac must be included in the flap and preserved. At times the sac is so spread out that it is impossible not to cross it; if this is the case, the margins are reconstructed after the operation with 8-0 silk. The incision is prolonged superiorly, along the superior petrosal sinus, but distanced by at least 1/2 cm for the reasons previously listed. Others (Kemink) prefer a single posterior incision or, if more space is needed, an L-shaped incision, which includes the superior and posterior openings but not the inferior one. Thus the risk of trauma to the endolymphatic sac is avoided, though the visual space in the angle is not as great as in a C-incision (Fig. 19-7).
- The dura is anchored with two 4-0 silk sutures and displaced anteriorly. It may also be replaced without suturing; it will stay in place.

VESTIBULAR NERVE SECTION

- In this phase, controlled ventilation and the administration of Mannitol help to reduce the cerebellar mass.
- A fenestrated Brackmann suction-irrigator is used. A cottonoid is placed lengthwise on the sigmoid sinus and is progressively advanced with suction and a Gimmick elevator. A continous flow of liquid from the suction-irrigator displaces the arachnoid fibers, facilitating the view of the underlying structures.
- The arachnoid bridles are opened with the dissector, enabling the spinal fluid to exit the lateral cistern. Then the cerebellum moves away from the temporal bone, falling back (Fig. 19-8). At this point the CN V may be seen above, the nerve bundle including IX-X-XI below and nerve VIII in the middle. Nerve VIII is generally found on a vertical line whose upper part is tangential to the superior part of the lateral semicircular canal. With the dissector, nerve VIII is carefully moved in an infero-superior direction to identify nerve VII. The facial nerve enters

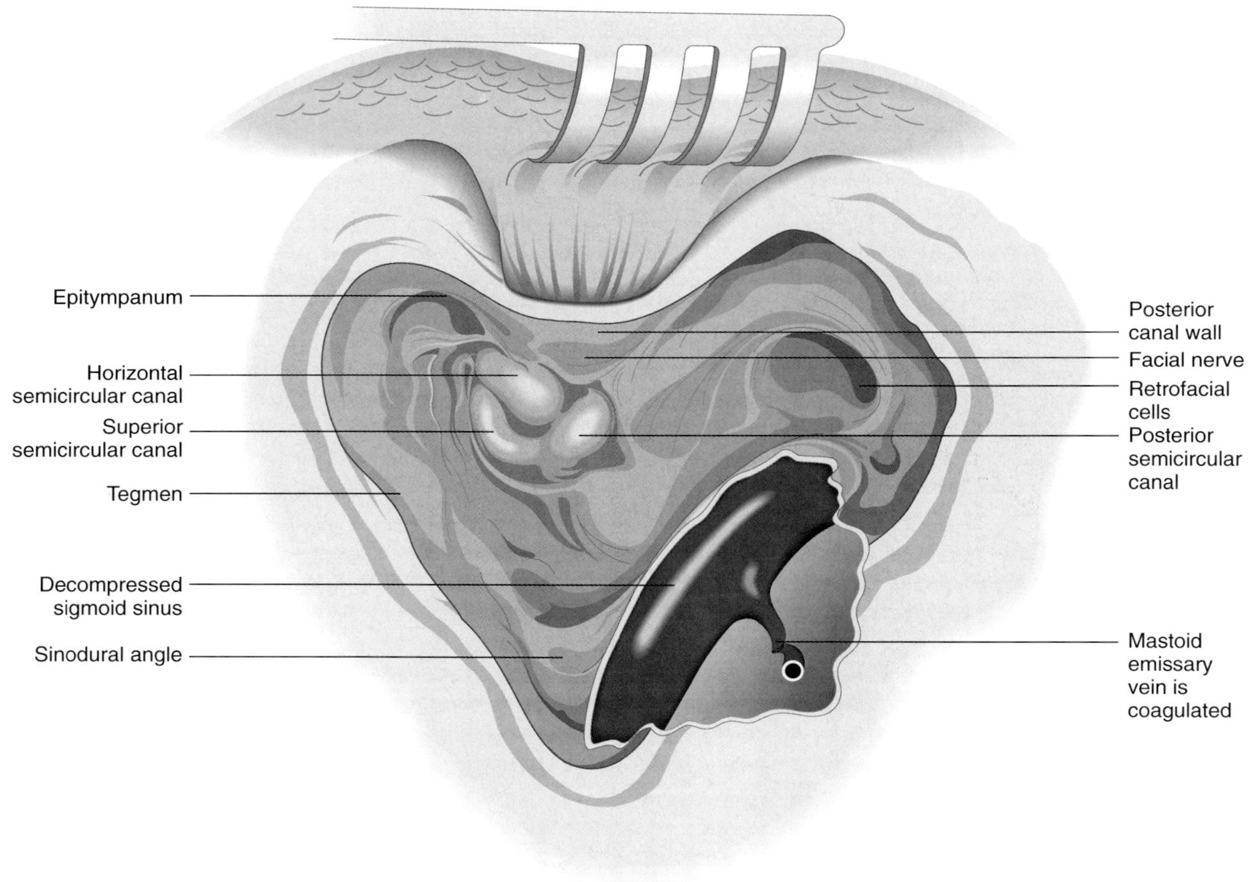

Fig. 19-4. The sigmoid sinus is exposed. The emissary mastoid vein is coagulated.

the caudal part medially from the pons and slightly caudally regarding the vestibulocochlear nerve, and is hidden by it. It is essential to know VII's position before sectioning the vestibular nerve. The AICA must also be identified. It often passes between the two nerves, at varying levels, and perpendicular to them (Figs. 19-9, 19-10, 19-11).

- At times the cerebellar floccule protrudes, hiding nerve VIII. At this point a delicate dissection may be performed from the nerve. If this is insufficient, a cottonoid may then be moved forward until the extremity is brought onto the floccule, using moderate suction compression.
- The vestibular nerve is superior and the cochlear nerve inferior. Finding the exact cleavage plane is the most important moment in this operation. The following tips may help: The cochlear nerve is larger than the vestibular nerve and slightly paler, due to its higher myelin content. An artery is frequently found along the line of nerve cleavage. Other landmarks may be found by observing the anterior surface of the nerves with a mirror, since it may be that the cleavage is better defined behind.
- A small sharp hook is used to enter superficially into the cleavage plane and the pia mater is separated above the nerve. The two nerves are separated, penetrating the separation plane with a blunt hook. With straight microscissors the nerve is incised layer after layer until only a few posterior fibers remain exposed. The latter are not cut but interrupted with a hook; in this way the risks of injuring the internal auditory artery (which lies behind nerve VIII) and the facial nerve are avoided (Figs. 19-12, 19-13).
- The total section of the vestibular nerve already performed is confirmed by the retraction of the two stumps well beyond the edge of the incision. It is as if a tense rubber band has been partially cut; the two margins remain close, but when the cut is completed, the two pieces of rubber move away.

It is not advisable to proceed beyond this section line. Up until 1990 the House Ear Institute performed a small notch of the cochlear nerve along with the vestibular section,because histological studies had demonstrated the existence of a transition area,where the vestibular nerve cells braided with those of the cochlear nerve. However

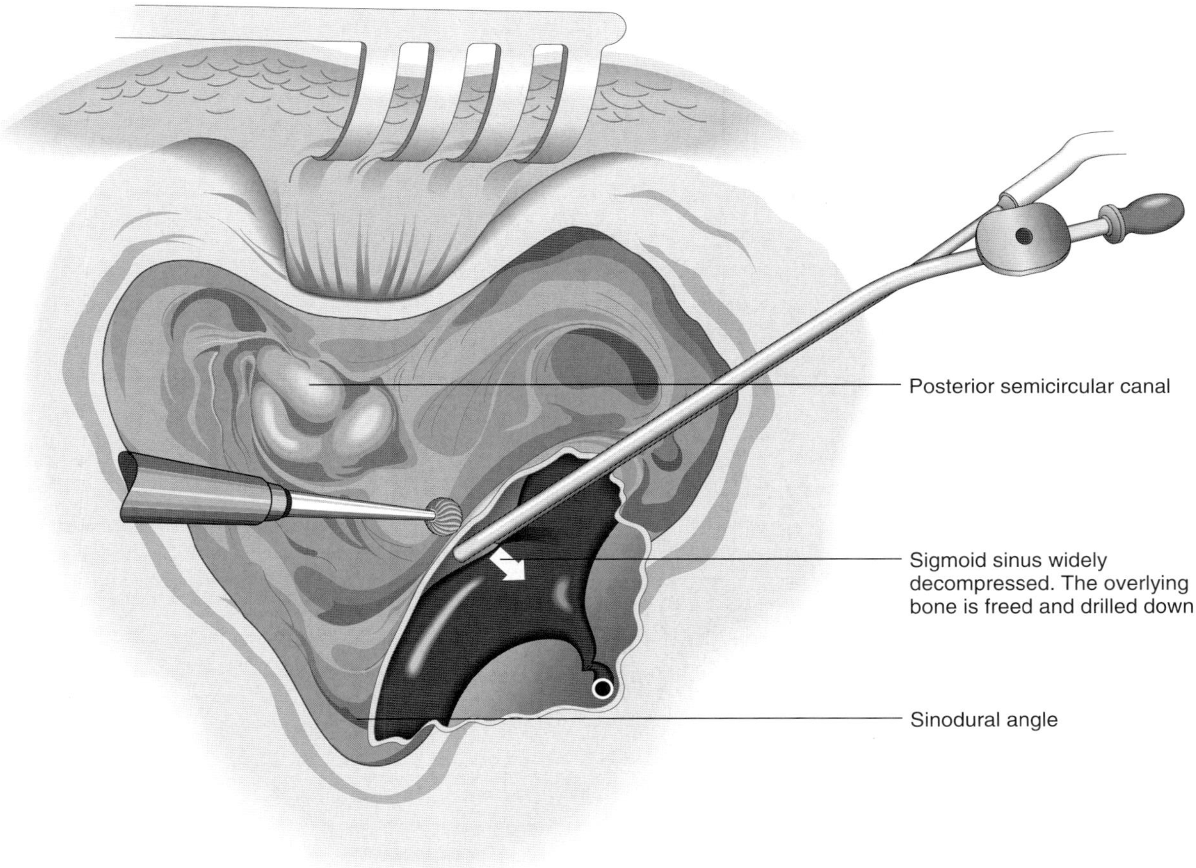

Fig. 19-5. The bony plate over the sigmoid sinus and the posterior fossa dura is drilled down.

Brackmann and Hitselberger's study demonstrated that with this technique the results of the vertigo tests were no better, while a higher incidence of hearing loss was reported (Fig. 19-14).
When the nerve section is completed, the facial nerve can be easily seen medially.

CLOSURE

- The dura is closed with interrupted 4-0 silk sutures. The mastoid cavity is filled with abdominal fat to seal possible deficits in the adherence of the flaps and to prevent liquor fistulas.
- The subcutaneous tissues are closed with interrupted 2-0 chromic catgut and the skin is closed with a 2-0 interrupted silk sutures. It is preferable to close with interrupted stitches rather than continuous, because, if infection occurs, the suture in the infected area may slip, without compromising the entire suturing. If this does occur, the incision is performed, followed by drainage, pus culture and appropriate antibiotic treatment.

COMPLICATIONS

Following the operation, hearing loss may occur (2%, McElveen), for various reasons:

- Natural progression of the original pathology (e.g. Mèniére's Disease).
- Interruption of the cochlear duct at the moment of dural incision.
- Accidental fenestration of the posterior semicircular canal.
- Interruption of the internal auditory canal, which lies posterior to the vestibular nerve.
- Tearing of the cochlear nerve fibers at the moment of the neurectomy (McElveen).

TIPS AND PITFALLS

- When the mastoidectomy has been completed, the bone of the posterior cranial fossa is drilled. In order to make bone removal less traumatic and easier, it is well to begin by skeletonizing the sigmoid sinus first superiorly (for identification) then posteriorly (to decompress it), and then anteriorly. The 14 or 12-caliber suction-irrigator is placed flat on the lateral sinus and exerts enough pressure to dissect the sinus from the overlying bone. The dura frequently adheres to the bone, so that, while maintaining

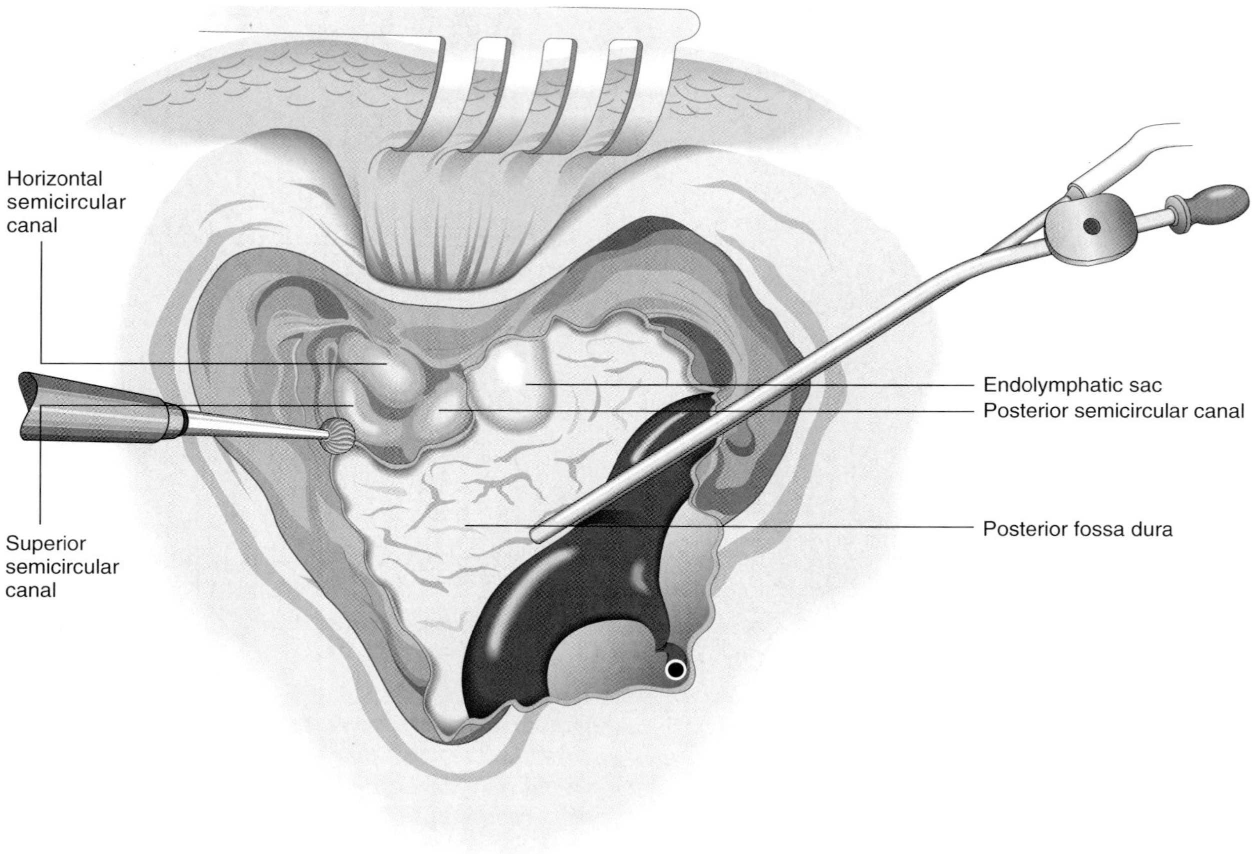

Fig. 19-6. The sigmoid sinus and the presigmoid dura have been exposed. Semicircular canals and endolymphatic sac can be seen.

pressure on the sinus with the suction, can be dissected with a House dissector. The suction-irrigator is moved forward into the gap between dura and bone to maintain the progress already obtained. The bone, thus liberated, is drilled with a large-diameter (4-5 mm) round or pear-shaped cutting burr. It is important to move quickly to reduce the risk of damaging the dura:

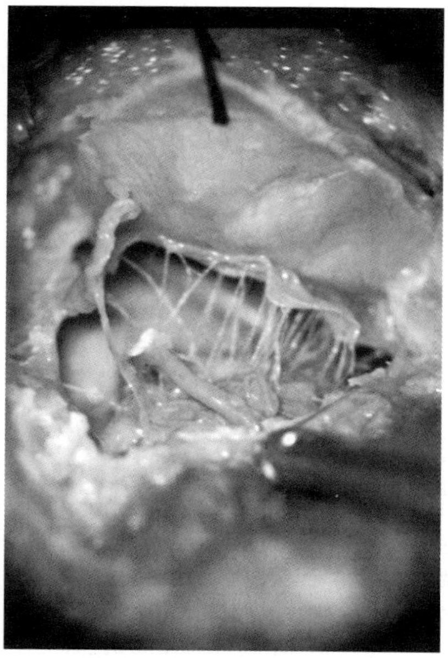

Fig. 19-7. The presigmoid dura is incised in a C shape based on the labyrinth. The arachnoid is opened, the CSF escapes.

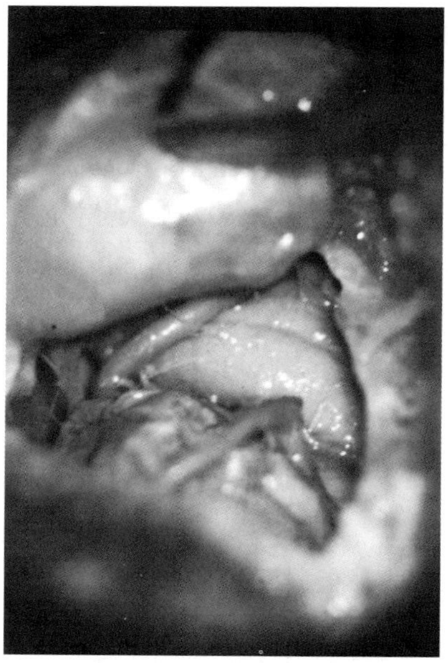

Fig. 19-8. The cerebellum comes into view. The flocculus can be seen.

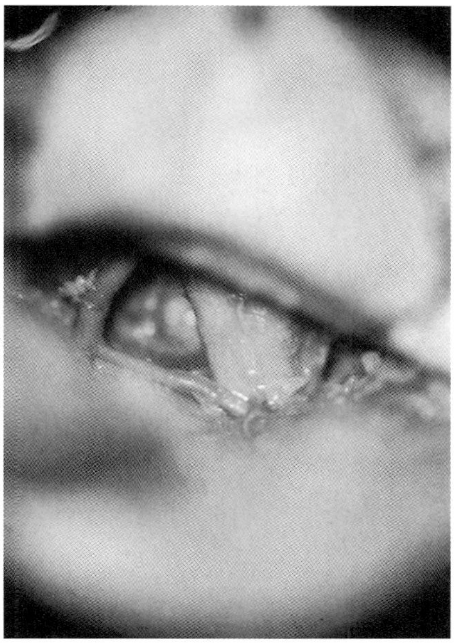

Fig. 19-9. The VIII CN is identified. AICA can be seen.

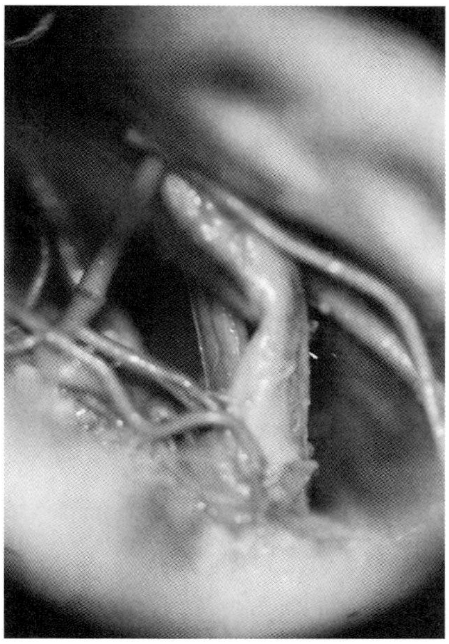

Fig. 19-11. The facial n. is identified by gentle inferior retraction of the vestibulocochlear n.

in fact, between this and the bone, a layer of free air remains. When the bone has been partially drilled, the surgeon can proceed medially in the same way by advancing the suction.

- At this point most of the bone between the sigmoid sinus and the labyrinth has been drilled with a cutting burr. It is important to leave a thin layer close to the posterior canal.

- It is also important to skeletonize the posterior canal without opening it; the canal is evident, but its posterior limits are indistinct. In order to get an idea of its borders and the depth of the canal, we advise pressing on the retrolabyrinthine dura (already exposed) with the suction or the dissector. We then note the thin layer of residual bone over the dura, while below we see bone, whiter and more compact, and deeper: this is the medial part of the canal, and this is its posterior limit. Now that we have the lateral and medial limits of the canal, it is easy and safe to remove the intermediate bone with a small diamond burr (2-3 mm) or if necessary with the House curette.

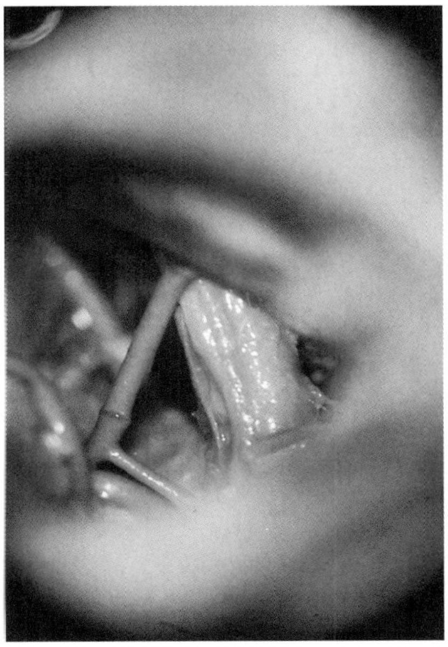

Fig. 19-10. Close-up view of 19-9.

In this way, the surgeon obtains the best conditions for the exposure of the anterior limits of the CPA with a retrolabyrinthine approach.

- The Donaldson line is a helpful landmark in surgery of the endolymphatic sac, and also indicates the superior vestibular nerve's direction, below the dura.

- When opening the dura, are used a Brackmann suction-irrigator and a dural elevator to slide along the anterior part of the petrous apex, then the "petrous ridge", and finally back to the cochlear-vestibular nerve.

- In a retrolabyrinthine approach, the dura must be thoroughly exposed. Care must be taken not to injure the superior petrosal sinus, found in the sino-dural angle.

- Once the cochlear-vestibular nerve has been identified, the surgeon may obtain a better view by moving his chair forward. In this way the an-

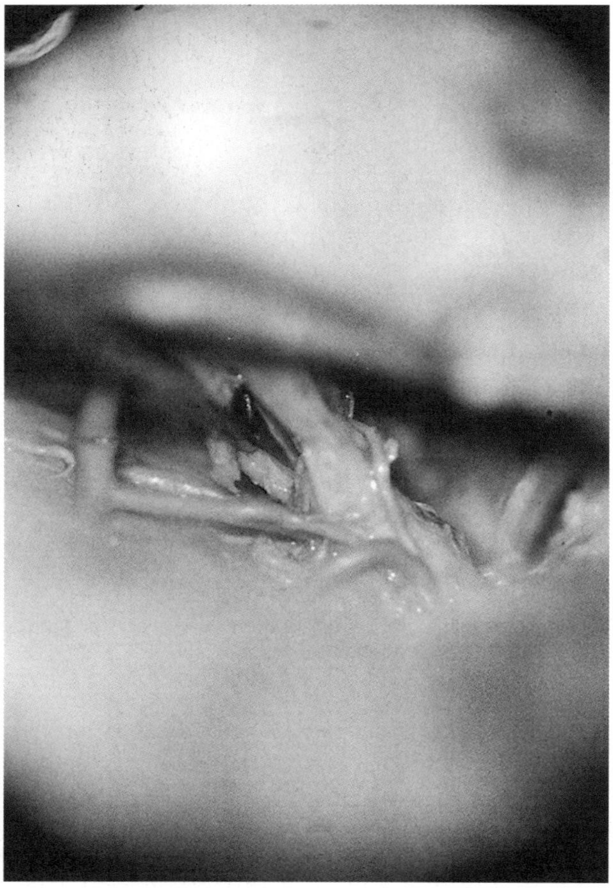

Fig. 19-12. The cleavage plane between the cochlear and vestibular nerve is identified. The vestibular fibers of the VIII CN are sectioned with care, so as not to injure the cochlear fibers and the underlying VII CN. The internal auditory artery, behind the cochleovestibular n., must not be injured, in order to preserve hearing.

gle between the visual axis and the line tangent to the sigmoid sinus becomes more acute. There is no view below the sigmoid sinus.

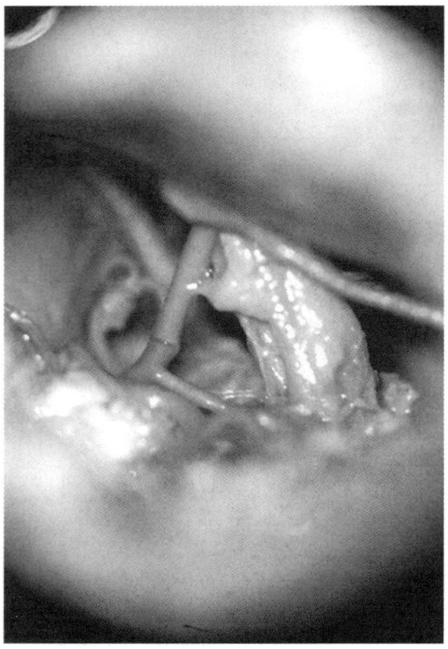

Fig. 19-13. Vestibular nerve is cut. The IAA, behind the stumps of the vestibular nerve, is preserved.

- In vestibular nerve section, the patient will completely recover from vertigo within 6 months. The less medicine administered, the quicker the recovery (the human body realizes what has happened and compensates accordingly).
- If the vertigo reappears more than 5 years after the execution of the endolymphatic shunt, it may mean that scar tissue has obstructed the incision of the sac. A revision of the shunt is indicated. In case of failure under five years, a section of the vestibular nerve must be performed. This "final weapon" does have a higher morbidity, but completely cures vertigo 95% of the time.
- When a section of the vestibular nerve is performed using either a retrosigmoid or retro-

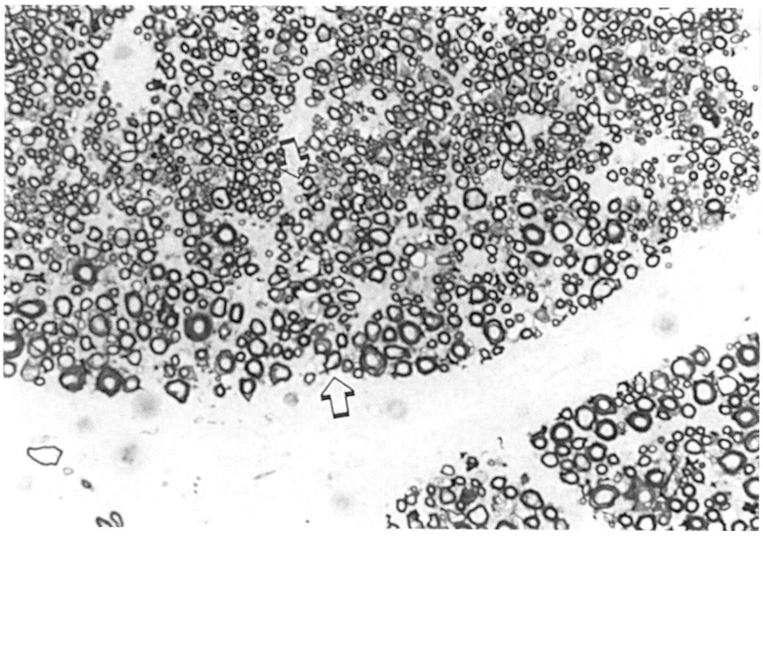

Fig. 19-14. Courtesy of Linthicum FH. Interface between cochlear nerve (small fibers) and vestibular nerve (large fibers). Note overlapping area between arrows. Toluidine blue X430

labyrinthine approach, a vascular loop touches the vestibulo-cochlear layer. The vessels may be found under the floccule, which must be displaced from nerve VIII in order to complete decompression. The vessels involved are usually arteries, but can at times be veins. In any case, besides the macroscopic situations in which a vessel rests upon or compresses nerve VIII, near the brainstem and close to nerve VIII is the most frequent site of unrecognized neurovascular conflicts. Thus it is well to section the vestibular nerve near the brainstem and then wrap the entry zone of the cochlear nerve with small fragments of autogenous muscle. The purpose of this maneuver is to prevent a reappearance of the neurovascular conflict and to provide vascular support to the cochlear nerve.

- In elderly patients, the means of compensation for posture maintenance (i.e the muscular-tendon receptors and sight) are less effective. Therefore we do not advise performing a bilateral section of the vestibular nerve, at any time, since the patient would have to depend on weakened resources.

Like the retrosigmoid approach, the retrolabyrinthine technique paves the way for other operations, besides the vestibular nerve section:

- Microvascular decompression of CNs V, VII and VIII (Janetta).
- Neurotomy of IX in the essential neuralgia or in the pharyngo-oral pain, e.g. for inoperable neoplasia.
- Retrogasserian neurotomy of nerve V in a trigeminal neuralgia (Hitselberger, Pulec).
- Removal of small extracanalicular acoustic neuromas.

RETROSIGMOID APPROACH FOR VESTIBULAR NERVE SECTION

The retrosigmoid approach provides an enlarged view of the posterior cranial fossa, from the cerebellar tentorium above to the foramen magnum below.

At the HEC we prefer to section the vestibular nerve using a retrolabyrinthine approach. In the rare cases of a very anteriorized sigmoid sinus, the retrolabyrinthine space is insufficient; thus a retrosigmoid approach is used.

On the other hand, a very posterior sigmoid sinus forces the retrosigmoid craniotomy to an overly posterior position. The cerebellum then occupies all the visual space and the problem of performing a significant retraction arises.

The problem is accentuated in the presence of a path inferior to the transverse sinus, especially in short-necked patients.

In these cases it is helpful to simultaneously decompress the retrolabyrinthine space, providing more visual space by bringing the sigmoid sinus further forward.

Even when a retrosigmoid approach is used in favorable conditions, we always perform a simultaneous retrolabyrinthine decompression.

POSITION OF THE PATIENT

The patient is put in a supine position, with his head turned to the side. The table is turned to a position opposite the surgeon (10-30°). This allows us to reduce the lateral torsion of the patient's head. Thus we avoid both injury to the cervical vertebrae and an alteration in the flow through the vertebral arteries, which would result in cerebellar edema.

SURGICAL TECHNIQUE

- An incision is made approx. 3 cm from the postauricular fold. This is on the same level and behind the mastoid tip, and superiorly is 1 cm above the limit of the temporal line.
- It is unnecessary to prolong the incision inferiorly. Otherwise we risk injuring the vertebral artery in its path behind the atlanto-occipital articulation and the arc of the atlas.
- The skin is cut; the cervical muscles are cut and separated anteriorly and posteriorly. The incision is perpendicular so as to preserve the nerves and the occipital vessels.
- The craniectomy, approx. 3 cm × 3 cm, goes from the posterior margin of the lateral sinus anteriorly to the inferior margin of the transverse sinus superiorly (Fig. 19-15).
- A simple cutting burr is used for bone removal. If necessary, a diamond burr may also be used, with a technique similar to that described for the craniotomy of the middle fossa (see chapter 32). A multifunctional drill may also be used (e.g. Midas Rex).
- Bleeding of the diploic osseous vessels is halted with bone wax. The open mastoid cells are sutured with bone wax.
- Mannitol is administered before the dural incision. The pre-pontine cistern is opened as well as the cisterna magna, if necessary. The spinal fluid flows out and the CPA space is opened. To retract the cerebellum, a self-retaining retractor may be used. We prefer the

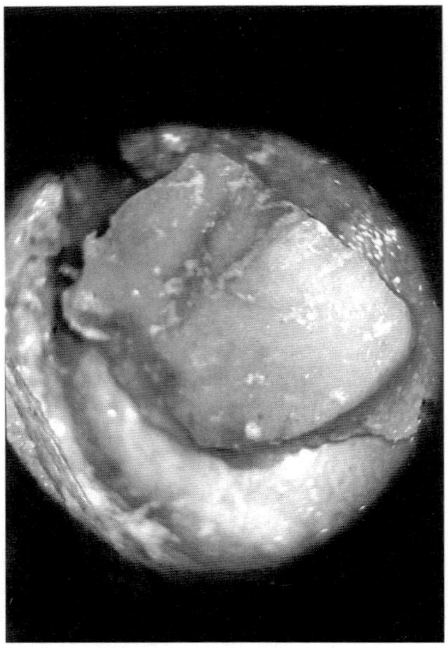

Fig. 19-15. Left ear. A posterior fossa craniotomy window of approx. 3 x 3 cm is made. The anterior limit is the sigmoid sinus, the superior limit is the transverse sinus.

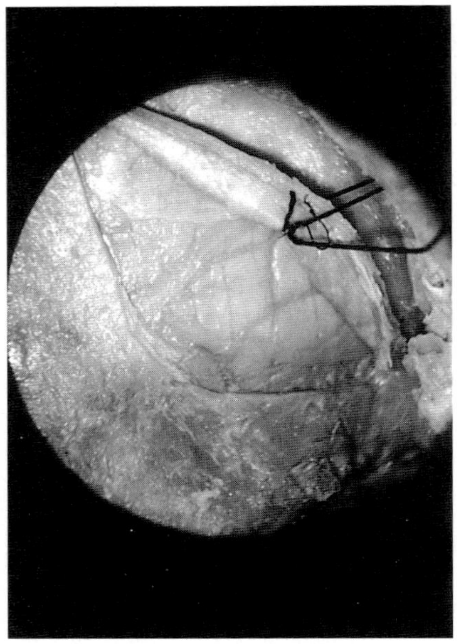

Fig. 19-17. The dural flap is elevated and suspended anteriorly with stay sutures.

simple suction-irrigator placed on a cottonoid which permits enough retraction for the simple sectioning of the nerve (see chapter 28) (Figs. 19-16, 19-17, 19-18, 19-19, 19-20, 19-21, 19-22, 19-23).

Combined retrolabyrinthine-retrosigmoid approach

When a retrosigmoid approach is to be performed, we prefer to combine it with a retrolabyrinthine approach, since in this way we can move the sinus forward and gain visual space between the cerebellum and the underlying nervous and vascular structures (Silverstein 1987) (Fig. 19-24).

A limited mastoidectomy is performed, exposing the sigmoid sinus.

The bleeding spots in the lateral sinus and in the emissary vein(s) are coagulated. The bleeding may also be halted with cellulose sponge (Surgicel) or bovine collagen (Avitene) placed on the bleeding spot and kept in place with a cottonoid.

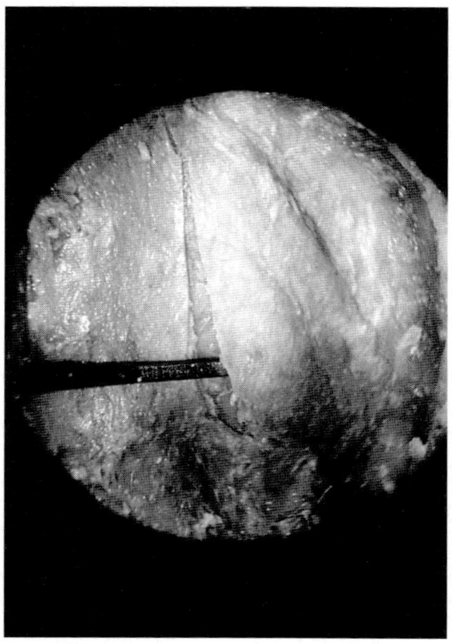

Fig. 19-16. The posterior fossa dura is incised and an anteriorly based dural flap is prepared.

Incision of the Dura

The dura is cut approx. 3 cm behind the sigmoid sinus. The incision is arc-shaped with anterior convexity. In this way, the incision follows the physiological curvature described at the beginning of the transverse sinus and the sigmoid sinus. Two or more sutures are placed in the dural margin and are anchored to the muscular tissue of the skin-muscle flap which was initially elevated.

TIPS AND PITFALLS

In rare cases (1 out of 299) the superior cerebellar artery (SCA)-a branch of the basilar artery-may penetrate in a perforation of the tentorium and exit, making a loop.

When the dura is incised and the cerebellum retracted, the artery may be torn. This can occur in the presence of rare variations in the arterial path, and gives rise to the possibility of cerebellum and/or pons infarction; death may ensue.

Fig. 19-18. The arachnoid of the cistern is lanced with a fenestrated suction-irrigator, CSF is aspirated and the cerebellum falls away medially.

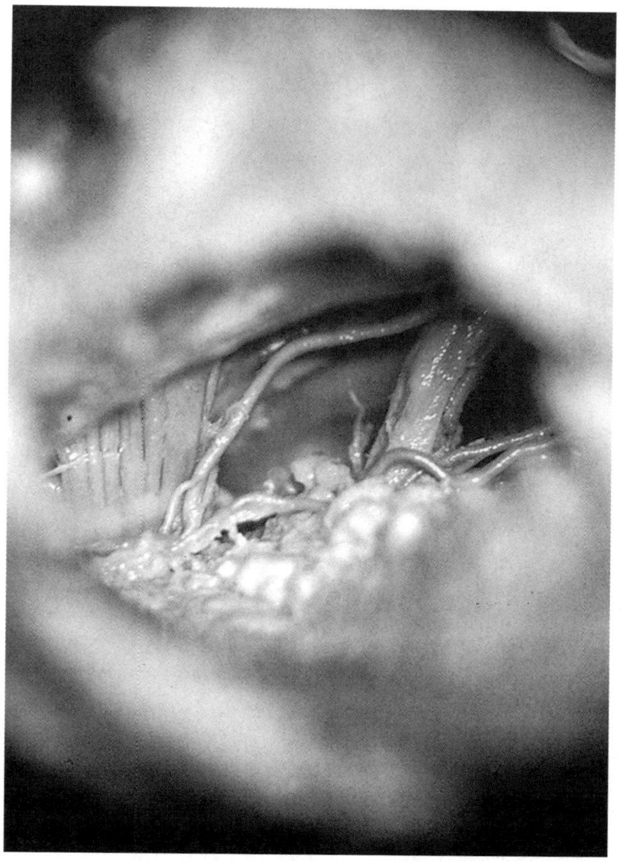

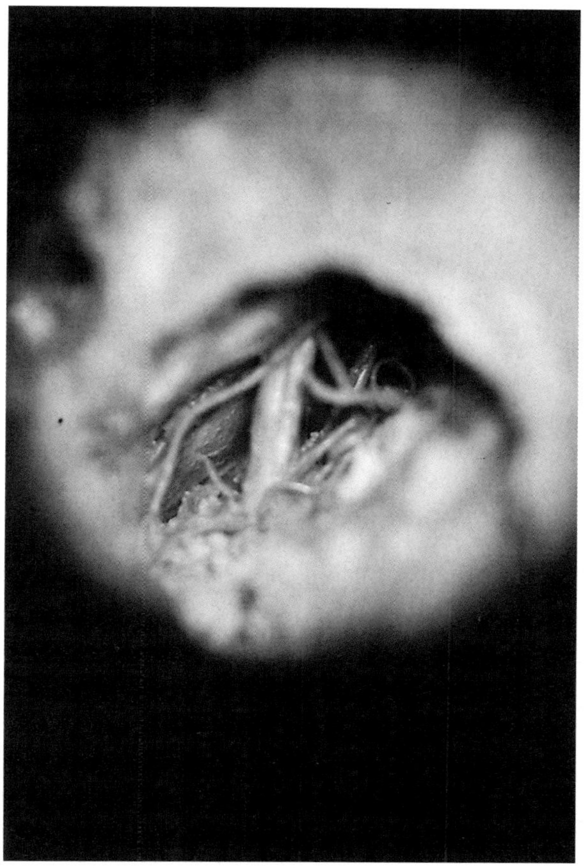

Fig. 19-19. The cochleovestibular nerve is identified. Branches of AICA are visible.

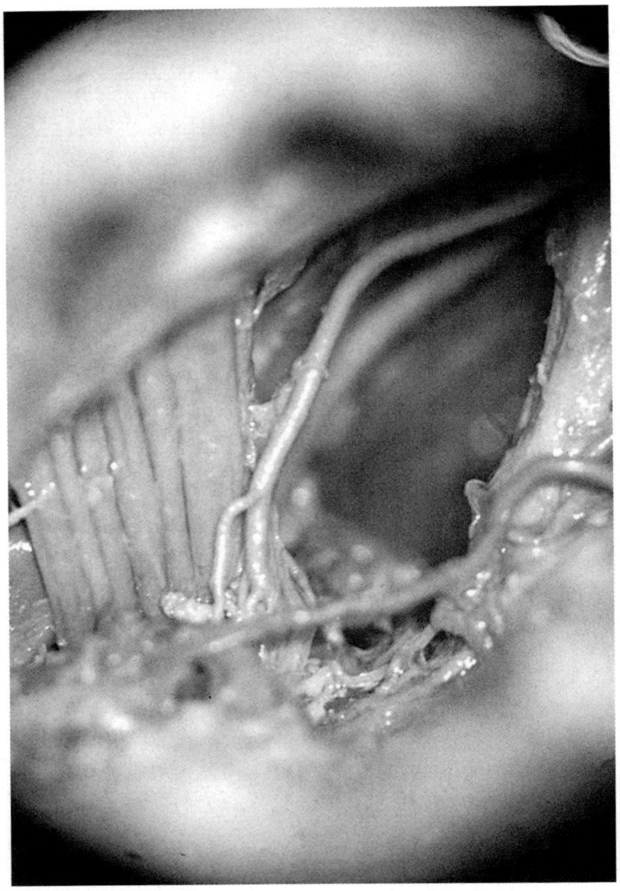

Fig. 19-20. IX-X-XI CNs are seen inferiorly. VIII CN is seen superiorly.

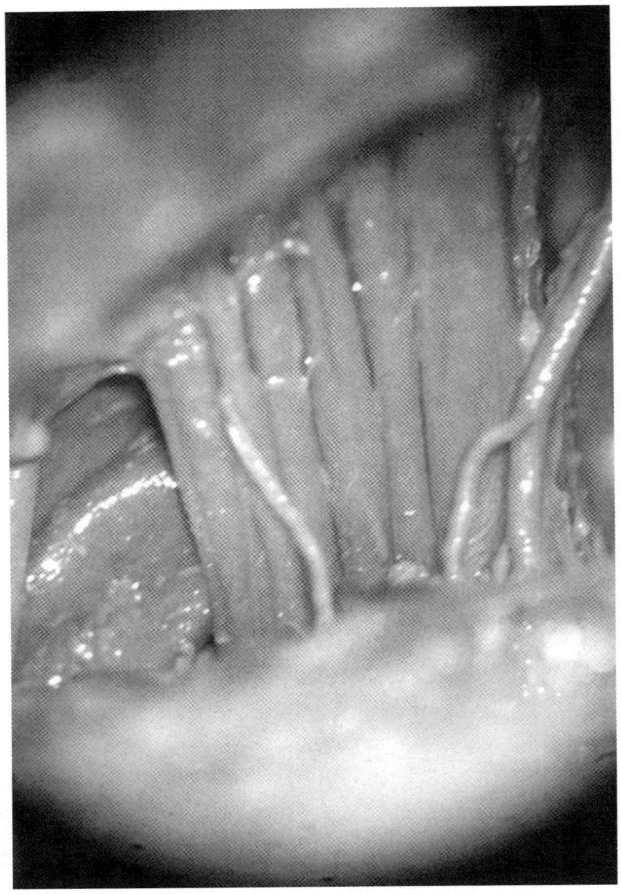

Fig. 19-21. Close-up view of IX-X-XI CNs.

VESTIBULAR NERVE SECTION WITH MIDDLE FOSSA APPROACH

- Until the IAC has been identified, the surgical approach is identical to the one used in removing intrameatal neuromas.
- The bone at the floor of the meatus must be thinned with a 1.5-2 mm diamond burr to safely identify Bill's Bar. If the procedure is followed correctly, the vertical crest may be seen through the overlying V-shaped dura.
- If the vertical crest cannot be identified, the lateral and posterior exposure is continued to the ampulla of the superior canal, until the superior vestibular canal is recognized. This guides us indirectly to the identification of the facial nerve (see chapter 32). The bone is thus completely removed from the IAC, and the dura is opened only at the end. In this way, normal CSF pressure is maintained until the opening of the dura, which pushes the facial and vestibular nerves against the dura and facilitates its identification.
- Superiorly, the craniotomy must be perpendicular to the temporal line, which generally corresponds to the middle cranial fossa floor.
- The IAC must be exposed at the fundus by at least 120°. It is important to expose the posterior margin of the IAC fundus, opposite the SSC and its ampulla, to thoroughly expose the superior vestibular nerve.
- When the entire length of the IAC has been exposed, the dura is opened with a 1-mm straight-angle hook. The point of the hook is directed as laterally as possible, over the dura covering the superior vestibular nerve (to the right in the right ear, to the left in the left ear). The dura is reflected downwards. The superior vestibular nerve is identified and sectioned with a neurectomy scalpel as laterally as possible, superior to Bill's Bar.
- Separating the nerve with a hook is not recommended since this maneuver leads to a trauma of the cochlear nerve or its vascularization.
- The dura of the meatus along the posterior margin of the IAC is cut in a latero-medial direction, to enlarge the field of vision. It is best to perform this incision after having sectioned

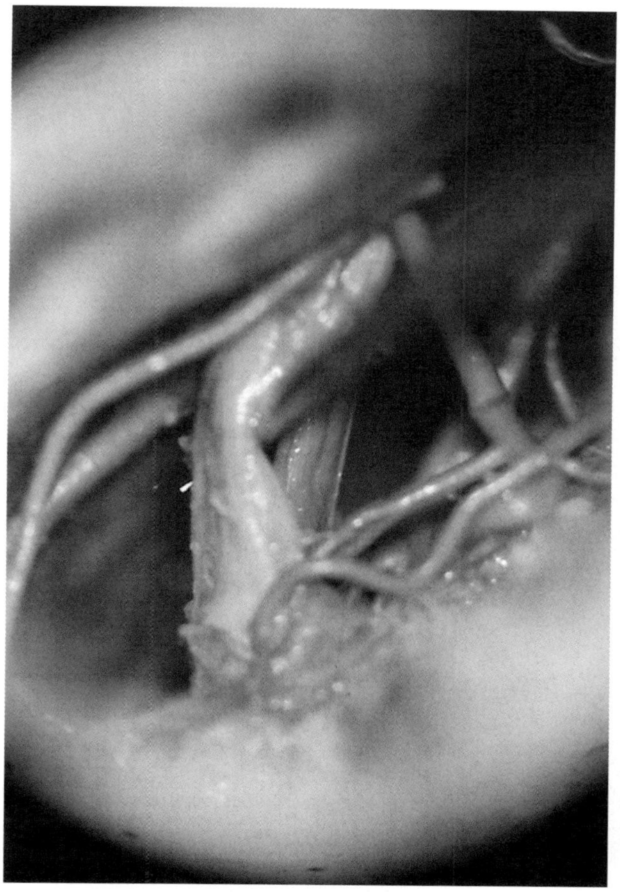

Fig. 19-22. The facial n. is identified by gentle retraction of the vestibulocochlear n.

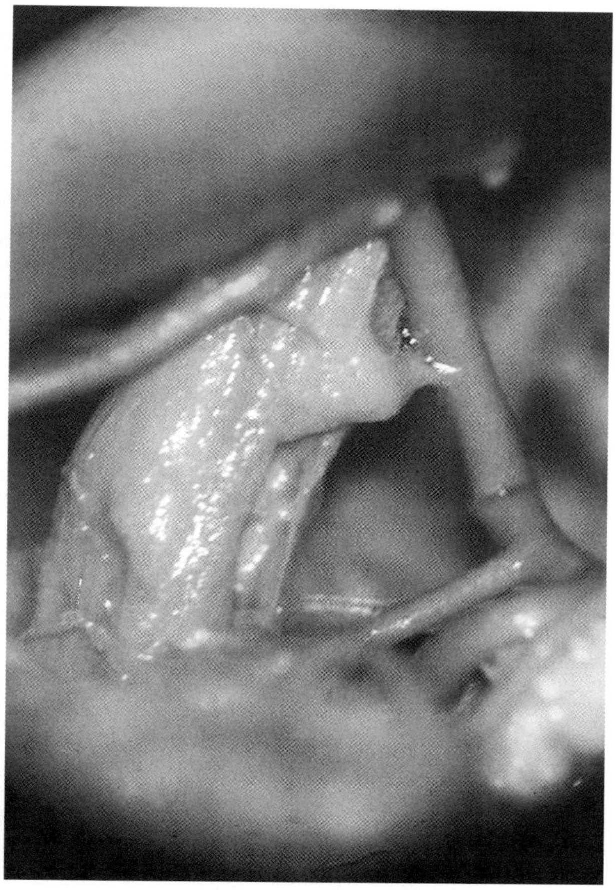

Fig. 19-23. Vestibular nerve is cut. Labyrinthine artery is seen behind the cochlear nerve.

the superior vestibular nerve (SVN). Thus, if the dura is inadvertently passed by with the scalpel and the nerve is hooked, traction is not transmitted to the cochlear nerve.

- The dura above the facial nerve is kept whole, to protect the nerve, which is only partially exposed.
- With a microsuction, the extremity of the SVN is grasped and pulled downward. In this way the inferior vestibular nerve (IVN) is evidentiated along with its two branches, the saccular and singular nerves, which are sectioned with a neurectomy knife. The microsuction is placed on the cut extremity of the IVN and the stumps are medialized, without being pulled. The vestibular facial anastomoses are clipped with neurectomy scissors. The neurectomy scissors are the least traumatic in sectioning. Even the knife does exert traction, although minimal. The slightest trauma in this site may lead to a lesion of the vestibular cochlear artery and/or the cochlear artery, resulting in hearing loss.
- The vestibular nerve is moved medially with the suction. On the medial surface of Scarpa's ganglion, an artery is revealed, which is coagulated with a fine-point bipolar cautery. Scarpa's nerve can be recognized because it represents an enlargement of the nerve and also because of its slightly darker and more yellowish coloration compared to the white of the nerve.
- At this point a pregangliar section of the nerve is performed. With the suction, the ganglion is medialized while it is sectioned with microscissors. The section must begin from the medial surface of the ganglion so that the cut moves progressively away from the facial nerve which is fully visible. To begin the section from the lateral surface of the nerve exposes the facial nerve and the underlying vascularization to risk.
- When the section is finished, the stump of the vestibular nerve is observed near the porus acusticus. The vertical crest masks the view of the horizontal crest, whereas the facial nerve covers the cochlear nerve.
- The internal auditory canal is closed with a fragment of temporalis muscle, which is stabilized with fibrin glue.
- If the tegmen has been opened, it is closed with a fragment of bone (see chapter 32, suggestion).

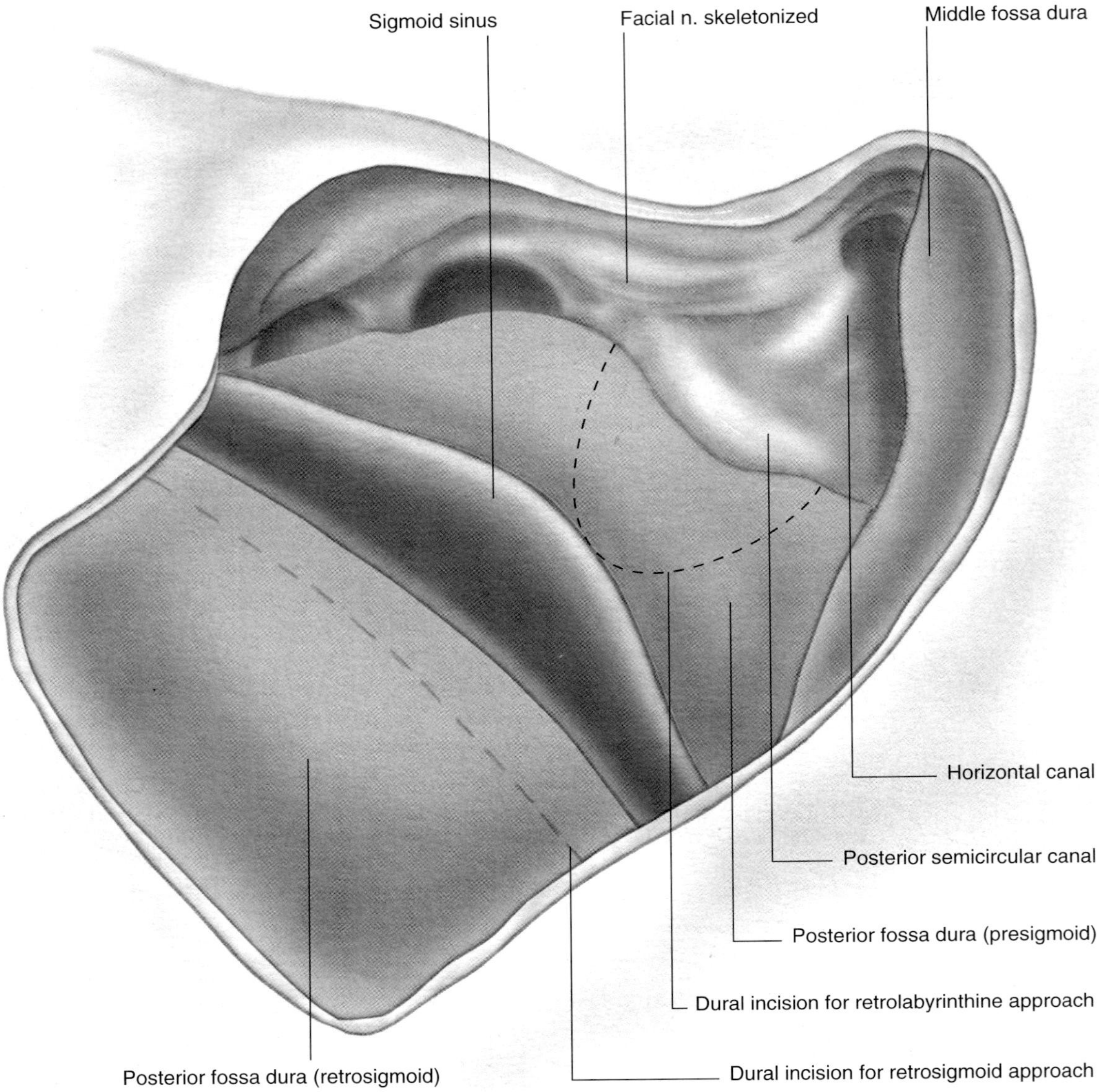

Fig. 19-24. Exposure of the presigmoid dura: retrolabyrinthine approach. Exposure of the retrosigmoid dura: retrosigmoid approach. Both exposures can be used in the combined retrolabyrinthine-retrosigmoid approach, proposed by Silverstein H.

REFERENCES

Belal A Jr. Retrolabyrinthine surgery: Anatomy and pathology. Am J Otol 7:29-33, 1986.

Brackmann DE, Hitselberger WE: Retrolabyrinthine surgery-a direct approach: technique and newer indications. Laryngoscope 88:286-297, 1978.

Dandy W: Effects on hearing after subtotal section on cochlear branch of auditory nerve. Bull John Hopkins Hosp 55: 240-243, 1934.

Dolan EJ, Tuckers WS, Rotenberg D, Chui M: Intracranial hypoglossal schwannoma as un unusual cause of facial nerve palsy. J Neurosurg 56: 420-423, 1982.

Fisch U: Neurectomy of the vestibular nerve. Surgical technique, indication and results in 70 cases. Acta Oto Rhino Laryngol Bel 25: 729-752, 1971.

Fish U: Vestibular neurectomy. In: Silverstein H. Norrel H (edit) Neurological surgery of the ear. Aesculapius Pub (Birmingham-alab) 144-149, 1977.

Glasscock M, Kyeton J, Christiansen S: Middle fossa vestibular neurectomy: An update. Otolaryngol Head Neck Surg 92: 216-220, 1984.

Hitselberger WE, Pulec JL: Trigeminal nerve (posterior root) retrolabyrinthine selective section. Arch Otolaryngol Head Neck Surg 96: 412-415, 1972.

Jones R, Silverstein H, Smouha E: Long-term results of transmeatal cochleovestibular neurectomy: An analysis of 100 cases. Otolaryngol Head Neck Surg 100: 22-29, 1989.

McDaniel A, Silverstein H, Norrell H: Retrolabyrinthine vestibular neurectomy with and without monitoring of 8th nerve potentials. Am J Otol (Supp) 23-6, 1985.

Parry RH: A case of tinnitus and vertigo treated by division of the auditory nerve. J Laryngol Otol 19:402, 1904.

Rosenberg S, Silverstein H, Norrell H, White D: Audio and vestibular function after vestibular neurectomy. Otolaryngol Head Neck Surg 104: 139-140, 1991.

Silverstein H, Norrell H, Haberkamp T, McDaniel A: The unrecognized rotation of the vestibular and cochlear nerves from the labyrinth to the brainstem: Its implications in surgery of the eighth cranial nerve. Otolaryngol Head Neck Surg 95: 543-549, 1986.

Silverstein H, Norrell H, Haberkamp T: A comparison of retrosigmoid IAC, retrolabyrinthine, and middle fossa vestibular neurectomy for treatment of vertigo. Laryngoscope 97(2): 165-173, 1987.

Silverstein H, Norrell H, Rosenberg S: An evolution of approach in vestibular neurectomy. Otolaryngol Head Neck Surg 102: 374-381, 1990.

Silverstein H, Norrell H, Rosenberg S: The resurrection of vestibular neurectomy: A 10-year experience with 115 cases. J Neurosurg 72: 533-539,1990.

Silverstein H, Norrell H, Smouha E, Jones R: Combined retrolab-retrosigmoid vestibular neurectomy: An evolution in approach. Am J Otol 10: 166-169, 1989.

Silverstein H, Norrell H, Smouha E, Jones R: Retrolabyrinthine or retrosigmoid vestibular neurectomy: Indications. Am J Otol 8: 414-418, 1987.

Silverstein H, Norrell H, Smouha E: Retrosigmoid-internal auditory canal approaches vs retrolabyrinthine approach for vestibular neurectomy. Otolaryngol Head Neck Surg 97: 300-307, 1987.

Silverstein H, Norrell H: Retrolabyrinthine surgery: a direct approach to the cerebellopontine angle. Otolaryngol Head Neck Surg 88:462-429, 1980.

Silverstein H, Norrell H: Retrolabyrinthine surgery: A direct approach to the cerebellopontine angle. In Silverstein H, Norrell H (eds): Neurological Surgery of the Ear, Vol II, Birmingham, AL, Aesculapius, 1979, p. 318.

Silverstein H, Rosenberg S: Intraoperative facial nerve monitoring. Otolaryngol Clin North Am 24: 709-725, 1991.

Silverstein H, Rosenberg S: Vestibular neurectomy via the posterior fossa. In Silverstein H, Rosenberg S (eds): Surgical techniques of the temporal bone and skull base. Philadelphia, Lea & Febiger, 1992, pp 175-194.

Silverstein H, Wanamaker H, Flanzer J, Rosenberg S: Vestibular neurectomy in the USA 1990. Am J Otol 13: 23-30, 1992.

Silverstein H, Wazen J, Norrell H, Hyman S: Retrolabyrinthine vestibular neurectomy with simultaneous monitoring of eighth nerve action potentials and electrocochleography. Am J Otol 5: 552-555, 1984.

Silverstein H, Norrell H, Snouha E, et al. Retrosigmoid-internal auditory canal approach vs. retrolabyrinthine approach for vestibular neurectomy. Otolaryngol Head Neck Surg 97:300-307, 1987.

Silverstein H: Cochlear and vestibular gross and histologic anatomy (as seen from the postauricular approach). Otolaryngol Head Neck Surg 92: 207-211, 1984.

Silverstein H: Microsurgical instruments and nerve stimulator monitor for retrolabyrinthine vestibular neurectomy. Otolaryngol Head Neck Surg 94: 409-411, 1986.

Silverstein H: Silverstein lateral venous sinus retractor. Otolaryngol Head Neck Surg 89: 303-304, 1981.

Silverstein H: Silverstein wrist rest. Otolaryngol Head Neck Surg 89: 305-306, 1981.

Silverstein H: Transmeatal labyrinthectomy with and without cochleovestibular neurectomy. Laryngoscope 86: 1777-1791, 1976.

Zini C, Mazzoni A, Gandolfi A, Sanna M, Pasanisi E: Retrolabyrinthine vs. middle fossa vestibular neurectomy. Am J Otol 9: 448-450, 1984.

20

Transcanal labyrinthectomy

A transcanal labyrinthectomy abolishes vertigo by destroying vestibular function.

It provokes hearing loss and thus must be reserved for patients with disabling vertigo: this is correlated with age, profession, recurrence of the episodes. Hearing in the contralateral ear must also be taken into consideration, as well as the patient's needs and residual hearing. In the past, the limit was set at 50 dB of hearing loss and 50% of speech discrimination. Today we recommend operating patients with serious or profound hearing loss, a speech reception threshold greater than or equal to 75 dB, and a speech discrimination score less than or equal to 20% (Nadol et al). The definition of non-usable hearing thus tends to be more and more restricted, due to the improvements in hearing aids developed and the evolving concept of the role of binaural hearing in central comprehension.

The clinical success of the operation is also positively influenced by good capacity for compensation. It is lower in elderly subjects with arthrosic alterations, obese or sedentary subjects, or subjects "weak-willed".

SURGICAL TECHNIQUE

- General anesthesia is used to prevent an acute vestibular response during surgery. If a second operation is performed, local anesthesia is recommended; the symptomatic response signals when the residual zone of the vestibule has been reached.
- The hair is cut 4 cm behind the auricle, in case it becomes necessary during surgery to pass to a postauricular approach.
- The patient is placed in a supine position, with his head turned as in a mastoidectomy; preparation is the same.
- A tympano-meatal flap is elevated with the apex 7-8 mm above the fibrous annulus (Fig. 20-1). Part of the posterior bony annulus is removed, with the operating table inclined toward the surgeon to provide the best visual angle possible, until the second part of the facial nerve, the footplate and the round window niche have been exposed.
- The incudo-stapedial articulation is disarticulated. The incus is removed and displaced into the epitympanum. The tendon of the stapes is clipped as close as possible to the promontory. The stapes is mobilized and removed in an anterior-posterior direction, to exert pressure on the posterior crus, the more robust of the two. The stapes is thus removed in its entirety, along with the footplate (Fig. 20-2).
- The oval window is enlarged anteriorly and inferiorly. In order to obtain an optimal exposure of the underlying vestibular organs, it is helpful to connect the oval window with the round window, drilling a part of the promontory. In this way the basal turn of the cochlea is exposed (Fig. 20-3).
- A 1 mm diameter diamond burr is used. The instrument nurse irrigates the field with a few drops and the bone debris is removed with a n. 18 suction, with the extremities pointed outside the oval window, so as not to aspirate the vestibular structures.
- The purpose of the operation is to completely destroy the neuroepithelium of the ampullae (the ampullary crests), and of the vestibule and saccule (the maculas). The utricle is not aspirated due to the danger of dislodging it; in general, it is retracted upward under the horizontal part of the facial nerve, making its subsequent complete removal more difficult. A 4 mm utricular hook with a whirlybird edge is used. The utricle is removed beginning at the superior part of the vestibule, with the hook lightly touching the medial part of the vestibule; care is taken not to break the cribriform area which corresponds to the superior wall of the internal auditory canal, to avoid a subsequent CSF fistula. At times the utricle is dislodged above and behind an en-

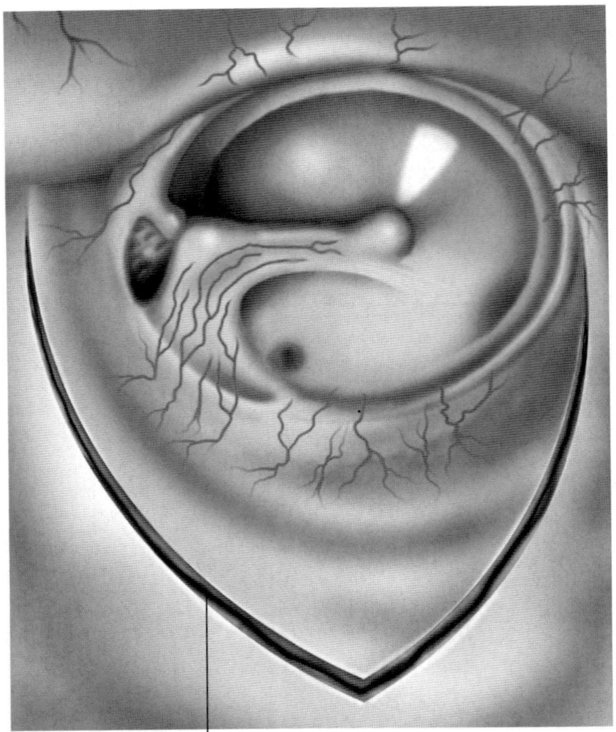

Fig. 20-1. Transcanal labyrinthectomy: the incisions.

larged saccule (e.g. by successive hydropsic crises) and its identification is made more difficult.

- Care must be taken not to damage the medial part of the horizontal tract of the facial nerve, which runs behind the oval window, with the hook.
- While removing the utricle, the crests of the lateral and superior canal ampullae are also removed. The bony walls of the two ampullae are scraped with the hook, after which the hook is brought into the ampulla of the posterior canal; here the ampullar crista and the posterior ampullary nerve are removed (Fig. 20-4).

CLOSURE

Once the vestibular organs have been destroyed, the vestibule is closed with fat taken from the earlobe. Another method is to use Streptomycin-soaked Gelfoam to destroy the residual neuroepithelium, followed by fat packing (Fig. 20-5). After packing, communication between the vestibule and the middle ear is occluded, thus preventing the risk of a CSF fistula. The cribriform bone of the medial wall of the vestibule makes up the lateral wall of the internal auditory canal. If an intraoperative fistula does occur, a profuse flow of liquor will be seen. The fistula is closed with fat and/or fascia. Fibrin glue may be helpful in closure.

POST-OPERATIVE PERIOD

- In the postoperative period, a vestibular reaction is seen, its intensity being directly proportional to the pre-operative vestibular function. Symptoms are controlled with suppressants, such as Dimenhydrinate or Prochlorpemazine or Promethazine hydrochloride or Droperidol. The immuno-suppressant treatment must be suspended as soon as possible, because it masks the organism's recognition of the structural modifications which have taken place, slowing compensation.

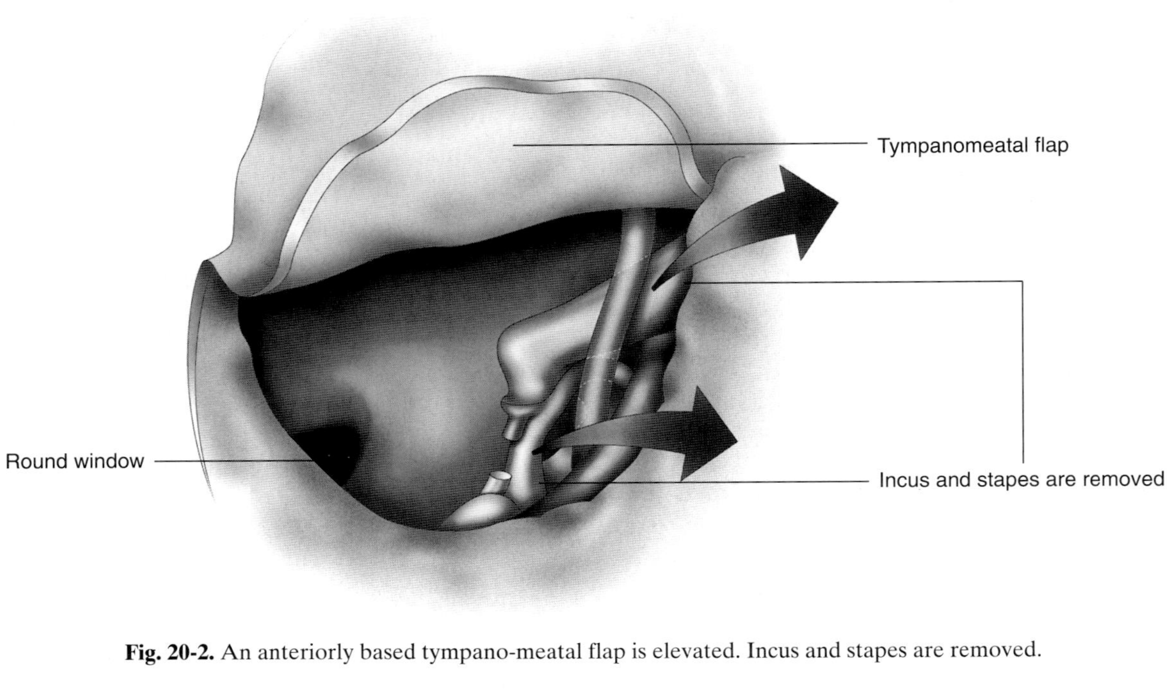

Fig. 20-2. An anteriorly based tympano-meatal flap is elevated. Incus and stapes are removed.

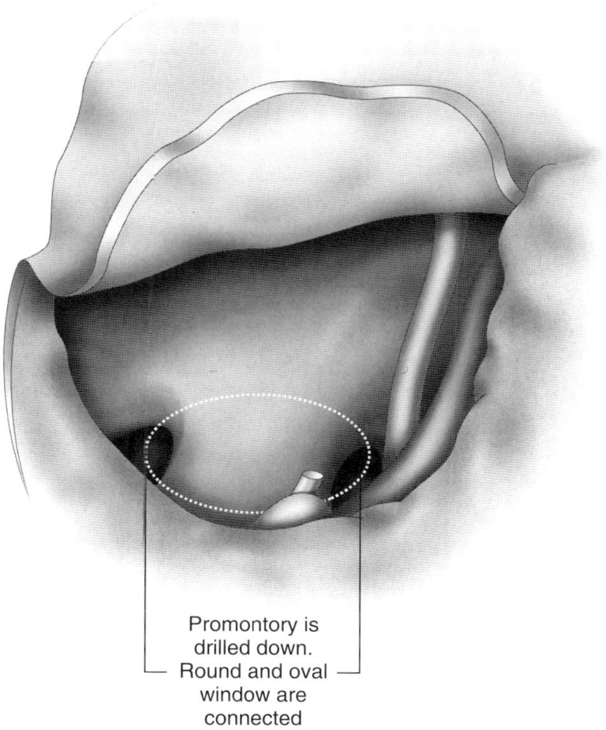

Fig. 20-3. Round and oval windows are connected with cutting burr.

- The patient is encouraged to resume a sitting position and walk as soon as possible, and can generally be released within a week. At the one month check-up the sense of instability is generally gone, as well as the spontaneous Ny. According to Fitzgerald-Hallpike, the caloric test will reveal a complete areflexia if a successful vestibular ablation has been performed.
- The opposite is not always true, however: a complete areflexia does not necessarily indicate a complete vestibular ablation. In the latter case it is the clinic which lead the following decisions.
- The persistence of vestibular symptoms requires a new surgical operation. A revision of the transcanal labyrinthectomy is not recommended, since scarring makes recognition of the vestibular tissue more difficult (Fig. 20-6). Thus a transmastoid labyrinthectomy is preferable, destroying the bony part of the vestibular organs, associated with a section of the vestibular nerve.

The transcanal labyrinthectomy can be extended deeper to obtain total vestibular ablation, by per-

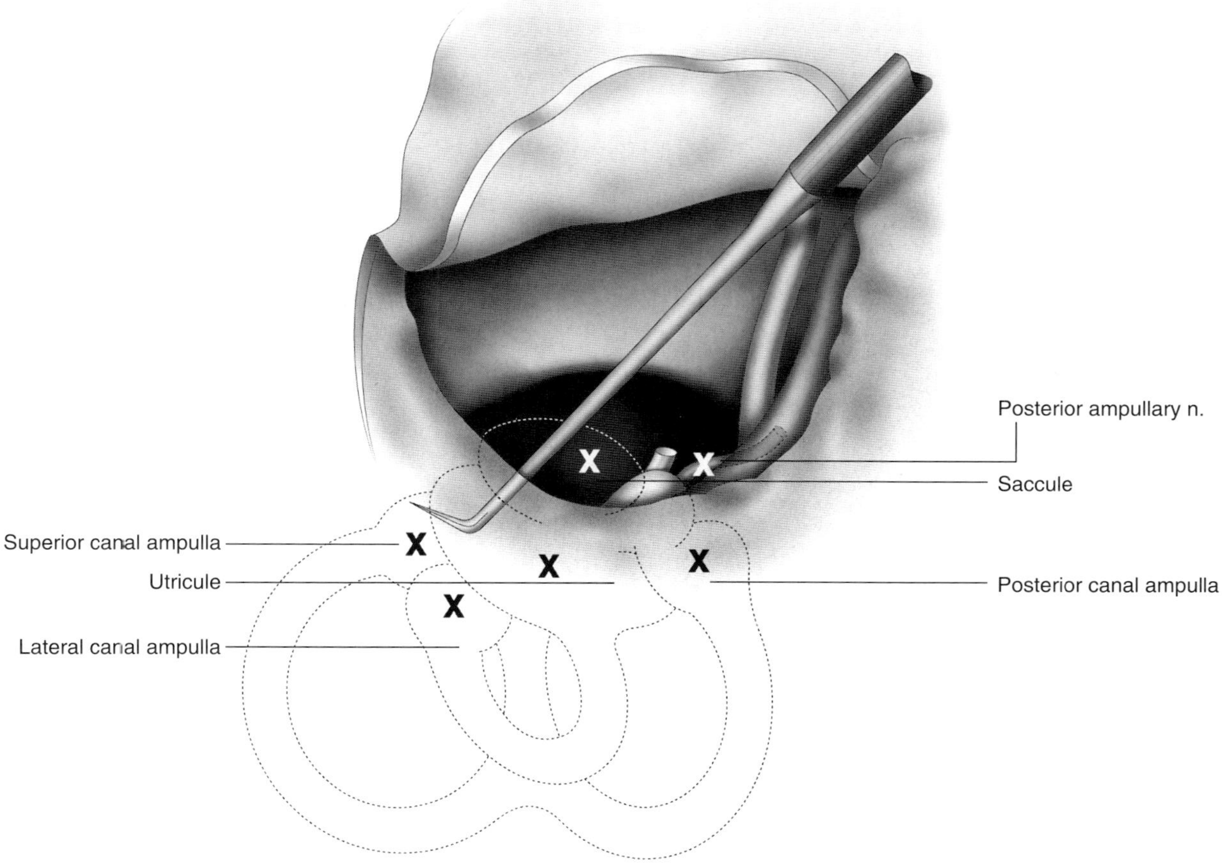

Fig. 20-4. The neuroepithelium of the five vestibular end organs (utricle, saccule, ampullae of the three semicircular canals) is destroyed with a hook (Adapted from Nadol JB and McKenna MJ).

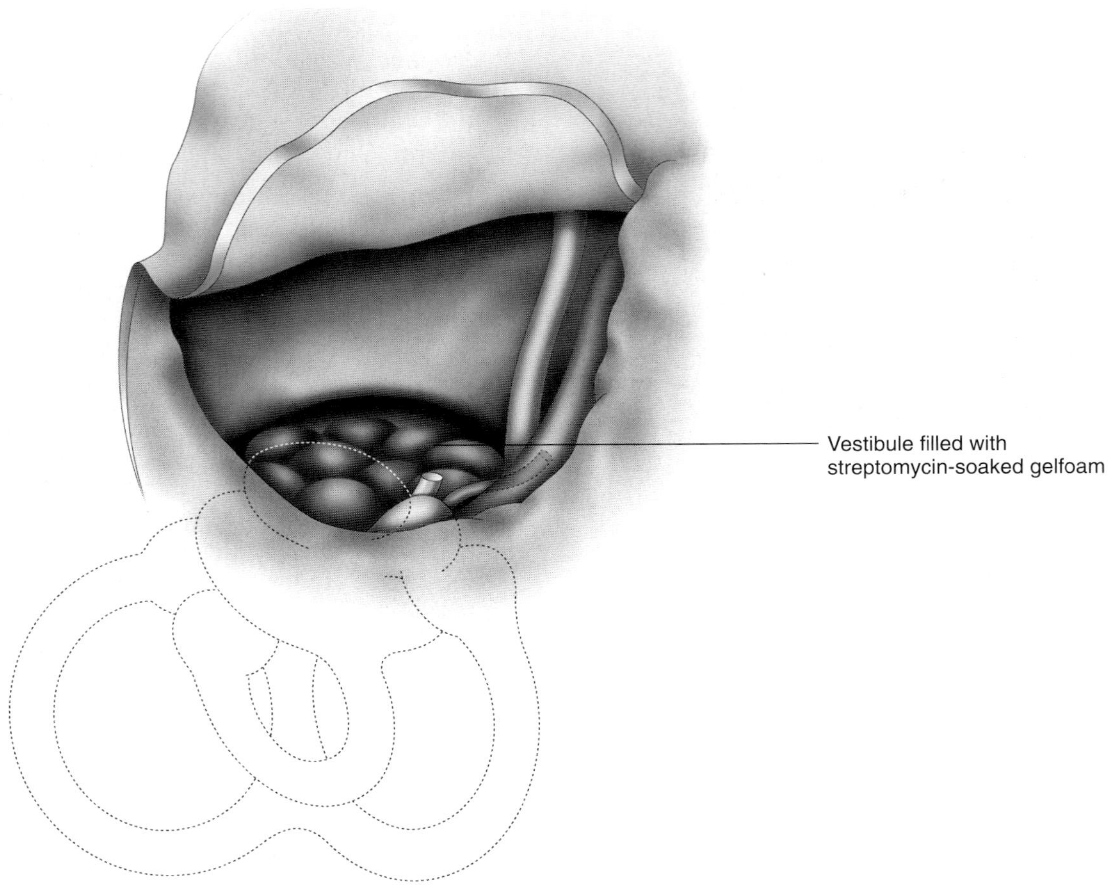

Fig. 20-5. The vestibule is packed with streptomycin-soaked Gelfoam (Adapted from Nadol JB and McKenna MJ).

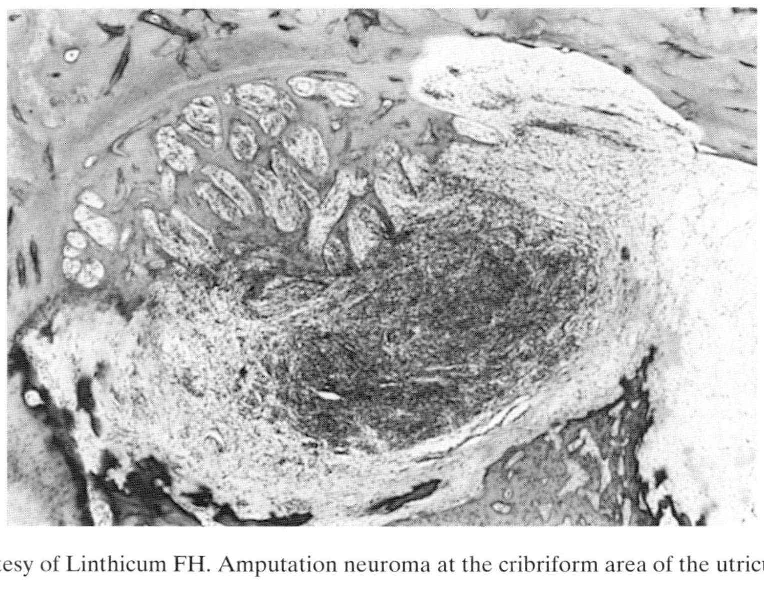

Fig. 20-6. Courtesy of Linthicum FH. Amputation neuroma at the cribriform area of the utricular nerve. X40.

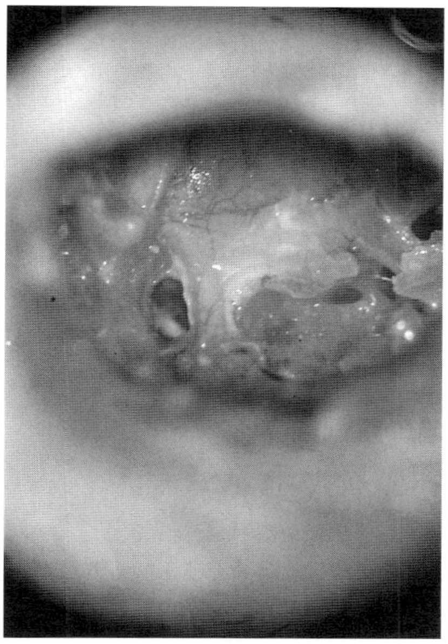

Fig. 20-7. The transcanal labyrinthectomy can be extended deeper to obtain total vestibular ablation, performing a transmeatal cochleovestibular neurectomy. A tympanomeatal flap is elevated through a transcanal approach. The stapes and incus are removed and the oval and round window are connected with a microdrill.

forming a *transmeatal cochleovestibular neurectomy*. This approach allows a more restricted exposure then the translabyrinthine vestibular neurectomy and places the facial nerve at greater risk (Figs. 20-7, 20-8).

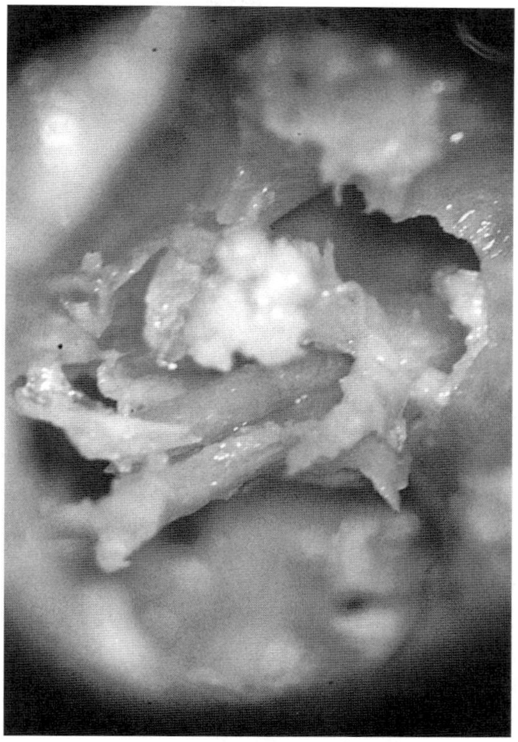

Fig. 20-8. The bone superior and inferior to the cochlear nerve is removed. The dura of the IAC is exposed and opened with a sharp hook, transecting the inferior vestibular nerve. The neural contents of the IAC are visualized. The superior vestibular nerve is separated from the deeper facial nerve. In the figure, in a clockwise motion, the inferior vestibular n. is anterior left, the cochlear nerve is anterior right, the superior vestibular n. is posterior right, the facial n. is posterior left.

REFERENCES

Ariagno RP: Transtympanic labyrinthectomy. Arch Otolaryngol Head Neck Surg 80: 282-286, 1964.

Armstrong BW: Transtympanic vestibulotomy for Mèniére's disease. Laryngoscope 69: 1071-1074,1959.

Belal A, Ylikoski J: Pathology as it relates to ear surgery. II. Labyrinthectomy. J Laryngol Otol 97: 1-10,1983.

Cawthorne T: Membranous labyrinthectomy via the oval window for Mèniére's disease. J Laryngol Otol 71: 524-527,1957.

Cawthorne TE: The treatment of Mèniére's disease. J Laryngol Otol 58: 63-71,1943.

Chen DA, Linthicum, RH, Rizer FM: Cochlear histopathology in the labyrinthectomized ear: Implications for cochlear implantation. Laryngoscope 98: 1170-1172,1988.

Crockett EA: The removal of the stapes for the relief of auditory vertigo. Ann Otol Rhinol Laryngol 12: 67-72,1903.

Dandy WE: Mèniére's disease: Its diagnosis and a method of treatment. Arch Surg 16: 1127-1152,1928.

Gacek RR: Transection of the posterior ampullary nerve for the relief of benign paroxysmal positional vertigo. Ann Otol Rhinol Laryngol 83: 596-605,1974.

Greven AJ, Oosterveld WJ: The contralateral ear in Mèniére's disease. Arch Otolaryngol Head Neck Surg 101: 608-612,1978.

Hammerschlag PE, Schuknecht HF: Transcanal labyrinthectomy for intractable vertigo. Arch Otolaryngol Head Neck Surg 107: 152-156, 1981.

Hilding DA, House WF: "Acoustic neuroma": Comparison of traumatic and neoplastic. J Ultrastruct Res 12: 611-623, 1965.

Jansen A: Referat uber die operationsmethoden bei den verschiedenen otitischen gehirukoneplikationen. Verh Dtsch Otol Gesell (Jena), 1895, p 96.

Kszeton JF, Abbott C, April M, et al: Cochlear implantation after transmastoid labyrinthectomy. Laryngoscope 99: 610-613,1989.

Lake R: Removal of the semicircular canals in a case of unilateral aural vertigo. Lancet i: 1567-1568,1904.

Lambert PR, Ruth RA, Halpin CF: Promontory electrical stimulation in labyrinthectomized ears. Arch Otolaryngol Head Neck Surg 116: 197-201,1990.

Lempert J: Lempert decompression operation for hydrops of the endolymphatic labyrinth in Mèniére's disease. Arch Otolaryngol Head Neck Surg 47: 551-570,1948.

Linthicum FH, Alonso A, Denia A: Traumatic neuroma. Arch Otolaryngol Head Neck Surg 105: 654-655,1979.

Milligan W: Mèniére's disease: A clinical and experimental inquiry. Br Med J 2: 1228,1904.

Nadol JB Jr: Positive "fistula sign" with an intact tympanic membrane. Arch Otolaryngol Head Neck Surg 100: 273-278,1974.

Paparella MM, Griebie MS: Bilaterality of Mèniére's disease. Acta Otolaryngol (Stockh) 97: 233-237,1984.

Pulec JL: Labyrinthectomy: Indications, technique and results. Laryngoscope 84: 1552-1573,1974.

Schuknecht HF: Ablation therapy for the relief of Mèniére's disease. Laryngoscope 66: 859-870,1956.

Schuknecht HF: Ablation therapy in the management of Mèniére's disease. Acta Otolaryngol Suppl (Stockh) 132: 1-42,1957.

Schuknecht HF: Behavior of the vestibular nerve following labyrinthectomy. Ann Otol Rhinol Laryngol 91 (5 Suppl 97): 1632,1982.

Schuknecht HF: Destructive labyrinthine surgery. Arch Otolaryngol Head Neck Surg 97: 150-151,1973.

Schuknecht HF: Destructive therapy for Mèniére's disease. Arch Otolaryngol Head Neck Surg 71: 562-572,1960.

Silverstein H, Smouha E, Jones R: Natural history versus surgery for Mèniére's disease. In Nadol JB Jr (ed): Second International Symposium for Mèniére's disease. Amsterdam, Kugler & Ghedini Publishers, 1989, pp 543-544.

Stockwell CW, Graham MD: Vestibular compensation following labyrinthectomy and vestibular neurectomy. In Nadol JB Jr (ed): Second International Symposium for Mèniére's disease. Amsterdam, Kugler & Ghedini Publishers, 1989, pp 489-498.

21

Posterior ampullary nerve section

Surgical theraphy of benign positional paroxysmal vertigo

Benign positional paroxysmal vertigo (BPPV), described by Barany in 1921, is characterized by brief recurring episodes of vertigo which are produced with backward head movements from an ortostatic position, or sideways movements from a supine position. It may also be provoked by movements such as bending forward, shaking the head, getting out of bed suddenly...

The most frequent cause is cranial trauma, often resulting from car accidents. Other causes are: viral labyrinthitis, vestibular neuronitis, chronic otitis media, and traumas transmitted to the inner ear during middle ear surgery.

The etiology proposed by Schuknecht hypothesized that the cause of inner ear debris formation was probably utricular otoliths. These debrises then reach the ampulla of the posterior semicircular canal and deposits on the dome. The dome is weighted down by calcium carbonate (cupololitiasis). The canal, usually sensitive only to a rotary acceleration, becomes sensitive to linear and gravitational acceleration as well. This is why during the Hallpike maneuver the particles deposited on the cupola move away, taking the dome with them, and causing nystagmus and vertigo.

The particles freely fluctuating in the endolymph also have a catalyzing role. During the Hallpike maneuver, they move away from the cupola and provoke a solid endolymphatic flow which dislodges it.

The Hallpike maneuver

- The patient, seated on the bed, is brought rapidly into a supine position, with the head down to a head-hanging position, turned to one side. Within 2-10 seconds nystagmic impulses are evoked lasting several seconds, along with vertigo and frequently nausea.
- Two to three minutes after the nystagmic waves have ceased, the patient is brought once again to a sitting position. After a few seconds, the nystagmus occurs again, this time in an inverse direction.
- The maneuver is repeated using the same technique but turning the head to the other side.
- The excitation of the oblique superior ipsilateral muscle and of the contralateral inferior rectus muscle in the lateral Hallpike position provokes nystagmus. Its rapid phase is always geotropic, while the slow phase is rotational in a clockwise direction on the right-hand side, and counterclockwise on the left-hand side. Upon returning to a sitting position, the nystagmus assumes an opposite direction, is less intense, and the intensity of the vertigo is lesser.
- The repetition of the maneuver provokes a reduction in the symptoms and the duration of the nystagmus, testifying to a peripheral pathology (Fig. 21-1).

  Parnes and Price-Jones reported favorable results with the particle repositioning maneuvres, effective on the free-floating particles wich are the most common cause of BPPV (Fig. 21-2)

SURGICAL TECHNIQUE

- The incision for the tympano-meatal flap is higher then that used for stapedectomy.
- The round window is exposed (Fig. 21-3). The anterior bone projection is removed with a 1 mm diamond burr. A mucous membrane is often seen, and is removed with a hook. Medially to the bone protrusion is the membrane of the round window. The membrane is dark gray in color and has a homogeneous structure. It is not recommended to touch the ossicles to observe the movement of the windows and obtain

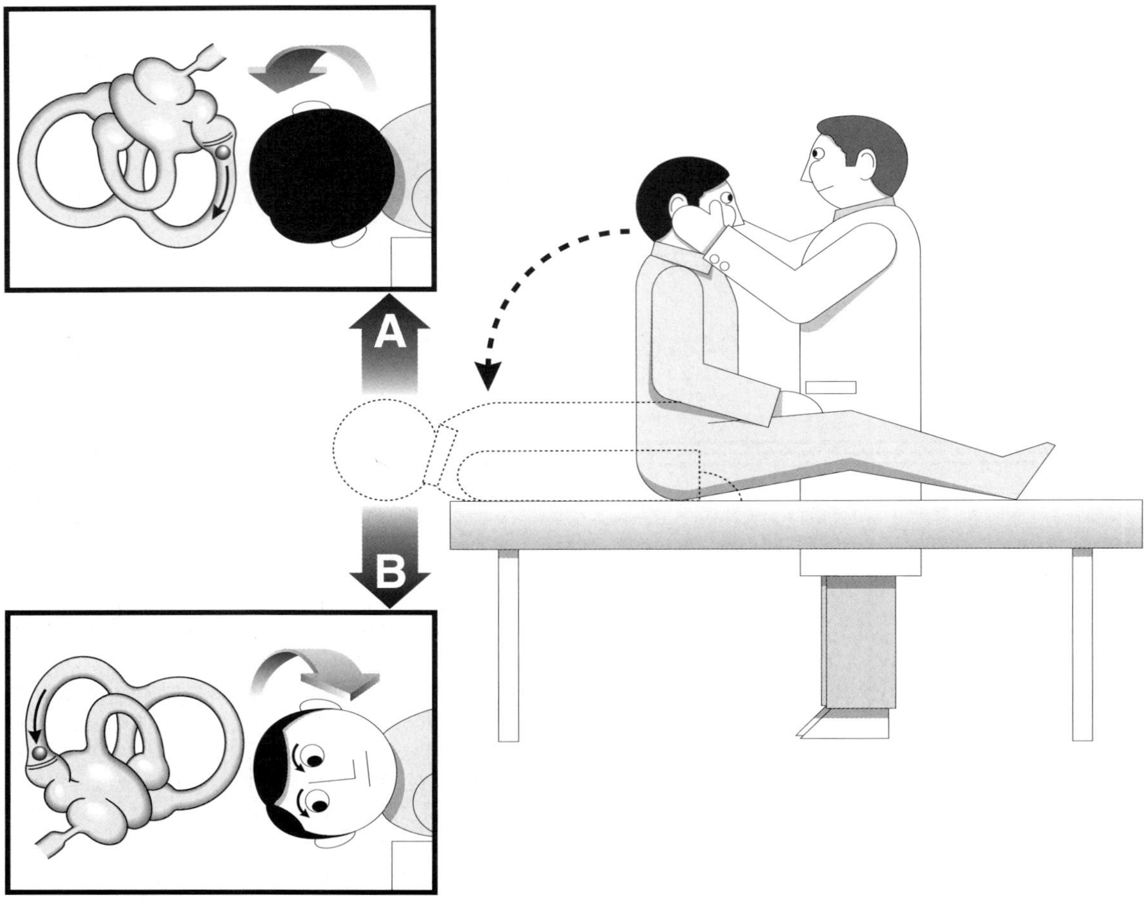

Fig. 21-1. Right ear affected. **A**: no vestibular response. **B**: when the involved ear is geotropic, cupular deflection causes depolarization. There is a latency of a few seconds, then rotatory nystagmus that builds to a crescendo and finishes over a period of approx. 30 sec. Vertigo subsides in 2-3 minutes. Nystagmus reappears when the sitting position is reassumed.

confirmation that the round window is the one in question; this is a completely antiphysiological movement and could damage the inner ear.

- A niche is dug with the burr posterior to the round window, near its superior margin (Fig. 21-4). The niche is deepened by approx. 2 mm. The nerve, which appears white due to its myelin fibers, is identified, thin. Sometimes the nerve cannot be identified. In this case, the niche is enlarged toward the round window membrane insertion and the nerve is sought further forward and from top to bottom, under the round window membrane insertion.
- The identification of the nerve is confirmed by the vestibular response and/or pain of the patient. The nerve lies in a bone canal and can be divided in three parts: the cribriform part, which exits the ampulla of the posterior canal; the intermediate part; and the canalicular part below the vestibular floor, nearing it to the inferior vestibular nerve. With a 0.5 mm hook the proximal extremity of the canal is explored. In this way the intermediate part of the nerve is destroyed. The maneuver must be delicate and repeated to interrupt all the nerve fibers. It is important not to proceed too proximal toward the canalicular tract, because of the risk of provoking a CSF fistula. Neither should we proceed too distally, because of the risk of injuring the ampulla of the posterior canal (Fig. 21-5).
- When the nerve has been completely interrupted, the posterior bony wall of the IAC is drilled to collect a small amount of bone dust which is then positioned inside the canal. In this way, the bone acts as a biological barrier and impedes regeneration of the nerve fibers. More bone dust is used to fill the gap left by the burr.
- The tympano-meatal flap is turned over. The dressing and the following phases are the same as in otosclerosis surgery.

TIPS AND PITFALLS

- If the hook is pushed too proximally towards the canalicular tract which lies under the vestibule, a CSF fistula may be provoked. Here, the nerve is

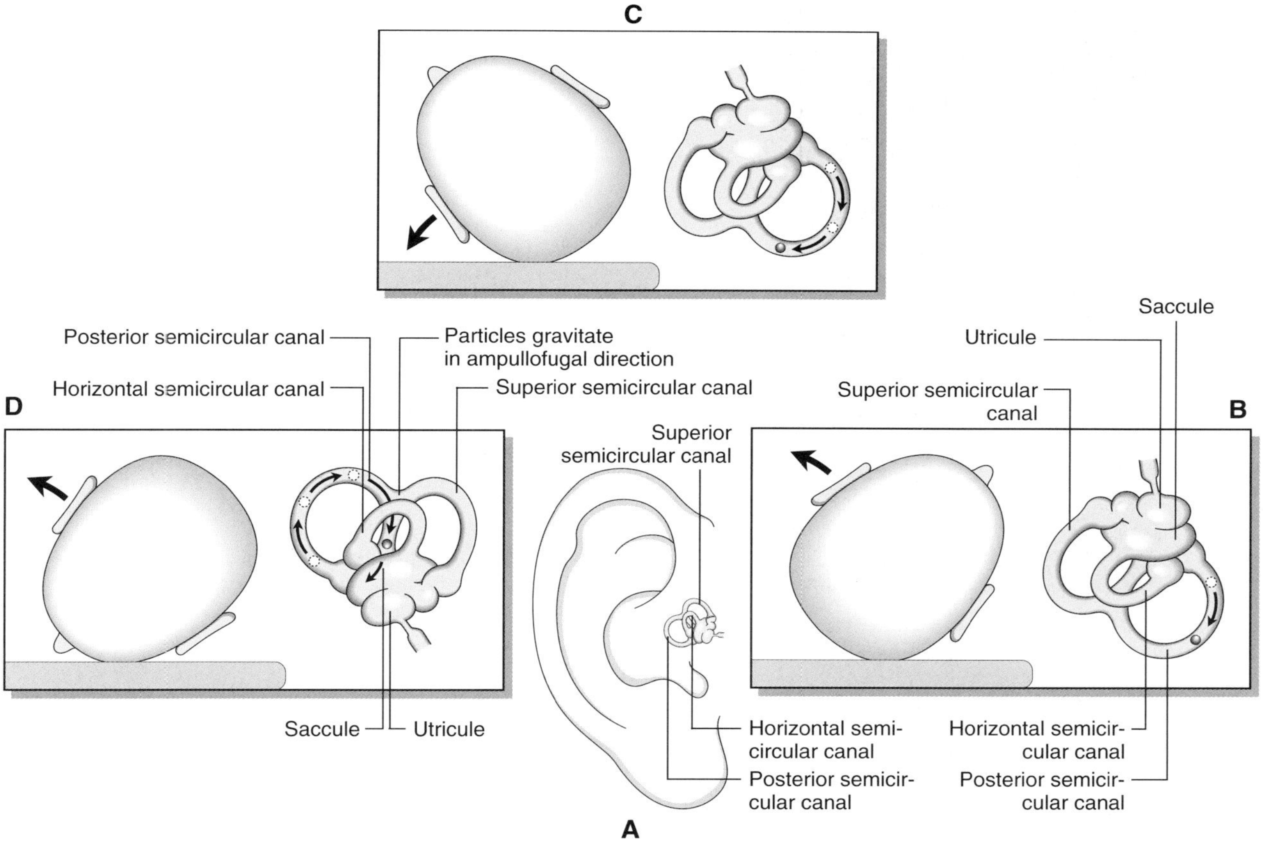

Fig. 21-2. A: Particle repositioning maneuver. Orthostatic position. **B:** Hallpike head position (3 minutes), then a steady continuous motion is performed (c-d). **C:** Middle position. **D:** Final position. Particles gravitate into utricule. (Adapted from Parnes L.).

surrounded by CSF. In this situation, it is sufficient to pack the fistula with adipose tissue.

- Since drilling is done nearby, the risk of damaging the round window and the cochlea with it is high. It is thus helpful to preserve a small bone bridge between the round window and the area where the drilling is being performed (Gacek).

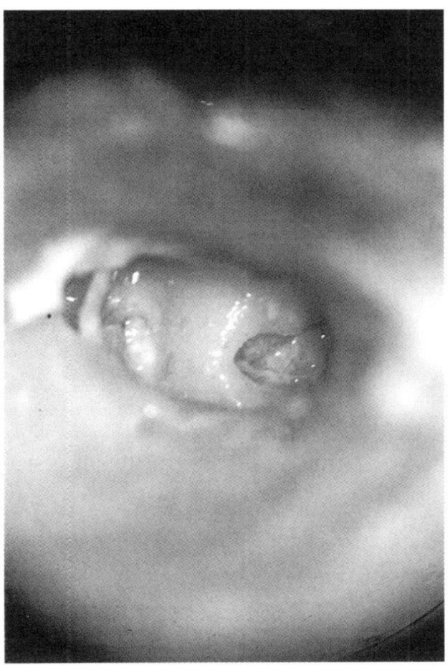

Fig. 21-3. The superior lip of bone of the round window niche is drilled away, exposing the round window membrane.

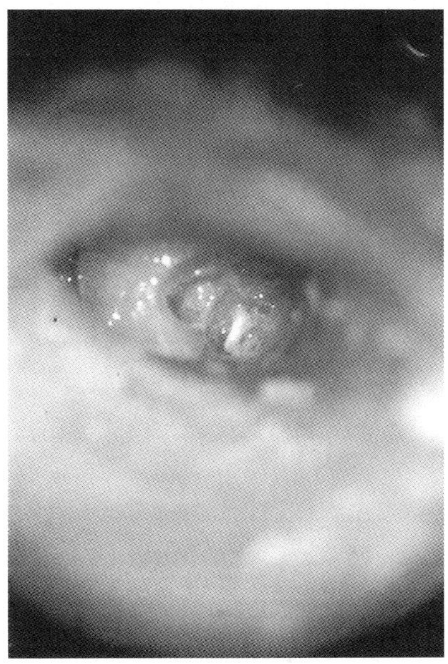

Fig. 21-4. The bone posterior and inferior to the round window membrane is drilled away. The posterior ampullary nerve (singular) is visualized.

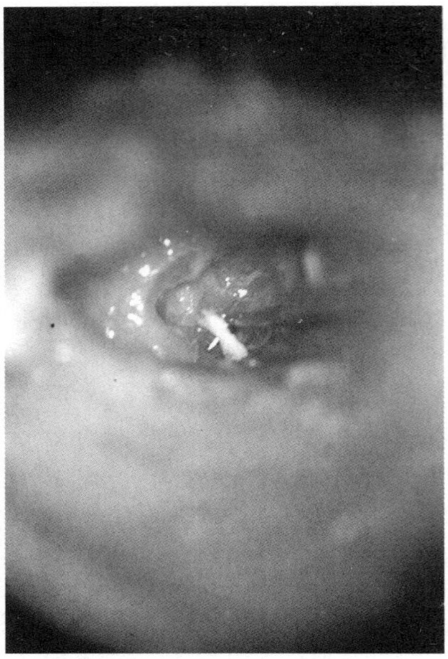

Fig. 21-5. The singular nerve is transected with a hook.

- Finding the singular nerve is difficult since its path varies, especially when the nerve lies under the insertion of the membrane in the round window. In cases where the nerve is not visible, we must go by the patient's reaction. When the hook touches the nerve, the patient will express pain and vertigo. This is possible only when using local anesthesia.

REFERENCES

Barany R: Diagnose non Krankheitserscheinungen im Bereiche des Otolithenapparates. Acta Otolaryngol (Stockh) 2: 434-437, 1921.

Barber HO: Positional nystagmus, especially after head injury. Laryngoscope 74: 891-944,1964.

Brandt T, Daroff RB: Physical therapy for benign paroxysmal positional vertigo. Arch Otolaryngol Head Neck Surg 106: 484-485, 1980.

Carmichael EA, Dix MR, Hallpike CS: Pathology, symptomatology and diagnosis of the organic affections of the eighth nerve system. Br Med Bull 12: 146-152,1956.

Gacek RR: Pathophysiology and management of cupulolithiasis. Am J Otolaryngol 6: 66-74, 1985.

Gacek RR: Singular neurectomy update. II. Review of 102 cases. Laryngoscope 101: 855-862, 1991.

Longridge NS, Barber HO: Bilateral paroxysmal positioning nystagmus. J Otolaryngol 7: 395-400, 1978.

McClure JA: Horizontal canal BPV. J Otolaryngol 14: 30-35, 1985.

Parnes LS, McClure JA: Posterior semicircular canal occlusion for intractable benign paroxysmal positional vertigo. Ann Otol Rhinol Laryngol 99: 330-334, 1990.

Schuknecht HF: Cupulolithiasis. Arch Otolaryngol Head Neck Surg 90: 113-126, 1969.

22

Occlusion of the posterior semicircular canal in benign paroxysmal positional vertigo

Parnes and McClure (1990) have proposed a new surgical technique for the treatment of BPPV. It is based on the non-ampullar occlusion of the posterior semicircular canal.

SURGICAL TECHNIQUE

- General anesthesia is used. A classical postauricular incision is made; periosteum is drawn from the mastoid region and the fascia of the temporalis muscle. With a large cutting burr (4 mm) the mastoidectomy is performed until the lateral semicircular canal is seen. By following it caudally, the posterior canal will be reached.
- It is unnecessary to expose the body of the incus; thus trauma to the ossicular chain is avoided. It is also unnecessary to skeletonize the mastoid tract of the facial nerve, though it is important to remember that the posterior semicircular canal is like an arrow, pointed towards the nerve immediately under its ampullar extremity.
- It is unnecessary to perform a very large mastoidectomy; the surgeon should not push too posteriorly towards the sigmoid sinus nor drill the cells of the tip, except in very small mastoids. A superior large and poorly aerated cavity should be avoided.
- The lateral canal has a smooth surface. It is found at the bottom of the aereal cavity of the antrum and is not covered by bone, thus it is easily identifiable. The posterior canal is slightly deeper than the lateral canal and more difficult to identify, since it is covered by mastoid bone. The more eburneous the mastoid, the more difficult it is to identify the canal; the spongier the mastoid bone, the easier it is to identify the depth of the canal through it. When nearing the canal, the overlying mastoid bone must be removed, using a cutting burr whose diameter is the same as the transverse diameter of the canal. The burr is allowed to run from forward to backward without pressure and without stopping. Thus the view is maintained and the anatomic curvature of the canal is followed. The anterior part of the canal is exposed with a smaller cutting burr, in order to avoid injuring the facial nerve.
- The posterior canal is completely skeletonized, and all the spongy bone is removed. Porous surfaces are no longer seen: just the compact white labyrinthic bone can be observed.
- At the center of the posterior canal there is an island of approx. 3 mm lengthwise and 2 mm across. A blue line is made of the canal in a central position under continuous irrigation, leaving only a thin layer of bone through which the membranous labyrinth can be seen. Then the flow of water is interrupted and the residual bone is removed with a straight-angle hook, until the labyrinth is exposed without being traumatized. Here aspiration must not be used, to avoid suction on the membranous labyrinth causing "dry ear" with subsequent hearing loss.
- Small pieces of bone are taken from the mastoid, placed on a teflon surface and mixed with a few drops of fibrin glue until a homogeneous plug is formed. This plug is inserted into the opening, reinforced with more glue and with a flap of temporalis muscle fascia covering the surgical area (Figs. 22-1, 22-2, 22-3, 22-4, 22-5).
- Other Authors begin the obliteration by inserting a flap of periosteum larger than the canal margins into the opening. The following steps

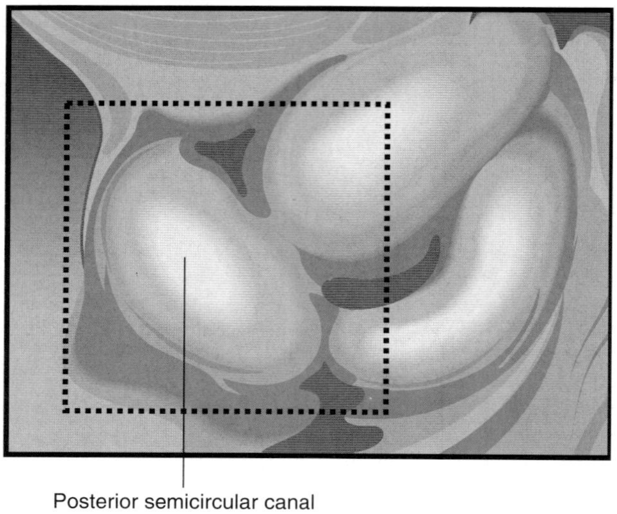

Fig. 22-1. Left ear. Limited mastoidectomy. The semicircular canals are exposed.

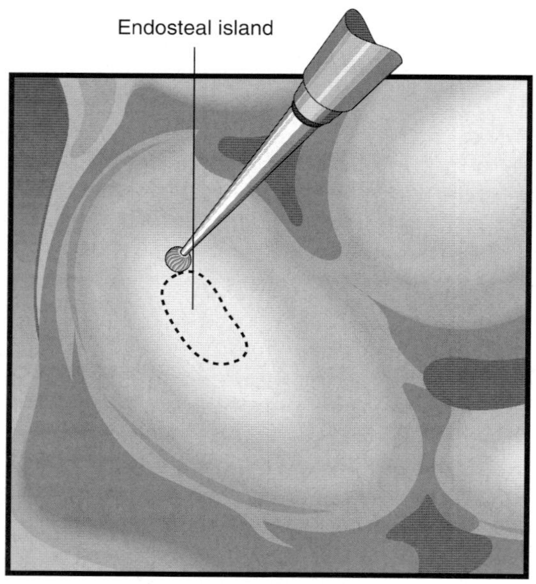

Fig. 22-2. A 3 mm. segment of the posterior semicircular canal, located along Donaldson's line (see chapter 18) is fenestrated down to the endosteum (Adapted from Parnes L).

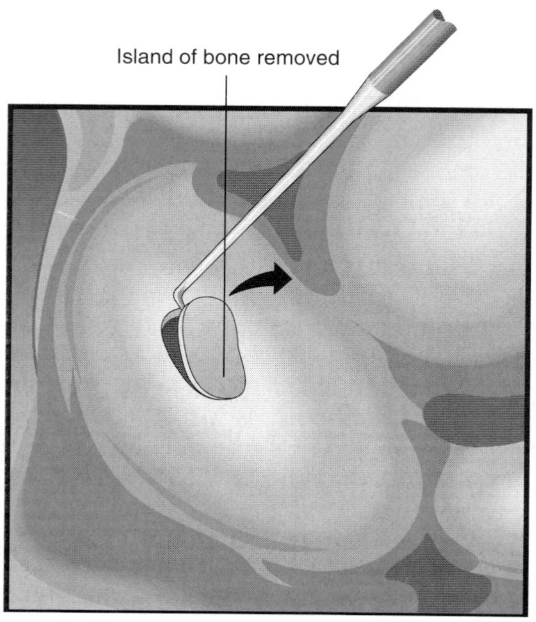

Fig. 22-3. The exposed endosteum is removed with a hook.

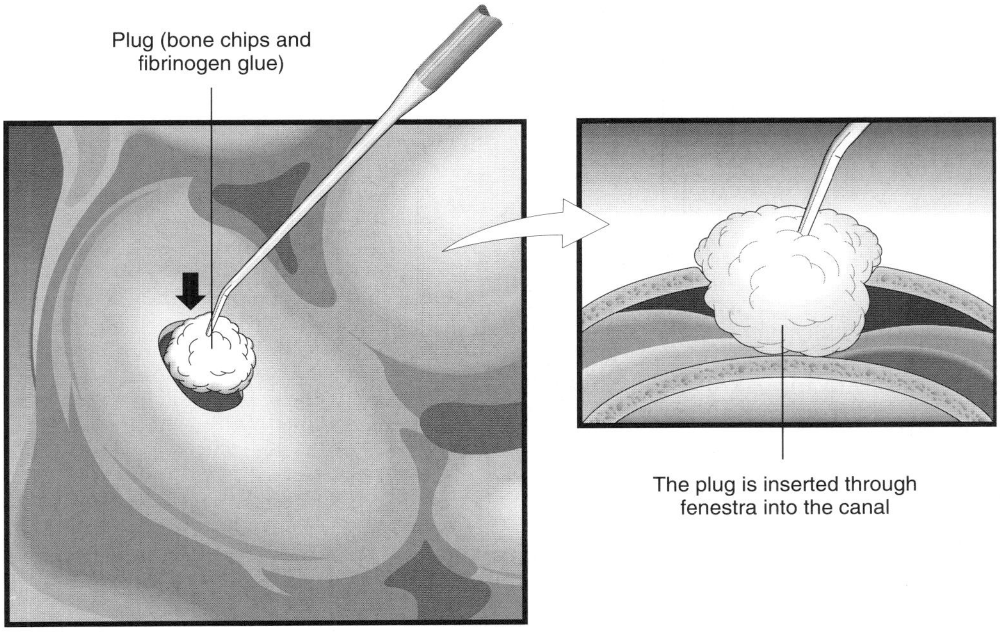

Fig. 22-4. Bone plug (bone paté plus fibrinogen glue) is prepared and inserted through the fenestra into the canal. The membranous labyrinth is compressed (Adapted from Parnes L).

are the same, using bone, glue, and strips of temporalis muscle (Balzan, Rutka).

- If well done, a transitory conductive hearing loss occurs without modification of the bony sheath. Hearing will return to normal within a few weeks.
- Patients are immediately freed of the position vertigo. The occlusion of the posterior canal creates a barrier to the free flow of endolymph; in this way the endolymph, which is not compressible, may not fluctuate and causes neither cupola movement nor subsequent vertigo.

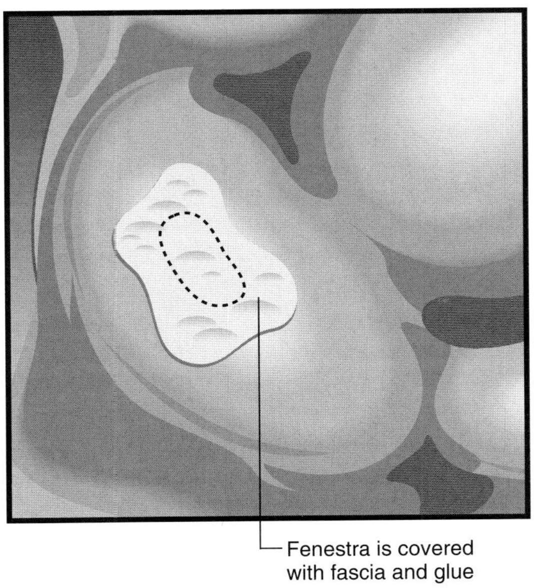

Fig. 22-5. The fenestra is covered with temporalis fascia and glue.

REFERENCES

Anthony P: Partitioning the labyrinth: Application in benign paroxysmal positional vertigo. Am J Otol 12: 388-393, 1991.
Baloh RW, Honrubia V, Jacobson K: Benign positional vertigo: Cllnical and oculographic features in 240 cases. Neurology 37: 371-378, 1987.
Baloh RW, Sakala S, Honrubia V: The mechanism of benign paroxysmal positional nystagmus. Adv Otorhinolaryngol 25: 161-166, 1979.
Barber HO, Leigh RJ: Benign (and not so benign) postural vertigo: Diagnosis and treatment. In Barber HO, Sharpe A (eds): Vestibular Disorders. Boca Raton, FL, CRC Press, 1988, pp 215-232.
Barber HO: Positional vertigo and nystagmus. Otolaryngol Clin North Am 6: 169-187,1973.
Brandt T, Daroff RB: Physical therapy for benign paroxysmal positional vertigo. Arch Otolaryngol Head Neck Surg 106: 484-485, 1980.
Cohen B, Suzuki J, Bender MB: Nystagmus induced bv electrical stimulation of ampullary nerves. Acta Otolaryngol (Stockh) 60: 422-436, 1965.
Epley JM: Singular neurectomy: Hypotympanotomy approach. Otolaryngol Head Neck Surg 88: 304-309, 1980.
Gacek R: Further observations on posterior ampullary nerve transection for positional vertigo. Ann Otol Rhinol Laryngol 87: 300-305, 1978.
Gacek R: Singular neurectomy update. Ann Otol Rhinol Laryngol 91: 469-473, 1982.
Gacek R: Transection of the posterior ampullary nerve for the relief of benign paroxysmal positional nystagmus. Ann Otol Rhinol Laryngol 83: 596-605, 1974.
Hall SF, Ruby RRF, McClure JA: The mechanics of benign paroxysmal vertigo. J Otolaryngol 8: 151-158, 1979.
Harbert F: Benign paroxysmal positional vertigo. Arch Ophthalmol Head Neck Surg 84: 298-302, 1970.
Katsarkas A, Outerbridge JS: Nystagmus of paroxysmal positional vertigo. Ann Otol Rhinol Laryngol 92: 146-150, 1983.
Lindsay IR, Hemenway WG: Postural vertigo due to unilateral sudden partial loss of vestibular function. Ann Otol Rhinol Laryngol 65: 692-706, 1956.

McClure JA, Lycett P: Vestibular asymmetry. Arch Otolaryngol Head Neck Surg 109: 682-687, 1983.
McClure JA, Rounthwaite J: Vestibular dysfunction associated with benign paroxysmal vertigo. Laryngoscope 87: 1434-1442, 1977.
McClure JA, Willett JM: Lorazepam and diazepam in the treatment of benign paroxysmal vertigo. J Otolaryngol 9: 472-477, 1980.
Meyerhoff WL: Surgical section of the posterior ampullary nerve. Laryngoscope 95: 933-935, 1985.
Money KE, Scott JW: Functions of separate sensory receptors of nonauditory labyrinth of the cat. Am J Physiol 202: 1211-1220, 1962.
Nedzelski JM, Barber HO, McIlmoyl L: Diagnoses in a dizziness unit. J Otolaryngol 15: 101-104, 1986.
Ohmichi T, Rutka J, Hawke M: Histopathologic consequences of surgical approaches to the singular nerve. Laryngoscope 99: 963-970, 1989.
Parnes LS, McClure JA: Effect on brainstem auditory evoked responses of posterior semicircular canal occlusion in guinea pigs. J Otolaryngol 14: 145-150, 1985.
Parnes LS, McClure JA: Free-floating endolymph particles: A new operative finding during posterior semicircular canal occlusion. Laryngoscope 12: 988-992, 1992.
Parnes LS, McClure JA: Posterior semicircular canal occlusion for intractable benign paroxysmal positional vertigo. Ann Otol Rhinol Laryngol 99: 330-334, 1990.
Parnes LS, McClure JA: Posterior semicircular canal occlusion in the normal hearing ear. Otolaryngol Head Neck Surg 104: 52-57, 1991.
Parnes LS, Price-Jones G: Particle repositioning maneuver for benign paroxysmal positional vertigo. Ann Otol Rhinol Laryngol 102: 325-331, 1993.
Schuknecht HF, Ruby RRF: Cupulolithiasis. Adv Otorhinolaryngol 20: 434-443, 1973.
Schuknecht HF: Pathology of the Ear. Cambridge, MA, Harward University Press, 1974.
Semont A, Freyss G, Vitte E: Curing the BPPV with a liberatory maneuver. Adv Otorhinolaryngol 42: 290-293, 1988.
Silverstein H: Singular neurectomy: A treatment for benign positional vertigo. In Brackmann DE (ed): Neurological Surgery of the Ear and Skull Base. New York, Raven Press, 1982, pp 331-335.
Spector M: Positional vertigo after stapedectomy. Ann Otol Rhinol Laryngol 70: 251-254,1961.
Stahle J, Terins J: Paroxysmal positional nystagmus. Ann Otol Rhinol Laryngol 74: 69-83, 1965.

23

Transmastoid labyrinthectomy

Transmastoid labyrinthectomy permits the total removal of the sensorineural epithelium of the vestibular apparatus, in cases of disabilitating vertigo and non-usable residual hearing (see chapter 20). It is a post-gangliar deafferentation and causes complete hearing loss.

SURGICAL TECHNIQUE

- The incision is the same as that of a normal mastoidectomy, approx. 1 cm behind the postauricular fold.
- The galea aponeurotica is dissected laterally to the temporalis muscle and is reflected forward in front of the ear. The periosteum-muscle flap is created according to the usual procedures (see chapter 28).
- Bone removal is limited to the supralabyrinthine cells until the antrum and the lateral semicircular canal have been identified. A cone-shaped cutting burr is utilized due to its large lateral cutting surface and the small size of its tip (see chapter 28). Once the lateral canal has been identified, it is enlarged posteriorly and superiorly with the burr until the superior and posterior canals are in evidence. A top-to-bottom motion is used so as not to reduce vision. Bone is removed from the intersinuso-facial cells so that a thin layer is left above the dura of the medial fossa, the sinodural angle, the sigmoid sinus and the dura of the posterior fossa (see chapter 28).
- The facial nerve is skeletonized to safely reach the vestibule. The lateral canal is opened and is followed posteriorly to open the posterior canal; the crus communis is identified between the posterior and superior canals and is followed until the superior canal is opened.

The superior canal is the deepest and the hardest to find. The following landmarks may be used to locate and open it when identification is difficult (e.g. in cases of eburneous mastoids):

- Crus communis, as mentioned,
- Exposure of the dura of the middle fossa along the tegmen antri to uncover the convexity of the canal, which is at times directly adherent to the dura. More frequently, it is separated by a thin bony sheath. Once the ampulla of the lateral canal has been identified, the surgeon drills 1 mm superior and posterior to it, until the ampulla of the superior canal is opened; the surgeon then proceed posteriorly by opening the canal.
- The subarcuate artery is usually found in the underlying circle of the lateral and posterior canals. When it bleeds, it is coagulated or closed with a diamond burr, without irrigation.
- The lateral canal is opened halfway, preserving its medial wall so as not to injure the external part of the second genu of the facial nerve. It is important not to drill beyond the ampulla of the posterior canal, since it is immediately medial to the facial nerve.
- The crus communis is followed anteriorly to the vestibule. Along the crus communis lies the endolymphatic duct, which goes from the endolymphatic sac to open in the medial part of the vestibule.
- The bone is thinned in a posterior-anterior direction over the facial nerve, to increase exposure of the vestibule. Here the utricle is observed behind and the translucent gray saccule in front. All the semicircular canals are completely connected using a large diamond burr. Then, all the residual elements of the membranous labyrinth in the semicircular canals, the utricle, and the saccule are removed, in order to eliminate any residual vestibular function. The vestibule appears empty; on its medial wall, the elliptic recess of the utricle is observed posteriorly and the spheric recess of the saccule anteriorly.
- In this way the post-gangliar postauricular labyrinthectomy is completed. The House Ear Institute reports observing traumatic neuromas in the temporal bone of patients operated with a transmastoid labyrinthectomy. The clinical data relating to the persistence of balance disturbances have been connected to this anatomical data.

- For this reason, we prefer the translabyrinthine approach for a vestibular neurectomy when a vertiginous patient shows the requisites for a hearing sacrifice (non-usable hearing). In fact, once a labyrinthectomy has been performed and the patient is already under general anesthesia, the anatomical and temporal space separating us from the opening of the IAC is very little. Thus the operation meets the goal of the complete vestibular function abolition.

REFERENCES

Brackmann DE, Green D: Translabyrinthine approach for acoustic tumor removal. Otolaryngol Clin North Am 25: 311-329,1992.

Brackmann DE: Fenestrated suction for neuro-otologic surgery. Trans Am Acad Ophthalmol Otolaryngol 84: 975, 1977.

Brackmann DE: Translabyrinthine removal of acoustic neurinomas. In Brackmann DE (ed): Neurological Surgery of the Ear and Skull Base. New York, Raven Press, 1982, pp 235-241.

Hitselberger WE, House WF: A warning regarding the sitting position for acoustic tumor surgery (Editorial). Arch Otolaryngol Head Neck Surg 106: 69, 1980.

Horowitz NH, Rizzoli HV: Postoperative complications of intracranial neurological surgery. Baltimore: William & Wilkins, 1982.

House WF, Luetje CM: Acoustic tumors, vols I and II. Baltimore: University Park Press, 1979.

House WF: Acoustic neuroma (Monograph). Arch Otolaryngol Head Neck Surg 80: 598-757, 1964.

House WF: Translabyrinthine approach. In House WF, Luetje CM (eds): Acoustic Tumors, Vol Management. Baltimore, University Park Press, 1979, pp 43-87.

House WF: Transtemporal bone microsurgical removal of acoustic neuromas. Arch Otolaryngol 80:597, 1964.

Rhoton AL Jr: Microsurgical anatomy of the brain stem surface facing an acoustic neuroma. Surg Neurol 25:326-339, 1986.

Rodgers GK, Luxford WM: Factors affecting the development of cerebrospinal fluid leak and meningitis after translabyrinthine acoustic tumor surgery. Laryngoscope 103:959-962. 1993.

Sterkers JM, Billet R: Petites tumeurs de l'acoustique. Diagnostic et cure precoces. Ann Otolaryngol (Paris) 89:323-339, 1972.

Sterkers JM, Desgeorges M, Corlieu P, Sterkers O: Ablation par voie translabyrinthique des volumineux neurinomes de l'acoustique. Ann Otolaryngol (Paris) 101:9-14, 1984.

Sterkers JM, Desgeorges M, Sterkers O, Corlieu P: Our present approach to acoustic neuroma surgery. Adv Otorhinolaryngol 34:160-163, 1984.

24

Translabyrinthine vestibular neurectomy

When medical treatment proves fruitless for a young Mèniére's patient with non-usable hearing, a translabyrinthine vestibular neurectomy is indicated.

This is the most complete and effective of all denervation procedures. This is because it associates a postgangliar interruption of the nerve (in the labyrinthectomy) with a pre-gangliar section, thanks to a vestibular nerve section.

- The preparation of the patient follows the usual criteria. The incision is approx. 3 cm. behind the postauricular fold.
- The elevation of the cutaneous-subcutaneous flap and the muscle-periosteal flap is done with the usual technique (see chapter 28).
- An enlarged mastoidectomy is performed. A thin layer of bone is left on the dura of the middle and posterior fossa. The cells of the mastoid tip are drilled until the digastric crest is seen. The sigmoid sinus is skeletonized while leaving a paper-thin bone layer which is later compressed and egg-shell broken. The sinus may thus be kept compressed by the suction-irrigator placed flat, allowing space for the view underneath. It is unnecessary to expose the dura of the retrosigmoid posterior fossa since a large depression of the lateral sinus is not needed, as it is in the translabyrinthine approach.
- The mastoid emissary is thus left undisturbed. The sino-dural angle is opened wide to allow a broad view of the labyrinthine block. The mastoid tract, which is the anterior dissecting limit of the facial nerve, is skeletonized. The labyrinthectomy is performed. In this situation it is not advisable to follow the rapid labyrinthectomy method (drilling the labyrinthine block with a large cutting burr after identifying the semicircular canal ampullae (see chapter 28, tips and pitfalls), because of the risk of leaving residual membranous tissue.
- The best and safest way to perform a labyrinthectomy is the classic technique. With a 2 mm cutting burr, the lateral canal is opened and followed posteriorly to open the posterior canal. The posterior canal is then followed to the confluence of the superior canal, where the two canals join in the crus communis, which is followed anteriorly to the vestibule. The posterior canal is completely opened up to the ampulla, under the facial nerve. Anteriorly, the lateral canal is opened to the ampulla. Immediately superior to the ampulla of the lateral canal, the ampulla of the superior canal is opened. The superior canal is then opened and followed along the tegmen antri. The opening of the vestibule is completed by drilling anteriorly under the mastoid tract of the facial nerve. The anterior aperture includes, in a cranio-caudal direction, the ampulla of the superior canal, the ampulla of the lateral canal, the elliptic recess of the utricle, and the ampulla of the posterior canal. Anterior to the utricle recess is the spheric recess of the saccule. A hook is used to remove all residual vestibular tissue from these structures. Thus the first part of the operation is completed: a postgangliar labyrinthectomy.
- *Opening of the internal auditory canal.* We must now identify the internal auditory canal. Unlike the translabyrinthine approach, this technique does not necessitate exposing the entire internal auditory canal, from fundus to porus, but rather it is enough to expose half of the canal, beginning at the fundus. The ampulla of the superior canal indicates the position of the superior vestibular nerve, which runs toward the sino-dural angle and runs along the superior margin of the canal. The inferior margin begins from the ampulla of the posterior canal and runs parallel to the superior margin. We also know that the canal is inclined in a posterior direction, medially and caudally and that the medial

vestibular wall is also the lateral wall of the IAC. Keeping the canal's position in mind, the bone is removed along its path, more medially than laterally, where the bone is thinner. Thus half of the internal auditory canal is skeletonized. The canal can be seen through a very thin layer of bone. It is bluish in color ("blue line") but differs from its appearance as a tumor site, when it has a reddish color. The ampulla of the superior canal is drilled to show the trunk of the superior vestibular nerve. Then the nerve is followed laterally to show the branches of the nerve which cross the cribriform area to reach the ampulla of the lateral and superior canals. The residual bone of the canal is removed with a diamond burr and the remaining bone fragments are removed with a hook.

- The canal must be exposed by approx. 180°. This wide exposure is necessary to avoid the dangers and difficulties present when working in restricted space. It also permits hemostasis if bleeding occurs, owing to the interruption of small vessels.
- The dura is incised towards the inferior margin of the internal auditory canal, where the facial nerve is the farthest away. The dura is then slightly hooked at the fundus of the canal and stretched downward. The closed end of Jacobson's microscissors may also be used for this purpose. The dura is also opened superiorly (Fig. 24-1).
- *The internal auditory canal* is now opened. The position of the superior and inferior vestibular nerves is confirmed by the contact with the facial nerve stimulator, if it is used. The superior vestibular nerve is separated with a hook exerting traction on the nerve. The tip of the hook is directed in a cranial to caudal position so as to hold the nerve in its curvature. The genu of the hook is then placed on the recess that accommodates the vestibular nerve, lateral to the fallopian canal. The nerve is separated by means of traction in a cranio-caudal direction, so that the movement is directed away from the facial nerve which is medial and slightly superior.
- Thus, the underlying facial nerve becomes visible. The vestibulo-facial fibers must be sectioned. Behind the superior vestibular nerve, the posterior wall of the fallopian canal (Bill's Bar) becomes evident.

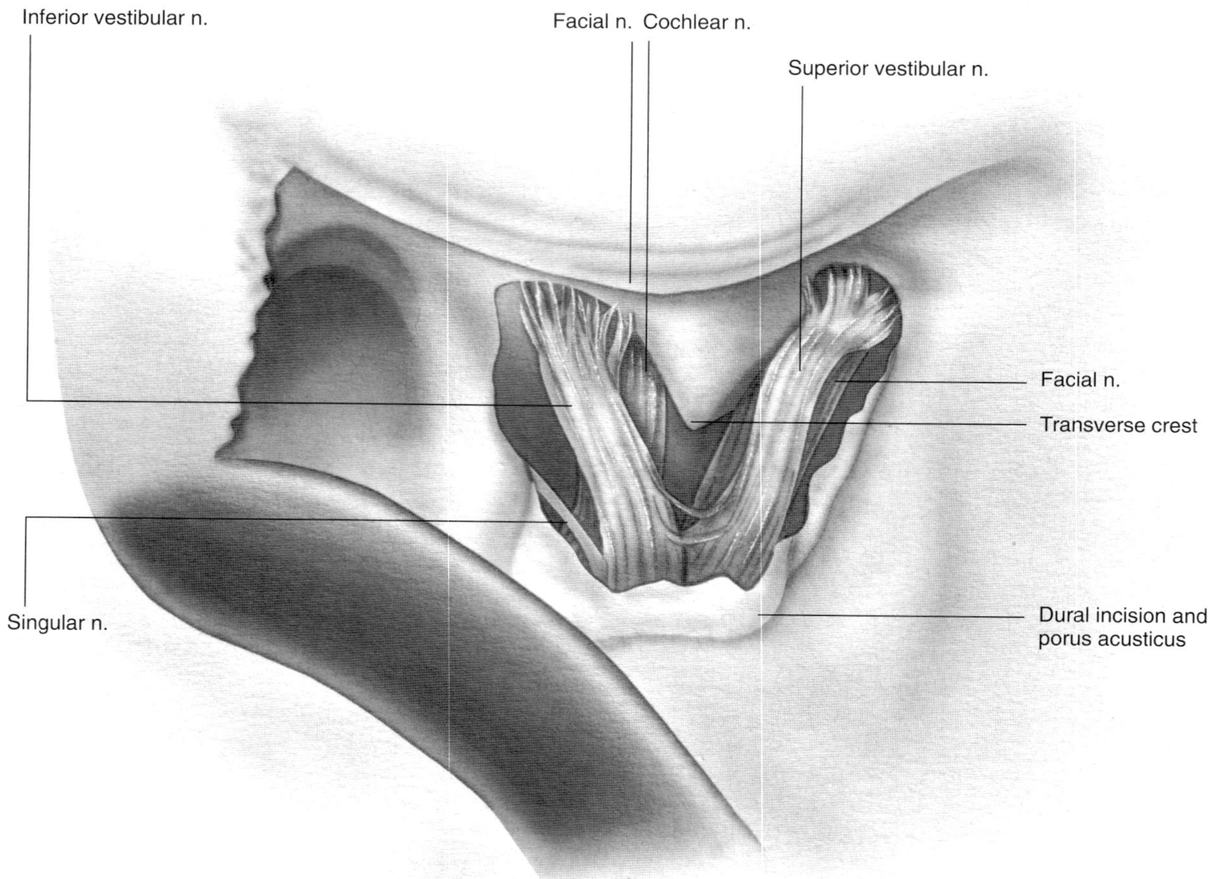

Fig. 24-1. Translabyrinthine vestibular neurectomy. The superior and inferior vestibular nerves, as well as the singular nerve, are avulsed. The fused vestibular nerves are sectioned medial to Scarpa's ganglion (adapted from Nelson RA).

- Inferior to the superior vestibular nerve, a bony crest (the transverse crest) divides the canal into a superior and an inferior part and laterally separates the superior vestibular nerve from the inferior vestibular nerve and medially, the facial nerve from the cochlear nerve.
- The inferior vestibular nerve is separated, in one of its terminal arborizations, from the cribriform area through which the ampulla enters from the posterior canal into the sac.
- The singular nerve is separated along with the inferior vestibular nerve. It is important that it be identified since it is frequently in an eccentric position. It originates in the ampulla of the posterior canal and reaches the trunk of the vestibular nerve a few mm medial to the fundus. If it is not identified, it may not be included in the section of the inferior vestibular nerve and it may cause failure of the surgery.
- The two stumps of the vestibular nerves are moved back. The position of the AICA is identified. It often describes a loop in the canal, between the vestibular nerves and the facial nerve. It must be carefully preserved.
- The two vestibular nerves unite in one single nerve approx. halfway down the IAC. At their junction a bulge is seen which corresponds to Scarpa's ganglion. The two nerves are sectioned medially to the ganglion. Thus a pregangliar vestibular section is performed.
- The cochlear nerve is identified and preserved. In this way the possibility of a future cochlear implant is left open, if it becomes. Even in cases of very intense tinnitus, the section of the acoustic nerve is not very helpful, since the process eventually becomes central.
- Hemostasis is controlled with a bipolar cautery and the application of bovine collagen (Avitene). The edges of the dural breach are closed with 4-0 silk. The closure of the flaps, the positioning and the permanence of the nasogastric drain, the urinary catheter and the abdominal drain follow the same technique as in the translabyrinthine approach (see chapter 28). Complications, such as the CSF fistula, are treated in the usual way.

REFERENCES

Horovitz NH, Rizzoli HV: Postopérative complications of intracranial neurological surgery. Baltimore: William & Wilkins, 1982.

House WF, Luetje CM: Acoustic tumors, vols I and II. Baltimore: University Park Press 1979.

House WF: Transtemporal bone microsurgical removal of acoustic neuromas. Arch Otolaryngol 80:597, 1964.

Linthicum FH, Alongso A, Denia A: Traumatic neuroma: A complication of transcanal labyrinthectomy. Arch Otolaryngol Head Neck Surg 105: 654-655, 1979.

Nelson RA, Brackmann DE: Clinical problems in diagnosis and documentation of Ménière's disease. Immunobiology, Histophysiology and Tumor Immunology in Otolaryngology. Proceedings of 2nd International Academic Conference, Utrecht, The Netherlands. Berkeley, CA, Kugler, 1987, pp 3-8.

Nelson RA: Labyrinthectomy and translabyrinthine nerve section. In Brackmann DE (ed): Neurological Surgery of the Ear and Skull Base. New York, Raven Press 1982.

Rhoton AL Jr: Microsurgical anatomy of the brain stem surface facing an acoustic neuroma. Surg Neurol 25:326-339, 1986.

Shelton C, Hitselberger WE, House WF, Brackmann DE: Hearing preservation after acoustic tumor removal: Long-term results. Laryngoscope 100: 115-119, 1990.

Sterkers JM, Billet R: Petites tumeurs de l'acoustique. Diagnostic et cure precoces. Ann Otolaryngol (Paris) 89:323-339, 1972.

Sterkers JM, Desgeorges M, Corlieu P, Sterkers O: Ablation par voie translabyrinthique des volumineux neurinomes de l'acoustique. Ann Otolaryngol (Paris) 101:9-14, 1984.

Sterkers JM, Desgeorges M, Sterkers O, Corlieu P: Our present approach to acoustic neuroma surgery. Adv Otorhinolaryngol 34: 160-163,1984.

25

Cochleosacculotomy

Cochleosacculotomy is an endolymphatic shunt procedure. The shunt of the endolymphatic sac is an operation that drains endolymph in excess into the mastoid (external shunt). The cochleosacculotomy is, on the other hand, a procedure which drains the endoymph internally, into the perilymphatic space (internal shunt).
The operation is based on several theoretical and experimental assumptions:

- It has been noted in animals and in the temporal bone of patients with Mèniére's disease that a fistula of the membranous labyrinth may be present without deafness. Fistulization may cause remission of even long-lasting symptoms.
- It has further been noted that the only way to create a persistent fistulization is to interrupt the cochlear duct (Schuknecht).

INDICATIONS
The elderly patient has a longer period of central compensation, so that convalescence lasts longer. Due to these patients' poor health, it is thus helpful to use a procedure which may be performed under local anesthesia. For the same reason, an intense post-operative symptomatology must not be present.
The cochleosacculotomy is indicated in the treatment of elderly patients with hearing loss but good vestibular function (shown in the ENG test).
This procedure has a high risk of sensorineural hearing loss, so it is reserved for patients with compromised hearing.

SURGICAL TECHNIQUE.

- The operation is performed under local anesthesia.
- The external auditory canal is infiltrated posteriorly and anteriorly with a 1% Lidocaine solution. The tympano-meatal flap is elevated in the same way as that described for a stapedectomy. The chorda tympani is avoided. The operating table is inclined as much as possible toward the surgeon. In this way views of the posterior mesotympanum and the round window are obtained.
- In rare cases the prominence of the bony annulus masks the view of the round window. This bony prominence is removed, in a maneuver similar to the stapedectomy, with a curette or a 3 mm cutting burr. The rare instance of a prominent jugular bulb requires the surgeon's intervention. A 3 mm straight-angle hook is inserted into the niche of the round window. The direction of penetration is inferior-superior, towards the oval window. It is necessary to slide with the hook touching the lateral wall of the cavum tympani, to safely cross the cochlear duct. At times the bony prominence of the subiculum, located between the oval window and the sinus tympani, impedes the introduction of the instrument or forces it in a direction medial to the lateral wall of the cavum tympani. In these cases, the subiculum is drilled.
- The hook, introduced in a superior direction, passes into the scala tympani, crosses the osseous spiral lamina (a thin bony structure is felt to yield), the cochlear duct, and the saccule. In general, the superior margin of the round window is approx. 3 mm from the inferior margin of the oval window and the saccule; the complete introduction of the instrument thus maintains the requisites of safety. If, on the other hand, the bony margin of the window is drilled, for an easier and better-aimed introduction of the instrument (see chapter 8), then the hook's progression must be slowed. The hook's progression is imagined visually along the lateral wall of the tympanic cavity, until the tip is brought just under the footplate of the stapes. If the hook passes posterior to the footplate and reaches a superior position, it perforates the saccule. If the footplate is crossed and passed by, the saccule and its maculas are perforated. In both cases, post-operative vertigo is the result.

- The hook is extracted and the perforation is closed with a bit of fat and a flap of perichondrium. The repositioning of the tympanomeatal flap and the dressing follow the same procedures as the stapedectomy.

RESULTS

One of the reasons for failure of an internal shunt is occlusion of the fistula by the membranous labyrinth, and thus occlusion of the endolymph flow. Schuknecht reports the control of vertigo in 70% of patients, with a worsening of the audiometric threshold in 35% of patients, including the 10% who presented profound sensorineural hearing loss following the operation. Silverstein et al and Dionne reported a similar percentage in the control of vertigo and a higher incidence of profound sensorineural hearing loss following the operation. Due to the elevated incidence of post-operative sensorineural hypoacusia, we consider cochleosacculotomy to be a destructive procedure. We reserve this procedure for elderly patients in precarious health, with poor residual hearing and good vestibular function.

REFERENCES

Cody DTR: The tack operation for endolymphatic hydrops. Laryngoscope 79: 1737-1744, 1969.

Cody DTR, Simonton KM, Hallberg OE: Automatic repetitive decompression of the saccule in endolymphatic hydrops (tack operation). Preliminary report. Laryngoscope 77: 1480-1501, 1967.

Committee on Hearing and Equilibrium: Report of Subcommittee on Equilibrium and its Measurement. Mèniére's disease: Criteria for diagnosis and evaluation of therapy for reporting. Trans Am Acad Ophthalmol Otolaryngol 76: 1462-1464, 1972.

Dohlman GF: On the mechanism of the Mèniére attack. Arch Otorhinolaryngol 212, 301-307, 1976.

Duval AJ III, Rhodes VT: Ultrastructure of the organ of Corti following intermixing of cochlear fluids. Ann Otol Rhinol Laryngol 76: 688-708,1967.

Fick IA van N: Decompression of the labyrinth. A new surgical procedure for Mèniére's disease. Arch Otolaryngol 79: 447-458, 1964.

Fick IA van N: Mèniére's disease: Aetiology and a new surgical approach: Sacculotomy: J Laryngol Otol 80: 288-306, 1966.

Kimura RS, Schuknecht HF, Ota CY, Jones DD: Experimental study of sacculotomy in endolymphatic hydrops. Arch Otorhinolaryngol 217: 123-137, 1977.

Kimura RS, Schuknecht HF: Effect of fistulae on endolymphatic hydrops. Ann Otol Rhinol Laryngol 84: 271-286, 1975.

Pulec JL: Mèniére's disease. The otic-perotic shunt. Otolaryngol Clin North Am 1: 643-648,1968.

Schuknecht HF, Bartley M: Cochlear endolymphatic shunt for Mèniére's disease. Am J Otol (Suppl): 20-22, 1985.

Schuknecht HF, Gulya AJ: Endolymphatic hydrops: An overview and classification. Ann Otol Rhinol Laryngol 92: (Suppl 106) 1-20, 1983.

Schuknecht HF, Neff WD: Hearing losses after apical lesions in the cochlea. Acta Otolaryngol (Stockh) 42: 263-274, 1952.

Schuknecht HF, Ruther A: Blockage of longitudinal flow in endolymphatic hydrops. Eur Arch Otorhinolaryngol 248: 209-217, 1991.

Schuknecht HF, Seifi A: Experimental observations on the fluid physiology of the inner ear. Ann Otol Rhinol Laryngol 72: 687-721, 1963.

Schuknecht HF, Sutton S: Hearing losses after experimental lesions in basal coil of cochlea. Arch Otolaryngol 57: 129-142, 1953.

Schuknecht HF: Cochlear endolymphatic shunt. Am J Otol 5: 546-548, 1984.

Schuknecht HF: Cochleosacculotomy for Mèniére's disease: Internal endolymphatic shunt. Op Tech Otolaryngol Head Neck Surg 2: 35-37, 1991.

Schuknecht HF: Cochleosacculotomy for Mèniére's disease: Theory, technique and results. Laryngoscope 92: 853-858, 1982.

Schuknecht HF: Mèniére's disease: A correlation of symptomatology and pathology. Laryngoscope 73: 651-665,1963.

Schuknecht HF: Pathology of Mèniére's disease as it relates to the sac and tack procedures. Ann Otol Rhinol Laryngol 86: 677-682, 1977.

Torok N: Old and new in Mèniére's disease. Laryngoscope 87: 1870-1877, 1977.

Tumarkin A: Otolithic catastrophe. A new syndrome. BMJ 2: 175-177, 1936.

26

Chemical elimination of vestibular function

Aminoglycosides like Amikacin, Dihydrostreptomycin, Gentamycin and Kanamycin are predominantly vestibulotoxins.

Among the aminoglycosides, Streptomycin has the greatest affinity for the vestibular receptors and the least for cochlear receptors (Tran).

Streptomycin's active mechanism consists, according to experimental studies (McGee and Olszewski) in a loss of the hair cells of the posterior labyrinth. In particular, the hair cells of the cristae, the utricule and the saccule are destroyed, without involving the nearby neurons of the first order (Takumida; Meza; Norris).

The vestibulotoxic side effects of the aminoglycosides Gentamycin and Streptomycin are used by many authors for therapeutic purposes.

Schuknect's experience (begun in 1950) is based on the intramuscular administration of Streptomycin in doses of 0.75 to 1.75 g. every 12 h (from 1.5 to 3.5 g/day), average dosage 1 g. every 12 h.

In all patients, control of the vertiginous crises was obtained and hearing was preserved. The total ablation of the vestibular system has led to chronic unbalance, ataxia due to alteration of the vestibulospinal reflex, and oscillopsia due to alteration of the vestibulo-ocular reflex.

To control these side effects, a subtotal treatment has been developed, based on the total accumulated doses.

INDICATIONS

Streptomycin treatment may be considered in patients with Mèniére's induced acute vertiginous crises in the following three situations (Monsell):

1. Mèniére's disease active in both ears, especially when the provoking ear has not been determined.
2. Mèniére's disease in the one hearing ear.
3. Mèniére's disease in the second ear, with the first already operated on with a conservative procedure, e.g. selective vestibular neurectomy.

ADMINISTRATION PROTOCOL

- 1 g of Streptomycin sulfate two times a day for 5 days, for a total dose of 10 g.
- Clinical evaluation, test of spontaneous reflexes, audiometry, study of vestibular function (caloric test, rotation test, post-urographic test).

Interruption of therapy when

Good response to therapy, with significant reduction or abolition of vertiginous crises, or when:

- Onset or worsening of acute vestibular alteration syndrome.
- Worsening of the vestibular-spinal reflex response.
- Reduction in vestibular response to instrumental tests.
- Hearing loss.

New (II) treatment cycle

If the vertiginous crises are not significantly reduced, hearing is unchanged and no reduction in vestibular function is shown:

- 1 g twice a day for 5 days, or 10 g in the second cycle and 20 g of total dosage.

Before undertaking a new therapeutic cycle, it must be taken into account that the effects of the Streptomycin may be slowed. After the first cycle it is thus recommended to wait for at least 3 months.

New (III) therapeutic cycle

- If no clinical improvement is shown and the instrumental data are unchanged, the dosage may be increased to 1 g a day for 5 days, for a total dosage of 5 g.

RESULTS

According to Langman's data, vertigo was controlled in 95% of cases within 18 months of treatment. After 9 years, 64% of the patients reported no reoccurrence of the vertigo. 60% of patients retained a slight unbalance and 16% of patients presented oscillopsia.

Perfusion of the lateral semicircular canal with Streptomycin

This operation is based on experimental work (Kimura et al) and on clinical studies by Shea and Norris. The purpose is to bring the pharmacological agent *in situ*, so that it exerts as selective an action as possible on the vestibular cells, and not on the cochlear cells.

SURGICAL TECHNIQUE

- A mastoidectomy is performed; the lateral semicircular canal is identified. With a House elevator or another blunt instrument, the mucosa is separated from the lateral canal. With a diamond burr and under continous irrigation the bone is thinned at the two margins of the semicircular canal, as close as possible to the ampullar extremity, until a double blue line and a thicker bone plate are delineated. The bone island is removed with a hook. This technique, derived from the fenestration technique, permits the opening of the canal with minimal trauma.
- The movement, performed in an anterior-posterior direction, must be cautious, with the tip of the hook raking the underlying bone surface, to avoid damaging the underlying membranous canal adhering to the plate of bone. The opening is approx. 1 mm in diameter.
- *Shea's technique.* The lateral membranous canal is measured with a micrometer. Approx. one-fourth of the canal has a greater amplitude than the norm (40 μm) and this is a sign of greater endolymph volume, especially when combined with the data of the ECoGh. In ears in which the membranous canal appears enlarged and the endolymph pressure to the ECoGh increased, with a needle mounted on a syringe of tubercoline the membranous canal may be punctured to release endolymph and 0.1 ml. of physiological solution containing 25 μg of Streptomycin/ml is slowly injected. The fenestration is then closed with a small Teflon sheet over which temporalis muscle fascia is placed.

Electrocochleography

This data is based on Shea's experience.

With a round silver electrode in the niche of the round window a base tracing is created (the normal SP/AP relationship).

Upon completion of fenestration, another test is performed. If the SP/AP relationship increases, this means an increase in the endolymphatic pressure and, especially when combined with the data of the enlargement of the membranous canal, justifies continuing surgery.

If the bony opening is covered with a Teflon lamina and pressed, the pressure of the endolymph diminishes as does the SP/AP relationship.

At the end of the operation a new test generally reveals a decrease in the SP/AP relationship, meaning that the endolymph pressure has returned to normal.

Results

The application of streptomycin to the labyrinth through the lateral semicircular canal, although effective in the control of vertigo, appears to cause a higher rate of hearing loss then does transtympanic or intramuscular application.

Intratympanic injection of Gentamycin

The purpose of this treatment is to abolish vestibular function selectively, without involving the contralateral ear. It is thus a treatment indicated in forms of unilateral Mèniére's Disease. It is an outpatient treatment and thus indicated for elderly patients and patients in poor health.

Preparation of the Gentamycin solution (Monsell 1995).

- 40 mg/ml solution with a PH 5.4., or
- Solution buffered to a PH of 6.4.

Injection

The patient is supine, with the ear to be treated facing upwards. A drop of phenol is used to anesthetize the central region of the tympanic membrane. A 27-gauge needle attached to a tubercoline syringe goes through the umbus region of the tympanic membrane and injects approx. 0.5 ml of solution into the middle ear. The patient must remain in a supine position, without swallowing or coughing, to prevent the fluid from flowing down the tubes, for at least 30'.

Administration

An intratympanic injection of 0.5 ml of Gentamycin (30mg/ml, pH 6.4) is made once a day until the first signs of ototoxicity are observed. 1 to 12 doses are given, with an average of 4-6 doses (Beck and Schmidt).

A different method, proposed by Cass, administers the dosage over a longer period of time, in the attempt to reduce the incidence of hearing loss.

An intratympanic injection is performed with 0.5 ml of Gentamycin (30 mg/ml, pH 6.4) once a week for four weeks (total dosage equal to 40-60 total mg). In cases of audiometric alteration seen at the weekly check-up, the treatment is interrupted. If the vertigo is not cured or if it recurs, other dosages may be administered. The preliminary data demonstrate that the control of the vertigo and the abolition of the vestibular response to the caloric test has been obtained, while hearing has been preserved.

Results

The treatment has proven to be effective and the vertigo has been controlled. In some cases, precocious hypoacusia may manifest after treatment. The current direction taken is to administer a total defined dosage of the drug, spacing the administration of the dosages further apart (Monsell). Neither oscillopsia nor chronic unbalance are seen, which are frequently present in patients treated with intramuscular Streptomycin, although the patient's tolerance of this treatment is comparatively lower.

REFERENCES

Alford BR: Mèniére's disease: Criteria for diagnosis and evaluation of therapy for reporting. Trans Am Acad Ophthalmol Otolaryngol 76: 1462-1464, 1972.

Beck C, Schmidt CL: Ten years of experience with intratympanically applied streptomycin (gentamicin) in the therapy of morbus Mèniére. Arch Otorhinolaryngol 221: 149-152, 1978.

Berg K: The toxic effect of streptomycin on the vestibular and cochlear apparatus. Acta Otolaryngol (Stockh) Suppl 157:177, 1951.

Blessing R, Schlenter W: Langzeitergebnisse der Gentamicin Therapie des Morbus Mèniére. Laringorhinootologie 68: 657-660, 1989.

Cass S, Bouchard K, Graham M: Controlled application of streptomycin to the round window membrane of the cat. Otolaryngol Head Neck Surg 103: 223, 1990.

Fouzler EP: Streptomycin treatment of vertigo. Trans Am Acad Ophtalmol Otolaryngol 52:239-301, 1948.

Goycoolea M, Carpenter A, Muchow D: Ultrastructural studies of the round-window membrane of the cat. Arch Otolaryngol 113:617-624, 1987.

Graham MD, Kemink JL: Titration streptomycin therapy for bilateral Mèniére's disease: A progress report. Am J Otol 5: 534-535, 1984.

Graham MD, Sataloff RT, Kemink JL: Titration streptomycin therapy for bilateral Mèniére's disease: A preliminary report. Otolaryngol Head Neck Surg 92: 440-447, 1984.

Henley CM III, Schacht J: Pharmacokinetics of aminoglycoside antibiotics in inner ear fluids and their relationship to ototoxicity. Audiology 27:137-147,1988.

Jahnke K: Transtympanic application of gentamicin with cochlea protection. In Nadol JB (ed): Second International Symposium on Mèniére's Disease. Amsterdam, Kugler & Ghedini, 1989.

Kawauchi H, DeMaria T, Lim D: Endotoxin permeability through the round window. Acta Otolaryngol (Suppl 457): 100-115, 1988.

Kimura RS, Iverson NA, Southard RE: Selective lesions of the vestibular labyrinth. Ann Otol Rhinol Laryngol 97:577-584, 1988.

Kimura RS, Lee K-S, Nye CL, Trehey JA: Effects of systemic and lateral semicircular canal administration of aminoglycosides on normal and hydropic inner ears. Acta Otolaryngol (Stockh) 111: 1021-1030, 1991.

Konishi S, Shea JJ: Experimental endolymphatic hydrops and its relief by interrupting the lateral semicircular duct in guinea pigs. J Laryngol Otol 89:577-592, 1975.

Konrad HR: Intractable vertigo: when not to operate. Otolaryngol Head Neck Surg 95:482-484, 1986.

Laitakari K: Intratympanic gentamicin in severe Mèniére's disease. Clin Otolaryngol 15:545-548, 1990.

Lange G: Gentamicin and other ototoxic antibiotics for the transtympanic treatment of Mèniére's disease. Arch Otorhinolaryngol 246: 269-270, 1989.

Lange G: Isolierte Medikamentose Ausschaltungeines Gleichgewichtsorganes beim Morbus Mèniére mit Streptomycin-Ozothin. Arch Klin Exp 191: 545-549, 1968.

Lange G: Transtympanic treatment for Mèniére's disease with gentamicin sulfate. In Vosteen K-H, Schuknecht HF, Pfaltz CR, et al. (eds): Mèniére's Disease, Pathogenesis, Diagnosis and Treatment. Stuttgart, Georg Thieme Verlag, 1981.

Langman AW, Kemink JL, Graham MD: Titration therapy for bilateral Mèniére's disease: Follow-up report. Ann Otol Rhinol Laryngol 99:923-926, 1990.

Lindeman H: Regional differences in sensitivity of the vestibular sensory epithelia to ototoxic antibiotics. Acta Otolaryngol 67: 177-189, 1969.

Lundman L, Bagger-Sjoback D, Holmquist L, Juhn S: Round window membrane permeability. Acta Otolaryngol (Suppl 457): 73-77, 1988.

Magnusson M, Padoan S: Delayed onset of ototoxic effects of gentamicin in treatment of Mèniére's disease. Acta Otolaryngol 111: 671-676, 1991.

McGee T, O]szewski J: Streptomycin sulfate and dihydrostreptomycin toxicity. Arch Otolaryngol Head Neck Surg 75:295-311, 1962.

Miller C, Odkvist L, Thell J, et al: Vestibular and audiologic functions in gentamicin-treated Mèniére's disease. Am J Otolaryngol 9: 383-391,1988.

Monsell EM, Brackmann DE, Linthicum FH: Why do vestibular destructive procedures sometimes fail? Otolaryngol Head Neck Surg 99: 472-479, 1988.

Monsell EM, Cass SP, Rybak LP: Aminoglycoside treatment for vertigo: Development and current status. Adv Otolaryngol Head Neck Surg 7: 174-188, 1993.

Monsell EM, Cass SP, Rybak LP: Chemical labyrinthectomy: methods and results. In Brackmann DE, Shelton C, Arriaga MA (ed): Otologic Surgery. Philadelphia, Saunders WB, 1995.

Monsell EM: Electrocochleographic recording in patients undergoing labyrinthotomy with streptomycin infusion. In Arenberg IK (ed): Surgery of the Inner Ear. Amsterdam, Kugler & Ghedini, 1991.

Nedzelski J, Schessel D, Bryce G, Pfleiderer A: Chemical labyrinthectomy: Local application for the treatment of unilateral Mèniére's disease. Am J Otol 13: 18-22, 1992.

Ohmori H: Mechano-electrical transduction currents in isolated vestibular hair cells of the chick. J Physiol 359:189-217, 1985.

Park J, Cohen G: Vestibular ototoxicity in the chick: Effects of streptomycin on equilibrium and on ampullary dark cells. Am J Otolaryngol 6:117-127, 1982.

Pender D: Gentamicin tympanoclysis: Effects on the vestibular secretory cells. Am J Otolaryngol 6:358-367, 1985.

Rybak LP: Ototoxic mechanisms. In Altschuler RA, Hoffman DW, Bobbin RP (eds): Neurobiology of Hearing. New York, Raven Press, 1986, pp 441-454.

Saijo S, Kimura R: Distribution of HRP in the inner ear after injection into the middle ear cavity. Acta Otolaryngol 97:593-610, 1984.

Sala T: Transtympanic administration of aminoglycosides in patients with Mèniére's disease. Arch Otorhinolaryngol 245: 293-296, 1988.

Sande MA, Mandell GL: Antimicrobial agents. In Gilman AG, Rall TW, Nies AS, Taylor P (eds): Goodman and Gilman's. The Pharmacological Basis of Therapeutics, 8th ed. New York, Pergamon Press, 1990, pp 1098-1116.

Schuknecht HF: Ablation therapy for the relief of Mèniére's disease. Laryngoscope 66:859-870,1956.

Schuknecht HF: Ablation therapy in the management of Mèniére's disease. Acta Otolaryngol (Stockh) Suppl 1132: 1-42, 1957.

Shea JJ, Norris CH: Streptomycin perfusion of the labyrinth. In Nadol JB (ed): Second International Symposium on Mèniére's Disease. Amsterdam, Kugler & Ghedini, 1989.

Shea JJ: Perfusion of the inner ear with streptomycin. Am J Otol 10: 150-155, 1989.

Silverstein H, Hyman SM, Feldbaum J, Silverstein D: Use of streptomvcin sulfate in the treatment of Mèniére's disease. Otolaryngol Head Neck Surg 92: 229-232, 1984.

Silverstein H: Streptomycin treatment for Mèniére's disease. Ann Otol Rhinol Laryngol 93 (Suppl 112): 44-88, 1984.

Smith B, Myers M: The penetration of gentamicin and neomycin into the perilymph across the round window membrane. Otolaryngol Head Neck Surg 87:888-891, 1978.

Subcommittee on Equilibrium: Mèniére's disease: Criteria for diagnosis and evaluation of therapy for reporting. AAO-HNS Bulletin, 6-7 July 1985.

Williams SE, Smith DC, Schacht J: Characteristics of gentamicin uptake in the isolated crista ampullaris of the inner ear of the guinea pig. Biochem Pharmacol 36:89-95, 1987.

Williams SE, Zenner H, Schacht J: Three molecular steps of aminoglycoside ototoxicity demonstrated in outer hair cells. Hear Res 30:11-18,1987.

Wilson W, Schuknecht S: Update on the use of streptomycin therapy for Mèniére's disease. Am J Otol 2: 108-111, 1980.

27

Surgical therapy of microvascular compression syndromes

Cranial nerves V-XI lie in the cerebellopontine angle. They proceed outward from the bulb and the pons, and in this tract the perineural sheath is absent. Conditions for nerve suffering may be present in the cerebellopontine angle, due to venous or arterial compression. The degenerative processes related to age are the most important predisposing causes. The arteriosclerotic processes typical of age provoke a lengthening and a hardening of the arterioles of the cranial base. These vessels become twisted and may compress the nervous structures, both in the segment crossing the cerebellopontine angle and in the junction between central and peripheral myelin (Sunderland).
Over the years the natural reduction of the cerebral mass provokes tension on the venous and arterial vessels, and may compress the nervous structures.

Our understanding of these problems began with Dandy's work in 1930 and continued with Gardner and Miklos in the 50's. The surgical application came into being thanks to Jannetta particularly, who performed the first vascular decompression in 1966 on a patient with hemifacial spasm.
This technique's validity has since been confirmed for various pathologies:

- Trigeminal neuralgia.
- Hemifacial spasm.
- Glossopharyngeal neuralgia.
- Invalidating positional vertigo.
- Tinnitus.

TRIGEMINAL NEURALGIA

- **V3**: The involvement of V3 is the most frequent cause of trigeminal neuralgia, which is manifested with pain in the inferior hemiface. Vascular compression is generally caused by the superior cerebellar artery.
- **V2**: Pain upon compression of V2, less frequent, is due to a vessel, usually venous, which compresses the nerve near Meckel's cave and goes from the trigeminal nerve (trigeminal vein) to the dura mater.
- **V1**: The agent which provokes the compression of V1 is usually a vessel acting on the caudal part of the nerve.

Symptomatology
Trigeminal neuralgia is a relatively rare pathology, manifested in 3.4 men and 5.9 women out of 100.000 (S. Katusic).

- The disease is manifested with acute and intense pain in the hemiface, in one or more of the distribution areas of the nerve, but more frequently in the second or third division. The crisis is initially provoked by mechanical stimuli (talking, eating, shaving, putting on make-up, brushing teeth) and thermal stimuli (cold wind). There may be intervals, even long ones, where the problem does not appear. In time, the crises become more frequent and less correlated to trigger events. One clinical variation is atypical trigeminal neuralgia, which is manifested with a diffused aching pain, without specific trigger areas.

- *Medical treatment*. Pharmacological treatment is based on baclofen, carbamazepine, fenitoin. This therapy may, in rare instances, resolve the problem, or, more frequently, it may make the painful stimulus tolerable for a long time and help patients fearful of surgery live with the pathology. There may be allergic reactions to these drugs. Side effects may appear to the carbamazepine, such as hepatic alterations, disturbances in memory and equilibrium, dermatitis. These events hasten the date of surgery.

Indications

The patient must be in good health to undergo a craniotomy, as well as being under 65 years of age and having a life expectancy of at least 5 years.

Pre-operative evaluation

The patients go through routine tests for general anesthesia, tonal audiometry, brainstem evoked potentials and MRI with gadolinium, to seek possible neoplasms. The angiography is not considered useful, nor is the angio MRI. Though the vessels are evidentiated, the position of the nerves is not detected with any precision. It is therefore preferable to avoid placing the patient at risk by performing this exam, though problems are rare.

The patient must use an antiseptic shampoo and shower the evening before surgery. One hour before surgery the hair is cut from half of the patient's head.

Surgical technique

- The patient is placed in a supine position with his head in a lateral position. Ten minutes before the incision, Mannitol is administered with a rapid infusion.
- The skin is infiltrated with xylocaine and 1:100.000 of adrenaline.
- The mastoid tip is palpated and the skin is incised approx. 1 cm behind the posterior margin of the mastoid. The incision is approx. 8 cm long, and goes to 1 cm below the mastoid tip. The incision must not be extended too inferiorly because of the risk of injuring the vertebral artery, nor must it be too posterior because of the danger of damaging the occipital nerve. The emissary veins are coagulated and their aperture into the bone is closed with bone wax.
- The craniectomy, approx. 3 cm × 4, must be done superiorly to the transverse sinus and anteriorly to expose the sigmoid sinus. The dura is incised approx. 4 mm behind the sigmoid sinus and behind the first 2 cm of transverse sinus. The dura is anchored anteriorly with 2-0 silk.
- A rectangular cottonoid is positioned along the cerebellum. With the back of the suction-irrigator delicate pressure is exerted on the cerebellum in a medial and posterior direction. To open the space in the posterior cranial fossa, we prefer to use the mere pressure of the suction-irrigator because, since it is not continuous, it does not present problems of cerebellar edema.
- If necessary, a self retaining blade may be used, e.g. the blade utilized by Fukushima, with the protection of an underlying cottonoid. In this case we position it only after reaching nerve V, to reduce the time it is used and thus the effects of compression on the cerebellum.
- The petrosal vein is found between the dura and the trigeminal nerve. It is generally in a paramedial position, though its position is variable. It is coagulated and separated. It is preferable to incise the vein only partially, control hemostasis and then complete it. In this way the surgeon avoids provoking bleeding from the stumps, and since they tend to retract, hemostasis may be difficult (R. Apfelbaum).
- We proceed above CNs VII-VIII, without incising the surrounding arachnoid and we reach nerve V superiorly.
- Using blunt instruments, the arachnoid is carefully separated both superior and inferior to the nerve, until it is completely exposed. The nerve is examined. It is important to keep in mind that the neurovascular conflict occurs at the level of the brainstem, whereas a pathology resulting from distal compression is rare. In the vast majority of cases, compression is due to one or more arterial vessels. In general, the superior cerebellar artery is involved. The arterial vessels are separated with a dissector and pushed away from the nerve. Between the two structures, teflon filaments are inserted, which unlike Gelfoam has the advantage of not being reabsorbable. The teflon is placed around the nerve, so as to protect as much of the surface as possible (three sides of a teflon square) and to avoid subsequent dislocation. The vessels must not be bent. The separation must be both anterior and posterior to the nerve. To control the situation anterior to the nerve, a Zini speculum may be used. In 15% of cases, compression is caused by venous structures; these may be separated from the nerve with the technique described or they may be separated and coagulated.
- Care must be taken to avoid injuring the nearby nerves: IV, VII, VIII. Nerve IV is thin and lies superior to nerve V, near the tentorium. The arachnoid bridles around n. V must be set aside delicately, one layer at a time, to avoid damaging the nerve, if it is found inside.
- Nerve VIII lies inferior to V. The registration of intraoperative auditory potentials decreases the possibility of lesion due to traction or nerve compression. In this approach, preserving the acoustic nerve also means preserving the facial nerve.

Results

In Apfelbaum's experience, 68.8% of 300 patients operated no longer required medical treatment after 10 years. 18.9% had to have medical treatment, though the dosages were significantly lower compared to those before the operation.

In 12.8% recurrences were seen of the aching crises, not dominated by medical therapy.
Results are generally better in patients who have never undergone destructive procedures. The relapses, when they occur, do so usually within 1 year (99%), due to a dislocation of the vessel from compression (Jannetta).
This treatment requires a craniotomy, and there is a risk of death (1%) or serious complications, such as cerebral infarction (0.6%) (Apfelbaum). The risk of hematoma to the cerebellum, if using the technique which minimizes or abolishes the use of the self-retaining retractor, is practically nonexistent.
On the other hand, compared to the treatment of neurolysis of the trigeminal nerve with a percutaneous approach, this technique has the advantage of being definitive in the vast majority of patients, while preserving the integrity of the nerve and not provoking torpidity, corneal anesthesia, or dysesthesia.

HEMIFACIAL SPASM

The hemifacial spasm is a rare pathology: 0.8 cases out of 100.000 (R.G. Auger).
It appears with contractions which generally begin in the muscles around the eye, and through the years extends to the face. In serious instances it may involve both sides of the forehead and the platysma muscle in the anterior region of the neck. In quiet periods no symptoms are present, though in time a slight weakness in the muscles of the hemiface may appear.
The involuntary closing of the eye may be very bothersome, especially in some professions, and may alter the quality of life.

Instrumental diagnosis
If a branch of the facial nerve is stimulated electrically and electromyographic potentials of the muscles innervated with a different branch than the nerve are recorded, a typical response is obtained, with a latency of 10 msec (A.R. Møller).
If the patient is made to blink, synkinesis takes place in the muscles of the lower half of the face. This is clinically evident, and also evident to the electromyographic recording.

Differential Diagnosis
The aberrant regeneration after Bell's palsy is manifested with similar physical signs, during the period of nerve regeneration. In this case, a history of a previous Bell's paralysis guides the diagnosis.
In facial myokymia, wave-like muscular movements are present, associated with a pathology of the brainstem and with other alterations of the cranial nerves.
The blepharospasm involves only the musculature of the eye, bilaterally, without progressing downwards to the facial muscle.
Nervous tics have a clear relationship with emotional state and involve several muscles, not just those unilaterally innervated by the facial nerve.

Surgical operation
- The hemifacial spasm does not clinically improve with medical treatment. Its symptomatology may reduce the working and relational capacity and become a serious handicap. In these instances, if the subject is under 65 years of age and in good health, surgery may be considered. The operation is the only rational and effective treatment, but it is a craniotomy and thus, risky.
- Surgery is performed with a retrosigmoid approach. The position of the facial nerve has been described (chapter 19).
- The arachnoid is delicately pushed superior to nerve IX. Medially, the exits of n. VII and VIII are found, from the choroid plexus of the lateral recess of the fourth ventricle. The vessels that can compromise the nerve are almost always arterial vessels. In 90% of cases it is a loop of the AICA or more rarely, of the PICA. Rare cases of vertebral arterial ectasy have been seen.
- The vessels are separated with a teflon fragment.

The complications in this operation are, in rare cases, a transitory facial palsy subsequent to the manipulation of the nerve and/or hypoacusia, the degree of which is proportional to the trauma exerted on the acoustic nerve. Following the technique that minimizes the use of a self-retaining retractor, the incidence of focal epilepsy and edema of the cerebellum are almost nil.

GLOSSOPHARYNGEAL NEURALGIA

Similar to trigeminal neuralgia, a neuralgia of the glossopharyngeal nerve may appear. This rare occurrence is caused by vascular compression.
It is manifested in very acute painful crises of the posterior part of the tongue and the pharynx, provoked by phonation and swallowing.
Medical treatment frequently controls the symptoms and surgery is rarely indicated.

Surgery
- The craniotomy procedures are the same. The mixed nerves are identified and nerve IX is followed to its exit.

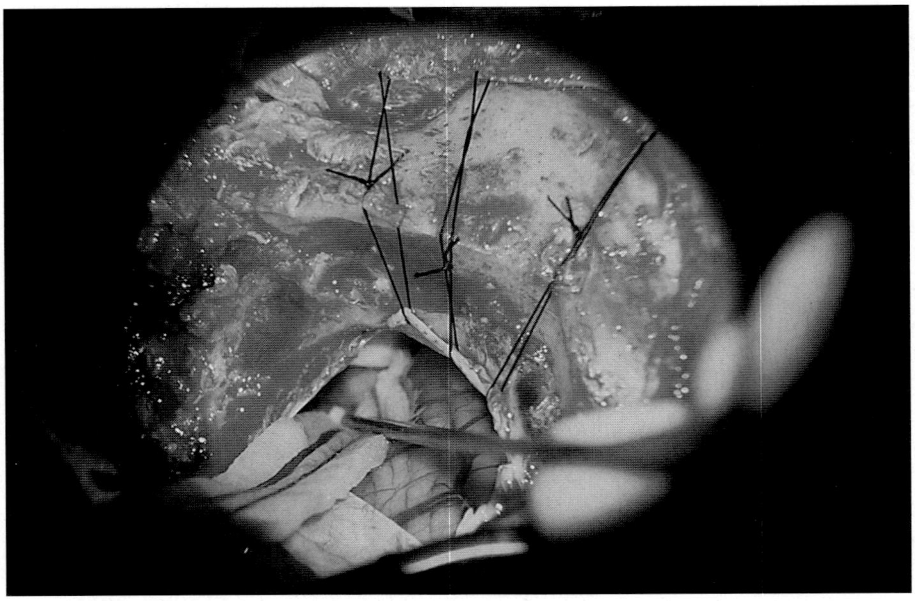

Fig. 27-1. Left ear. A partial mastoidectomy is performed and the sigmoid sinus is exposed. A retrosigmoid craniectomy, approx. 2.5 cm × 4 cm is performed. The dura is opened in a C shape. An anteriorly based dural flap is prepared, elevated and suspended anteriorly with stay sutures. For a wide anterior exposure it is important, that the base of the dural flap be lateral enough to reach the edge of the sigmoid sinus.

- The nerve exits from the medulla between the olive and the inferior cerebellar peduncle, in three or four roots which converge to form the nervous trunk. The vagus nerve is inferior. The nerve, initially covered by the floccule, goes from the jugular tubercle of the occipital bone, bends downward, crosses the jugular fossa, and emits the tympanic nerve, before exiting through the jugular foramen. Decompression is performed as described above.

VASCULAR COMPRESSION OF THE VESTIBULAR NERVE

Janetta J and Møller AR demonstrated that vascular compression of the vestibular nerve may provoke specific alterations of equilibrium, nausea, and vertigo. They named this phenomenon Disabling Positional Vertigo (DPV).

Diagnosis

The patient is afflicted by a frequent sensation of rotation and nausea, and shows instability typical of intoxication, with an added tendency toward deviation and falling towards the afflicted side. Rapid rotations are difficult and the nausea and vertigo increase with physical activity and decrease with rest. The symptoms are aggravated when the head and the body are in certain specific positions. The patient also has the sensation of constant head movement, like a pendulum and when assuming an ortostatic position the patient

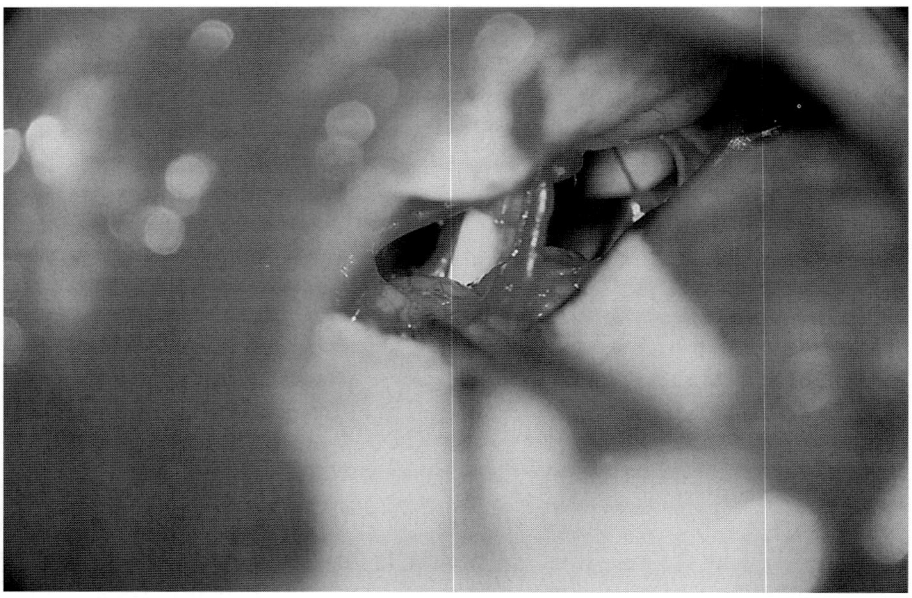

Fig. 27-2. The arachnoid is opened with sharp dissection and the cerebellum is gently depressed with the rod of a fenestrated suction-irrrigator, protected by a cottonoid. The vestibulocochlear nerve with the offending vessel is identified.

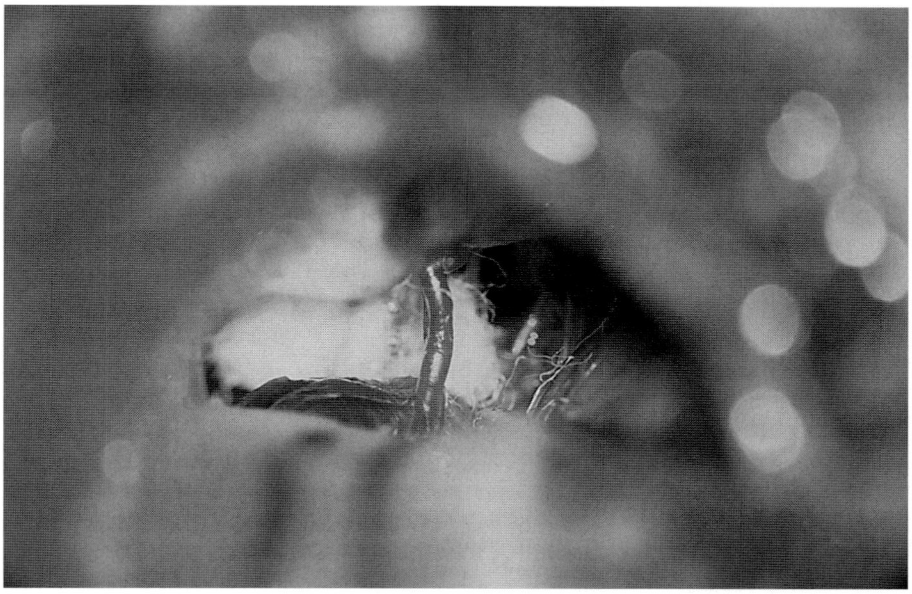

Fig. 27-3. The artery is mobilized and held away from the nerve with shredded Teflon felt.

has the impression that the floor moves up and down.

Therapeutic response: benzodiazepine is effective, whereas vestibular suppressing drugs are useless and may worsen the symptoms (Møller).

- The blood vessel exerting compression on the vestibular nerve may exert compression on other nerves of the posterior cranial fossa as well. The involvement of the intermedius nerve (branch of the facial nerve) provokes an acute otalgia (neuralgia of the geniculate ganglion). The involvement of the facial nerve is further manifested with a slight contraction of the orbicularis oculi muscle from one side.
- The involvement of the trigeminal nerve causes a transitory torpidity and pain in the hemiface, generally in the area of distribution of V2.
- The symptomatology of the perilymphatic fistula has elements similar to the DPV, but is differentiated by its acute and traumatic onset (barotraumas).
- Vestibular neuronitis appears with recognizable signs: the vertigo is acute, worsens with head movements, is associated with vegetative phenomena, and the caloric response of the affected side is reduced or absent. In a period varying from a few days to 5-6 months the symptoms disappear.

Mèniére's disease (see chapter 17) and Benign Paroxysmal Vertigo (see chapter 21-22) appear with symptomatology and instrumental data that permit a precise differential diagnosis.

Instrumental diagnosis

A tonal audiometric examination is performed, as well as a vocal audiometry, tympanometry, BERA and ENG. The audiometric tonal exam shows small hearing losses (dip) in the frequency from 1500 to 2000Hz. With the auditory evoked potentials an ipsilateral increase is seen in the interval I-III or else the interval III-V may be prolonged contralaterally (Janetta PJ).

Therapy

Microvascular decompression of the vestibulocochlear nerve (Figs. 27-1, 27-2, 27-3).

REFERENCES

Adornato DC, Gildenberg PL, Ferrario CM, et al: Pathophysiology of intravenous air embolism in dogs. Anesthesiology 49:120, 1978.

Apfelbaum RI, Duncalf D, Phillips PL: Is central venous catheterization necessary for neurosurgical procedures in the sitting position? Presented at the annual meeting of the American Association of Neurological Surgeons, New York, 1980.

Apfelbaum RI, Kirk M, Terra AM: Microvascular decompression of the trigeminal nerve for the treatment of trigeminal neuralgia. J Neurosurg Nurs 10:77,1978.

Apfelbaum RI, Neurosurgical applications of video techniques. Clin Neurosurg 28:246, 1981.

Apfelbaum RI: Surgery for tic douloureux. Clin Neurosurg 31:351, 1984.

Cushing H: The major trigeminal neuralgias and their surgical treatment based on experiences with 332 gasserian operations. Am J Med Sci 160:157, 1920.

Dandy WE: The treatment ot trigeminal neuralgia by the cerebellar route. Ann Surg 96:787, 1932.

Frost EA: Anesthesia for neurosurgical procedures in the sitting position. Weekly Anesthesiology Update, Lesson 4, vol 1, 1977.

Gardner WJ, Sava GA: Hemifacial spasm-a reversible pathophysiologic state. J Neurosurg 19:240, 1962.

German WJ: Surgical treatment of spasmodic facial tic. Surgery, 11:912, 1942.

Hakanson S: Trigeminal neuralgia treated by the injection of glycerol into the trigeminal cistern. Neurosurgery, 9:638, 1981.

Hitselberger WE, Pulec JL: Trigeminal nerve (posterior root) retrolabyrinthine selective section: operative procedure for intractable pain. Arch Otolaryngol 96:412-415, 1972.

Janetta PJ: Treatment of trigeminal neuralgia by suboccipital and transtentorial cranial operations. Clin Neurosurg 24:538, 1976.

Jannetta PJ, Abbasy M, Maroon J, et al: Etiology and definitive microsurgical treatment of hemifacial spasm. J Neurosurg 47:321, 1977.

Jannetta PJ: Observations on the etiology of trigeminal neuralgias, hemifacial spasm, acoustic nerve dysfunction, and glossopharyngeal neuralgia. Definitive microsurgical treatment and results in 117 patients. Neurochirurgia (Stuttgart) 20:145-154, 1977.

Jannetta PJ: Arterial compression of the trigeminal nerve at the pons in patients with trigeminal neuralgia. J Neurosurg 26:159, 1967.

Jannetta PJ: Microsurgical approach to the trigeminal nerve for tic douloureux. Prog Neurol Surg 7:180,1976.

Jannetta PJ: Observations on the etiology of trigeminal neuralgia, hemifacial spasm, acoustic nerve dysfunction and glossopharyngeal neuralgia. Definitive microsurgical treatment and results in 117 patients. Neurochirurgia 20:145, 1977.

Lunsford LD, Apfelbaum RI: Choice of surgical therapeutic modalities for treatment of trigeminal neuralgia: Microvascular decompression, percutaneous retrogasserian thermic or glycerol rhizotomy. Clin Neurosurg 32:319, 1985.

Lunsford LD: Treatment of tic douloureux by percutaneous retrogasserian glycerol injection. JAMA 248:449, 1982.

Mizuno N, Akimoto C, Mochizuki K, Matsuschima R: Experimental studies of efferent fibers in the hypoglossal nerve in the cat: a scanning electron microscopic observation in the lingual mucosa following transsection of the nerve, and a degeneration study with silver impregnation methods. Arch Histol Jpn 35: 99-113, 1973.

Nugent GR: Technique and results of 800 percutaneous radiofrequency thermocoagulations for trigeminal neuralgia. Appl Neurophysiol 45:504, 1982.

Rasmussen P, Riishede J: Facial pain treated with carbamazepine (Tegretol). Acta Neurol Scand 46:385,1970.

Scoville WB: Partial extracranial section of seventh nerve for hemifacial spasm. J Neurosurg 31:106, 1969.

Siegfried J: 500 percutaneous thermocoagulations of the gasserian ganglion for trigeminal pain. Surg Neurol 8:126, 1977.

Tew JM, Keller JT: The treatment of trigeminal neuralgia by percutaneous radiofrequency technique. Clin Neurosurg 24:557, 1976.

White JC, Sweet WH: Pain and the neurosurgeon; medical treatment of trigeminal neuralgia. Springfield, III, Charles C Thomas, 1969, p 169.

28

Translabyrinthine approach to acoustic neuromas

I have never seen a tumor too large for the translabyrinthine approach.

HITSELBERGER W.

PATIENT'S POSITION

N.B. Orientation (anterior, posterior, medial, lateral...) in this text always refers to the surgical position.

The patient is supine, with his head turned to the side. Some surgeons lower the headrest of the table, especially in middle ear surgery, so that the patient's head is lower than his body, thus improving the surgeon's view of the external auditory canal and tympanic membrane.

We prefer a table without a headrest, to avoid torsion of the neck when the headrest is lowered and to avoid possible alterations in the carotid and vertebral axis flow. The risk of lesions to the cervical rachis, bone or nerve, is reduced by not using the headrest. Further more, it is best not to elevate the head, so that the view of the posterior wall of the IAC is improved.

The patient's movements are controlled by the operating table. It is therefore advisable to be completely familiar with it.

- The patient is placed on the side opposite the surgeon. This gives the surgeon room to rest his arms by the patient's head.
- To lower the head with respect to the body, the table must be inclined in the infero-superior position. The price to pay is probably slightly more bleeding than would occur with the headrest.
- Sterile drapes are positioned. We use irrigating solution liberally during the bone work, and plastic drapes are taped to the patient's head to avoid contamination through water and blood running onto the patient's head and hair. For the same reason we use modified retractors with suction on the posterior blade, to remove excess irrigating solution and blood from the wound.
- The facial nerve stimulator electrodes are positioned (see chapter 41).
- The patient wears elastic stockings and a cushion is placed under his knees to reduce the risk of thrombosis. The stockings are removed when the patient is ready to walk.
- After inducing anesthesia, a nasogastric probe is inserted. It is left in place, in aspiration, for 24 hours. The stomach thus remains empty in patients who may present post-operative vomiting. It also immediately identifies a gastric hemorrhage due to stress-induced ulcers.
- After inducing anesthesia, a urinary catheter is inserted and left in place until the patient enters the intensive care unit.

PREPARATION OF THE SURGICAL AREA

The patient is asked to wash his hair with an antiseptic shampoo the evening before the operation. Immediately before the operation, while the patient is still in the ward, the hair is cut in the postauricular and temporal area. It is useful to wait until the last minute to cut hair to avoid folliculitis and possible risks of local surface infection. The skin is washed with povidone-iodine (Betadine) and the surgical area is covered with a sterile plastic drape. Sterile drapes are placed around the operating area and on the body of the patient. These are held in place with plastic adhesive strips.

ACOUSTIC NEUROMAS

The three main surgical approaches for the treatment of acoustic neuromas are:

- The translabyrinthine approach.
- The retrosigmoid approach.
- The middle cranial fossa approach.

CLINICAL DIAGNOSIS

The diagnosis of a tumor of the cerebellopontine angle is obtained principally through audiometric tests (liminal and supraliminal), vestibular tests, BERA, radiologic images (MRI with gadolinium, HRCT with contrast enhancement). These techniques are not discussed in this text.

SOME NEUROLOGICAL CLINICAL DATA

An ophthalmoscopic examination makes it possible, in larger tumors, to identify the first signs of increased intracranial pressure, such as: blurring at the edges of the optical disk, vein swelling, lack of venous pulsation. More delayed signs are the disappearance of the margins of the optical disk, reductions in the number of vessels, small hemorrhaging areas (Hitselberger W).

Examination of V
The distribution area of the trigeminal nerve may be anesthetized. The cheecks are softly touched bilaterally and the patient's sensation is compared. The most precocious clinical sign is the reduction of corneal response, which is measured with an aesthesiometer or, more simply, with the pressure of the tip of a cotton swab on the external margin of the cornea.

Examination of VII
With a simple blunt hook, we can look for a reduction in sensitivity in the posterior part of the external auditory canal, compared to the contralateral canal.

Examination of IX
The sensitivity of the posterior part of the tonsillar fossa is reduced. This is shown by touching it with a cotton swab.

These symptoms are precocious and can be observed in common clinical practice. A delayed observation of a patient with tumor of the posterior cranial fossa affecting the cerebellum, brain stem, or cranial nerves will reveal more serious clinical results and will require the investigation of these systems.

PATIENT SELECTION

The average incidence of acoustic neuromas is 9.4 per million inhabitants per year, but anatomical studies of the temporal bones have shown that the number of clinically verified tumors appear to be far fewer than the actual incidence of the pathology.

The majority of neuromas must be operated upon, since their growth in the posterior cranial fossa will lead to hearing loss, paralysis of CN VII, compression of the brainstem, and death.

It is advisable to observe the growth of small intracanalar tumors or those near the CPA with MRI. If the tumor does not grow, in the absence of vestibular and facial deficit, and in the presence of unilateral hearing loss, the operation can be postponed, while continuing radiological controls. If a tumor growth is noted that can be expressed in mm/year, we know that growth will continue. Thus the growth rate can be predicted, and an operating date can be set. If attempting to preserve hearing, the size of the tumor and the operating date will be instrumental in deciding the success rate in middle fossa operations.

In elderly patients, the general state of health must be considered as well as the patient's age, the size of the tumor, the deficits caused, and the rate of tumor growth. For example, a patient aged 65 with an intracanalar tumor, with unilateral sensorineural hearing loss and no other signs of deficit, and a growth rate of less than 1 mm/year can be expected to have a tumor slightly larger than 1 cm in diameter at the age of 75. Since the life expectancy for men (in Italy) is 75 years, the value of an operation in this particular case is questionable.
We use the following procedures:

THE RETROSIGMOID APPROACH
Tumors up to a maximum of 1.5 cm in diameter
Unaffected IAC base
Good hearing (see Chapter 20).

THE MIDDLE FOSSA APPROACH
- Tumors up to 1 cm, contained in the IAC
- Unaffected IAC base
- Good hearing.

THE TRANSLABYRINTHINE APPROACH
- Good hearing in the contralateral ear
- Tumors larger then 1 cm.

THE TRANSLABYRINTHINE APPROACH TO ACOUSTIC NEUROMA

The following are the objectives in acoustic neuroma surgery, in descending order:
1. Save the patient's life.
2. Remove the tumor.
3. Avoid alterations to the brain stem and cerebellum.
4. Preserve the cranial nerves.

The translabyrinthine approach has the following advantages:

- The patient's supine rather than seated position reduces the risk of complications, such as air embolisms and cardiocirculatory disturbances. The surgeon's position is more comfortable.
- No pressure on the cerebellum is necessary.
- Ample space. Even the largest neuromas can be removed by this method. Hemostasis is facilitated.
- Easy identification of the infralabyrinthine part of the facial nerve, in the point not generally affected by the tumor. In the unusual event that this part is also affected, the nerve can be followed "a la demande", up to the geniculate ganglion, to the tympanic part, and to the mastoid part. This approach affords a complete view of the nerve from the brain stem to the stylomastoid orifice and, if necessary, to the intraparotid part.
- Rapid and direct access to the surgical area in case of post-operative hemorrhages.
- The major disadvantage to this approach is hearing loss (Figs. 28-1; see Fig. 32-16).

INCISION

- 5-10 ml of 0.5% lidocaine and 0.01% adrenalin are injected in the postauricular region.
- The incision begins high up, above the temporalis plane, and continues back to the helix of about 3 cm, ending in a curved line at the mastoid tip. The incision must never be too far forward because this would limit the view of the posterior cranial fossa (Fig. 28-2).
- The incision can be made with a cutting current which does not burn the skin as long as it is kept moving, and, at the same time, allows for hemostasis. With this instrument, the skin, subcutaneous layer, temporalis muscle, and periosteum are cut.

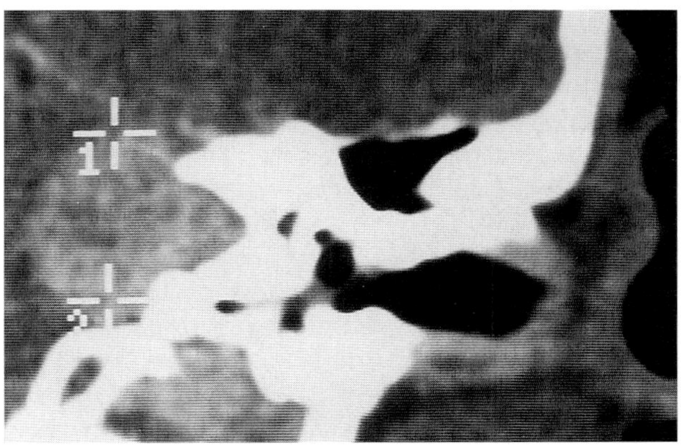

Fig. 28-1. HRCT. Acoustic neuroma.

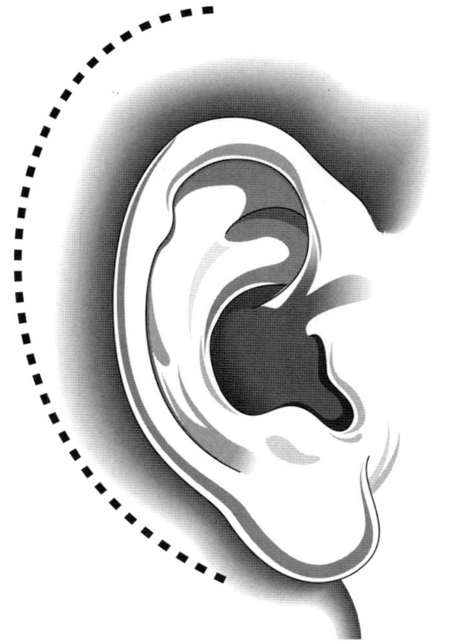

Fig. 28-2. Skin incision.

Some surgeons prefer to prepare a flap of muscle tissue and periosteum, based anteriorly. In this case, it is preferable to first cut the skin with a scalpel, detach it from the muscular layer, and then prepare the flaps with a cutting current.
The curved postauricular incision is made from the temporalis plane to the mastoid tip, 4 cm posterior to the auricle. An incision this far back allows adequate exposure of the sigmoid sinus and the dura of the posterior retrosigmoid fossa. The incision is also posterior to the operating cavity and reduces the risk of cerebrospinal fluid leakage.

- In both techniques, the detachment is completed with a Lempert elevator. The mastoid bone is thus exposed as follows: the upper part up to the middle cranial fossa, the lower part up to the mastoid tip, the anterior part up to the bony external auditory canal, the posterior part up to the occipital bone.
- To stabilize the flaps of the operating field, self-retaining retractors can be used. In general, one large Weitlaner retractor with the valves open in an antero-posterior direction is sufficient. A second supero-inferior retractor can be used to hold back the temporalis muscle. The advantage of the self-retaining retractor is that the force applied can be progressively regulated, thus exposing the bony area as required. The aspiration tube helps to absorb surplus water (Figs. 28-3, 28-4).
- Another method for holding the flaps in place is to use elastic bands with hooks, or silk sutures. The advantage of this method is that it does not limit the view of the operating field, particularly along the posterior cranial fossa.

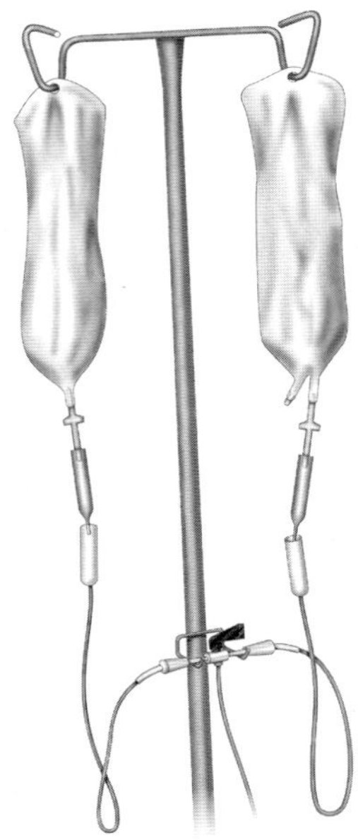

Fig. 28-3. Two bags of irrigant solution connected to the delivery system.

MASTOIDECTOMY

A postauricular incision is made approximately 3 cm behind the postauricular fold. The aponeurotic galea is detached laterally at the temporalis muscle and the ear is folded forward. A flap of periosteal muscle is prepared by cutting in an anterior-posterior direction along the temporalis plane up to the mastoid tip. The resulting triangular flap based anteriorly is detached with the Lempert elevator, moved to scrape the bone. The cutaneous and periosteal muscle incisions are asymmetrical, to facilitate closure on irregular planes and prevent the loss of cerebro-spinal fluid. The flap is held with a large self retaining retractor so that it remains in an anterior position.

A radical mastoidectomy is carried out according to the method already described, so that the following landmarks are exposed:

- Anteriorly: the external bony auditory canal.
- Anteriorly-superioly: the antrum, the semicircular lateral canal, the incus body.
- Superiorly: the tegmen tympani of the middle cranial fossa.
- Posteriorly: the sinodural angle, the compact bone lamina above the sigmoid sinus and 1-2 cm of cortex in back of the sigmoid sinus.
- Inferiorly: the mastoid tip, the digastric crest and the jugular bulb below (Figs. 28-5, 28-6).

IDENTIFICATION OF THE THIRD SEGMENT OF THE FACIAL NERVE

- At this point, the third segment of the facial nerve is skeletonized, based on landmarks of the lateral canal, the posterior canal, the incus body and the digastric crest. This is a propitious moment, due to the ample space created in an anterior-posterior direction.
- This allows the nerve to be skeletonized, working with the back of the burr in a posterior-anterior direction. The posterior canal and its ampulla is like a finger pointing to the second genu of VII, and terminates 1-2 mm from the nerve: a good landmark. We follow the canal to arrive at the nerve. At this point in time, the canal must not be opened. If this should inadvertently occur, it need not be considered a complication,

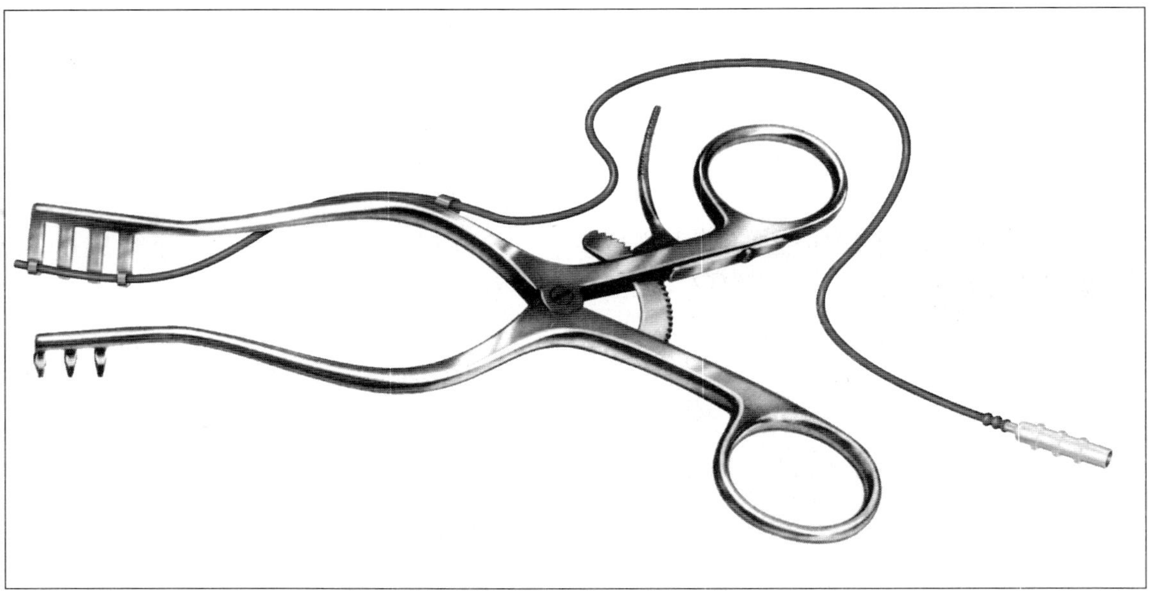

Fig. 28-4. Modified Weitlaner retractor. The suction on the posterior blade of the retractor removes excess irrigation fluid and blood from the wound.

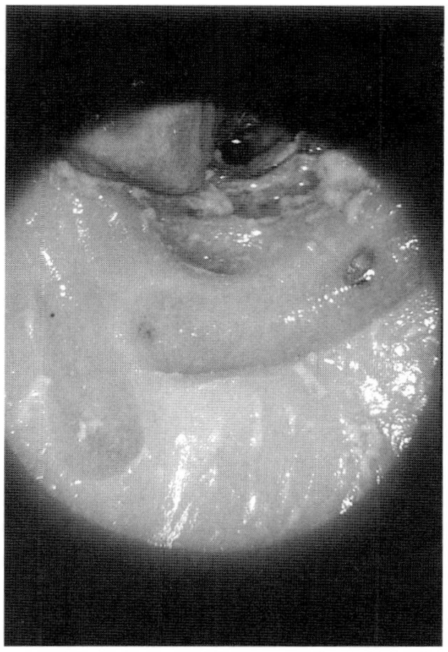

Fig. 28-5. Right ear. Initial cut on the mastoid bone.

since a labyrinthectomy is to be performed. It is also possible to completely skeletonize the third part of VII after the labyrinthectomy, to utilize as much space as possible. We believe that the sooner the landmarks and the structures to save are identified, the more rapid the successive part of any operation will be. The identification of VII is fundamental because it represents the anterior dissecting limit. In fact, if too much bone is left on the third part of the facial nerve, it is not possible to adequately visualize the IAC floor (Fig. 28-7).

- The bone is cut above the sigmoid sinus, working first with a finishing burr, then with a 5-7 mm diamond burr. The residual bone is very thin and the blue sinus can be seen through it. With the rod of the suction-irrigator, the thin bone layer is compressed to produce minute fractures. The bone fragments are removed from back to front with a House dissector, until the underlying sinus is visible. In the same way, the posterior part of the lateral sinus is exposed. The bone layers above the sinus are not detached from front to back, since this would obstruct the visual field and lead to uncontrollable tension in the blood vessel walls, possibly causing perforations. This part of the sinus is preferably exposed with a large diamond burr. Posterior to the sinus, 1-2 cm of the dura of the middle cranial fossa are exposed, working first with a large cutting burr and then with a large diamond burr (5-7 mm).

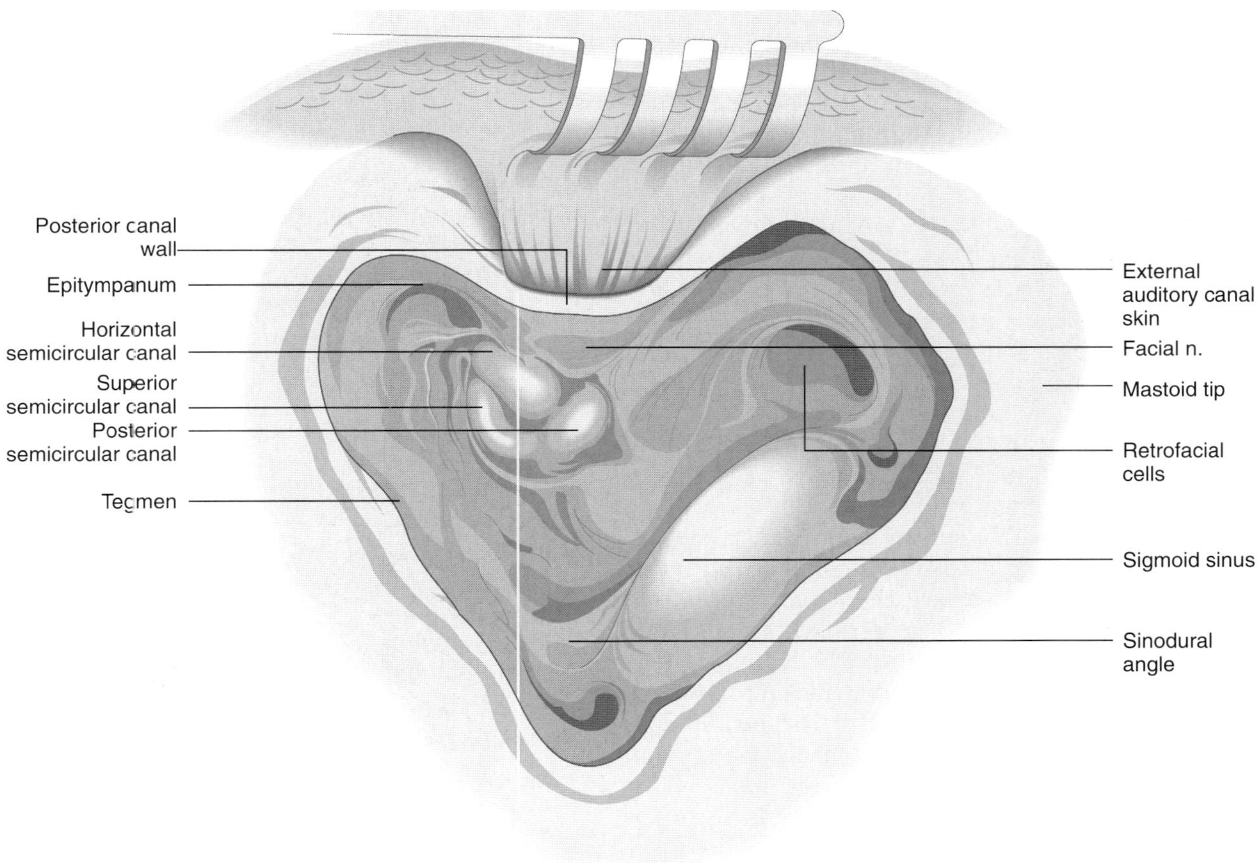

Fig. 28-6. Complete mastoidectomy.

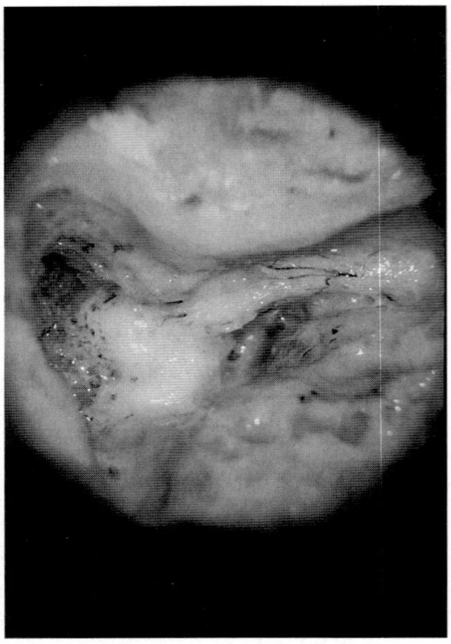

Fig. 28-7. Horizontal and posterior semicircular canals are exposed. The third part of the facial nerve is skeletonized: it is the anterior limit of the dissection.

- It is fundamental to remove a great deal of bone, especially in large tumors, in order to thoroughly expose the surgical area. Thus, it is possible to compress the sinus and the dura of the middle and posterior fossa in order to increase visibility below, without encountering bone resistance at the back.
- The emissary mastoid vein(s) lead(s) to the posterior edge of the sinus, connecting the latter with the veins of the external part of the cranium. The emissary mastoid vein can be found again in the surgical field when the dura of the posterior fossa is exposed. When it is deep within the sinus, it can be preserved; more often, it is near the surface, and prevents adequate exposure of the sinus and posterior dura. In this case, it must be coagulated with a bipolar cautery as far as possible from the sinus, and sacrificed.
- The upper part of the sinus is detached from the overlying bone, then compressed gently with a suction-irrigator (12") while the overlying bone is cut with a cutting burr. Step by step, the whole sigmoid sinus is exposed. An island of bone can be left above the sinus. This was recommended by W. House to provide a resting place for the suction-irrigator, which compresses the sinus and aspirates below during progressive phases of the operation (Bill's Island). It also serves to protect the sinus from the traumatic action of the rotating shaft of the burr. The sino-dural angle and the dura of the posterior and middle cranial fossa are also exposed. The venous structures now visible are the sigmoid sinus, with its upper part near the entrance of the transverse sinus and the lower part near the jugular bulb and the superior petrosal sinus. The superior petrosal sinus runs along the angle formed by the dura of the middle and posterior cranial fossa. At this point the shadow of the jugular bulb is seen through the bone.

THE JUGULAR BULB

- The position of the jugular bulb may vary. When it is high, it may reach the ampulla of the semicircular posterior canal. At other times it may be as low as the level of the digastric crest. In this last case, it may not be necessary to expose it, but we prefer to do so because it gives us a reliable landmark for our dissection. Also, the best way to avoid damaging anatomical structures is, of course, to identify their positions.
- When the bulb is low, it is sufficient to identify the blue shadow of the jugular bulb through the bone. When it is high, it is exposed with a diamond burr, leaving a very thin layer of bone. Sometimes this does not suffice to expose the lower part of the internal acoustic canal. The bone layer is then fractured into small fragments by exerting downward pressure. The bulb is depressed and kept in situ with bone wax. If blood oozes from the microfractures, Surgicel and bone wax are applied (Fig. 28-8).
- The surgical field is shaped like an inverted cone and gives the surgeon an ample view. On the average, the semicircular canals are still in-

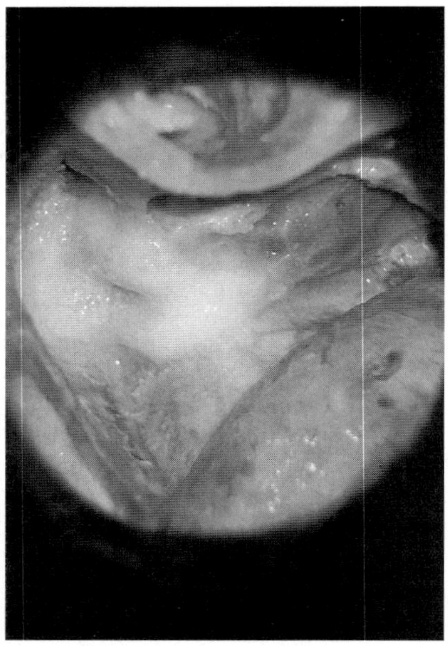

Fig. 28-8. Right ear. High jugular bulb that reduces the exposure of the lower part of the internal acoustic canal. The bone layer is then fractured into small fragments by exerting downward pressure. The bulb is then depressed and kept in situ with bone wax. If blood oozes from the microfractures, Surgicel is applied followed by bone wax.

tact. Above them, about 1 cm of bone is preserved over the meninx of the middle and superior fossa, to protect from traumas caused by burr slippage during the labyrinthectomy to follow.

- The labyrinthectomy is performed with a 4-6 mm cutting burr. The canals (fenestration) are opened beginning with the lateral canal, which is followed back to the posterior canal, finally reaching the superior canal. The lateral canal is completely opened, and followed back to the posterior canal. Then the superior canal is completely opened. At this point, the common crus of the posterior and lateral canals is visible, as are the ampullae of the three canals (Fig. 28-9). The incision must not go beyond the ampulla of the posterior canal because the facial nerve runs alongside. The ampulla of the semicircular superior canal must be preserved because it is the key to the subsequent identification of the superior vestibular nerve. To speed the process, the labyrinthine block can be cut with a large cutting burr, though not before identifying the ampullae of the semicircular canals (Figs. 28-10, 28-11, 28-12, 28-13).
- The ampulla of the lateral canal, at the upper pole of the elliptical recess of the utricle, guides us to the superior ampulla just above. The ampulla of the posterior canal is found under the mastoid position of the facial nerve and at the lower pole of the elliptical recess.
- The anterior wall of the lateral canal is preserved since the third part of the facial nerve is on the other side, with its skeletonization to be completed.
- A blood vessel is seen inside the circle formed by the upper and horizontal canals; this is the subarcuate artery. It is coagulated with a bipolar cautery.
- On the crus communis floor there is the endolymphatic duct, which is lighter in color than the surrounding bone. It passes under the posterior semicircular canal and enters into the endolymphatic sac, located in a dural duplication of the posterior fossa. Anteriorly it opens into the medial vestibular wall.

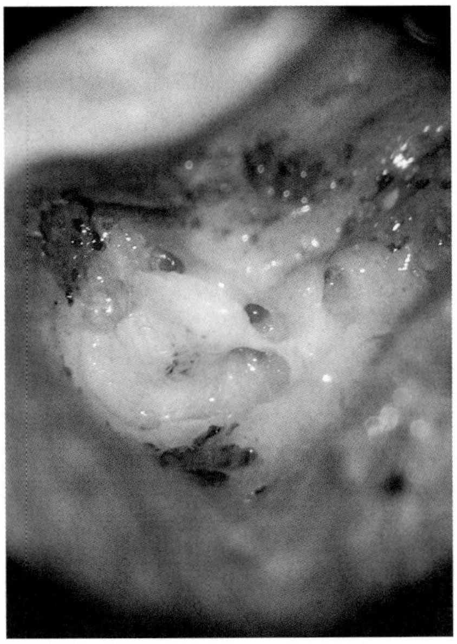

Fig. 28-9. Fenestration of the semicircular canals. The horizontal semicircular canal leads to the posterior canal that leads to the common crus and the superior canal. The anterior wall of the horizontal canal is kept intact, as a protection for the external genu and horizontal portions of the facial nerve.

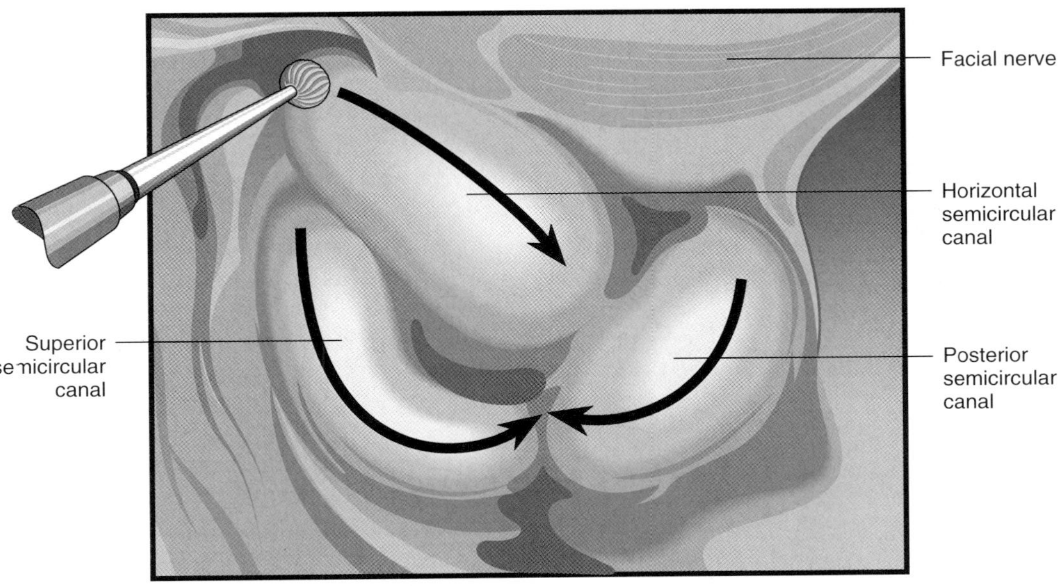

Fig. 28-10. Fenestration of the semicircular canals. The horizontal semicircular canal leads to the posterior canal that leads to the superior canal.

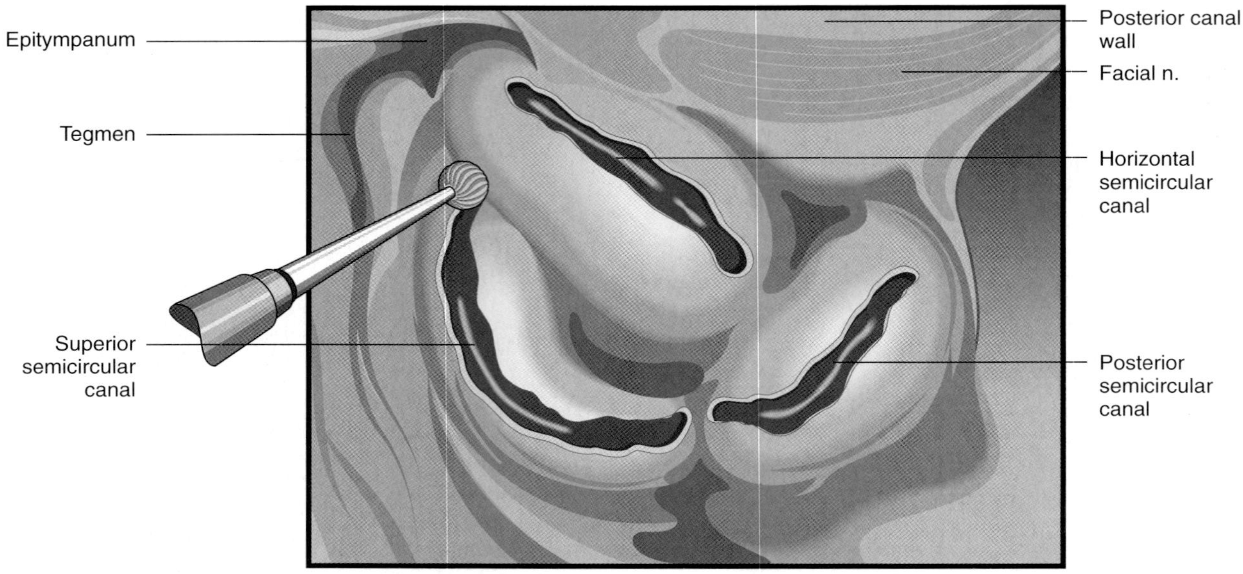

Fig. 28-11. Fenestration of the semicircular canals.

- The labyrinthectomy proceeds anteriorly to the vestibule. The posterior utricle and the anterior saccule are aspirated. The anterior vestibule is then opened wide. The roof of the vestibule consist of the posterior part of the medial wall of the tympanic cavity, where the stapes footplate is located.
- When introducing a diamond burr into the vestibule, it is important to be aware of the superior facial nerve, which crosses the roof of the vestibule. On the other hand, it is fundamental to adequately expose the vestibule, since the medial wall of the vestibule is also the lateral wall of the fundus of the internal auditory canal. The exposure of the vestibule is therefore essential to the identification of nerves VII and VIII at their entrance into the IAC (Figs. 28-14, 28-15, 28-16).

THE COCHLEAR DUCT

- A diamond burr is used to identify the origin of the superior vestibular nerve from the ampulla of the superior semicircular canal. This is essential, since this is the superior limit before coming to the facial nerve. The cutting burr proceeds with respect to this landmark near the porus acusticus. The posterior cranial fossa is pressed, thus liberating the overlying bone which is treated with the burr and freeing the porus of the canal. If the underlying dura is not completely

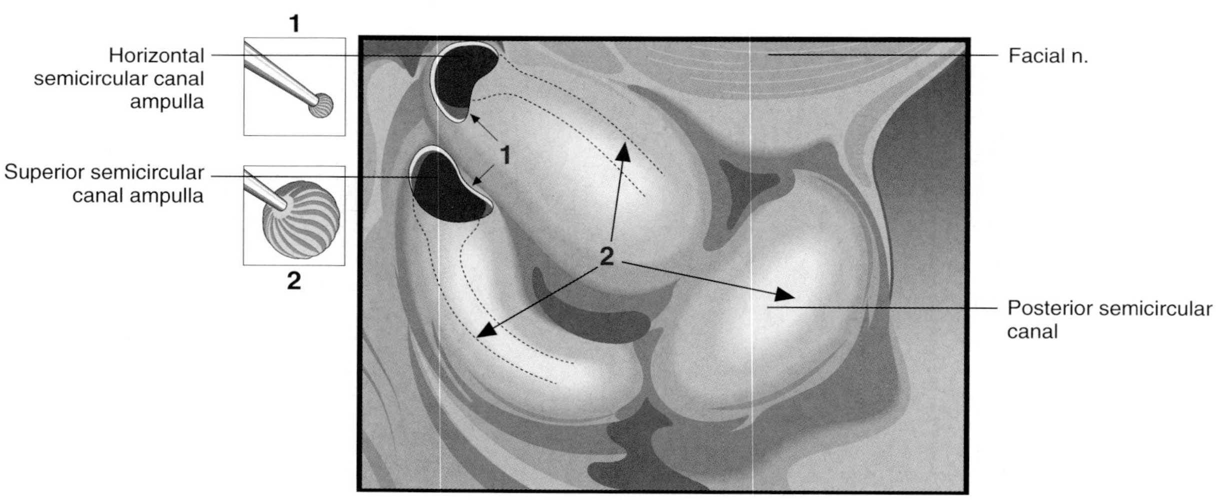

Fig. 28-12. The horizontal and superior semicircular canal ampullae are opened first, with a small cutting burr. The labyrinthectomy is then performed with a large cutting burr. We always preserve the ampulla of the superior semicircular canal, for easier identification of the superior vestibular nerve in the following stages. Opening of the medial wall of the superior ampulla shows the superior vestibular nerve as it enters the labyrinth.

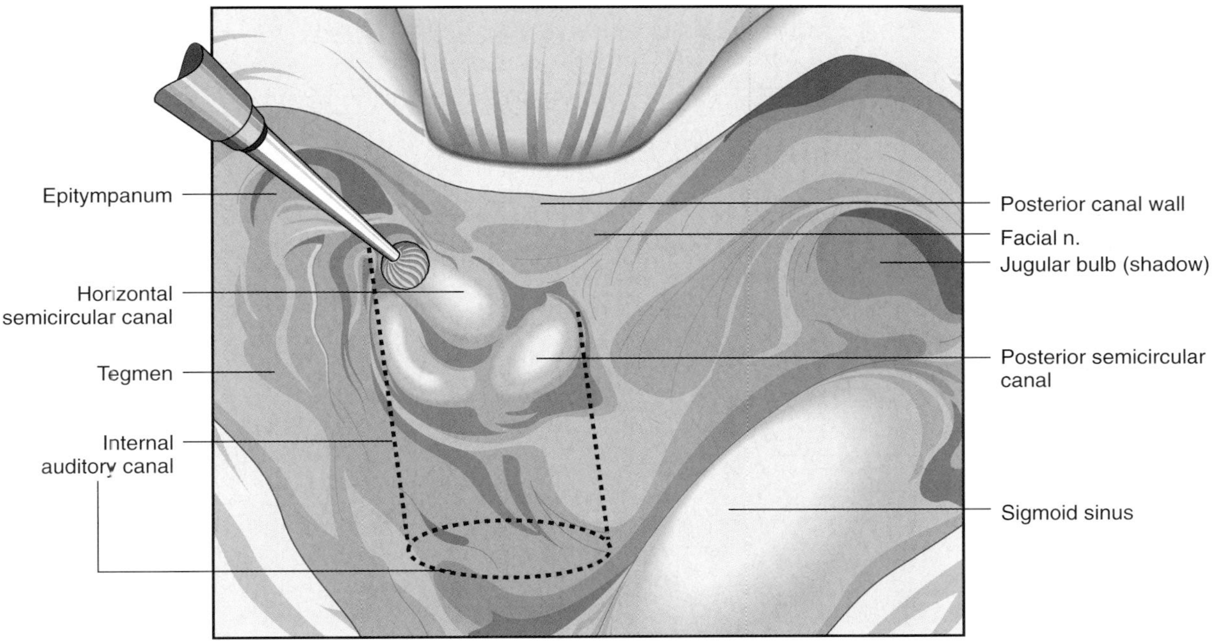

Fig. 28-13. The internal auditory canal.

separated from the bone, a safety margin of bone must be left in place, and removed later with a diamond burr. This is virtually the rule near the superior margin of the porus acusticus, due in part to the fact that the surgeon sees the bony floor of the dura in a horizontal position, and therefore has a limited view.

- Bone is removed with a cutting burr, until a bony skeleton is defined at the IAC. The bone between the IAC and the jugular bulb is removed.
- The dissection is extended forward up to a small white hole; this is the cochlear aqueduct, from which the spinal fluid flows. The dissection must be carried neither forward nor medially because of the danger of damaging nerve IX. The latter exits the cranium and descends along the medial and superior aspects of the

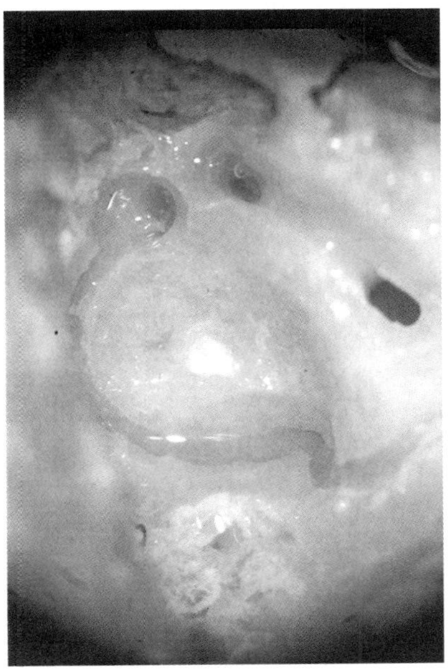

Fig. 28-14. The semicircular canals are completely opened. The subarcuate artery penetrates the labyrinthine bone in the center of the circle inscribed by the superior and horizontal semicircular canals.

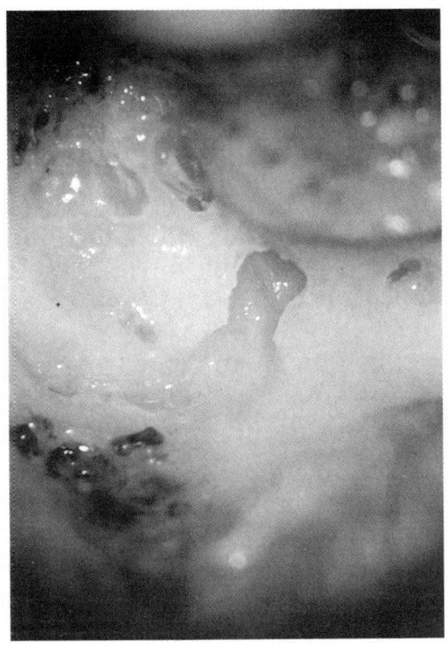

Fig. 28-15. The semicircular canals are completely connected, the bone over the facial nerve is thinned to provide good access to the vestibule, the vestibule is opened. The medial wall of the vestibule is the lateral wall of the IAC.

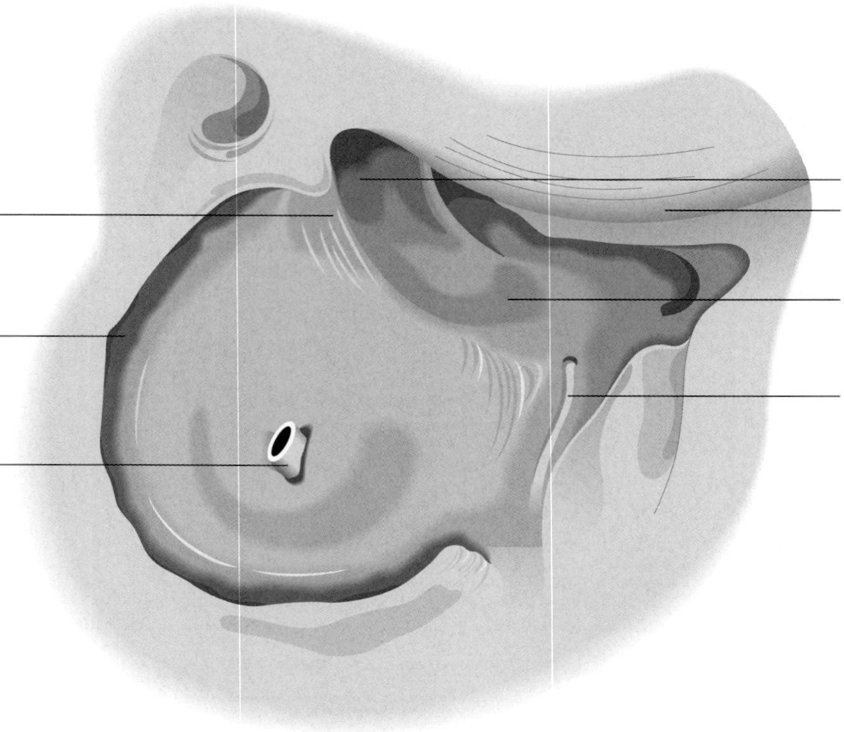

Fig. 28-16. Postauricular labyrinthectomy. The vestibule is opened. The medial wall of the vestibule is the lateral wall of the internal auditory canal fundus.

jugular bulb. Other nerves which could be damaged by an extended downward dissection are X and XI. Below the cochlear duct is the jugular bulb. To identify it, it is sufficient to note its bluish shadow through the bone.

The bordering structures are as follows:

Superior: dura of the middle posterior fossa plates, superior petrosal sinus.

Posterior: dura of the posterior fossa plates and sigmoid sinus.

Anterior: third part of the facial nerve, entrance of the vestibular nerve (superior in the IAC), cochlear aqueduct.

Inferior: jugular bulb.

Inside the field is the IAC, covered by a thin plate of bone.

- At this point a diamond burr is used. The residual plates of bone are removed in the deepest part of the middle and posterior fossa. The residual bone is removed from the posterior part of the IAC and its fundus. A small diamond burr (1, 1.5 mm) may be used to remove the bone of the fundus, by drilling canals superior and inferior to the IAC. The bone is then dislodged from the dura with a House elevator and removed with a common forceps.
- The dura of the IAC is now outlined predominantly at the meatus. When moving on to the superior part, it is important to be careful of the facial nerve which lies just underneath the dura. It is therefore wise to drill superiorly to the IAC, exposing it almost 270 degrees.
- The drill must turn in the direction going from the IAC to the dura of the middle fossa. Otherwise bone fragments may be captured by the burr and pushed into the IAC, damaging nerve VII. The possibility of damaging the facial nerve in this phase is greater in small tumors, since the burr may easily damage the facial nerve which lies just underneath the dura. In large neuromas the cancerous tissue mediates between dura and nerve, acting as a buffer to the trauma of the burr. Extreme care must always be taken. In rare instances, in larger tumors, the nerve may be pushed upward into contact with the dura of the IAC.
- A thin plate of bone is left on the presumed path of nerve VII. It is carefully dissected from the dural plane, moving the nerve along with it, and is removed with the burr or with forceps. The IAC is then exposed as much as possible, up to approximately 270 degrees. This is important because the space that is gained anteriorly in this phase will later allow for a better surgical exposure of the tumor's anterior margin (Fig. 28-17).
- We then move on to the superior part of the IAC (the fundus). At this point, the superior vestibular nerve has already been identified. Below, a

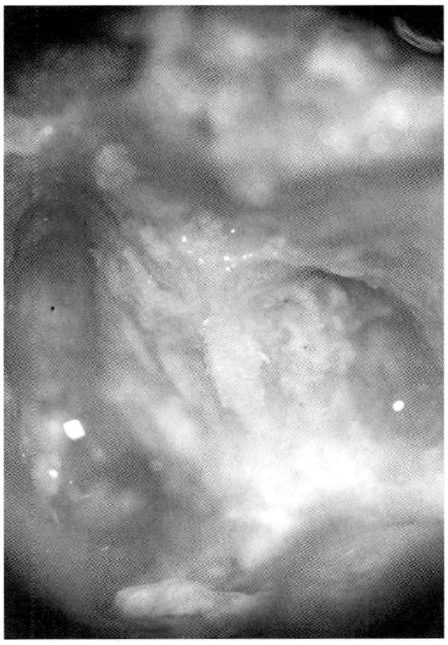

Fig. 28-17. The dura of the internal auditory canal is exposed. The transverse crest comes into view.

bony ridge, called the transverse or falciform crest, is identified (see chapter 6). With respect to the falciform crest, in the surgical position in the IAC, the superior vestibular nerve is posterior-superior, the inferior vestibular nerve and the singular nerve are posterior-inferior, the facial nerve with the intermediate nerve is anterior-superior and the cochlear nerve is anterior-inferior. This anatomic division does not correspond, however, to the true surgical view, which shows posteriorly the facial, the superior vestibular and the inferior vestibular nerves; anterior, but not visible, is the cochlear nerve.

IDENTIFYING THE FACIAL NERVE AT THE FUNDUS OF THE IAC

- Once the superior vestibular nerve has been identified, the labyrinthine part of the facial nerve may be sought by drilling 2 mm anteriorly and superiorly to the ampullar exit of the vestibular nerve (Fisch). The direction of the dissection must be upward and downward. It must be parallel to the nerve, and not perpendicular to it, in order to avoid trauma to the nerve trunk. The facial nerve, several millimeters from the meatal foramen, is then identified. A bony crest (the vertical crest or Bill's bar), separates the facial nerve from the superior vestibular nerve. This crest is the posterior limit of the fallopian canal.
- Another method is to insert a blunt hook under the point where the vestibular nerve exits the ampulla and find Bill's bar (William House).
- It is very important to identify both the nerve near the meatal foramen and Bill's bar, since this maneuver permits the identification of the facial nerve where it is not involved with the tumor. In rare cases, the tumor may involve the nerve even at this level. With this method it is possible to follow the nerve to the geniculate ganglion and proceed along the fallopian canal, finally reaching the landmark of healthy nerve.
- Intraoperative electrical stimulation of the facial nerve, combined with neurophysiological monitoring, is of great help to the surgeon in the safe identification of the facial nerve before it becomes visible surgically.

OPENING THE DURA

- We now have an operating field with the dura of the middle fossa exposed superiorly, as well as the superior petrosal sinus. Posteriorly we see the dura of the posterior fossa and the sigmoid sinus; anteriorly there is the third part of the facial nerve and the superior part of the internal auditory canal, with the vertical crest and the facial nerve, the internal auditory canal, and inferiorly the jugular bulb.
- Any residual bony sheath is removed.
- The blood vessels are coagulated.
- A U-shaped incision is made on the dura with microscissors. The incision begins immediately superior to the jugular bulb. Another incision descends inferior to the superior petrosal sinus. The two incisions are joined at the porus. The dura is first elevated with a hook, then a small hole is made from which CSF exits, and finally it is opened with a No. 11 Bard-Parker knife blade or with the tip of Jacobson scissors. The underlying arachnoid should not be violated, to avoid bleeding before gaining adequate exposure. We then proceed in a downward motion in the attempt to see what is under the dural surface, avoiding cutting cerebellar arteries or veins, especially the petrosal vein. This vein lies behind the surgical field, in the pontine region, but it may be lateralized in large tumors. It is important to take care not to injure any vascular loops of the AICA, which may be found lateral to the porus, nor the facial nerve which may be near the porus or even along the superior surface of the tumor (Fig. 28-18).
- The inferior incision must be made first. Since the dura is thicker here, due in part to the presence of the endolymphatic sac, this incision is easier to perform in conditions of dural stability.
- The dural flap is then brought back to protect the cerebellum. The incision must have an opening back far enough to permit posterior exposure of the tumor and the area of contact with the cerebellum. In large tumors or in the presence of a very anteriorized sigmoid sinus, the tumor may

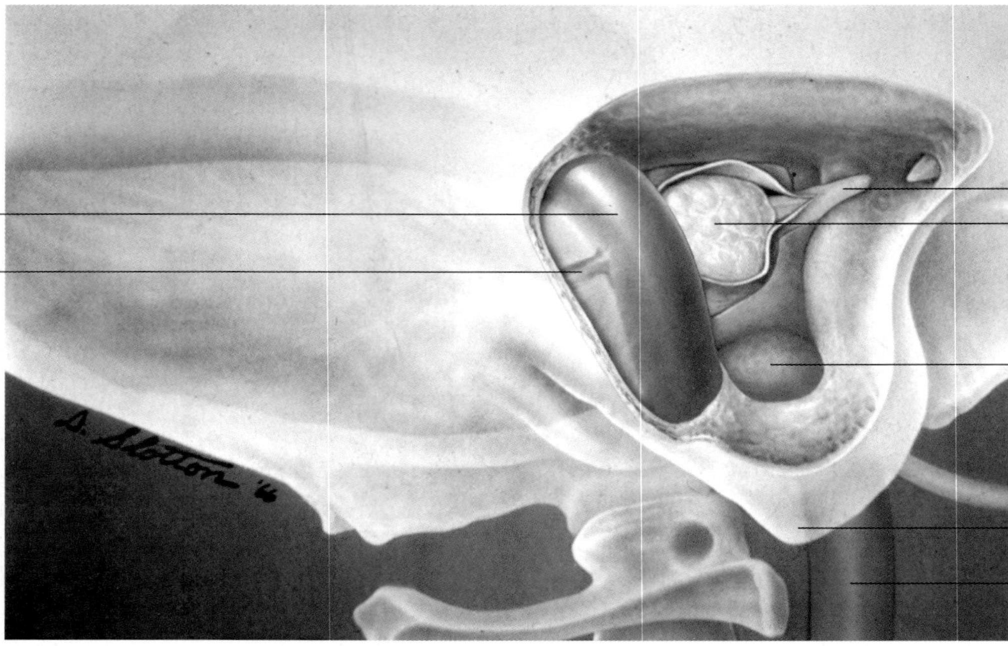

Fig. 28-18. Posterior fossa dura has been opened, the tumor is exposed.

extend posterior to the sigmoid sinus. The cerebellum, compressed, may not then be identified. In these rare instances, a surgical view of the posterior margin of the tumor may be obtained by opening the dura behind the sigmoid sinus. Thus a translabyrinthine-retrosigmoid approach is performed. The transsigmoid approach is not recommended, since it requires an unnecessary vascular sacrifice. The residual dura covering the IAC is removed with a hook, penetrating below to the falciform crest (Fig. 28-19).

IDENTIFICATION OF THE FACIAL NERVE

After the dura is opened, the falciform crest (transverse crest) may be seen. It separates the inferior vestibular nerve from the superior vestibular nerve. The vertical crest (Bill's bar) may also be noted, dividing the superior vestibular nerve from the facial nerve (Fig. 28-20). The nerve is thus identified and its position is confirmed by the facial nerve stimulator (Figs. 28-21, 28-22, 28-23).

OPENING OF THE CISTERNS

The cisterns of the posterior cranial fossa are, from top to bottom: the cerebellar cistern, the cerebello-pontine cistern and the cerebello-medullary cistern. The tumor compresses the three cisterns proportionately depending on its size. The cerebellopontine cistern is the first to be involved. The arachnoid membrane of the tumor is in contact with the arachnoid of the cisterns. Below, near the foramen magnum, is the cisterna magna.

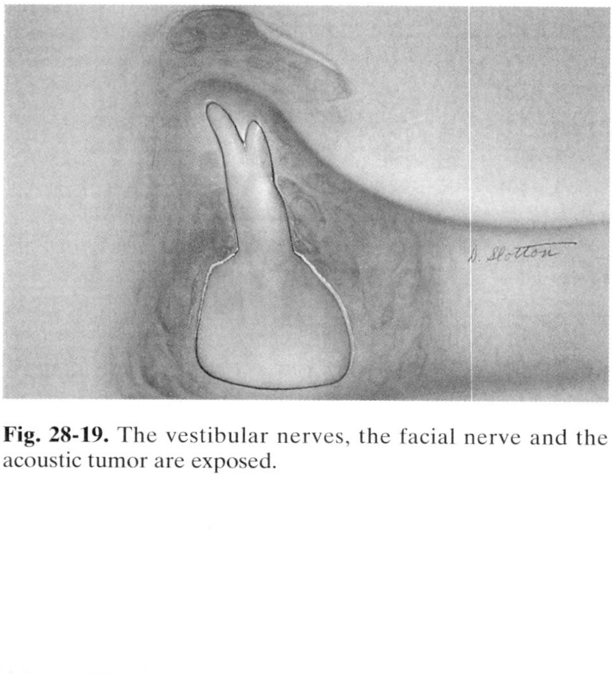

Fig. 28-19. The vestibular nerves, the facial nerve and the acoustic tumor are exposed.

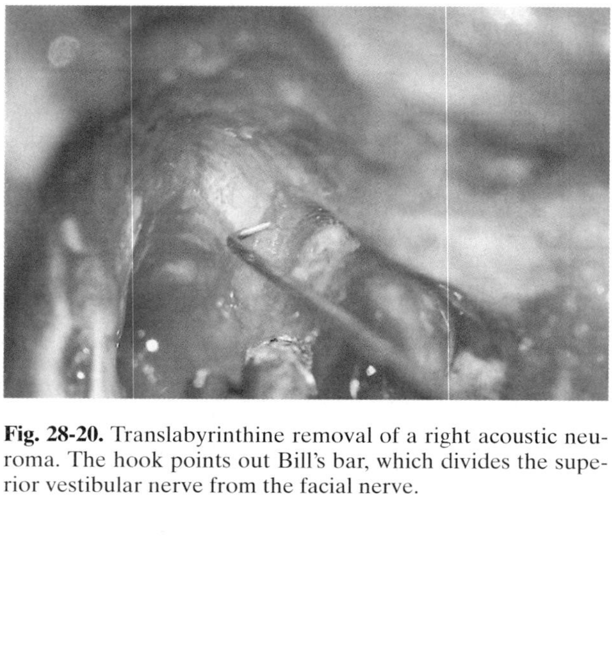

Fig. 28-20. Translabyrinthine removal of a right acoustic neuroma. The hook points out Bill's bar, which divides the superior vestibular nerve from the facial nerve.

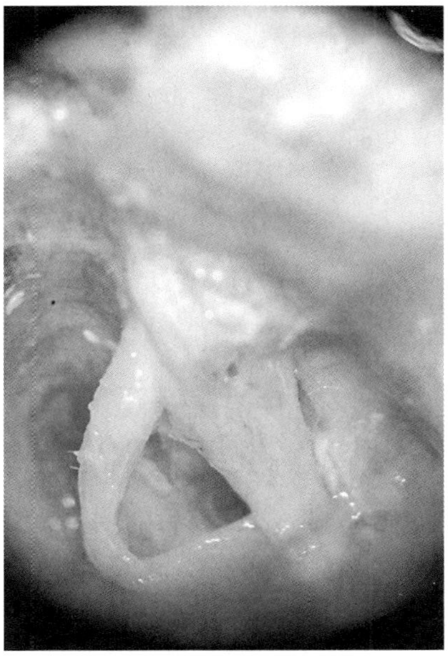

Fig. 28-21. The dura of the IAC is incised along the inferior border of the canal, far away from the facial nerve which is anterior inferior.

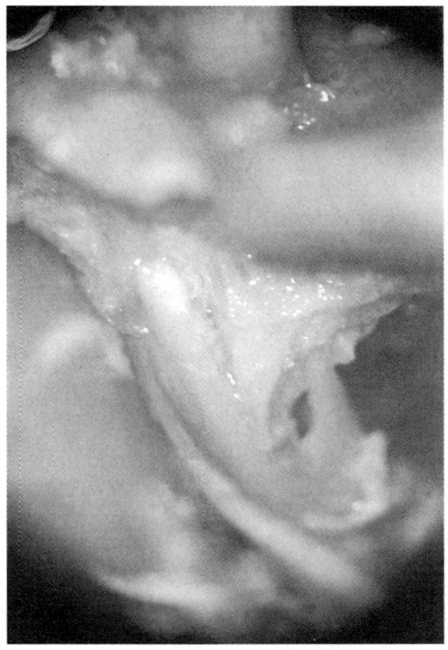

Fig. 28-23. IAC of a right temporal bone. Facial nerve, Bill's bar, superior vestibular n., transverse crest, inferior vestibular n. are exposed.

LIQUOR DRAINAGE

- A dissector is introduced along the inferior margin of the tumor and the arachnoid is opened using slight pressure, or, if necessary, with a hook. It is important to be careful not to damage the mixed nerves, a loop of the AICA, or the vagus vein, which proceeds posteriorly.
- Thus the CSF exits, freeing up room in the posterior cranial fossa. In large tumors, the dissector is advanced towards the foramen magnum, in order to open the cisterna magna and release as much liquor as possible.
- In some very large tumors (over 5 cm in diameter), the tumor herniates across the breach after the opening of the dura and impedes liquor drainage. It is then essential to proceed with a partial intracapsular gutting.
- On the posterior plane of the tumor we often find a cyst full of yellowish CSF, with a high protein content. The growth of the tumor causes the porus to close two arachnoid layers like the neck of a sack. This is called a "herald cyst" because in the suboccipital approach it is the first indication of the presence of a tumor. The cyst is opened.

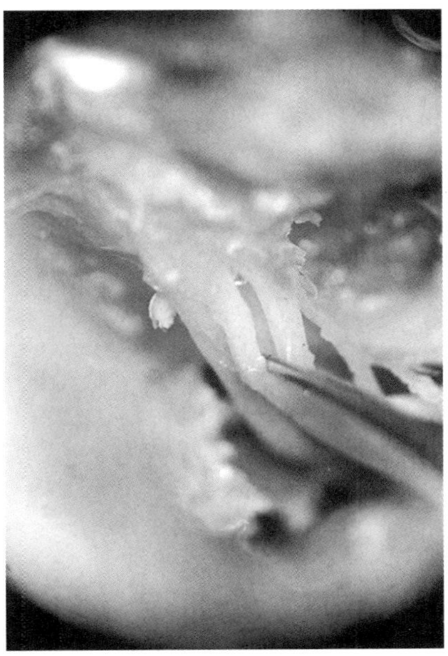

Fig. 28-22. IAC of a right temporal bone. Facial nerve, Bill's bar, superior vestibular n., transverse crest, inferior vestibular n. are exposed.

IDENTIFICATION OF THE CLEAVAGE PLANE

It is fundamental to remain in the plane between the capsule and the arachnoid. Along with the arachnoid, most of the venous and arterial vessels are displaced. These vessels originate by the internal arteries and veins and by the subarcuate artery, as do the dural vessels. When necessary, they are coagulated with a bipolar cautery, which does not carry the risk of retrograde thrombosis to the AICA. If a correct cleavage plane is not developed between the arachnoid and the tumoral capsule, bleeding will be heavier.

The internal auditory arteries are the only vessels which cross the arachnoid and capsular plane, to vascularize the tumor. They originate in the AICA. They are coagulated.

THE POSTERIOR SURFACE OF THE TUMOR

- The cleavage plane is identified between the posterior surface of the tumor and the cerebellum. A cottonoid is placed upon it to stabilize it. This also serves to protect that portion of the cerebral surface not shielded by the dural flap.
- The posterior surface of the tumor is evaluated and the arachnoid of the capsule is removed with a House elevator, to ensure that there are no nerves on the capsule. The facial nerve stimulator is also used. The tumor capsule is then opened and intracapsular dissection begins. The dissection may be performed with forceps and a Brackmann fenestrated suction-irrigator (Fig. 28-24). The suction-irrigator stabilizes the tumor, and some pieces are removed with forceps. The suctioning action exerts posterior traction, counterbalancing the forceps which push anteriorly. When the isolated part of the tumor is grasped with the forceps, the posterior traction is balanced by the tip of the irrigator.
- It is very important to neither pull nor push the tumor because a spasm of the AICA may be provoked, causing ischemia of the brainstem.
- If the tumor is pushed forward, the facial nerve in front may also be damaged. It is therefore important to steady not only the facial nerve, but also the vestibular nerves and the arachnoid. This helps to maintain the solidity of the whole. To reduce bleeding, a bipolar cautery may be used, followed by the forceps; thus part of the tumor is necrotized, and then removed.
- The intratumoral removal may also be performed with a rotating House-Urban dissector, or with an ultrasonic suction aspirator (Cavitron or Surgitron) (Fig. 28-25). These are utilized in the removal of medium-to-large tumors. In smaller tumors, their use may place the nervous and vascular structures at risk. First, fragments of the tumor are grasped with a Weil forceps,

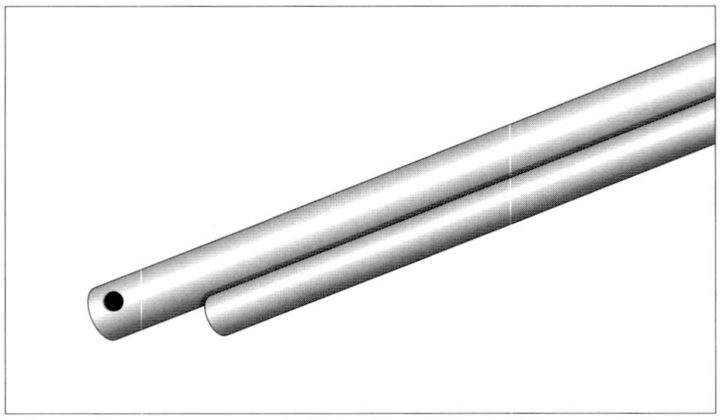

Fig. 28-24. Brackmann fenestrated suction irrigator.

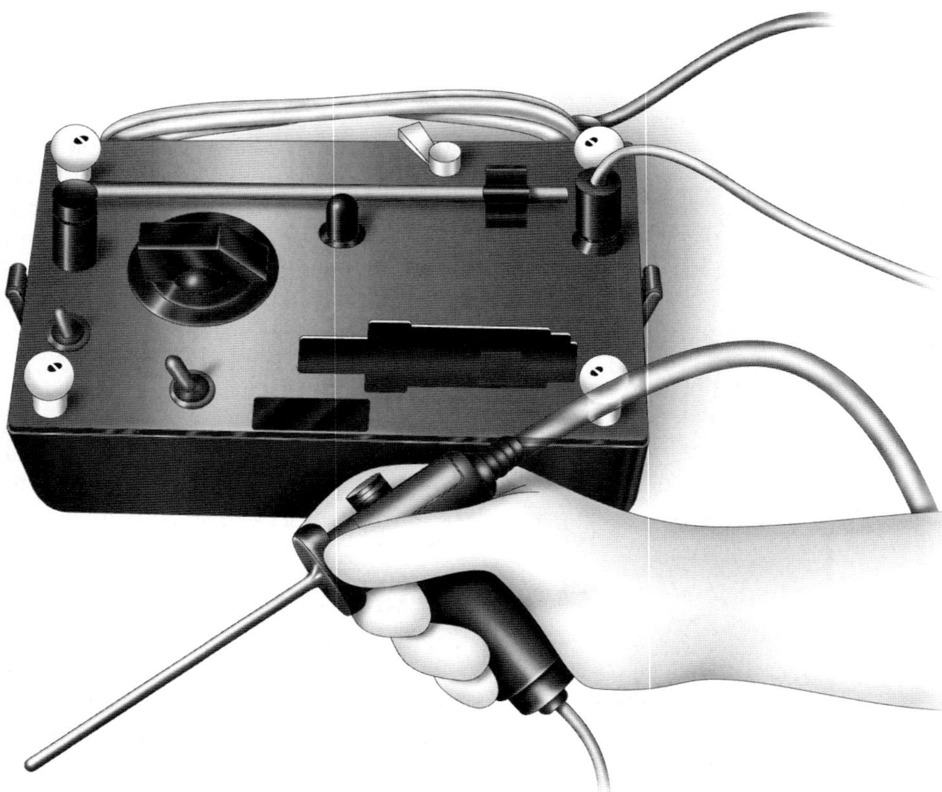

Fig. 28-25. House Urban suction dissector. A suction tube with an inner rotating tube that sucks the tumor into the opening of the tube, where the inner rotating cannula clips it off.

then fragments are aspirated. The gutting of the tumor must begin from the postero-superior part, adjacent to the tentorium. Gutting inside the capsule does not risk damaging important nerves and vascular structures, which are extracapsular. The House-Urban and ultrasonic aspirators have a greater capacity to remove not capsulated soft tissue. However, the tumor removal must take place under constant visual control. Vascular anomalies must also be kept in mind; in W. House's experience, out of thousands of translabyrinthine operations, one case of AICA with an intracapsular course within the soft cancerous tissue was seen. On the other hand, in meningiomas, the intratumoral course of neuro-vascular structures is common.

- At this point, the tumor has been almost completely gutted. The surgeon has more room to work, since the cisterns are emptied of liquor and the volume of the tumor is significantly reduced. The capsule is followed inferiorly. The cleavage plane is identified below between the capsule and the brainstem.

IDENTIFICATION OF THE FACIAL NERVE AT THE PONS

- The exiting point of the vestibulo-cochlear nerve at the pons is approx. 9 mm medial to the midline. Medially to it the facial nerve and the nervus intermedius (Wrisberg) are identified exiting from the pons approx. 11 mm medial to the midline. Two points of the facial nerve can be recognized: one at the fundus, and one at the pons. The nerve's path between these two points varies, and depends on the size of the tumor and the pressure exerted by the tumor during growth. The same method may always be used to identify VII above the fundus, in tumors of any size. Its identification, however, is more difficult at the pontine exit, particularly in large tumors. The exit is an anatomically stable point, but the mass of the tumor may spread the nerve onto the capsule, wrap it in arachnoid, and flatten it onto the brainstem. Even in these cases, the nerve must be identified. This can be accomplished by reducing the tumor's mass (Figs. 28-26, 28-27).
- The tissue of the choroid plexus exiting the foramen of Luschka and the floccule are immediately posterior-inferior to nerves VIII and VII. These nerves exit the brainstem at the lateral end of the ponto-medullary sulcus, just above the glossopharyngeal nerve.
- The large vessels are then separated from the capsule and the AICA is preserved. The small perforating vessels are carefully coagulated near the tumor. The proximal stumps of the injured vessels are found on the pons where coagulation becomes risky if the vessel is reopened. It is therefore preferable to leave the stump in place as long as possible. It is unnecessary to coagulate the very small vessels, since once cut, they coagulate spontaneously.
- The intracapsular gutting of the tumor proceeds. The inferior part is lifted so that the cleavage point with the brainstem may be identified. Nerves VIII and VII may be identified by lifting the tumor from the bottom. VII is in an anterior-inferior position at about 2 mm from VIII. Its identification is confirmed with the facial nerve stimulator. The plane is stabilized by positioning a cottonoid between the two surfaces. It is now safe to remove part of the tumor capsule, significantly reducing its dimensions.
- Inferior to the tumor are the mixed nerves.
- Nerve IX may be conserved. In the larger tumors it is flattened onto the capsule and may be clipped; one landmark is the medial projection of the cochlear duct.
- If pressure is placed on nerve X, bradycardia will ensue. The surgical procedure must be in-

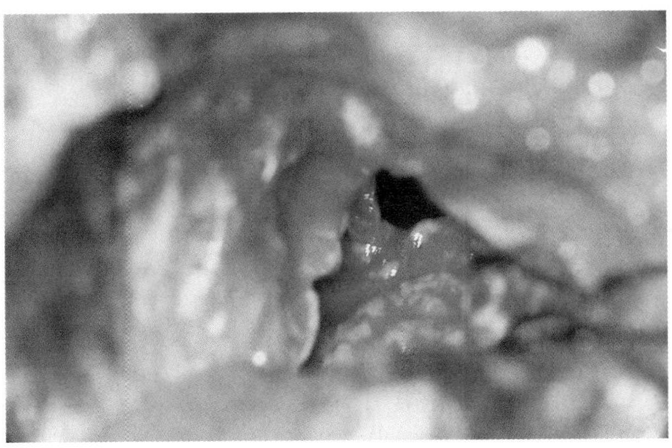

Fig. 28-26. The facial nerve is identified at the brain stem. Tumor is separated from the facial nerve (not vice-versa!).

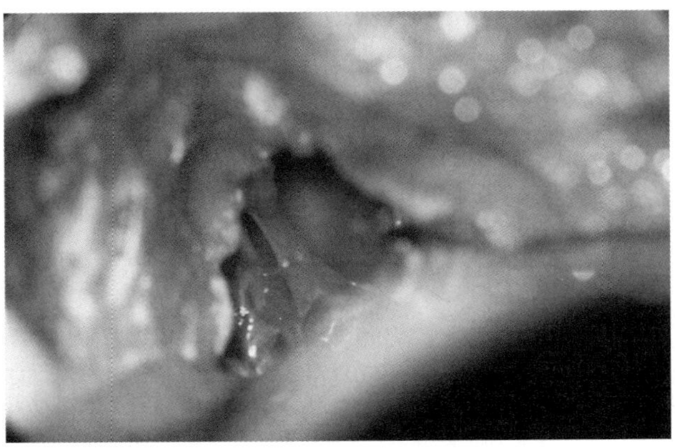

Fig. 28-27. Tumor is completely removed. The facial nerve is intact.

terrupted, and conditions must return to normal before resuming surgery.
- Superiorly, nerve V is identified.

THE ANTERIOR SURFACE OF THE TUMOR

The tumor has been defined both posteriorly and inferiorly. We thus move on anteriorly. This dissection is the most delicate, for the following reasons:
- The facial nerve always proceeds anteriorly, if only in part.
- The petrosal vein and its branches proceed anteriorly and superiorly to the superior petrosal sinus. The AICA may proceed anteriorly.
- Many vessels reach the tumor both from the dura of the porus and the posterior fossa. Bleeding from these vessels provokes problems in hemostasis because of the proximity of the facial nerve.
- The presence of nerve VII makes using cottonoids problematic when following the cleavage plane. In any case, this dissection is necessary since it increases the tumor's mobility. The anterior part of the tumor is gutted intracapsularly. The capsule can be checked with the stimulator on the superior and inferior surfaces of the tumor, to ensure that nerve VII is not present. Part of the capsule may be removed to improve the anterior surgical view.

THE ANTERIOR AND SUPERIOR SURFACES

The operating table is moved away from the surgeon, to improve his view of the lateral part of the IAC.
- The previous dissections were performed while maintaining the anterior structure: the capsule, the arachnoid, the two vestibular nerves, and the facial nerve. The structure thus has a solidity meant to preserve the facial nerve during the previous maneuvers; now is the moment to break it down.
- The fundus is completely exposed. It is very important to have adequately exposed the vestibule in the drilling phase, since its medial wall is also the lateral wall of the fundus of the internal auditory canal. If the tumor does not reach the fundus (10% of cases) the inferior and superior nerves as well as the facial nerve are clearly visible. If, on the other hand, the tumor reaches the fundus, the inferior vestibular nerve, where the tumor almost always originates, is not recognizable. Identification of the superior vestibular nerve may also be difficult, but the two bony crests guide us; immediately superior to the transverse crest is the superior vestibular nerve, then the vertical crest, and, superior to it, the facial nerve. The vertical crest is also the posterior wall of the fallopian canal.
- A hook is inserted into the vestibular nerve canal to remove the nerve. The underlying facial nerve is thus further exposed.
- A cleavage plane is developed between the nerve and the arachnoid surrounding the tumor anteriorly. The inferior vestibular nerve is also sectioned by means of traction with the hook and is reflected posteriorly. The tumor is now mobile in the lateral section of the internal auditory canal and it is moved back. The acoustic nerve is preserved if it can be separated from the tumor. This leaves open the possibility for future cochlear implants. Blunt instruments are used, such as the Gimmick elevator, in order to separate the anterior dural adherences, which are almost always at the level of the porus acusticus. Sometimes the McElveen's dissector can be used, since it has a superior cutting edge. There is the risk of injuring the AICA, which may form a loop in the IAC between VII and VIII, and generally rests on the anterior surface of the cochlear nerve.
- Superiorly and medially, the trigeminal nerve is visible as a large white structure. Inferiorly we can identify nerve IX. More caudally are the other mixed nerves, X and XI. If, while working on the tumor, pressure is placed on nerve X, a slowing of the cardiac rhythm may occur. In this case it is necessary to wait before resuming surgery.
- A plane is observed between the facial nerve and the arachnoid anteriorly, and the tumor capsule posteriorly (Fig. 28-28). This plane is followed by separating the facial nerve from the arachnoid with a hook and microscissors. Straight Jacobson's scissors are used in this phase so that the cutting surface may be more easily viewed, with no blind spots. This procedure is very delicate, since excessive pressure on the tumor may damage the facial nerve. In this phase, magnifying lenses are utilized (40X). The arachnoid is progressively separated from the nerve while proceeding in a lateral-medial direction. With the deepening dissection, difficulties generally increase, since the nerve tends to become progressively thinner. In the cerebello-pontine angle, the nerve is not surrounded by epineurium. It is frequently crushed and flattened onto the tumor capsule, especially in larger tumors. Following the nerve may be problematic. It is essential to remain in the cleavage plane between tumor and nerve. If the plane is lost while entering the cancerous tissue, it becomes very difficult to recover.
- Vessels are found spaced along the dissection plane; they should be preserved if possible, but at times they bleed. The proximity of the facial nerve makes hemostasis difficult and risky.

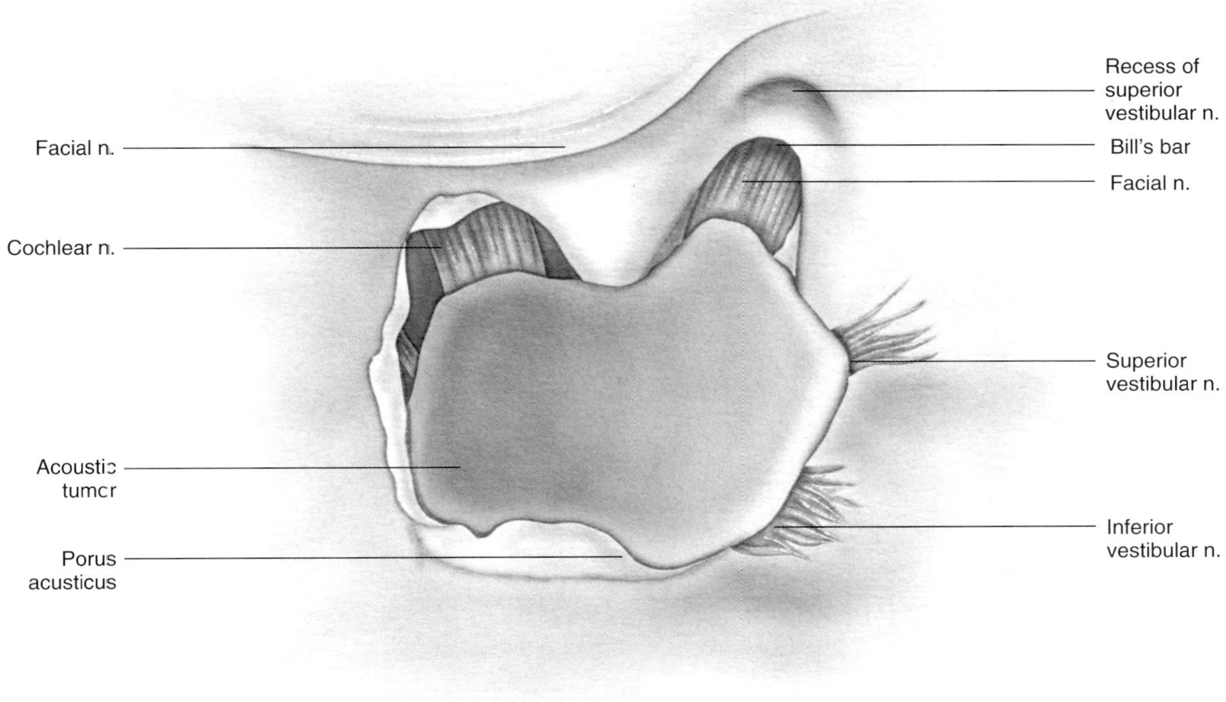

Fig. 28-28. Vestibular nerves are avulsed. The tumor, along with the facial nerve, is separated from the facial nerve.

Many vessels, coming from the dura of the porus, penetrate into the tumor and are coagulated.

- The facial nerve is followed to the brainstem. Now that the nerve's path is known, most of the tumor can be safely removed, leaving only a small residual part on the brainstem. A cleavage plane is developed between the tumoral capsule and the brainstem. The dural adherences (not very resistant in this phase) are clipped. The vessels are dissected from the surface of the tumor and the fundus is lifted from the brainstem. The great reduction in tumor mass allows the separation plane with the brainstem to be viewed. In large tumors the trunk is dislocated from the median line and compressed, and there are adherences which make the development of a cleavage plane more difficult. The adherences, even in the most difficult cases, are usually rather weak. The tumor is removed from the facial nerve.
- All the vessels that can be separated from the tumor are preserved, while the others are coagulated. Many veins are trapped between the tumor and the brainstem. Coagulation of the bleeding extremities is a delicate operation and should be done with a bipolar cautery. A low intensity of coagulation as well as continuous irrigation should be used, because of the proximity of the pons. Rarely, and only in the large vessels, are clips utilized. Care must be taken not to damage the AICA, which in rare instances may be trapped between the tumor and the brainstem.

COAGULATION

After the tumor has been removed, the cottonoids are also removed. Thus their action of coagulation by compression ceases. The cerebello-pontine angle is irrigated with a physiological solution, enabling the surgeon to remove any blood clots and note bleeding vessels. Hemostasis may be difficult because of the presence of the vessels on the brainstem; it is necessary to use a low current bipolar cautery with a narrow tip and continuous irrigation, in order to avoid damage to the facial nerve or overheating. In smaller vessels a tiny piece of Surgicel may be used; in the large vessels, clips must be used. It is important not to leave too much Surgicel in the cerebello-pontine angle, since it later tends to increase in volume and may cause symptoms of brainstem compression.

CLOSURE

- Abdominal fat is harvested and cut into 3-4 cm-long cone-shaped strips. These are preserved in an antibiotic solution (penicillin).
- The incus is removed, exerting traction on its body with a hook (Fig. 28-29). Two small flaps of Surgicel are placed in the attic, along with

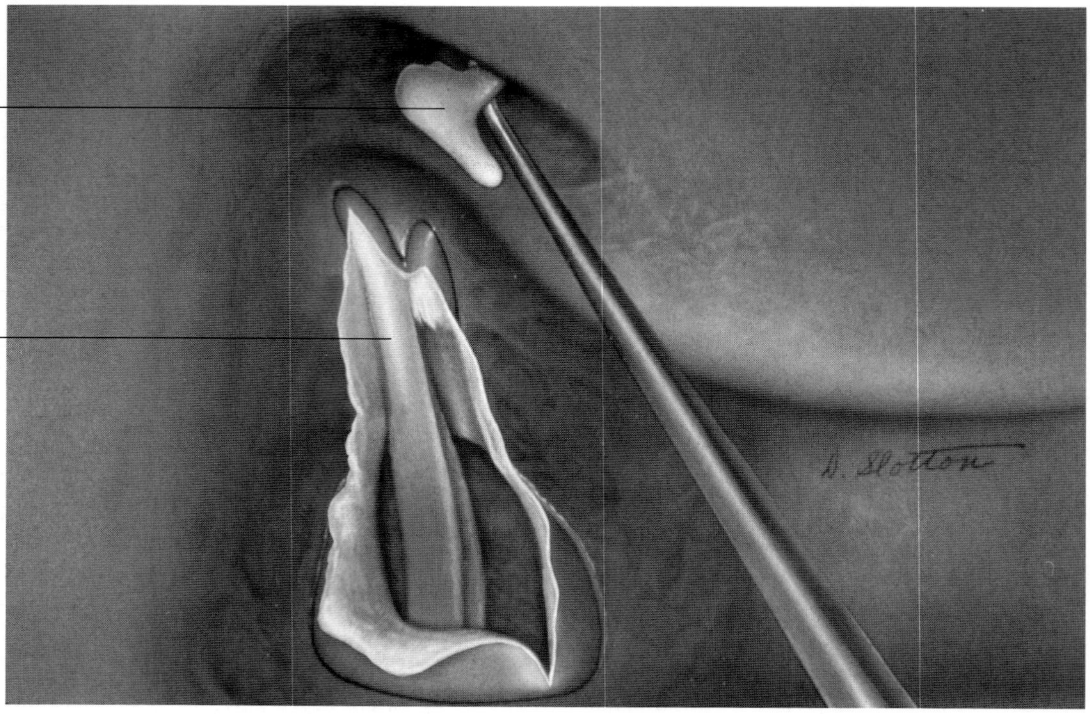

Fig. 28-29. Closure involves the use of abdominal fat. The incus is removed and the middle ear is packed with muscle, to prevent CSF leak through the nose, via the ET.

fragments of temporal muscle. In this procedure, it is important to avoid provoking tympanic lesions. The obliteration of the attic is necessary in order to prevent the CSF in the dural breach from reaching the tube, with consequent rhynoliquorrea and the risk of septic contamination. Some AA (Glasscock, Ekwall,) open the facial recess, remove the malleus and the incus, and close the ostium tubaricus (with bone, bone wax, muscle, ...). Sanna has noted that in transcochlear surgery, where the ET orifice is routinely closed, the incidence of CSF leaks is significantly lower, when compared with the translabyrinthine approach.

- The edges are closed with a 4-0 silk suture; the suture may not be complete, causing substance loss at the end of the operation. The strips of fat are inserted 0.5-1 cm into the dural breach. The partial suturing of the dural flaps reduces the risk of the fat penetrating into the cerebello-pontine angle, which would give rise to the possibility of facial nerve trauma and pressure on the brainstem, with possible ischemic complications. The cone shape permits the insertion of many points into the breach. The strips then spread to occupy a larger space then the mastoid space. It has been noted that the use of several strips of fat (rather than one single piece) for the obliteration reduces the incidence of CSF leaks.
- The fat is positioned so that it protrudes approx. 0.5 cm from the mastoid cortex. The limb is repositioned; the muscular-periosteum layer is then closed with Vycril 0 and the subcutaneous layer is closed with Vycril 3-0. The suture of the muscular plane is similar to that performed in middle ear surgery. The muscular-cutaneous flap, sutured in an adhering manner, keeps the fat compressed so as to occupy all the spaces. It is better to err on the side of too much fat than too little; the excessive fat protruding from the sutured lips of the wound may be removed by simply rubbing with a gauze strip.

Steril-Strips are then placed on the edges of the wound.

The external closure may be enforced with 2-0 silk. External silk guarantees a tighter closure of the skin flap and a greater compression of the underlying fat. When not using external silk, the muscular planes are joined with chromic catgut 0 and the subcutaneous planes with Vicryl 3-0. The closure of the abdominal wound is similar; here a drain is also positioned.

In the intraoperative site a urinary catheter is positioned, as well as a nasogastric tube. The tube is left in place post-operatively, in order to keep the stomach empty (nausea and vomiting may occur). The day after surgery the nasogastric tube is removed, along with the abdominal drain and the urinary catheter. Both the dressing and the Steril-Strips should be kept on for 7 days. If there is CSF leakage, the dressing must be reinforced, preferably with a silk bandage.

The patients are encouraged to remain in a sitting position, with their feet on the floor, and to assume a sitting position in a chair the first or second day after surgery. They should walk as soon as possible (even the day after surgery) with assistance.

VARIATIONS IN THE FACIAL NERVE'S PATH

Intrameatal variations

Usually, the facial nerve is found on the medial (anterior) surface of the tumor, along with the acoustic nerve. At times the nerve is quite high up. It is very rare to find the nerve on the lateral surface (posterior) of the tumor. The acoustic nerve may undergo similar variations in its course even if it is almost never dislocated superiorly, but rather inferiorly.

Extrameatal variations

Extrameatal variations are frequent. In general, the nerves run along the medial surface of the tumor. If the tumor becomes wedged between the two nerves while growing, it tends to displace the facial nerve superiorly and the acoustic nerve inferiorly. In rare instances, the nerves may run along the lateral surface of the tumor. The modifications in the path may be of only one nerve or others associated with it. The difficulty in following the path of the facial nerve increases depending on the size of the tumor; the greater the variations in the nerve's path, the greater the reduction of the surgical view. Thus, identification of the nerve at the trunk is more difficult. The nerve's size is reduced due to crushing by the tumor.

VARIATIONS IN TECHNIQUE

The method described by Tos and Thompsen does not take into account the identification of Bill's bar and the facial nerve. The possibilities offered by the facial nerve stimulator provide adequate safety during dissection. The tumor is gutted and the capsule is removed. The anterior barrier is preserved, including the arachnoid, the vessels, and the acoustic nerve. The AICA anterior to the facial nerve is safeguarded. The facial nerve remains hidden anteriorly.

Advantages

- The anterior barrier is solid. The tumor may be manipulated with less risk of injuring the facial nerve. (In the last part of the classical dissection, the facial nerve is the only residual structure anterior to the tumor).
- It is unnecessary to dissect the capsule from the nerve. Rather, the capsule should be dissected from the arachnoid. This means that the trauma undergone by a nerve crushed by a medium to large tumor, especially on the porus and in the CPA, may be very slight.
- There are fewer problems in dissection.

Limits

- If the nerve is not identified at the fundus and at the trunk, no estimation of the nerve's path between these two points is possible, nor can it be followed from where it is known to be to where it is not.
- The operation is easier to perform and the risks of damaging the nerve are fewer, because the trauma inflicted is less. However remote the facial nerve is considered to be during the operation, it is nevertheless quite near, and the best way to preserve it is to identify its location.
- Identifying the facial nerve in the points described is fundamental when the nerve has an anomalous path, otherwise it may be damaged very easily.
- The difficulties in staying in the correct cleavage plane may lead to leaving residual tumor in place.

COMPLICATIONS

The emissary mastoid vein is isolated in the superior and lateral surface and coagulated as far as possible from the sigmoid sinus. If it is injured close to the sigmoid sinus, heavy bleeding will occur. Generally this may be controlled by means of bipolar coagulation. If this is not sufficient, the edge of a large flap of Surgicel is placed in the breach. The flap must never be small, since it could be absorbed and embolized.

Treatment of surgical complications

VII NERVE LESIONS (see chapter 12-15).

The translabyrinthine approach satisfies three safety requirements:

1) No cerebral compression
2) No gasseous embolism
3) Possibility of a rapid decompression in case of postoperative hemorrhage.

The retrosigmoid approach satisfies the second and partially satisfies the first requirement. The suboccipital approach satisfies none of the above requirements.

PREOPERATIVE HYDROCEPHALUS

Voluminous lesions of the posterior fossa may obstruct the fourth ventricle, altering the normal circulation of the CSF. The patient presents ataxia, headache, papilloedema. The CT and the MRI demonstrate dilated ventricles and flattened cortical sulcus. If the operation is postponed, hernia of the tentorium may occur, with death resulting. The operation removes the tumor and resolves hydrocephalus. Some AA prefer to decompress the ventricular system before the operation, using a ventricular-atrial or ventricular-peritoneal shunt.

VENOUS BLEEDING

Venous bleeding in ear surgery may be profuse and prove problematic for the surgeon. In any case, it is a low-pressure oozing, and may be controlled temporarily without great difficulty by means of an extraluminal dressing. Familiarity with the repair technique and steady nerves help to definitively resolve the problem.

- Once the intracapsular gutting of the tumor has been performed, the arachnoid membrane is carefully dissected from the tumoral capsule, taking the arterial vessels, branches of the cerebellar arteries and the venous vessels along with it.
- The sacrifice of the venous vessels must be as moderate as possible. At times some petrosal veins must be sacrificed, especially in the presence of large tumors. It is necessary to act as conservatively as possible. This is because the extended occlusion of these veins, which provide the venous drainage from the cerebellum and from the brainstem, has been known to provoke hemorrhaging edema of these structures.
- The venous lesions do not provoke embolization, since the venous pressure in a supine patient is superior to the atmospheric pressure.

MASTOID EMISSARY VEIN

At the beginning of the operation, 1 cm of bone is always removed posterior to the sigmoid sinus. Here the mastoid emissary vein begins, entering postero-laterally to the sinus, in its upper third. Occasionally there may be several mastoid veins. These must almost always be sacrificed in order to allow an adequate decompression posterior to the sinus. The vein is skeletonized with a cutting burr, and is then exposed using a diamond burr in its upper two-thirds. It is then coagulated and cut as far as possible from its entrance into the sigmoid sinus, in order to avoid provoking a hole in the sinus. The distal bone foramen is occluded with bone wax.

SIGMOID SINUS

Besides the situation described above, the sinus may be damaged by the burr or by bone fragments perforating the wall.
In the case of a lesion to the sigmoid sinus, the procedure is as follows:

- A small hole is coagulated with a bipolar cautery. The coagulation must not be on the bleeding hole, but rather must move along a line. A prolonged coagulation in the same point may in fact increase the size of the perforation.
- If this is not sufficient, the breach is packed. The sinus is completely exposed, removing the residual bone fragments with a diamond burr or with a dural dissector. Troublesome bleeding is reduced by using a dissector to place pressure on the breach. One single flap of Surgicel is positioned extraluminally. It must be large enough to prevent embolization. If this does not suffice, the Surgicel is positioned intraluminally. The excess of Surgicel is then trimmed with microscissors, in order to reduce the visual obstacle to a minimum. Bone wax is then positioned in order to avoid dislodging the Surgicel during surgery.
- Another possibility is to place hystoacril glue around the Surgicel.
- If the problem is still not solved, it is necessary to use a transfixed silk stitch, closing while crossing with the suture even a fragment of adipose tissue or muscle.
- If very heavy bleeding occurs, it is helpful to raise the patient's head with the table, in order to reduce pressure.
- If these measures are insufficient, it is necessary to proceed with the ligation of the sigmoid sinus (see chapter 16).

SUPERIOR PETROSAL SINUS

A lesion of the superior petrosal sinus may generally be controlled by means of bipolar coagulation and occluded with Surgicel. If bleeding continues, bone wax may be placed over the Surgicel. If difficulties arise, the sinus must be isolated laterally and medially to the perforation. Superiorly, small holes may be made in the dura at the edges of the sinus and clips are applied across the holes. Inferiorly, Surgicel is used to pack. If the intraluminal dressing proves inadequate, the petrosal sinus is elevated from the underlying bony sulcus and Surgicel is positioned between the two structures.
The two most difficult points for a lesion of the superior petrosal sinus are near the IAC and the sigmoid sinus.

- If the internal auditory canal has already been opened, the lesion at this level makes hemostasis risky for the facial nerve.
- A lesion of the superior petrosal sinus near the sigmoid sinus may provoke a leak in the latter.

JUGULAR BULB

- If the jugular bulb is accidentally opened, the breach is plugged with a flap of Surgicel, which may be either external or partially internal. It must always be sufficiently large to prevent its being embolized in the venous circle in the right side of the heart and proceeding to the lungs, where it could provoke a serious infarction. The dressing must be immediate, since much blood may be lost by aspirating indiscriminately in the search for the breach, which must still be plugged in exactly the same way. Once packed, a decision must be made. If the hemostasis appears adequate and the breach is not large enough to fear Surgicel embolization, the excess of Surgicel is cut off with microscissors and bone wax is positioned above.
- If the size of the breach presents risks, on the other hand, the jugular vein must be tied in the throat, to be able to freely pack inside the jugular bulb when necessary. The cut is prolonged along the anterior margin of the sternocleidomastoid muscle, up to the level of the hyoid bone. The muscle is partially separated from the mastoid tip and folded posteriorly. Inferiorly the lateral process of C1 may be touched. The posterior margin of the digastric muscle is retracted superiorly with a retractor. The jugular vein is identified anterior to the lateral process of C1. The accessory nerve is identified. This nerve usually passes posteriorly over C1, lateral or medial to the jugular (lateral in two-thirds of cases). It is necessary to identify the nerve in order to avoid including it in the ligation, which must be double and should be done with two no. 2 silk threads.
- The ligation of the jugular vein protects against embolization. At this point small flaps of Surgicel may be inserted into the breach. It is important not to use too much Surgicel, since it tends to increase in volume. This will exert pressure on the mixed nerves, and may result in their paralysis. A combination of Surgicel and Avitene may also be used. The latter has a smaller mass. The occlusion of the jugular bulb and the jugular vein causes an increase in intracranial venous pressure, and swelling of the brain. The following phases of the operation are therefore complicated due to the decrease in space in the CPA.
- Ligation of the jugular vein and intraluminal packing of the sinus do not prevent retrograde bleeding, since the jugular bulb receives blood from other collaterals, such as the inferior petrosal sinus and the condylar vein.

PETROSAL VEIN

- The petrosal vein enters into the superior petrosal sinus superior to the level of the internal auditory canal. The flap of dura of the posterior cranial fossa, reflected posteriorly, is generally sufficient to keep this vein out of the surgical field. Otherwise, the vein must be identified and removed from the tumor and compressed under a cottonoid.
- The vein may be damaged by stretching or by surgical errors. In this case, hemorrhage is profuse. As a preventative measure, the superior petrosal sinus must at this point be occluded. In the CPA, neither Gelfoam nor Surgicel is recommended, since they obscure vision and when removed, leave the operating field bloodier than before. It is better to compress the vein on the breach with the back of a suction-irrigator (Brackman) held in the left hand (for right-handed surgeons). Bleeding is momentarily reduced and the aspirator removes the excess blood, thereby permitting the surgeon to safely occlude the vessel, by means of electrocoagulation or with neurosurgical clips.
- In the presence of large acoustic neuromas, the patient may show hydrocephalus before the operation. Some maintain that the preoperative treatment of hydrocephalus brings the patient to the operating table in better conditions (Borgesen, Tos). Thus, in the case of a marked hydrocephalus, they resort to an external ventricular drain or a high-pressure shunt of the CSF. In the case of a slight hydrocephalus, they resort to a simple shunt of the CSF.

In over 3000 operations at the House Ear Institute, no patient has ever undergone a shunt. It is the removal of the tumor which resolves the hydrocephalus.

ARTERIAL BLEEDING

ANTERIOR-INFERIOR-CEREBELLAR ARTERY

- The anterior-inferior cerebellar artery (AICA) supplies the lateral section of the pontine tegmen. If the AICA is coagulated without adequate anastomosis of the posterior inferior cerebellar artery (PICA) or of the superior cerebellar artery (SCA), a terminal infarction of the lateral part of the pontine tegmen will occur, with necrosis of the pons and cerebellar brachia and death. Blood pressure control centers are found in this region, as well as control centers for cardiac rhythm and respiration.
- The small branches of the AICA do not supply blood to vital zones. When necessary, they may be coagulated. Complications may be entirely absent or cerebellar edema may take place, but never death.

- The AICA must always be recognized and separated from the tumor's surface. Its bright red color differentiates it from the dark red veins.
- If in doubt, the vessel may be momentarily closed with the tip of a bipolar cautery. The arteries will expand, while the veins will not.

POSTERIOR INFERIOR CEREBELLAR ARTERY

When coagulation is performed with the PICA, death may occur in 5% of cases. The PICA medial branch supplies the cerebellar hemisphere and the inferior vermis, while the lateral branch supplies the inferior cerebellar surface and its lateral border.

The occlusion of this artery causes a medullary syndrome (Wallemberg's Syndrome) with controlateral hemiparesis, hemianesthesia, ipsilateral ataxia, nystagmus and Horner's syndrome. The chances for recovery in these cases are much better than in AICA occlusion.

PERFORATING ARTERIES

Small arteries, called perforating arteries, emerge from the basilar artery like the teeth of a comb, near the vertebral arteries. If they are coagulated, hemiplegia may occur.

BLEEDING

- CPA neuromas are highly vascularized. At the turn of the century, neurosurgeons spoke of the CPA as "the bloody angle", due in part to the difficulty of preserving the vessels without the aid of the surgical microscope. All vessels that can be preserved and separated from the tumor must be. Frequently the vascular walls, especially the venous ones, break and give rise to profuse bleeding. The amount of lost blood must always be checked, by subtracting the volume of irrigating solution utilized from the total quantity of liquid present in the aspirator containers.
- A loss greater than 500 cc may cause hypovolemia, with tachycardia and hypotension. These modifications may have a masking effect. For example, they may mask bradycardia induced by the pressure on the vagus nerve, or the bradycardia and hypertension resulting from ischemia of the AICA.

Blood transfusions are then performed as needed.

CEREBELLAR ALTERATIONS

At the entrance of the dura, particular care should be taken to avoid damaging the underlying vessels. In medium and large tumors, these are usually cerebellar vessels, since the cerebellum's surface is pushed against the medial surface of the dura by the tumor. The vessels are set aside and only coagulated in rare cases. The cerebellum is protected by the dural flap brought posteriorly.

CEREBELLAR EDEMA

One of the main advantages of the translabyrinthine approach is that adequate space and an ample view are had even in the largest tumors, so that posterior pressure on the cerebellum is rarely required. However, continuous pressure, such as that made by a blade mounted on a Yasargill shaft, does exert a damaging action. We use one or more cottonoids to protect the cerebellum, and pressure is exerted only when necessary with the dorsum of a suction-irrigator. Its extremity continues the surgical procedure. Due to its nature, it is a temporary pressure (intermittent) and therefore not harmful.

CEREBELLO-PONTINE ANGLE ALTERATIONS

- When the tumor must be dissected from the brainstem, rather weak adherences are found. In any case, both the pressure and traction exerted while operating on the tumor may provoke ischaemia of the brainstem causing modifications in the vital signs. The modifications in heartbeat precede respiratory modifications by a few minutes. Bradycardia may also be caused by pressure on the vagus nerve. Compression of the AICA may cause alterations in the cardiac rhythm and blood pressure.
- ECG and blood pressure monitoring enable the surgeon to note these modifications at the outset. At this point the surgical procedure must be interrupted, the cottonoids removed (since they may exert pressure on the vessels) and the surgeon must wait. When the vital parameters have returned to normal, the operation may be resumed in part of the tumor far from the "trigger zone".
- If the alterations in vital signs appear once more upon returning to the trigger zone, the tumor must be reduced as far as possible by working on the other parts, and the operation must be terminated. The decreased size of the tumor permits an improved vascularization of the brainstem. The second operation, after 6-12 months, is thus easier to perform and more resolutory.

CRANIAL NERVES LESIONS

Besides VII and VIII, other nerves in the operating field are: V, VI, IX, X, XI.

- Nerve V is found in a superior position in the operating field. Generally, the tumor can be easily separated from the nerve and it is rarely injured. In cases of facial paralysis, the preservation of V is important in order to preserve corneal sensitivity and prevent corneal damage.
- Nerve IX may be damaged during the bone phase. Therefore it is important to recognize the cochlear duct and to avoid drilling anteriorly or inferiorly. Nerve IX exits the cranium just underneath the cochlear duct, runs medially to the jugular bulb and enters into the pars nervosa of the jugular foramen.
- Nerves IX and X may be damaged when working on the inferior part of the tumor. The compression of X will provoke bradycardia which can be serious.
- Nerves IX, X, and XI lie in the pars nervosa of the jugular foramen. If a breach in the jugular bulb must be plugged, a lesion of the contiguous nerves may occur (see above).
- A lesion of IX and X may lead to respiratory pneumonia. It is a good idea to leave a nasogastric tube in place in the first 24 hours after surgery.

POSTOPERATIVE THERAPY

VENTRICULAR HEMORRHAGE

Intraventricular hemorrhaging is a rare but very serious event. It should be suspected in cases of intraoperative difficulty in stopping bleeding or if the patient does not awaken after surgery.
In this case, a CT must immediately be performed. If there is intraventricular bleeding, an external ventricular drain must be put into place.

MENINGITIS

- Postoperative meningitis is a complication which occurs in 2-4% of cases; HEI: 2.9% (Rodgers). No correlation has been found between meningitis and CSF leaks. Meningitis usually appears in the first week but may also appear even after 20 days. The later its appearance, the more likely its bacterial origin. One predisposing cause is a CSF fistula. The patient shows rigidity in the neck, headache and fever. The liquor extracted with a lumbar syringe confirms the diagnosis (leukocytes, hypoglycemia). The white blood cell count is over 100. A culture is also taken to find any aerobic or anaerobic bacteria. The antibiotic treatment can be modified based on the results of the cultures. One effective therapy is the endovenous infusion of 4 gr/day for 10 days of cefotriaxone. The lumbar injection is repeated after 5 days of treatment. The therapy is protracted until the white blood cell count goes below 100 and the population proves predominantly monocytic.
- Prophylactic antibiotic therapy does not significantly change the incidence of this complication and is not recommended. On the contrary, it may give rise to silent infections, favoring suprainfections. In cases where the pathology is absent, its only function is to create resistence.

POST-OPERATIVE HEMATOMA

A post-operative hematoma of the CPA may be diagnosed clinically and radiologically. The following symptoms may be observed:
- Decreased state of consciousness.
- Increase in arterial pressure.
- Slowing of the arterial pulse.
- Dilatation of the pupils.
- Respiratory depression.

If the symptoms worsen, with a progressive reduction in the state of consciousness, a diagnosis may be made with an emergency CT. The CT enables us to differentiate the possible causes: an hematoma and an hydrocephalus.
If a rapid loss of consciousness occurs, there is no time for the CT. In this case the incision must be immediately reopened and the fat removed. The clot is then aspirated. The plugging of the dural breach with fat enables an extremely rapid decompression in cases of post-operative hemorrhage, and is one of the main advantages of this technique.
This type of complication may cause death very rapidly, within 30 minutes of the manifestation of the first symptoms.
More importantly, in cases of hemorrhaging in the cerebellopontine angle, the decompression procedure must be immediate.

SPINAL FLUID LEAKS

Spinal fluid leaks may occur postauricularly or, twice as often, nasally. The current frequency at the HEI is 6.8%. No correlation has been yet made between the patient's age, the size of the tumor, and the operating time (Rodgers G.K.). The liquor can be distinguished from the mucous because it is not viscous, limpid, or positive to a glucose test. The risk of fistulas lies in the possibility of suprainfections. In case of postauricular fistulas, the stitches are replaced and the dressing is tightened.
In the case of rhynoliquorrea the patient is put to bed, with his head in a raised position. Diuretics are administered (e.g. acetazolamide). If needed, cough suppressants are administered as well. The dressing is reinforced. If this is insufficient, daily lumbar injections may be given or a subarachnoid lumbar catheter may be put in place, to lower the liquor pressure.
If all these measures prove fruitless, the patient is reoperated on within three days.

The incision is reopened in the same point and the dressing is reinforced in points of possible leakage:

- The dural breach.
- Communication between meatus and epitympanum.
- Communication between meatus and tympanic cavity through the oval window where the stapes is dislocated. In particular, the stapes may have been dislodged during the packing of the cavum through the epitympanum at the end of the operation.

The dressing of the epitympanum and of the cavum tympani is reinforced with new Surgicel and muscular tissue. The communication with the CPA is occluded with more fat.

Technical modifications to reduce the incidence of CSF.

Hardy's technique

In Hardy's casebook, 13% of 100 patients operated translabyrinthically showed CSF. Here the closure procedure is modified: the eustachian tube is closed with fat, the middle ear is closed with bone paté and the posterior canal and the aditus are closed with fascia lata and fibrin glue. The mastoid cavity and the petrosal apex, full of fat, are sealed with fibrin glue. In the last 58 patients, no CSF leak was verified.

Pulec technique

J.L. Pulec, in 100 consecutive cases of neuromas operated translabyrinthically, observed only one case (1%) of a "CSF leak" in a patient operated both with a middle fossa and with a translabyrinthine approach.

- During surgery, care must be taken to preserve the external auditory canal. Once the tumor has been removed, the facial recess is opened, penetrating between the fibrous annulus of the tympanic membrane and the facial nerve. The chorda tympani may be removed if more space is required. The chorda tympani is (along with the greater petrosal nerve) one of the two dividing branches of the intermediate nerve, which is often sacrificed when removing the tumor.
- The bone surrounding the posterior suspensory ligament of the incus should be respected. With a Yankauer curette, we transverse the facial recess until reaching the opening of the tube. The mucosa covering the upper half of the tubotympanum (1/2 cm deep) is removed while taking care not to injure the ossicular chain or the tympanic membrane. A strip of fibrous tissue is removed (approx. 1 × 1/2 × 1/2 cm) from the lower part of the temporal muscle insertion, inserted into the tubotympanum, and pressed with a Yankauer curette or a Rosen dissector. The osseous area previously scratched tends to form adherences with the fibrous tissue introduced.
- A muscle fragment (1 × 1 × 1 cm) drawn from the temporalis muscle is positioned in the middle ear to obliterate the cavum tympani and the facial recess. Another small piece of muscle is placed in the posterior epitympanum to close the attic. Abdominal fat is harvested and molded into one single cone-shaped piece. The small end enters partially into the posterior fossa. The wider end has a lateral diameter greater than that of the dural breach, and prevents the fat from slipping into the endocranium. The fat must protrude from the cavity approx. 1 cm, so that the skin suture may obtain a compression effect.

According to Pulec, the presence of fibrous tissue in the tube, preventing the liquor fistula from forming in the eustachian tube for approx. 3 weeks, enables an arachnoid membrane to form around the fat placed in the petrosal apex. In this way a definitive natural barrier is made which could not otherwise occur in the presence of an immediate postoperative fistula. The significant reduction of CSF leaks, due to the occlusion of the tube, is confirmed as well by Sanna and Mazzoni in the transcochlear technique for clival tumors. In this operation the tube is systematically closed and the incidence of CSF leaks is significantly reduced compared to the translabyrinthine technique.

- For aesthetic reasons, abdominal fat may be removed by means of an elliptical incision in the lower abdomen, so as to be invisible even in a bikini. The skin is excised, in order to prevent an ugly depression (Pulec).
- The excess abdominal fat drawn is placed in a dry, sterile container, and is then sealed, labelled, and frozen at -20 F.

If stored under these conditions, the fat may be used for up to a year. If a revision of the dural breach closure is needed for a particular patient, his own fat may be reused, saving time and avoiding the necessity of a new abdominal incision (Pulec).

FEVER

A slight rise in body temperature (up to 38° C) is common in the first 2-3 days after surgery. If the fever does not diminish or tends to increase, possible causes must be evaluated. The possibility of an intracranial abscess should be considered, especially if the patient's response to antibiotics is unsatisfactory. A CT enables the diagnosis of the site of the abscess, though it is very difficult to the identify a superficial abscess in the area packed with fat and muscle. Abscess drainage enables the fever's rapid remission.

HEADACHE
Headache is a common occurrence, appearing in one out of four patients within three days after surgery. It may have a vascular cause, or it may be due to muscle contractions or bandage pressure. A symptomatic therapy is sufficient.

AUDITORY PROSTHESIS
After the removal of a neuroma with a translabyrinthine approach, hearing loss will occur. The patients are asked to consider the possibility of a CROS prosthesis. The sooner they begin the process after recovery from the wound, the better their chances of adapting will be.

COAGULATION OF INTRAOSSEUS VESSELS
The simplest method of coagulating a small intraosseous vessel is by using a diamond burr, without irrigation. If a cutting burr is used, the same effect may be obtained by rotating it counterclockwise, without having to twice change the burr. It is important to keep in mind, however, that the chances of bone hemostasis are inversely proportional to the cutting capacity of the instrument. Cutting capacity, in decreasing order, is the following: cutting burr, finishing burr, inverse rotation of cutting burr, inverse rotation of finishing burr, diamond burr.

VII-XII
If anastomosis is performed post-operatively, and the patient walks and eats without difficulty, problems in swallowing following the operation are resolved in a few days.

Suggestions for practice on a cadaver

Tympanoplastic surgery with mastoidectomy, decompression of the facial nerve and jugular bulb

- Mastoidectomy preserving the posterior part of the canal: Skeletonization of the sigmoid sinus, the middle fossa and the sino-dural angle. Skeletonization of the digastric crest. In this way we can learn to identify the facial nerve in every point of its mastoid path, from the horizontal canal to the stylomastoid chain.
- Open the facial recess while preserving the ossicular chain.
- Dissect the chorda tympani. Open the facial recess enough to see the pyramidal process, the stapes, the cochleariform process, the tensor tympani tendon and the opening of the eustachian tube. Decompress the facial nerve from the stylomastoid foramen at the geniculate ganglion.
- Identify the cochleariform process, the cog, and study the relationship of the second genu of the facial nerve with the lateral semicircular canal and the oval window. Identify the endolymphatic sac and study its lumen and its relationship with the posterior and lateral semicircular canals. Perform an enlarged facial recess. Identify the fibrous annulus and follow it inferiorly and anteriorly up to the temporomandibular articulation. Remove the bone above the jugular bulb and identify the bony part between the jugular bulb and the internal carotid artery. Open the jugular bulb with a n. 15 knife and study the draining of the inferior petrosal sinus and its relationship with the cranial nerves IX, X, and XI.

Postauricular labyrinthectomy and translabyrinthine section of the eighth nerve

- Labyrinthectomy: open the labyrinthine part of the three semicircular canals. Study their ampullae, the common crus and their relationships with the facial nerve. Identify the subarcuate nerve, and the maculae of the utricle and saccule. Before opening the dura, identify the vertical crest called "Bill's bar". Identify the cochlear aqueduct.
- Section the superior vestibular nerve. Identify the singular nerve, then identify the cochlear nerve and follow it to its entrance in the modiolus. Perform a total facial decompression, including the labyrinthine part. Section the greater petrosal nerve and dissect the facial nerve from the fallopian canal, reflecting it posteriorly. Drill the fallopian canal and study the stapes muscle, its volume and its relationship with the facial nerve. Drill the promontory. Study the turns of the cochlea and their relationships with the middle ear structure. Study the cochlear nerve's entrance into the modiolus. Remove the cochlear turns and study the cochlear relationship with the internal carotid artery. Follow the internal carotid artery and study its relationship with the eustachian tube and with the second division of the V nerve.

Middle fossa approach

- Study the relationships between the temporal line and the level of the middle fossa; perform a craniotomy of 4 cm, two-thirds anteriorly to the external auditory canal and one-third superior and posterior to it. Identify the dura and the meningeal artery. Identify the superior petrosal sinus. Identify the arcuate eminence. Follow the meningeal artery forward until reaching the

foramen spinosum, and identify the greater superficial petrosal nerve. Identify the facial hiatus. Study the anatomy of the greater superficial petrosal nerve and the geniculate ganglion and its relationship with the foramen spinosum. "Blue line" the superior semicircular canal. Follow the facial nerve in the internal auditory canal.
- Study the internal auditory canal. Identify "Bill's bar" and the facial nerve and their relationships with the ampullae of the superior semicircular canal and the cochlea. Study the ossicles and the tympanic membrane. Open the eustachian tube to the isthmus. Remove the tensor muscle from the tympanum and study the relationships between the eustachian tube and the carotid artery. Open the carotid canal to study the artery. Remove the mastoid tegmen and follow the nerve into the middle ear. Remove the top of the temporo-mandibular articulation and study its anatomy, including the cartilage.

TIPS AND PITFALLS

- I have never seen a tumor too large for the translabyrinthine approach, since the underlying pressure pushes the tumor into the surgical field (W. Hitselberger).

- If a preoperative prophylactic therapy is to be utilized, an antiobiotic must also be used which can cross the hemato-encephalic barrier (e.g. Ceftixozime or Cefotriaxone 2 gr. i.v.).

- When working on the bone, it is advisable to use a slightly larger suction-irrigator than necessary. In this way, the swirling motion of the water, which impedes vision, is reduced. The field is also cleaner of bone fragments due to the greater aspirating capacity. Our objective during the bone work is to work through a thin veil of clear water.

- The burr must work with convexity, not with the tip. In the first position it removes the bone more rapidly and is more stable; in the second it is very unstable and may slip in undesirable directions.

- The burr is directed from front to back to avoid blind spots in front of the burr.

- Pear-shaped burrs with pointed ends are useful in the bone removal phase of middle and posterior cranial fossa exposure. The lateral resting surface is longer than that of a round burr. Thus its action is more rapid and stable. Using a large-diameter burr has its advantages. While drilling in restricted space (such as during exposure of the epitympanum and the incus body), we can drill with its point, which is no bigger than that of a round 1 mm burr.

- The falciform crest is perpendicular to the vestibule and originates below the vestibule. The falciform crest faces the surgeon, whereas the transverse crest faces the tegmen.

- If problems arise in identifying Bill's bar, the upper part of the fallopian canal may be drilled. When drilling close to the facial nerve, there must be abundant and continuous irrigation with water. When irrigation is insufficient, the nerve can become overheated and injured.

- Removing the posterior half of the bone covering the dura of the middle fossa makes it easier to expose sino-dural angle.

- Before opening the dura, the bone removal phase must be terminated, the blood vessels coagulated, and the field irrigated with saline solution to remove residual bone dust.

- To reduce the incidence of post-operative infection, prophylactic therapy may be administered using a third-generation cephalosporin, which can cross the hematoencephalic barrier. This preventative treatment is not unanimously supported; according to W. House, the drug may mask an infection, upon which a suprainfection may nest, especially in the presence of a CSF leak.

- Hyperventilation may be performed at the beginning of the mastoid phase in order to reduce intracranial pressure and encourage retraction of the cerebellum, (up to a end-tidal di 20 mm Hg.) and Mannitol (a diuretic) may be administered intravenously.

- The jugular bulb is medial to the mastoid part of the facial nerve.

- When the jugular bulb is high enough to prevent an accurate inferior skeletonization of the IAC, it must be decompressed. It is exposed and then pressed with a flap of Surgicel, over which bone wax is placed. Using the burr in a medial to lateral direction, the bone over the jugular bulb may be mobilized and moved down, decompressing the bulb, which is then stabilized with bone wax.

- In a small mastoid when restricted space is available, the dura of the posterior cranial fossa may be incised. This is done posterior to the sigmoid sinus, before removing all the bone. When the liquor gushes out, the cerebellum is decompressed.

- When the sigmoid sinus is prolapsed, the emissary mastoid vein must be coagulated in order to more easily decompress the sinus.

- When drilling is ended and before opening the dura, the field is irrigated with an irrigating perette containing Bacitracin (250 ml of dextrose 5% with 50,000 U of Bacitracin, in a physiologic solution). Irrigation has the dual purpose of removing all bony residue before the incision of the dura, and to disinfect. The sac containing the antibiotic is then connected to the suction-irrigator used in the tumor removal. The antibiotic solution may not be used during drilling because it produces foam. The area is repeatedly rinsed with the irrigating perette before the obliteration of the mastoid and closure of the incision.

- A large enough lesion of the sigmoid sinus will cause a great deal of blood to be lost in a short time, rapidly obscuring the surgical field. When blood loss begins, the instinctive reaction is to use the aspirator we are holding in the opposite hand from that which has caused the damage with the drill. In all but very small lesions, this is insufficient. The best instrument to use at this point is one we all have: our finger! Placing the finger on the lesion, the hemorrhage is momentarily stopped, while the instrument nurse prepares the instruments necessary for hemostasis (see Chapter 11).

- Bleeding of the superior petrosal sinus is frequent, due to its fragility. A small plate of bone may be left on it, and removed at the conclusion of the labyrinthectomy.

- Following the dura of the posterior cranial fossa during bone drilling provides a landmark for the cleavage plane to be followed, so that we don't have to drill blindly.

- Bipolar coagulation is preferable to monopolar coagulation when coagulating on the dura, in the presence of blood vessels or a dural laceration. Monopolar coagulation may provoke a breach in the dura.

- Generally the ampulla of the posterior canal is not adequately drilled, since it is below the facial nerve. It is important, however, to do so, since the inferior vestibular nerve and the singular nerve originate there. It is also important to thoroughly drill the bone in the angle between the middle fossa superiorly, the superior and lateral ampullae of the canal posteriorly, and anteriorly, the facial nerve. If bone is only partially removed, it will not be possible to thoroughly drill the ampullae.

- During the bone removal phase in the translabyrinthine technique, it is wise to keep the ampulla of the superior semicircular canal in sight. Later, while drilling above the ampulla in a latero-medial direction, the arborization of the superior vestibular nerve can be identified.

- One effective means of performing the labyrinthectomy is to begin by exposing the lateral sinus, and then go deeper by following the dura of the posterior and middle fossa as a cleavage plane.

- To begin with, the posterior section of the sigmoid sinus is exposed, since slight posterior bleeding is acceptable. Bleeding is bothersome anteriorly, where the surgical field is located. In this phase at least 1 cm of the dura of the posterior cranial fossa is seen, behind the sigmoid sinus. If serious lesions to the sinus occur there, the way is opened for its ligation.

- To free the overlying bone when the sinus is compressed, it is important to first remove the bone up to the top of the sinus. Thus the surgical plane is from top to bottom, with no impediment to the view of the underlying field. If, on the other hand, the bone is not removed to the top, the working angle is unfavorable and there is a risk of damaging the sinus. (Fig. 28-30).

- When the sigmoid sinus is exposed, bleeding may occur during bone removal. Coagulation may be attempted, but at times the bone may be coagulated instead. It is therefore preferable to first remove the bone, completely expose the dura, and then coagulate.

- When drilling the bone behind the facial nerve, bleeding may occur. This originates, not in the facial nerve, but in the underlying stapedial muscle and the two arteries supplying blood to the third tract of the facial nerve.

- The second genu of the facial nerve is on the same level as the concavity of the semicircular canal, immediately anterior to it. The facial nerve is preserved by maintaining the anterior wall of the lateral canal.

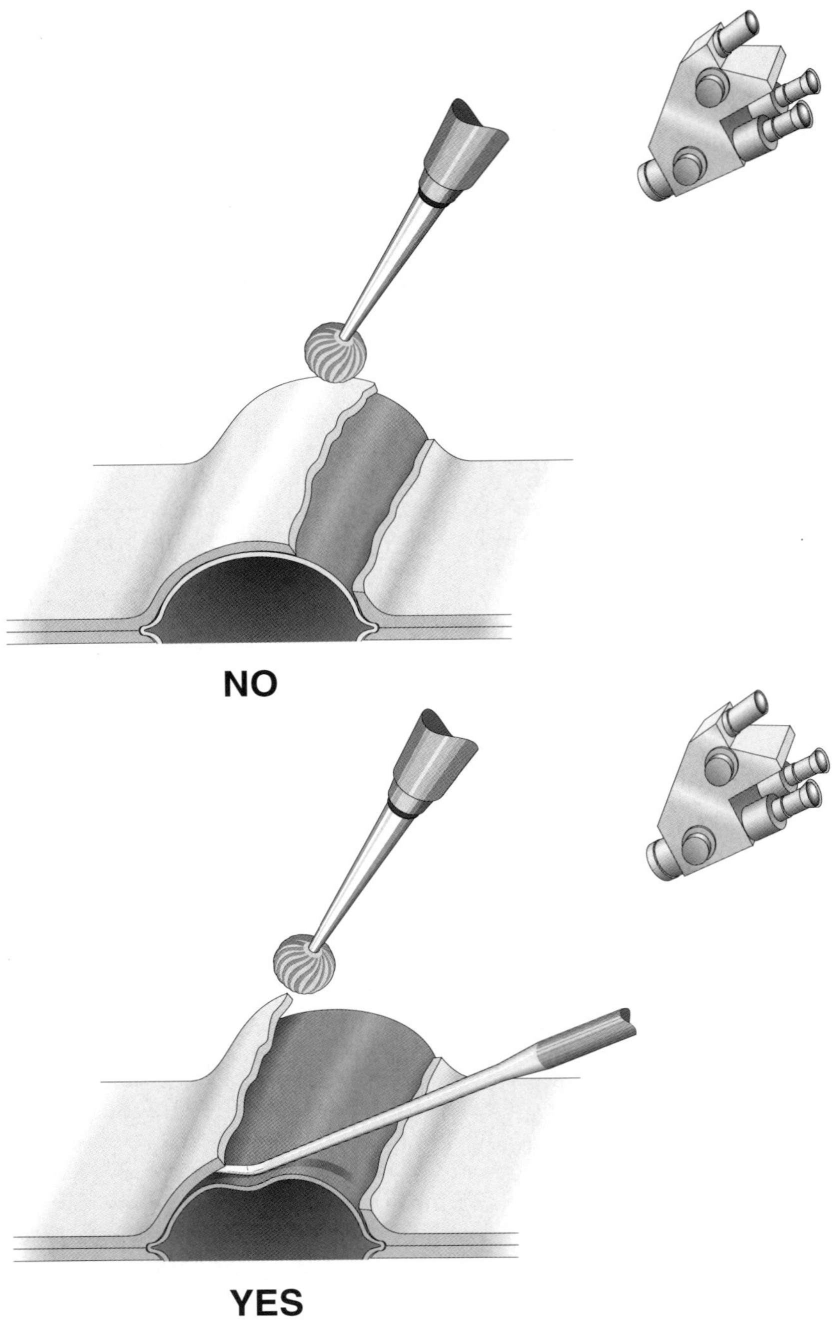

Fig. 28-30. How to obtain a favorable working angle to decompress the sinus and the posterior fossa dura.

- *Lesion points of the VII n.* In the mastoid phase, the third segment of the facial nerve is skeletonized. This is the anterior dissecting limit. The surgeon looks for the nerve and concentrates on it, and lesions of n. VII are rarely provoked in this phase. The vestibule is opened widely since its medial wall represents the lateral wall of the IAC. If a cutting burr is used, the facial nerve may be damaged, since it lies laterally. Merely touching the facial nerve with a cutting burr is enough to provoke a facial paralysis. It is preferable to use a small diamond burr. The risks are greater since here the surgeon's attention is not on the nerve, but rather on the vestibule.

- Besides the dura of the posterior fossa, it is also helpful to expose the dura of the middle fossa. This provides a better working angle. The dura is no longer compressed by an inflexible wall of bone, so it resumes elasticity and the liquor pressure is also reduced. The bone removal better exposes the superior margin of the IAC, forming an acute angle with the dura of the middle fossa, and giving the sino-dural angle more flexibility.

- It is not always necessary to remove bone near the jugular bulb, except when the bulb is very high (it can reach the ampulla of the posterior canal). We must keep in mind, however, that the cochlear aqueduct is usually near the jugular bulb. We also recommend opening the mastoid field wide enough to give the best exposure possible. A reduced exposure (on the IAC) means drilling in a hole, causing problems with the suction-irrigator, and allowing less space for the drilling and the tumor.

- The anterior-superior limit for removing the bone surrounding the IAC and showing Bill's bar is just posterior to the short process of the incus located above. Bone removal should not proceed anteriorly because of the danger of injuring the geniculate ganglion.

- The lateral extremity of the IAC is Bill's bar, which is also the most reliable landmark in identifying the facial nerve where it is not infiltrated by the tumor.

- To evidentiate Bill's bar, drill in the projection zone, immediately above (2 mm) and anterior (2 mm) to the vestibular nerve. In this area, the drilling should be done in a latero-medial direction. If drilling is performed in a superior-inferior direction, it is very easy to drill the vertical crest. The diamond burr must have a diameter superior to that of the facial nerve. If its diameter is equal or inferior to that of the facial nerve, it may slip inside the two exposed bone margins and damage the nerve. If its diameter is greater, it will not pass the lateral bone margins, and in any case it cannot act on the entire surface of the nerve.

- The anterior drilling is extended by passing with the burr under the horizontal tract of VII and opening the vestibule wide. The SSC ampulla is drilled, working in the vestibule.

- One method of skeletonizing the IAC at the porus is to remove bone from the dura of the posterior fossa up to the porus, and then to drill canals inferior and superior to the IAC, to evidentiate the dura. A diamond burr is used. Thus defined, the dura of the bone plate is dissected from top to bottom with a House elevator, and then removed with forceps. The bone at the edges of the IAC must be removed first, since it is thicker. The lateral part must be removed at the end, at the fundus.

- When skeletonizing the IAC, it is essential to drill in the same direction as the nerve rather than perpendicular to it, to reduce the risk of neural lesions. When drilling along the superior margin of the IAC, we are very close to the facial nerve. It is then useful to open the dura inferiorly to the sigmoid sinus. Thus the CSF flows out, the endocranial pressure decreases, and the nerves (previously crushed against the dura) recede.

- The facial nerve can be identified at the lateral end of the IAC medial and inferior to the ampulla of the superior semicircular canal.

- Great care must be taken when removing bone from the IAC so as not to damage the facial nerve just below. When bone is drilled on the dura of the middle fossa or the IAC superiorly, it is important not to let the drill slip and damage the nerve, either by entering into the IAC or by projecting bone fragments into it. The burr must rotate away from the facial nerve (i.e. clockwise in left ear, counterclockwise in right ear).

- If the bone is removed in proximity to delicate anatomical structures, (e.g. superior and inferior to the IAC), the risk of burr slippage can be reduced by carefully tracing a furrow, and then working with the burr in the sulcus.

- A greater skeletonization of the IAC, even 270 degrees, will improve the view of the CPA.

- When drilling bone of the middle or posterior fossa, it is helpful to use the suction-irrigator to place pressure on the underlying dura. In this way a cleavage plane is created by separating the dura from the overlying bone. The overlying bone may thus be safely removed with a cutting burr. However, it is important to never press with the burr on the bone. The burr must rest lightly and run without pressure, as if there were no bone to sustain it. Otherwise, when the bone suddenly ends, the burr's pressure will no longer be counterbalanced, and may injure the dura and the underlying structures.

- There is another means of exposing the dura of the middle fossa. A canal is created with the burr, exposing the dura on three sides: superior, inferior, and medial. The exposed bone is lifted with a House elevator and with the dural dissector, and is removed. The principle is analogous to the operation performed with the IAC. It is important to remove the bone covering the middle fossa to better decompress the underlying structures.

- When dissecting bone from the dura of the posterior fossa, it must always be done in a back to front direction. Dissecting the bone in an anterior-posterior direction is incorrect since the cleavage plane is hidden from view, and dural lesions may result.

- The burr must be kept in constant movement, parallel to the structures to be exposed. If the burr remains stable on the bone covering the dura or the vascular structures (petrosal sinus, sigmoid sinus, jugular bulb), it will cause a perforation. By keeping the burr moving, irregularities are avoided. A homogeneous and even work surface must always be used.

- To expose the sino-dural angle, the following procedure may be followed: The sigmoid sinus is exposed superiorly to the beginning of the transverse sinus. The superior part of the dura of the middle fossa is exposed. The two exposed surfaces are then joined by drilling the bone in between.

- It is also possible to perform a labyrinthectomy by opening first the ampullae of the lateral canal and the superior canal. The SSC ampulla lies above the lateral one, but it is easier to reach. It is reached by first opening the anterior part of the SSC, which leads to the ampulla. Once these two landmarks have been reached, the labyrinthectomy is performed with a large cutting burr.

- When the dura of the internal auditory canal has been opened, a Brackmann suction-irrigator should be used. It does not provoke trauma to the structures that it aspirates because of its lateral fenestration. The flow of water may also be used in some cases as an extremely delicate means of separating the facial nerve from the surrounding structures. This instrument can also be utilized as a dissector, to move the tumor as necessary, while the other hand uses microscissors.

- If the facial nerve still cannot be identified after opening the fundus of the IAC, the superior vestibular nerve can be identified. The facial nerve will be found immediately superior to it.

- When opening the ampulla of the superior semicircular canal and seeking the vestibular nerve, drilling may be either too low or too high. This is because the correct position of the ampulla is momentarily lost. At this point it may be useful to partially identify the IAC, though leaving the bone in place superiorly. The view of the canal is a guide, since we know the paths of the nerves within it. The falciform crest divides the fundus of the canal into an upper and a lower half. In the upper half, the facial nerve is superior and medial to the superior vestibular nerve, which is inferior and lateral. The virtual path of the nerves within the IAC guides us in difficult cases in identifying the nerves at their lateral extremes.

- One idea is to combine the retrosigmoid and translabyrinthine approaches. The purpose would be to pair the ample CPA exposure obtained in the suboccipital technique with the advantages of the internal auditory canal exposure and the facilitated identification of the facial nerve inherent to the translabyrinthine approach. In this way, the surgeon can work both anteriorly and posteriorly to the sigmoid sinus. Thus, we gain a greater control of the anterior and posterior extension of the large tumors. For an even wider field, a ligation and section of the sigmoid sinus may be performed (with suboccipital, translabyrinthine, and transsigmoid approaches).

- The facial nerve is very resistant to stretching and twisting. In fact, there may be a normally functioning facial nerve even in the presence of very large tumors. Total facial paralysis is rare and is observed only in the largest tumors. An anomaly in the microvascularization of the nerve may be at the base of the progressive neural dysfunction (W.A. Bucheit).

- Trigeminal nerve involvement is rare and is only seen in tumors larger than 3 cm. In its upward growth, the tumor may reach CN (cranial nerve) V. The first symptom is a decrease in the corneal reflex, which will eventually lead to a total loss of the reflex.

- In the CPA, it is preferable not to use cotton substances which adhere to the cerebellum and may cause irritation. Merocel is a better choice and can be aspirated.

- A neuroma or a meningioma may grow downward, involving the jugular foramen and compromising nerves IX, X and XI, with consequent hoarseness, dysphagia, and dysphonia. The symptoms of ataxia, from compression of the cerebellum and of the cerebellar peduncle, appear later. Lastly, papilledema and hydrocephalus may appear, along with symptoms of brainstem compression and symptoms of the pyramidal bundle. The first symptom to appear is without doubt a unilateral hearing loss, with or without tinnitus. The disease's progression leads to complete hearing loss on the side of the le-

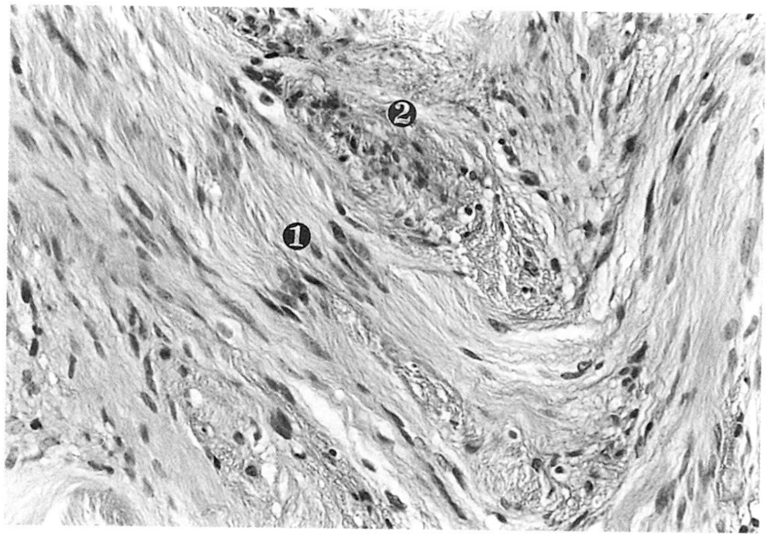

Fig. 28-31. Courtesy of Linthicum FH. Acoustic tumor containing dense and Antoni type I and vacuolar and Antoni type II tissue. Palisading of the nuclei (1) and Verocay bodies (2) are visible. ×430.

sion. This symptom is more and more frequently the cause leading the patient to seek a specialist. The improvement of health conditions and therefore prevention, along with the competence in the execution of auditory evoked potentials and the possibilities offered by new diagnostic techniques for images (MRI with Gadolinium) mean that the specialist is more and more responsible for the first diagnosis. The diagnosis of tumors in their initial state (while they are still small) will continue to move surgical therapy toward the goal of preserving hearing, which is rarely achieved today (Figs. 28-31, 28-32, 28-33).

- Next to neuromas, meningiomas are the most frequent tumors of the cerebello-pontine angle. They often originate in the superior and anterior parts of the IAC and are thus associated with precocious facial nerve involvement. Rarer and slower to appear is acoustic nerve involvement and a simultaneous hearing loss. Given its origins, the meningioma often involves CN V, causing facial weakness and tic-like symptoms. When symptoms of trigeminal involvement appear before the hypoacusia, diagnosis is oriented towards meningioma or, more rarely, a tumor of the trigeminal nerve (A. Buchheit).

- Meningiomas originating in the upper part of the cerebello-pontine angle may provoke the symptoms listed above, but they are differentiated from neuromas by precocious trigeminal nerve involvement. When the tumor grows towards the tentorial furrow, early signs of hydrocephalus and an increase in intracranial pressure (with papilledema) may be seen. With these symptoms, signs of involvement of the upper part of the pons and of the midbrain may be noted, causing an altered function of the CNs III, IV, VI (Buchheit, Rosenwasser).

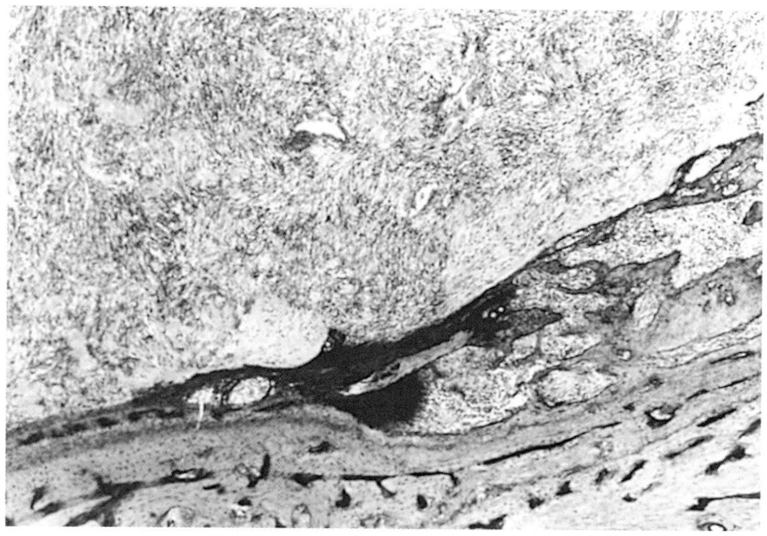

Fig. 28-32. Courtesy of Linthicum FH. Vestibular schwannoma arising from the utricular nerve.

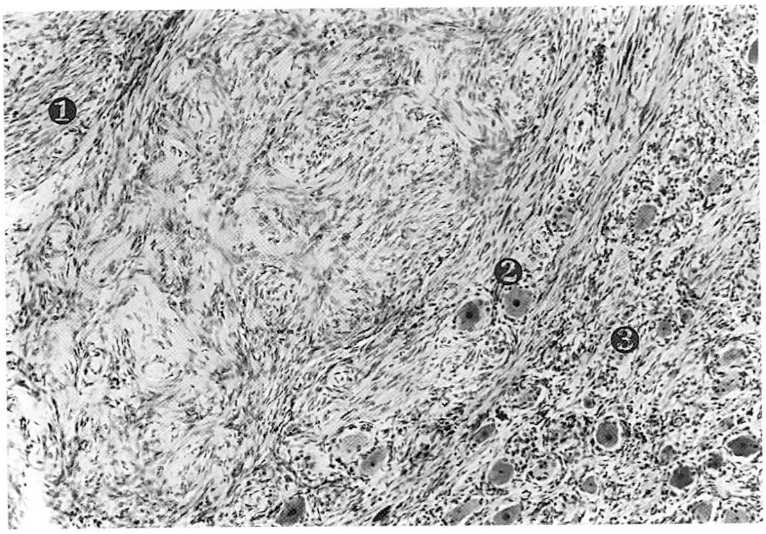

Fig. 28-33. Courtesy of Linthicum FH. Neurofbromatosis II. The tumor is pleomorphic containing remnants of schwannoma (1), ganglion cells (2), and meningioma (3). ×120.

- Metastases may involve the IAC, either selectively or as a systemic diffusion. We have observed the first case of selective bilateral metastasis in the CPA from a pleural adenocarcinoma (presented at the 2nd International Conference on Acoustic Neuroma Surgery, april 1995). The patient was operated twelve months before the onset of symptomatology for an adenocarcinoma of the left lung, with no limphonodal metastases. A metastatic work-up was considered in this patient, without detecting any metastases. The most distinctive feature was the short and aggressive course of symptoms: bilateral facial nerve paralysis (House-Brackmann 5); right anacusis and left profound sensorineural hearing loss (Figs. 28-34, 28-35, 28-36).

- The subarcuate artery indicates the vertex of the IAC.

- While removing a tumor, curved Jacobson microscissors are used to see what is being cut at all times. The incision must never be perpendicular to the facial nerve, but rather lengthwise to it. The scissors may then be used inferiorly with superior concavity, and superiorly with inferior concavity (Fig. 28-37). Both curved and straight Jacobson scissors may also be used to dissect and separate the arachnoid, the vessels, and the tumor capsule.

- The superior petrosal sinus represents the tentorium margin.

- If a bony island is left on the sigmoid sinus (Bill's Island) it is important not to leave osseous spurs on the margins. The pressure on the bone may in fact cause them to penetrate into the sinus and cause a lesion. If Bill's Island is not used, the bony spurs must still be removed to avoid traumatizing the sinus when it is compressed.

- When the jugular bulb is very low, it need not be exposed. When it is intermediate, the blue shadow under the bone is sufficient to identify it. When it is high, it must be exposed. When possible, some bone should be left on the jugular bulb. The walls of the jugular bulb are very thin and may easily be injured. The wall of the sigmoid sinus, however, is much more resistant.

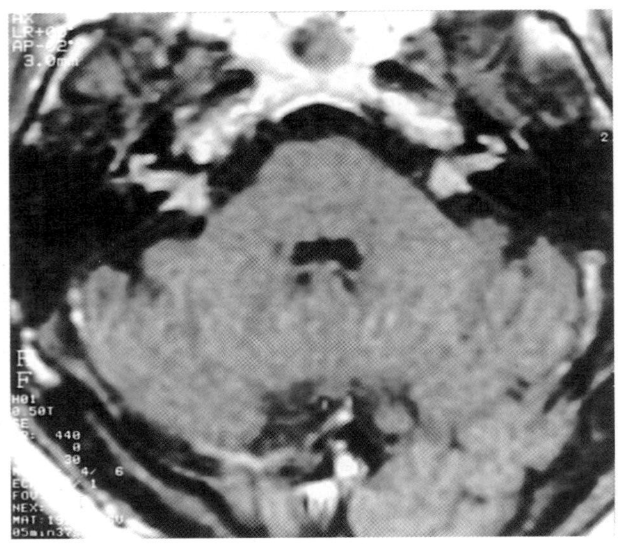

Fig. 28-34. In the review of the MRI there are some radiologic signs that could have excluded the hypothesis of bilateral neurinoma and suggest a secondary localization.The cisternal component of the mass in both sides has a wide basis of implant and describes an obtuse angle with the axis of the IAC and the temporal pyramid. Furthermore, neither IAC is enlarged. The other hypothesis of bilateral meningioma could have been excluded for the deep penetration of the lesions in the IAC.

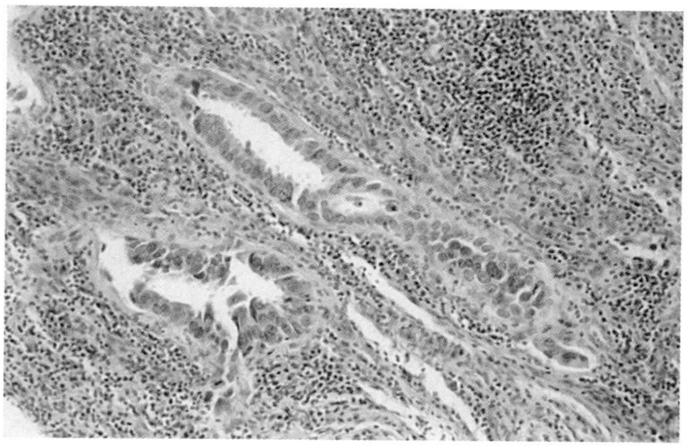

Fig. 28-35. Right cerebellopontine angle tumor. Elongated neoplastic glands composed by cells with mild atypia are deeped in a stroma reach of lymphocytes and small vessels. Some mytoses are seen. × 200. (Carbone A).

- When the dura of the posterior cranial fossa is opened to enter into the CPA, the maximum diameter of the opening can be measured with the tip of a Gimmick elevator, which is 11 mm long.

- Neither the Urban mechanical aspirator nor ultrasonic suction-aspirators must ever be used on small tumors, due to the proximity of nerve VII and the AICA.

- The intracranial part of VII is not surrounded by epineurium. When the IAC is opened, the slightest stimuli, inevitable when working on the tumor, are transmitted to the nerve. Therefore a transitory paralysis is quite frequent.

Once the nerve has been identified at the level of Bill's bar, in medium to large tumors with CPA extension, careful and thorough intracapsular gutting must be performed as follows:

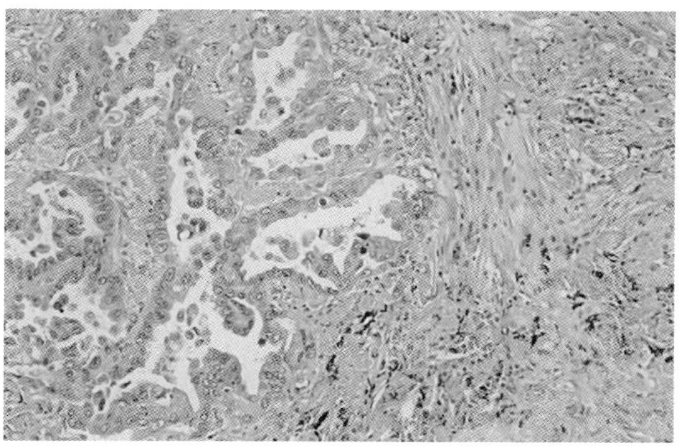

Fig. 28-36. Lung tumor. Well developed and irregurarly shaped glands (left side) and hyalinized stroma are reach in black pigment (anthracosis). Cellular atypia is from mild to moderate.

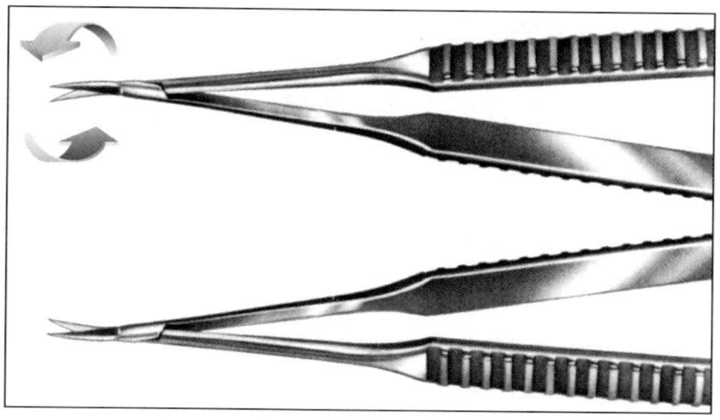

Fig. 28-37. Scissors for dural incision and tumor dissection.

- The tumor's mass is reduced so that it can be easily mobilized and allow an approach from all directions, anterior, posterior, superior, inferior, lateral, medial.
- The emergence of the facial nerve at the pons, previously hidden by the tumor's mass, may now be identified. The entrance at the fundus of the IAC is already known. The identification of these two points helps to imagine the path of the nerve from one point to the other.
- The facial nerve usually runs medial to the tumor. With the reduction in mass, the pressure it places on the nerve is also reduced. The residual structure tends to collapse gradually, taking the facial nerve with it towards the surface. In this way, the nerve's angle of deviation is reduced. Lengthened in the years of the tumor's compressing growth, the facial nerve is now longer than normal and thus less vulnerable to breakage during stretching.
- When the inferior pole of the tumor is moved away from the brainstem, in a backward to forward motion, the neuroma seems adherent due to the stabilizing action exerted by the cochlear nerve. Nerve VIII should be preserved whenever possible, to enable a future cochlear implant. The cochlear nerve, on the other hand, is sacrificed when this aids in a complete resectioning of the tumor. Here too, nerve VIII is kept whole at least until most of the intracapsular emptying has been completed. The traumatic action of dissection, with pressure and traction, is thus contrasted not only by the facial nerve, but also by the arachnoid membrane and by the cochlear nerve. Thus the possibility of injury to VII is reduced. When these precautions are not taken, however, nerve VII may break due to the tumor's weight.

- Due to reduced space, dural adherences are formed with the tumor's surface around the porus acusticus. This is a critical point in the preservation of the facial nerve, both in this and in the retrosigmoid technique. If the procedure of complete separation from the nerve capsule is followed (W. House) rather than that of preserving the anterior curtain (M.Tos), it is very important to remove the dural adherences and perform the cleavage from the superior surface of the tumor only after the facial nerve has been identified and followed to the intracanal part.

- Whenever possible, the cochlear nerve should be preserved when removing the tumor, to leave open the possibility for future cochlear implants, altough the destruction of the vascularization may provoke cochlear ossification (see Chapter 41).

- The tumor is separated from the facial nerve in a medial to lateral and a lateral to medial motion, passing several times from one position to another, while attempting to follow the plane with the tumor. This is seen frequently in smaller tumors, but only very rarely in medium to large tumors. In the latter, the cochlear nerve should be identified whenever possible at the brainstem. This is an important landmark in identifying n. VII, which exits medially to VIII. It is also helpful to preserve the cochlear nerve as long as possible, to exert less traction on VII.

- For the removal of the tumor and the preservation of the facial nerve, the guidelines are: to identify the facial nerve at the lateral extreme of the IAC outside the capsule; then, to empty the tumor while staying *inside* the capsule. Losing the capsule poses risks, due to the possibility of injuring the vascular and nervous structures behind.

- If the tumor is large enough to reach the prepontine cistern or to rest on the clivus, the transcochlear approach (see chapter 37-38) becomes necessary in order to obtain an adequate anterior view.

- Particularly in large tumors, it is helpful to identify n. VII at the lateral surface of the IAC. Then, the mass of the neuroma is reduced intracapsularly. From this point on, every theory on dissecting methods has a limited value since these are not always reproducible. We therefore advise not to advise! The tumor is treated posteriorly, anteriorly, superiorly, inferiorly, reducing it from every angle which appears propitious. It is essential to reduce the tumoral mass while remaining inside the tumoral capsule. The AICA lies outside the tumoral capsule, and may be injured. Later the VII becomes visible at the trunk and at the fundus.

- When the tumor has been gutted and nerve VII has been identified at the trunk, the dissection must not assume a latero-medial direction because this may lead to a trauma of VII nerve. The VII in the CPA is not covered by perineurium and is frequently crushed by the capsule by the growth of the largest tumors. At this point in the operation, neither the vestibular nerves nor the arachnoid nor the acoustic nerve (frequently impossible to preserve) medially counterbalance the weight of the tumor and the surgical maneuvers. The dissection of VII from the tumoral capsule thus assumes a medial to lateral direction. The last part of the dissection may be extremely difficult due to the many adherences. If a section does take place, it is usually here. To separate the nerve from the residual tumor, Sterkers uses a Beaver knife with a 67 blade. Close to the nerve it is less traumatic to cut than to dissect. The disposable blade is extremely sharp. While cutting it is important to push towards the tumor and not the nerve.

- All the vessels that can be dissected from the tumor's surface should be spared. Some vessels, however, must be coagulated. They must be moved away from the tumor and coagulated far from it. If they are coagulated on the tumor, they remain attached to it and mask the underlying plane.

- The vessels feeding into the tumor are coagulated before being cut. When they are very small, it is pointless to coagulate them, since once cut the blood coagulates internally and closes the opening.

- What to do for intraoperative bleeding of the vessels that supply the tumor? It is pointless to spend hours in the attempt to stop bleeding. The best way to stop bleeding is to remove the tumor. To reduce blood loss, it is necessary to go directly to the center of the tumor (W. Hitselberger).

- To separate the tumor from the facial nerve, we begin in a lateral to medial direction. Once the nerve has been identified, we always work in a medial to lateral direction, since all procedures going from lateral to medial cause trauma to the facial nerve.

- In a tumor of the CPA, facial paralysis is always slow to occur, and is preceded by sensory-neural hearing loss and at times tinnitus. The motor nerves are in fact much more resistant than the sensory nerves.

- The initial dissection of the tumor follows a lateral to medial direction, like the tumor's growth. This enables the surgeon to separate the tumoral capsule from the arachnoid, the adherences, and the surrounding vessels.

- In the translabyrinthine approach, where the anatomy is either normal or at least presents no marked variations due to tumor growth, the lateral branch of the AICA is in contact with VIII and medial to it.

- The vertebral artery is medial to the mixed nerves. In general the former unites with the controlateral artery to form the basilar artery at CN VIII entrance in the brainstem.

- The AICA generally reaches the bridge between n. VII and VIII.

- The tumor must be dissected from the nerve, and not vice versa.

- Small vessels run in the facial nerve towards the tumor. In cleaving the tumor from the nerve, these vessels may be damaged. If they must be coagulated, it is important to do so as far from the nerve as possible, near the tumor. When aspirating near the facial nerve, it is important not to aspirate directly, but rather over a merocel.

- When a mechanical House-Urban or ultrasonic suction-aspirator is used to gut the tumor, it is important to keep in mind the level at which surgery is being performed, to avoid damage to the brainstem. It is then necessary to dissect part of the capsule until we have identified the level reached. This process is repeated, gutting and checking several times, until the medial part of the tumor can be safely decompressed inside the capsule.

- When larger arterioles are to be coagulated, they must be coagulated not just twice and then dissected in the middle, but rather four times altogether. In the first case, if the patient has a pressure increase, the clot will be pushed through the lumen and the artery will open . In the second case, for opposite reasons, this does not occur (Fig. 28-38).

- In removing the tumor from the internal auditory canal, it is important to keep in mind that the AICA or one of its branches may reach the fundus of the IAC.

- A notable reduction in liquor pressure may be obtained by opening the cisterna magna. This may be done with a Friar dissector with blunt edges. The instrument is extended downwards, medial and inferior to the cochlear duct. The cisterna magna is not visible in the labyrinthine approach, but a sudden and intense spurt of liquid signals its presence.

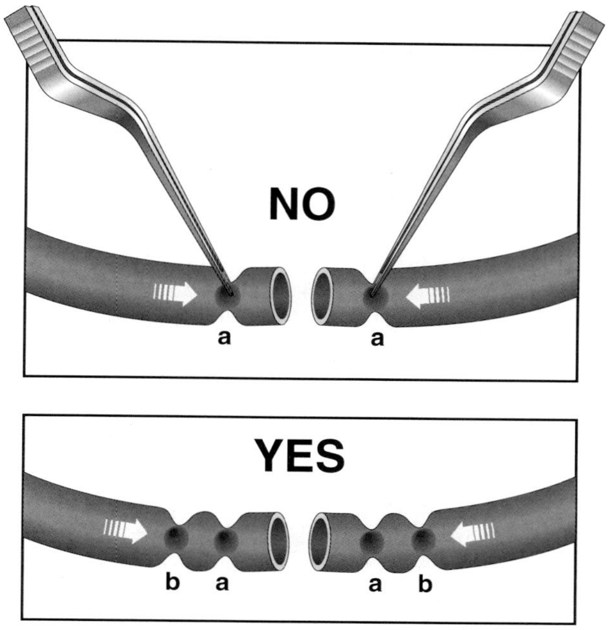

Fig. 28-38. The arteries should be preserved. When needed, double coagulation avoids the risk of reopening of the vessel.

- In cystic tumors, medial cysts in contact with the facial nerve make preservation of the facial nerve difficult. The nerve is crushed by the cyst and the identification of a cleavage plane is problematic.

- In highly vascularized tumors adhering to the brainstem, small flaps of Surgicel may be left in place at surgery's end. It is important not to use too much, since the Surgicel tends to swell and may increase intracranial pressure.

- In some cases, the facial nerve is dislocated anteriorly and in contact with the edges of the porus. Dissection proves very difficult, since any pressure on the tumor pushes nerve VII against the margins of the IAC, traumatizing it.

- The translabyrinthine approach enables us to expose the facial nerve even in its petrous segment. This is useful in the rare cases (2%) when the tumor originates in the facial nerve and spreads to the bone along the facial canal. Here the true origin and the extension of the tumor may not be revealed with a retrosigmoid or suboccipital approach. The possibility of exposing the intrapetrosal facial nerve and mobilizing it is an advantage if a termino-terminal anastomosis or a neural graft becomes necessary. In fact, a longer distal segment is available to work with (King).

- The translabyrinthine approach is particularly adaptable. It may extend along the middle fossa, dividing the superior petrosal sinus and the tentorium. This takes place in meningiomas extending from the cerebello-pontine angle through the tentorium and into the middle fossa. The translabyrinthine approach may be modified into a transcochlear approach: the facial nerve is dislodged from its canal, repositioned posteriorly, and the cochlea and the petrosal apex are drilled. This approach is indicated in epidermoid cysts of the petrosal apex, and in meningiomas of the petrous apex and of the clivus (see chapter 37-38).

- The translabyrinthine technique uses a direct approach to the tumor and enables the surgeon to work in a comfortable position. The main disadvantages of other approaches are the risk of embolization and hypotension in a sitting position, and damage to the arm which is under the patient in a lateral position.

- The meatal dura is very thin and thus impossible to preserve as part of a flap. It should be removed with a hook or the tip of curved Jacobson scissors.

The dissection of the tumor may be pursued in four directions:

- From the front, or the meatal side, along the facial nerve;
- From above, along the tentorium, the petrosal vein and, deeper down, the trigeminal nerve;
- From behind, along the anterior surface of the cerebellum and the midbrain;
- From below, along the cistern of the bulb and nerves IX, X, and XI (King).

- When the tumor is to be cleaved by proceeding upwards to deflect it downwards, the arachnoid of the neoplasia is elevated, while avoiding the tentorium and the AICA. The trigeminal nerve appears when entering into the cistern surrounding it. It is deep, and superior to the emergence of nerves VII and VIII. It is white, and clearly recognizable due in part to its size compared to the other cranial nerves. It runs along the subarachnoid space and enters into Meckel's cave.

- Medium-to-large tumors, even when touching the trigeminal nerve, are generally easily dissected. The dissection may thus be careful and blunted, without manipulating the nerve. Thus, no loss of sensitivity will appear in the face at a later date.

- In smaller tumors (1-1.2 cm), dissection may be almost exclusively anterior while separating the tumor from the nerve (but never the contrary). In medium to large tumors, this step is preceded by the intracapsular gutting, so that the neoformation is brought to the conditions of a small tumor. A plane is developed between nerve and tumor, beginning from the identification of the facial nerve at Bill's Bar, and proceeding medially. In this phase, an enlargement of 16X or 25X must be used. A Brackmann fenestrated suction-irrigator is used to avoid suction dangerous to the nerve. Not even a tiny bit of the tumor must be left on the facial nerve during dissection, since this will lead to a progressive increase of the tumoral mass on the nerve, to the point where the cleavage plane is completely lost. This last dissection is very delicate since the nerve, in itself more delicate in its path into the brainstem (due to its lack of a perineural sheath), is also structurally weakened by the tumor's compressing effect. It frequently loses its cylindric shape to assume the appearance of a strip spread on the tumoral capsule. The dissection is greatly aided by the continuous irrigating flow. Besides maintaining the field free of blood, this acts as a delicate dissector, facilitating recognition of the transition margin between nerve and tumor. The above also applies to the technique of complete tumoral excision, without preserving the anterior arachnoid curtain.

- When performing a posterior dissection, we proceed deeper medially along the arachnoid, until this practically disappears and the midbrain is seen. Frequently, the floccule masks the emergence of the cochlear nerve and the underlying facial nerve from the trunk. A slight pressure with a cottonoid on the floccule shows the emergence of the cochlear nerve. This is similar to the procedure used in sectioning the vestibular nerve with a retrolabyrinthine technique.

- If identification of the facial nerve at the brainstem proves difficult, the acoustic nerve may be identified and displaced upwards or downwards. Medial to it is the facial nerve.

- Total tumor removal is the goal whenever possible. Intraoperative changes in blood pressure and pulse are not unusual when the surgeon is working around the IX and X cranial nerves: in most cases it is sufficient to remove the packing around the tumor and stop surgical manipulation for a few minutes until the normal parameters resume. When blood pressure changes persist, the brainstem can be irreversibly damaged and the cerebellum and brainstem may swell. In rare cases (3%) a subtotal removal is preferred and the procedure is terminated. The patient is treated radiologically and, if necessary, surgery can be repeated.

- The House-Urban suction dissector is very effective in reducing the tumoral mass during the intracapsular gutting. It is inexpensive and relatively small and lightweight compared to other aspirators and ultrasounds. The rotating House-Urban suction-dissector is very useful in medium and large tumors. It consists of two concentric rods, the smaller of which fits perfectly in the larger. Each has an opening at the end. The internal rod is made to rotate by an electric motor found in the handpiece while the aspiration acts on its center. When the two openings coincide, the tumor is aspirated into the lumen of the rod and then amputated by the rod's rotation.

- The technique is as follows: the arachnoid is dissected from the capsule, which is then penetrated. Part of the tumor is bitten off with Takayashi forceps, after which the tissue mass is reduced several times with a House-Urban suction-dissector. When using the Takayashi forceps, it is important not to grasp the tumor too tightly. In this way, even if the capsule inadvertently breaks, the risk of injuring surface vessels is lowered. When the House-Urban suction-dissector is used, the suction-irrigator is held in the left hand. This is meant to stabilize the tumor, thus avoiding traction or pushing. This also applies when using Takayashi forceps, which can damage nervous and vascular structures. The aspirator acts as an aspirator and dissector, and allows a continuous flow of saline solution. The House-Urban aspirator acts as dissector and as an aspirator. The surgeon thus uses five different instruments simultaneously (King).

- Jacobson's microscissors may also be used in the intracapsular emptying of the tumor, along with the suction-irrigator. Straight scissors are used to separate the facial nerve from the capsule, but in the intracapsular emptying they should be curved, since they must act in a spherical plane. This is made possible by their curvature.

- Another useful instrument is the round knife. This is normally used for the incision of the skin of the external auditory canal in tympanotomy (e.g. for the stapedectomy). With this knife a large fragment of tumor may be cut with a circular movement, and later removed with Yasargill forceps. In large tumors this procedure is repeated several times. It is important to remember that the tumor is displaced more in this procedure than when sectioning it with Jacobson scissors, since the latter only touches the tumor with the cutting arms, while the round knife has the side effect of pushing. This is due to the blade's edge (they are not disposable knifes) and to the same bit which will eventually touch the tissue. If this procedure is used, it is important to carefully stabilize the tumor with the suction-irrigator.

- A non-saline Ringer solution is used to irrigate. The irrigating solution used during bone removal is at room temperature. It must prevent the burr's action from overheating the bone, since this effect is also transmitted to the facial nerve, with subsequent lesion. The diamond burr has a heating action much greater than that of the cutting burr. When operating in the CPA, the temperature of the solution must be lukewarm, to provide less stimulus to the facial nerve, which is not covered by perineurium in the CPA. If a cold solution is used, the facial nerve stimulator will register peaks of nerve irritation. Besides provoking nerve suffering (even if slight) this disturbs the surgeon intent on identifying VII, triggering the acoustic monitoring of the facial nerve monitor. Once the IAC has been adequately skeletonized, the irrigating liquid is replaced with a 0.25% Bacitracin solution in saline solution.

- We do not use Surgicel for small hemorrhaging spots. If excessive bleeding occurs, the anesthesiologist may be asked to maintain the systolic pressure at around 80 mmHg. This level of hypotension may be maintained for quite a while, but given the length of the operation, it is not recommended to go below it.

- After surgery, the cottonoids are removed one by one. Thus, if bleeding does occur, the origin is known, and another cottonoid is placed on it or it is immediately coagulated.

- Closure should be delayed for at least 30 minutes. The field is irrigated copiously with saline solution, to free it from coagulants and facilitate identification of the small blood vessels. They appear with a red line in the clear water. When in doubt, a bit of bovine collagen may be left on the pons, for future hemostatic action.

- We do not consider an incomplete removal of the tumor to be useful. Once the dura is opened and the tumor is manipulated, all possible complications must in any case be dealt with.

- *Bleeding*. During removal of the tumor, heavy bleeding may occur. If the bleeding spots are not easily identifiable and coagulable, it is advisable to proceed with tumor removal. Cottonoids may be placed between the tumor and the pons, while avoiding nerve VII. When the tumor has been removed, the cottonoids are removed one at a time. Thus we can check sites of possible bleeding under each cottonoid more precisely.

- If it proves difficult to stop bleeding, the patient's head may be raised temporarily, reducing the endocranial pressure.

- When coagulating, water is used. This enables a more precise identification of the opening of the bleeding vessels, since a line of blood can be seen more easily in the clear water. Furthermore, water is a good conductor, so the coagulation is more effective.

- When using needleholders in postauricular suturing, it is preferable that the surgeon not insert his fingers into the eyes of the instrument. Thus the procedure is much faster due to increased rapidity in handling.

- In the intraoperative period, after anesthesia is induced, a urinary catheter and a nasogastric tube are inserted. The nasogastric tube is left in aspiration post-operatively, in order to keep the stomach free (nausea and vomiting may occur). The day after surgery, the nasogastric tube, the abdominal drain, and the urinary catheter are removed. The dressing is left on for 7 days. In cases of liquor fistulas, the dressing must be reinforced, preferably with silk bandages.

- When the patient awakens from anesthesia, his corneal sensitivity must be evaluated. If nerve V has been injured, there will be corneal anesthesia which may lead to ulceration if the eye is not protected. If the corneal reflex is diminished, the eye must be covered with a protective glass monocle and bathed in artificial tears. If the reflex is absent or is present along with facial paralysis, with the facial nerve intact, a tarsorrhaphy can be performed together with physical therapy. If the facial nerve is not intact, tarsorrhaphy must be performed after the anastomosis of the facial nerve and possibly static facial support technique (see chapter 14-15).

- The patient may show signs of post-operative vertigo. It is not advisable, however, to administer antivertiginous drugs in the first 24 hours after surgery. This is because the vertigo is not the most pressing problem. The drugs also diminish the level of consciousness, falsifying the Glasgow scale data.

- The patients are encouraged to sit up, with their legs outside the bed, as soon as possible after surgery. They are then encouraged to sit in a chair, and to begin walking as soon as possible, with assistance.

SOME NOTIONS ON TUMOR GROWTH AND THERAPY

Improvements in anesthetic and surgical technique have greatly reduced surgical risk. Some categories of patients remain at risk: those with cardiovascular or lung disease, or elderly patients with a limited life expectancy.
When the decision is made not to operate, the patient is observed (wait and see) with an MRI check every year, to ensure that no change in the symptomatology appears.
Patients over 70 with tumors smaller than 2.5 cm are generally observed with radiologic tests.
Patients over 70 with tumors larger than 2.5 cm are usually operated, since the tumor's growth increases the intraoperative risk of injuring the facial nerve and compromising the central nervous system. In any case, respect for the patient's wishes has led us to observe one patient who has had a 4 cm-large neuroma since the age of 65. The patient has acute hearing loss but no signs of central nerve damage, and in 5 years there has been no tumor growth whatsoever.
We believe that the onset of internal necrosis, initially absent or slight but growing with the tumor, is a factor in volumetric homeostasis in this tumor. Studies to evaluate the growth of "large" tumors (greater than 3 cm), are needed but are made difficult by the current tendency towards surgical treatment.

After surgery, the patients have MRI check-ups after 1, 3 and 5 years, to diagnose any residual tumor.

A modification in the translabyrinthine approach has been proposed to preserve hearing. (McElveen 1991).
Modifications in the normal translabyrinthine procedure are as follows:
The semicircular bone canals are fenestrated with a diamond burr and continuous irrigation. The residual bone is then removed with a small curette while maintaining the integrity of the underlying membranous canals. The membranous labyrinth, denuded of its perilymph, collapses; it is then closed with bone wax at the ampullated

end of the canals, the lateral end of the lateral semicircular canal and at the crus communis. The other steps are similar to the translabyrinthine operation.

REFERENCES

Al-Mefty O, Fox JL, Smith RR: Petrosal approach for petroclival meningiomas. Neurosurgery 22:510-17, 1988.

Allan AF: Pneumatization of the temporal bone. Ann Otol Rhinol Laryngol 78:49-64, 1969.

Babu RP, Sekhar LN, Wright D: Extreme lateral transcondylar approach: technical improvements and lessons learned. J Neurosurg 81:49-59, 1994.

Benecke JE Jr, Tubergen LB, Miyamoto RT: Transmastoid labyrinthectomy. Am J Otol: 7:41-43, 1986.

Brackmann DE: Fenestrated suction tips for neuro-otologic surgery. Trans Am Acad Ophthalmol Otolaryngol 84:975, 1977.

Cohen NL: Retrosigmoid approach for acoustic tumor removal. Otolaryngol Clin North Am 25:295-310, 1992.

Coker NJ, Jenkins HA, Fisch U: Obliteration of the middle ear and mastoid cleft in subtotal petrosectomy: indications, technique and results. Ann Otol Rhinol Laryngol 95: 5-11, 1986.

Daspit CP, Spetzler RF, Pappas CTE: Combined approach for lesions involving the cerbellopontine angle and skull base: experience with 20 cases-preliminary report. Otolaryngol Head Neck Surg 105:788-796, 1991.

De la Cruz A: The transcochlear approach to meningiomas and cholesteatoma of the cerebellopontine angle. In:Brackmann DE. ed. Neurological surgery of the ear and skull base. New York: Raven Press, 353—60, 1982.

Fisch U, Mattox D: Microsurgery of the skull base. New York: Thieme, 1988.

Fisch U: Otochirurgische Behandlung des Akustikusneurinoms. In Plester, D, Wende, S, Nakayama, N: Kleinhirn-Bruckenwinkel-Tumoren. Springer, Berlin 1978 (pp.196-214).

Fisch U: Transmastoidaler translabyrintharer Zugang zum inneren Gehorgang. In Naumann, H.H: Kopf- und Halschirurgie. vol.III. Thieme, Stuttgart 1976 (pp.500-535).

Fisch U: Vestibular and cochlear neurectomy. Trans Amer Acad Ophthalmol Otolaryngol 78: 252-255, 1974.

Glasscock ME, Hays JW: The translabyrinthine removal of acoustic and other cerebellopontine angle tumors. Ann Otol Rhinol Laryngol 82:415-27, 1973.

Hirsch BE, Cass PS, Sekkar LN, Wright DC: Translabyrinthine approach to skull base tumors with hearing preservation. AT Otol 14: 533-543, 1993.

House WF, Luetje CM, eds: Acoustic tumors. Baltimore: University Park Davis, 1979.

House WF: Transtemporal bone microsurgical removal of acoustic neuromas. Arch Otolaryngol 80:599-756, 1964.

Kemink JL, Telian SA, Graham MD, Joynt L: Transmastoid labyrinthectomy: reliable surgical management of vertigo. Otolaryngol Head Neck Surg 101:5-10, 1989.

Koos WT, Spetzler RF, Land J: Color atlas of microneurosurgery. Stuttgart: Thieme, 1993.

Mazzoni A: Internal auditory artery supply to the petrous bone. Ann Otol Rhinol Laryngol 81:13-21, 1972.

Mazzoni A: Internal auditory canal: arterial relations at the porus acusticus. Ann Otol Rhinol Laryngol 78:794-814, 1969.

Mazzoni A: The subarcuate artery in man. Laryngoscope 80:69-79, 1970.

Naguib M, Saleh E, Cokkeser Y, Aristegui M, Landolfi M, Taibah A, et al: The enlarged translabyrinthine approach for removal of large vestibular schwannomas. J Laryngol Otol 108:545-550, 1994.

Pellet W, Cannoni M, Pech A: A widened transcochlear approach to jugular foramen tumors. J Neurosurg 69:887-94, 1988.

Pellet W, Cannoni M, Pech A: Otoneurosurgery. Berlin: Springer, 1990.

Poe D, Tarlov EC, Gadre AK: Translabyrinthine drillout from suboccipital approach to acoustic neuroma. Am J Otol 14:215-219, 1993.

Sanna M, Zini C, Gamoletti R, Landolfi M, Shaan M, Piazza F: Hearing preservation: a critical review of literature. In: Tos M, Thomsen J. Acoustic neuroma. Amsterdam: Kugler, 631-638, 1992.

Sanna M, Zini C, Mazzoni A, Gandolfi A, Pareschi R, Pasanisi E, et al: Hearing preservation in acoustic neuroma surgery. Am J Otol 8:500-506, 1987.

Sterkers JM: Acoustic neurilemmoma: otologic approaches. In: Sekhar LN, Janecka IP, eds. Surgery of cranial base tumors. New York: Raven Press, 715-725, 1993.

Tos M, Hashimoto S: Anatomy of the cerebellopontine angle visualized through the translabyrinthine approach. Acta Otolaryngol 108:238-245, 1989.

Tos M, Thomsen J: Translabyrinthine acoustic neuroma surgery: a surgical manual. Stuttgart: Thieme, 1991.

Vernick DM: Labyrinthectomy. In: Nadol JB, Schuknecht HF eds. Surgery of the ear and temporal bone. New York: Raven Press, 275 -280, 1993.

29

Retrosigmoid approach

- The position of the patient's head is the same as in the translabyrinthine approach.
- The facial nerve stimulator electrodes are positioned. The electrodes for the recording of evoked potentials are positioned, if they are to be utilized. We always use them when removing a neuroma with the retrosigmoid approach. If there is not usable hearing (see chapter 32), we always use the translabyrinthine approach.
- Skin incision, craniotomy, incision of the dura (Figs. 29-1, 29-2, 29-3).
- A self-retaining retractor with a wide blade is positioned on the cerebellum. Retraction must be minimal and the blade must not be allowed to slip and injure the mixed nerves. Once positioned, it must not be moved.
- The tumor must be attacked at the IAC, since here, the locations of VII and VIII are known. Thus, there is a landmark to follow in the tumor gutting to follow. If this delicate operation is performed at the beginning, the problem of bleeding is avoided. The integrity of the arachnoid membranes also prevents bone dust from penetrating into the subarachnoid spaces (Fig. 29-4).
- The porus acusticus is identified. An incision is made on the posterior wall, and a triangular flap of dura with its vertex on the fundus is dissected (Fig. 29-5).
- The bone of the IAC posterior wall is removed in a triangular shape with a suction-irrigator and a diamond burr. It is important not to penetrate into the semicircular canals which are immediately posterior to the lateral end of the IAC; otherwise, hearing loss will ensue. Thus bone removal should begin at the porus, to outline the base of the triangle. The IAC dura is identified medially, where the semicircular canals are not present, and followed laterally. In this phase, the burr must be maintained on the dura, up to the lateral end, for approx. 5-6mm, and must not be allowed to slip to the edges of the dura (Fig. 29-6).
- The underlying dura must not be left, so as not to damage the nervous structures. The dura is carefully opened to avoid injuring the AICA, which may loop in the IAC and/or the underlying nerves.
- At the fundus of the IAC, the transverse crest may be seen, along with the superior and inferior vestibular nerves and, antero-superiorly, the facial nerve (Fig. 29-7).
- The capsule's surface is stimulated to verify that it does not cover a facial nerve unidentified by the microscope due to its small size and thinness.
- The capsule is incised in a medial position, to prevent the blood from flowing from above and obscuring the underlying field. The intracapsular gutting of the tumor is initiated in the same way as in the translabyrinthine approach (Fig. 29-8).
- In large tumors, when the mass has been significantly reduced, the fundus is elevated and nerve VII is identified at the brainstem (see chapter 28).
- Intracapsular gutting is then performed, as described in chapter 28 (Fig. 29-9).
- The tumor must be gutted as carefully as possible. In this way, pressure on the internal capsule and the neural structures is reduced. An incomplete removal is revealed in a higher adherence to the nervous structures, due in part to the parenchyma acting as a brake inside the capsule. The cerebral pulses will eventually dislodge and reveal the residual parenchyma, which is removed (Rhoton).
- Cutting instruments must not be used near the internal limiting structure of the capsule, and the tumor must be dissected from the capsule with blunt instruments, to prevent injury of extracapsular structures.
- At the end of this phase, the capsule is thin and translucent. The pia-arachnoid membrane is dissected from the capsular surface. The continuous flow of the suction-irrigator is helpful. As

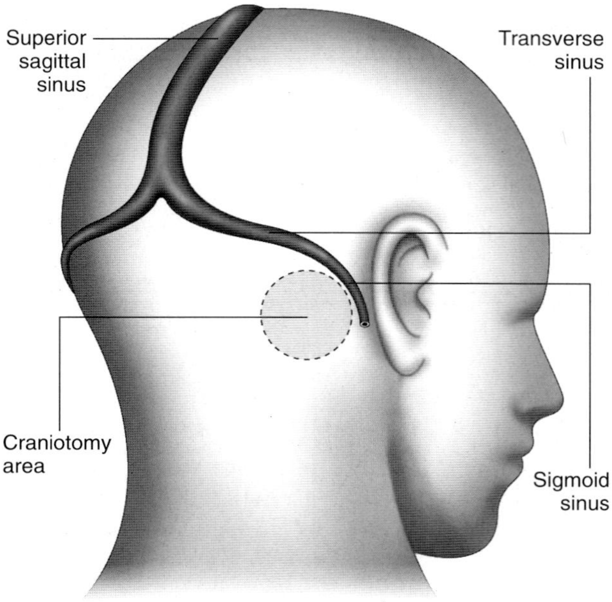

Fig. 29-1. Retrosigmoid approach. The craniectomy.

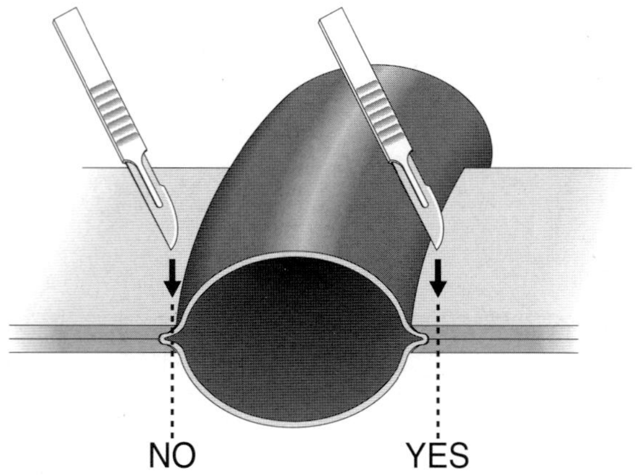

Fig. 29-3. In the retrosigmoid approach, the posterior fossa dura is incised behind the sigmoid sinus. The dural incision should not be too close to the sigmoid sinus, since the sinuses are not rounded, but the edges slope down in the dura.

always in microsurgery, it is very important to adopt the most conservative approach possible. All possible vessels are spared. These are the perforating arteries and the branches of the cerebellar arteries. These branches are separated from the capsule. Some small vessels are neural vessels (Figs. 29-10, 29-11).

- For the importance of preserving venous and arterial vessels, see chapter 28.
- When a craniotomy is performed and the posterior meatal margin of the internal auditory canal is drilled, mastoid cells are frequently opened. If mastoid cells are left open, the liquor may pass through the mastoid and from here to the cavum tympani, the tube and the rhynopharynx: this is rhynoliquorrea. These are closed with bone wax, while the osseous breach of the IAC is sealed with a fragment of suboccipital muscle.

In the presence of a tubal obstruction, signs of a serous otitis may be present. These may include bulging of the eardrum and vertigo due to com-

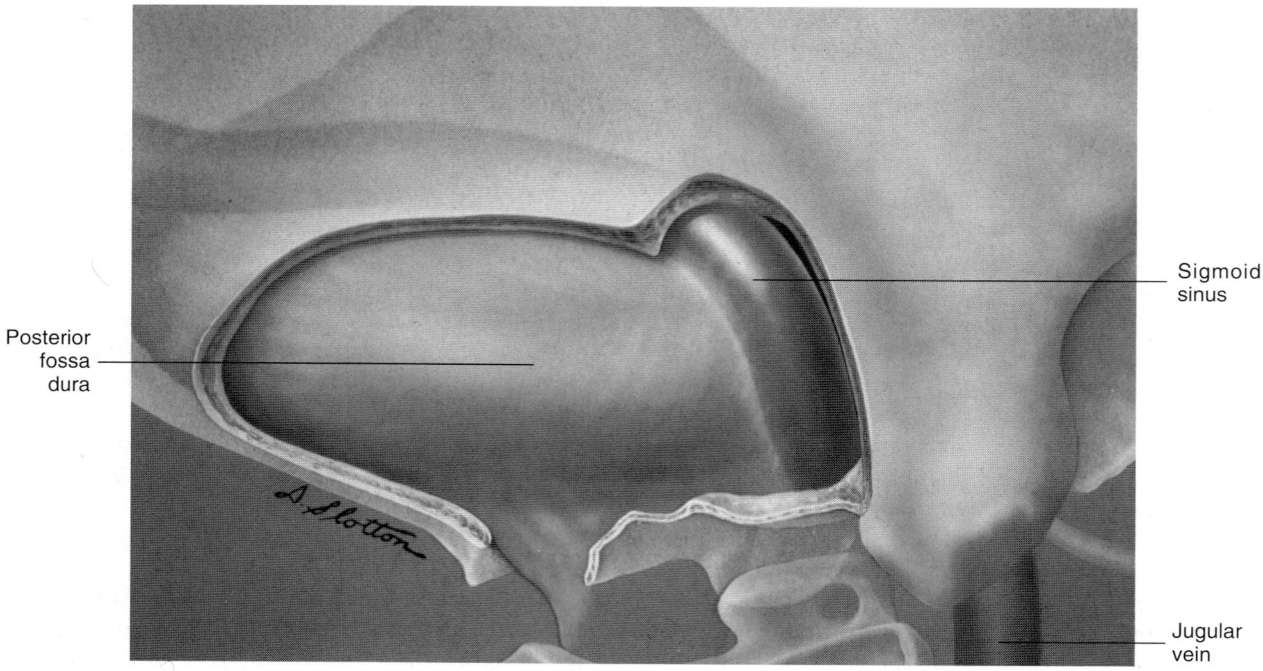

Fig. 29-2. Retrosigmoid approach. The craniectomy.

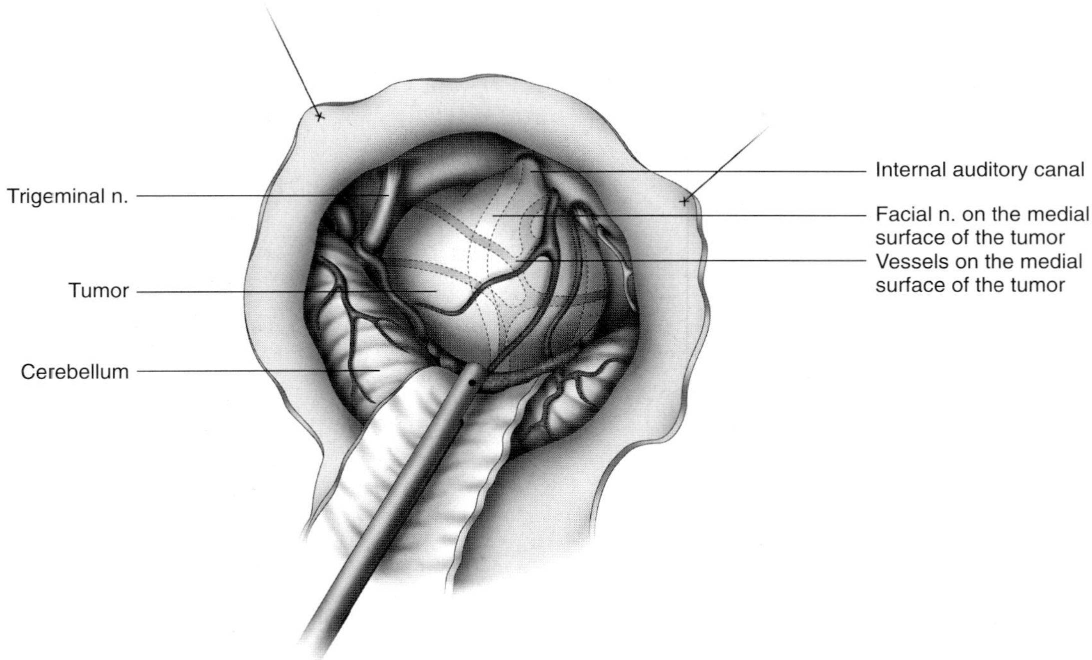

Fig. 29-4. Dura has been incised. The tumor is exposed.

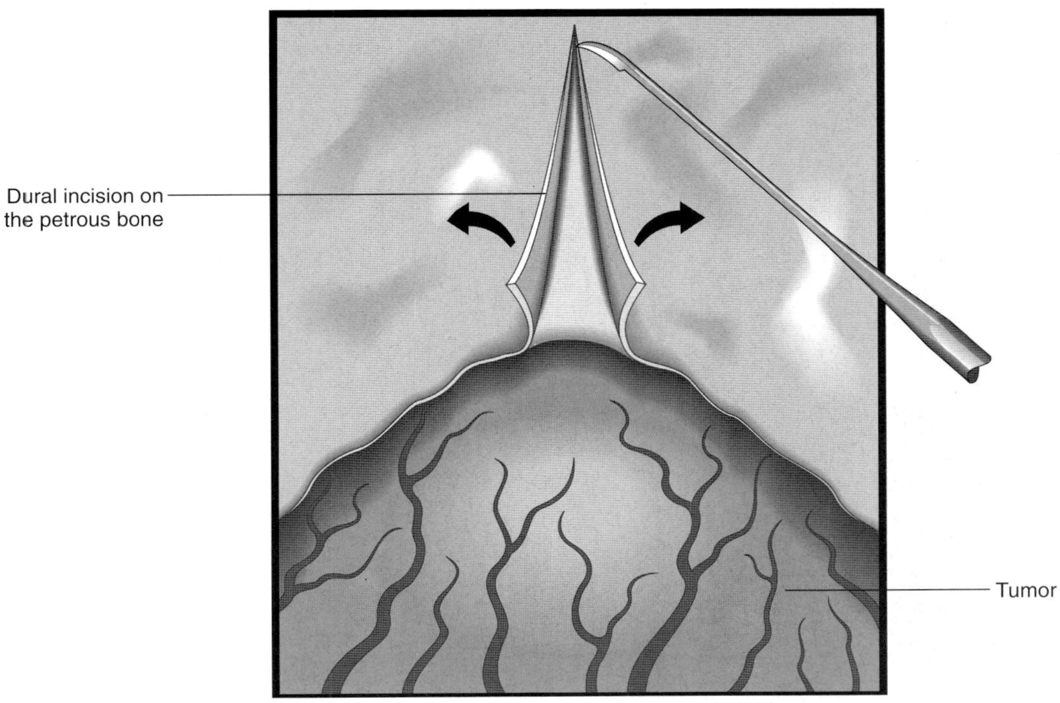

Fig. 29-5. The porus acusticus is identified and a V shaped dural incision is created.

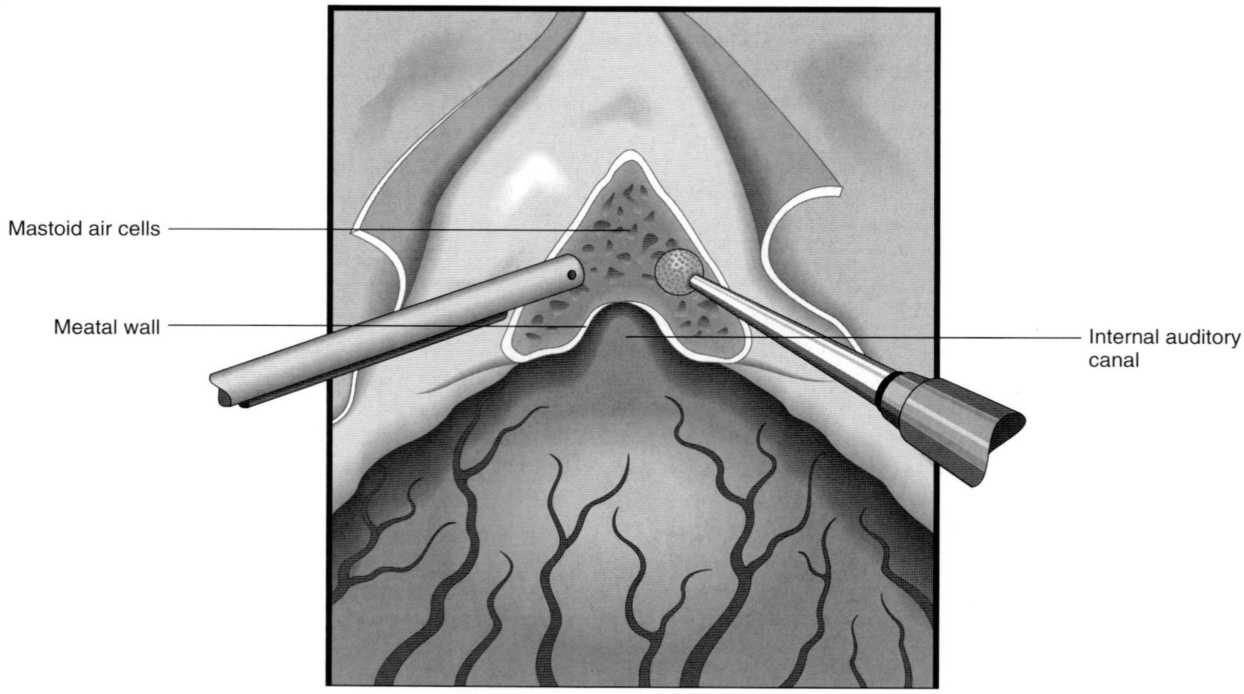

Fig. 29-6. The bone over the IAC is drilled with a diamond burr, medially to laterally.

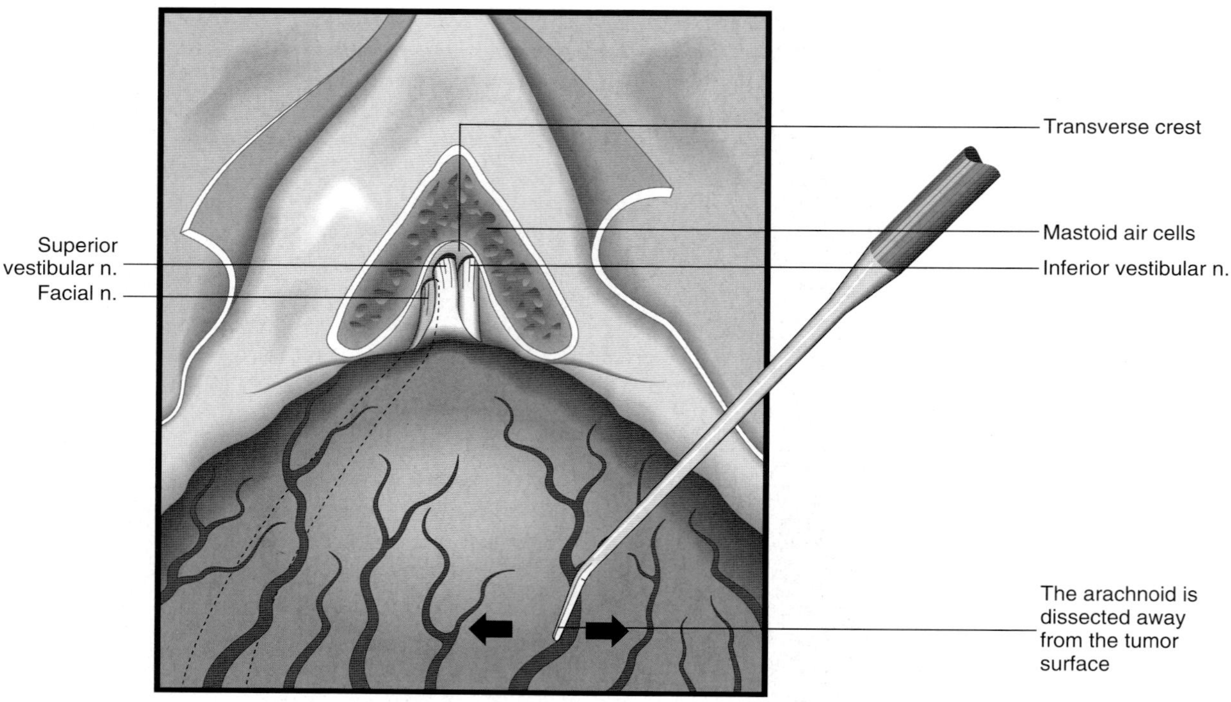

Fig. 29-7. The IAC dura is exposed and incised. The vestibulocochlear nerve and the facial nerve are exposed. When the tumor reaches the fundus of the IAC, the lateral-most extension of the tumor is reflected medially and the nerves are identified. The capsule is touched with the probe of the facial nerve stimulator. When no response is obtained, the arachnoid is dissected away from the tumor surface.

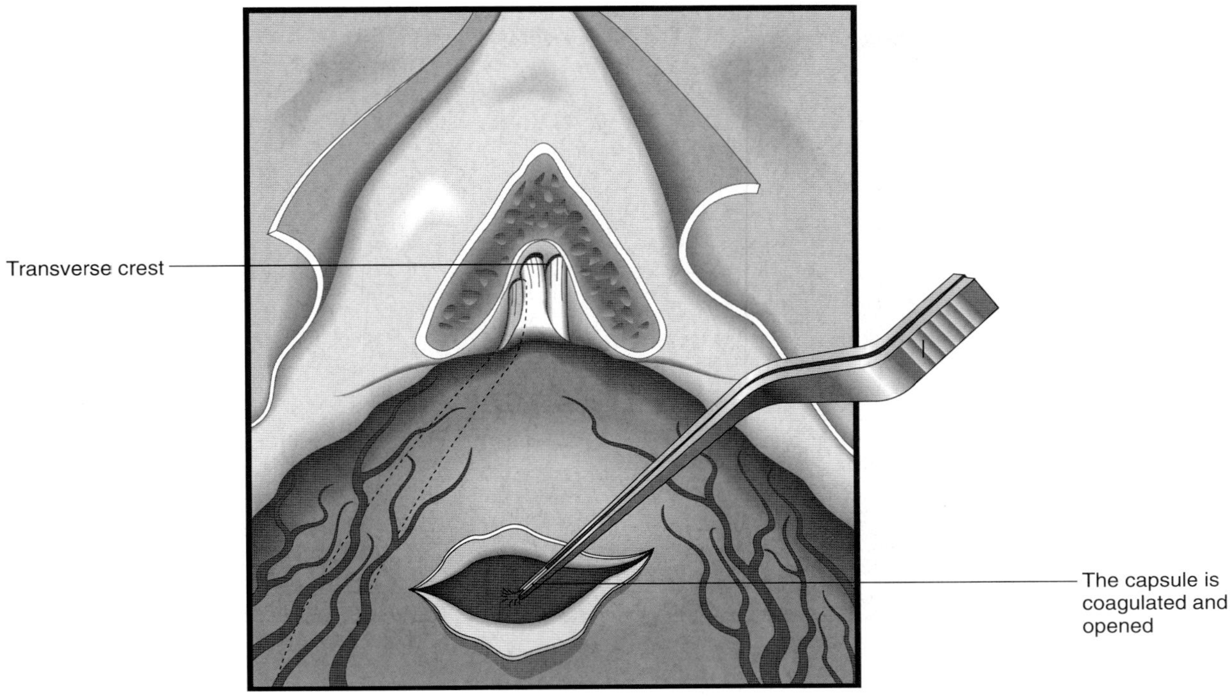

Fig. 29-8. The capsule is coagulated and opened.

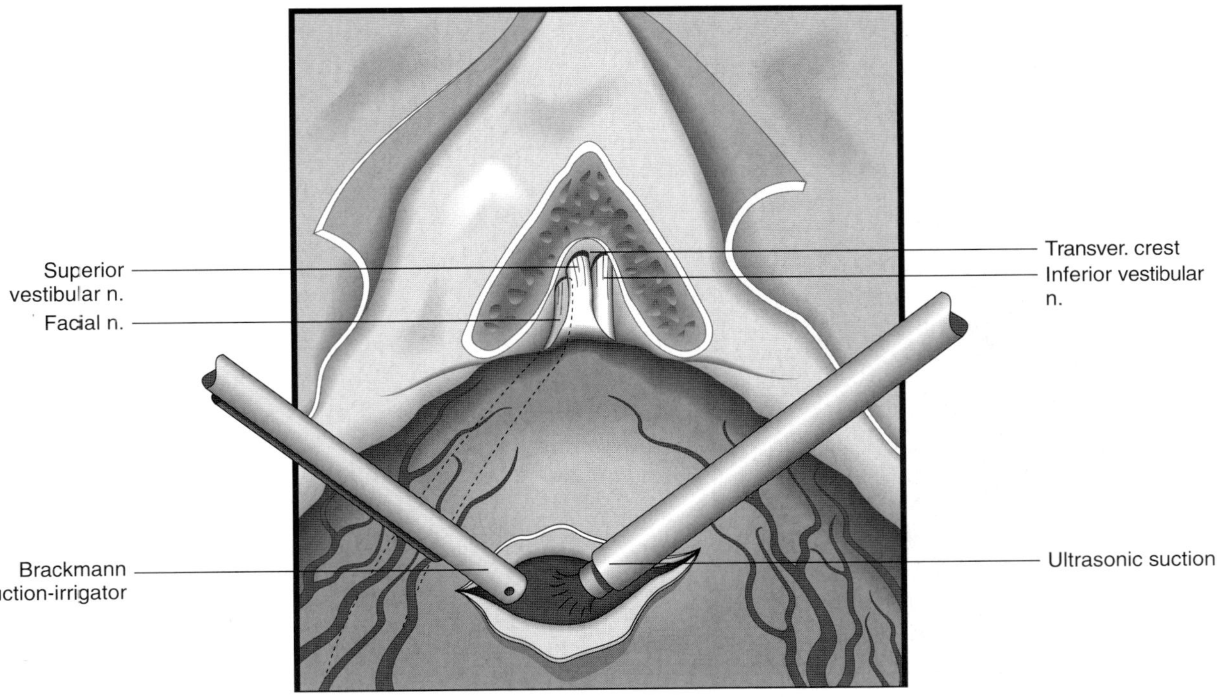

Fig. 29-9. An intracapsular debulking is performed.

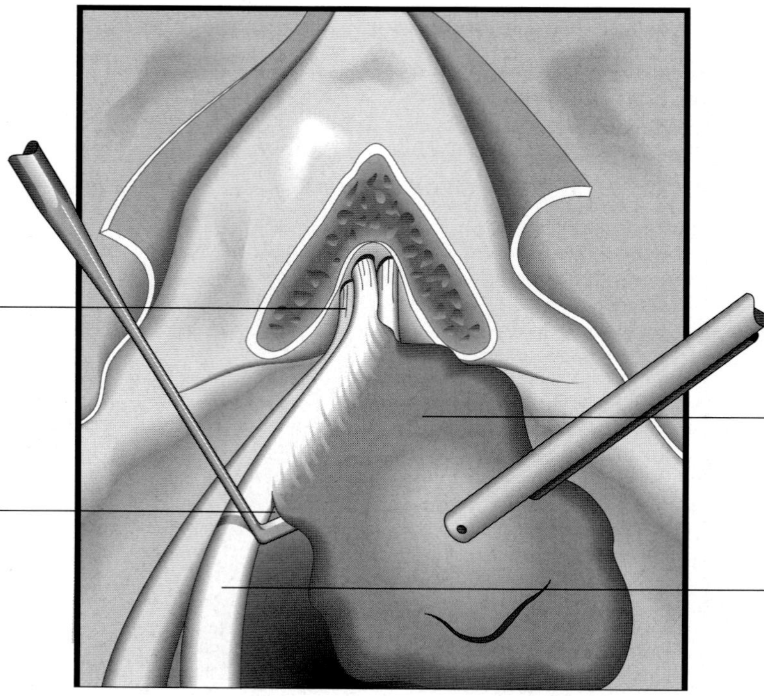

Fig. 29-10. Tumor is dissected away from the VIII CN in a medial to lateral direction, to avoid disruption of the filaments of the nerve passing through the lamina cribrosa.

pression of the footplate of the underlying vestibular structures.

- The dura is closed with a watertight suture. If there are dural lacerations, interrupted sutures may be used and, if necessary, a dural graft.

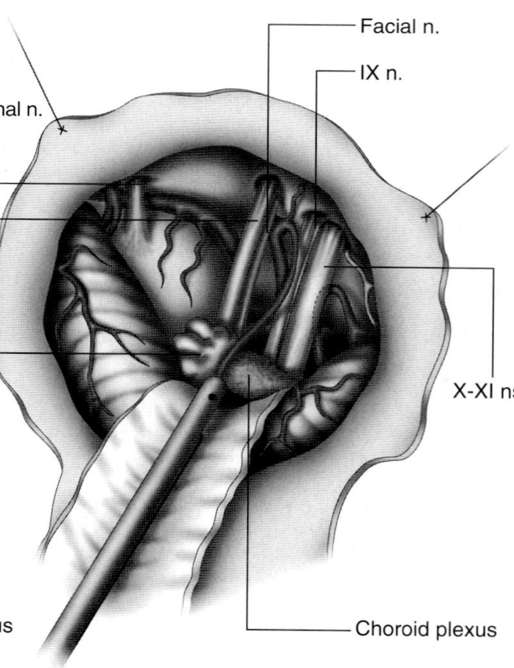

Fig. 29-11. Complete tumor removal. The neural structures of the CPA have been preserved.

COMPLICATIONS

- An edema of the cerebellum may be provoked by an overly long and intense retraction, which can completely obscure the underlying visibility.
- Hematomas of the posterior fossa present a mortal risk due to the rapid compression of the brainstem.
- When the head is raised and the veins are retracted, the false impression of a correct hemostasis may be had. To avoid the subsequent risks, it is advisable to perform repeated Valsalva maneuvers and jugular compression before suturing the dura.
- If a CSF fistula occurs, the cautionary procedures for a translabyrinthine procedure are adopted (see chapter 28, complications). If the fistula persists, a continuous spinal drain may be adopted. If the problem is still not resolved, it is necessary to reoperate with a flap of fascia anchored with fibrin glue. A cisternography with a water-soluble contrast agent may consent a precise diagnosis on site.

The use of intraoperative auditory evoked potentials is very helpful when attempting to preserve hearing. Some rules to follow:

- Make several interruptions during the IAC drilling.
- Avoid bipolar coagulation.
- Avoid pulling in one direction for a long time.
- Change the action zone frequently.

REFERENCES

Atkinson J: The anterior cerebellar artery. Its variations, distribution, and significance in the surgery of cerebello pontine angle tumours. J Neurol Neurosurg Psychiatr 1949.

Atlas MD, Harvey C, Fagan PA: Hearing preservation in acoustic neuroma surgery: A continuing study. Laryngoscope 102: 779-783, 1992.

Baer S, Tos M, Thomsen J, Hughes G: Synopsis on: Grading of facial nerve function after acoustic neuroma treatment. Acoustic Neuroma. In Tos M, Thomsen J (eds): Proceedings of the First International Conference on Acoustic Neuroma. Copenhagen, August 25-29, 1991. New York, Kugler Publications, 1992, pp 993-995.

Beatty CW, Ebersold MJ, Harner SG: Residual and recurrent acoustic neuromas. Laryngoscope 97: 1168-1171, 1987.

Camins MB, Oppenheim JS: Anatomy and surgical techniques in the suboccipital transmeatal approach to acoustic neuromas. Clin Neurosurg 38: 567-588, 1992.

Cohen NL, Hammerschlag P, Berg H, Ransohoff J: Acoustic neuroma surgery: An eclectic approach with an emphasis on hearing preservation. Ann Otol Rhinol Laryngol 95: 21-27, 1986.

Cohen NL, Ransonoff J: Hearing preservation, Posterior fossa approach. Otolaryng Head and Neck Surg 92/2: 176-183, 1984.

Cohen NL: Retrosigmoid approach for acoustic tumor removal. Otolaryngol Clin North Am 25: 295-310, 1992.

Ebersold MJ, Harner SG, Beatty CW, et al: Current results of the retrosigmoid approach to acoustic neurinoma. J Neur 901-909, 1991.

Glasscock ME III, Hart MJ, Vrabec JT: Management of bilateral acoustic neuroma. Otolaryngol Clin North Am 5: 449-469, 1992.

Haines JH, Maroon JC, Janetta PJ: Supratentorial intracerebral hemorrhage following posterior fossa surgery. J Neurosurgery 49, 881, 1978.

Hamer SG, Beatty CW, Ebersold MJ: Retrosigmoid acoustic neuroma: Experience 1978-1988. Otolaryngol Head Neck Surg 103: 40-45, 1990.

Harders A, Gilbach J, Weigel K: Supratentorial space occupying lesions following infratentorial surgery: Early diagnosis and treatment. Acta Neurochir (Wien) 74: 57, 1985.

Hinton AE, Ramsden RT, Lye RH, Dutton JE: Criteria for hearing preservation in acoustic schwannoma surgery: The concept of useful hearing. J Laryngol Otol 106: 500-503, 1992.

Hitselberger WE, House WF: A warning regarding the sitting position for acoustic tumor surgery. [Editorial] Arch Head Neck Surg 106: 69, 1980.

Jackler RK, Pitts LH: Selection of surgical approach to acoustic neuroma. Otolaryngol Clin North Am 25: 361-387, 1992.

Kemink JL, Langman AW, Niparko JK, Graham MD: Operative management of acoustic neuromas: The priority of neurologic function over complete resection. Otolaryngol Head Neck Surg 104: 96-99, 1991.

Krause F: Zur Freilegung der hinteren Felsenbeinflache und des Kleinhirns. Beitr Klin Chir 37: 728-764, 1903.

Lang J Jr, Samii A: Retrosigmoidal approach to the posterior cranial fossa. An anatomical study. Acta Neurochir (Wien) 111: 147-153, 1991.

Lang J: Clinical anatomy of the posterior cranial fossa and its foramina. New York, Thieme, 1991.

Lye RH, Pace-Balzan A, Ramsden RT, et al: The fate of tumour rests following removal of acoustic neuromas: An MRI Gd DTPA study. Br J Neurosurg 6: 195-201, 1992.

MacDonald CB, Hirsch BE, Kamerer DB, Sekhar LN: Acoustic neuroma surgery: Predictive criteria for hearing preservation. Otolaryngol Head Neck Surg 104: 128, 1991.

Mangham CA: Complications of translabyrinthine vs suboccipital approach for acoustic tumor surgery. Otolaryngol Head Neck Surg 99: 396-400, 1988.

McKenna MJ, Halpin C, Ojemann RG, et al: Long-term hearing results in patients after surgical removal of acoustic tumors with hearing preservation. Am J Otol 13: 134-136, 1992.

Moffat DA: Synopsis on near-total, subtotal or partial removal. Acoustic Neuroma. In Tos M, Thomsen J (eds): Proceedings of the First International Conference on Acoustic Neuroma. Copenhagen, August 25-29, 1991. New York, Kugler Publications, 1992, pp 983-984.

Nassif PS, Shelton C, Arriaga MM: Hearing preservation following surgical removal of meningiomas affecting the temporal bone. Laryngoscope 102: 1357-1362, 1992.

Pool JL: Suboccipital surgery for acoustic neurinomas: advantages and disavantages. J Neurosurg 24: 483-492, 1966.

Rhoton AL Jr, Tedeschi H: Microsurgical anatomy of acoustic neuroma. Otolaryngol Clin North Am 25: 257-294, 1992.

Rhoton AL: Microsurgical anatomy of the brainstem surface facing an acoustic neuroma. Surg Neurol 25: 326-339, 1986.

Rhoton AL: The suboccipital approach to removal of acoustic neuromas. Otolaryngol Head Neck Surg 1: 313-333, 1979.

Samii M, Janetta PJ: The cranial nerves. Springer-Verlag, 1981.

Samii M, Matthies C, Tatagiba M: Intracanalicular acoustic neurinomas. Neurosurgery 29: 189-198; Discussion 198-199, 1991.

Sanna M, Gamoletti J, Tos M, Thomsen J: Synopsis on: Hearing preservation following acoustic neuroma surgery. Acoustic Neuroma. In Tos M, Thomsen J (eds): Proceedings of the First International Conference on Acoustic Neuroma. Copenhagen, August 25-29, 1991. New York, Kugler Publications, 1992, pp 985-987.

Schessel DA, Nedzelski JM, Rowed Feghali JG: Headache and local discomfort following surgery of the cerebellopontine angle. Acoustic Neuroma. In Tos M, Thomsen J: Proc the First International Conference on Acoustic Neuroma. Copenhagen August 25-29, 1991. New York, Kugler Publ 1992, pp 899-904.

Seiler RW, Zurbrugg HR: Supratentorial intracerebral hemorrhage after posterior fossa operation. Neurosurgery 18: 472, 1986.

Selesnick SH, Jackler RK: Clinical manifestations and audiologic diagnosis of acoustic neuromas. Otolaryngol Clin North Am 25: 521-551, 1992.

Shelton C, Hitselberger WE, House WF, Brackmann DE: Long term results of hearing after acoustic tumor removal. Acoustic Neuroma. In Tos M, Thomsen J (eds): Proceedings of the First International Conference on Acoustic Neuroma, Copenhagen, August 25-29, 1991. New York, Kugler Publications, 1992, pp 661-664.

Shelton C: Hearing preservation in acoustic tumor surgery. Otolaryngol Clin North Am 25:609-621, 1992.

Silverstein H, Morrell H, Smouha E, Jones R: Combined retrolab-retrosigmoid vestibular neurectomy. An evolution in approach. Am J Otol 10: 166-169, 1989.

Slavit DH, Harner SG, Harper CM Jr, Beatty CW: Auditory monitoring during acoustic neuroma removal. Arch Otolaryngol Head Neck Surg 17: 1153-1157, 1991.

Smith PG, Leonetti JP, Grubb RL: Management of cerebrospinal fluid otorhinorrhea complicating the retrosigmoid approach to the cerebellopontine angle. Am J Otol 11: 178-180, 1990.

Thedinger BS, Whittaker CK, Luetje CM: Recurrent acoustic tumor after a suboccipital removal. Neurosurgery 29: 681-687, 1991.

Wiet RJ, Teixido M, Liang JG: Complications in acoustic neuroma surgery. Otolaryngol Clin North Am 25: 389-412, 1992.

Wigand ME, Haid T, Goertzen W, Wolf S: Preservation of hearing in bilateral acoustic neurinomas by deliberate partial resection. Acta Otolaryngol (Stockh) 112: 237-241, 1992.

Yasargil MG, Smith RD, Gasser JC: Microsurgical approach to acoustic neurinomas. Adv Tech Standards Neurosurg 4: 93-129, 1977.

Yingling CD, Gardi JN: Intraoperative monitoring of facial and cochlear nerves during acoustic neuroma surgery. Otolaryngol Clin North Am 25: 413-448, 1992.

30

Transcranial translabyrinthine approach

The translabyrinthine-retrosigmoid approach was developed in the attempt to combine the advantages of the translabyrinthine and retrosigmoid approaches. This means, however, performing two separate operations, with the consequent expense of time and the redoubled possibility of liquor fistulas.

The transcranial translabyrinthine approach was proposed by J.G. Feghali and A.B. Kantrowitz.

- A retrosigmoid approach is performed and the medial surface of the temporal bone is exposed, where the vestibular aqueduct is identified and palpated, and followed to the utricle. The bone separating the vestibular aqueduct from the posterior surface of the IAC is drilled, leaving a thin plate of bone to protect against trauma to the IAC nervous systems.
- The bony aperture is opened downwards, while avoiding injury to the jugular bulb and the mixed nerves. The labyrinthine aperture is opened further back and the vestibular aqueduct is sectioned. The aperture into the utricle is enlarged and the ampullae of the three semicircular canals are identified. Drilling over the ampullae, the transverse crest is identified. The vertical crest (Bill's bar) is identified just above and medial to the transverse crest.
- Thus the lateral limiting structure of the IAC has been identified. The medial limiting structure is easily identified with the suboccipital approach. The thin residual bone plate may now be removed, exposing the intracanalicular part of the tumor. Here, the identification of the transverse crest and the vertical crest permits the safe identification of the superior and inferior vestibular nerves of the facial nerve.

In short, the transcranial translabyrinthine approach combines the rapid and easy access of the suboccipital approach with the advantages of the translabyrinthine approach:

- Direct approach to the IAC fundus. In the suboccipital approach, on the other hand, the IAC is frequently insufficiently exposed, and at times part of the tumor is left in place.
- Stable bone landmarks: semicircular canals, cochlear aqueduct, utricle, transverse crest and vertical crest.
- Possibility of identifying the facial nerve where it is generally not invaded by the tumor, following a definite landmark such as Bill's Bar. Thus the nerve may be followed from a point of certainty, laterally, until the meatal porus is reached. Here the facial nerve is more at risk than in the suboccipital approach, since the nerve has not been identified. These advantages are obtained with no significant modifications in the general approach, the incisions, or the patient's position (Feghali JC, Kantrowitz AB).

REFERENCES

Cannoni M, Pech A, Pellet W, Zanaret M, Triglia JM: Les procidences veineuses et meningees au cours des voies trans-labyrinthiques elargies. Ann Oto Laryng (Paris) 103: 303-308, 1986.

Daspit CP, Spetzler RF, Pappas CTE: Combined approach for lesions involving the cerebellopontine angle and skull base: experience with 20 cases-preliminary report. Otolaryngol Head Neck Surg 105:788-796, 1991.

George B, Dematons C, Cophignon J: Lateral approach to the anterior foramen magnum. Surg Neurol 29:484-90, 1988.

Hakuba A, Tsujimoto T: Transcondyle approach for foramen magnum meningiomas. In: Sekhar LN, Janecka IP, eds. Surgery of cranial base tumors. New York: Raven Press, 1993: n-n.

Hakuba A, Nishimura S, Jang BJ: A combined retro-auricular and preauricular transpetrosal-transtentorial approach to clivus meningiomas. Surg Neurol 30:108-16, 1988.

Jackler RK: Overview of surgical neuro-otology. In: Jackler RK, Brackmann DE, eds. Neuro-Otology. Baltimore: Mosby, 651 -84, 1993.

Jackson CG, Glasscock ME, McKennan KX, et al: The surgical treatment of skull base tumors with intracranial extension. Otolaryngol Head Neck Surg 96:175, 1987.

Jackson CG: Surgery of skull base tumors. New York: Churchill Livingstone, 1991.
Kawase T, Toya S, Shiobara R, Mine S: Transpetrosal approach for aneurysms of the lower basilar artery. J Neurosurg 63:857-61, 1985.
Kinney SE, Hughes GB, Little JR: Retrolabyrinthine transtentorial approach to lesions of the anterior cerebellopontine angle. Am J Otol 13:426-30, 1992.
Mann WJ, Amedee RG, Gilsbach J, Pemeczky A, Wolfensberger M: Transsigmoid approach for tumors of the jugular foramen. Skull Base Surg 1:137-41, 1991.
Saleh E, Naguib M, Aristegui M, Cokkeser Y, Russo A, Sanna M: Surgical anatomy of the jugular foramen area. In: Mazzoni A, Sanna M, eds. Skull base surgery Update, 1. Amsterdam: Kugler, 1995 pp. 3-8.
Saleh E, Naguib M, Aristegui M, Cokkeser Y, Sanna M: The lower skull base: anatomical study with surgical implications. Ann Otol Rhinol Laryngol 104:57-61, 1995.
Saleh E, Taibah A, Achilli V, Aristegui M, Mazzoni M, Sanna A: Posterior fossa meningioma: surgical strategy. Skull Base Surg 4:209-219, 1994.
Samii M, Ammirati M: The combined supra-infratentorial presigmoid sinus avenue to the petro-clival region: surgical technique and clinical applications. Acta Neurochir 95:6-12, 1988.
Samii M, Draf W: Surgery of the skull base. Berlin: Springer, 1989.
Sekhar LN, Estonillo R: Transtemporal approach to the skull base: an anatomical study. Neurosurgery 19:799-808, 1986.
Sekhar LN, Schramm VL, Jones NF: Subtemporal-preauricular infratemporal fossa approach to large lateral and posterior cranial base neoplasms. J Neurosurg 67:488-499, 1987.
Sen C, Sekhar LN: Extreme lateral transcondylar and transjugular approaches. In: Sekhar LN, Janecka I, eds. Surgery of cranial base tumors. NewYork: RavenPress, 389-412, 1993.
Sen C, Sekhar LN: An extreme lateral approach to intradural lesions of the cervical spine and foramen magnum. Neurosurgery 27:197-204, 1990.
Sen C, Sekhar LN: The subtemporal and preauricular infratemporal approach to intradural structures ventral to the brain stem. J Neurosurg 73:345-354, 1990.
Thedinger BA, Glasscock ME, Cueva RA: Transcochlear transtentorial approach for removal of large cerebellopontine angle meningiomas. Am J Otol 13:408-415, 1992.
Velut S, Jan M: Anterior petrosectomy during approach to the petroclival area. In: Schmideck HE, ed. Meningiomas and their surgical management. Philadelphia: Saunders, 435-450, 1991.

31

Transotic approach

The transotic approach was introduced by Fisch essentially for treatment of CPA tumors. It differentiates from the translabyrinthine approach in its more anterior extension and thus, wider surgical access to the tumor.

Incision

See Figure 28-2.

Closure of External auditory canal

A blind sac closure of the EAC is performed. See chapter 16.

Subtotal Petrosectomy

A complete mastoidectomy is performed. The facial nerve is exposed at the second genu, close to lateral semicircular canal. A thin plate of bone is left in place. Once the position of facial nerve is known, the removal of the laterally placed external bone canal is easier and faster.

The tympanic bone is drilled out. Tympanic membrane and ossicles are removed. The tensor tympani muscle and bone medial to it are removed.

The facial nerve is exposed from the first genu to the stylomastoid foramen, where it blends with the stylomastoid periosteum.

The jugular bulb and the horizontal internal carotid artery are exposed. These structures appear through the thin plate of bone remaining. The complete infralabyrinthine compartment is opened. The limits of the surgical field are: Sigmoid sinus: (posterior limit); ICA (anterior limit); Middle fossa dura (superior limit); Jugular bulb and mastoid tip (inferior limit).

The posterior dissection is carried out as in the translabyrinthine approach.

The cochlea is drilled away. Bone under the facial nerve is drilled out. The facial nerve is left suspended in the field with only a thin plate of bone underneath.

The tympanic part of the facial nerve is followed with diamond burr and suction-irrigation up to the meatal foramen. Once the meatal foramen is identified, the dissection is carried out as anteriorly as the geniculate ganglion permits. This anterior exposure allows a complete visualization of the facial nerve in its fralest part.

The removal of the tumor is carried out as in the translabyrinthine approach (Chapter 28).

At the end of the procedure the ET orifice is closed with bone wax and a muscle plug sealed with fibrin glue. This prevents rhynoliquorrea. The closure of ET is possible through a facial recess approach, although there is limited space.

REFERENCES

Rousseaux M, Lesoin F, Petit H, Jomin M: Les kystes arachnoidiens de l'angle ponto-cerebelleux. Neurochirurgie 30: 119-124, 1984.

Albin MS, Babinski M, Maroon JC, Jannetta PJ: Anesthetic management of posterior fossa surgery in the sitting position. Acta Anes Scand 20: 117-128, 1976.

Albin MS, Benegin L, Dujovny M, Bennet MH, Jannetta PJ: Brain retraction pressure during intra-cranial procedures. Surg Forum 26: 499-500, 1975.

Altinors N, Senveli E, Erdogan A, Arda N, Pak I: Craniopharyngioma of the cerebellopontine angle. J Neurosurg 60: 842-844, 1984.

Bataini J, Pontvert D, Jaulerry C, Brunin F, Gaboriaud G, Scherrer A: Tumeurs du glomus jugulaire. Possibilites de la radiotherapie. Neuro-chirurgie 31: 377-380, 1985.

Bonnal J, Louis R, Combalbert A: L'abord temporal transtentoriel de l'angle ponto-cerebelleux. NeuroChir (Paris) 10/1: 3-12, 1964.

Bonnal J: La chirurgie conservatrice et reparatrice du sinus longitudinal superieur. Neuro-chirurgie 28: 147-172, 1982.

Borovich B, Doron Y: Recurrence of intra-cranial meningiomas: The role played by regional multicentricity. J Neurosurg 64: 58-63, 1986.

Brackmann DE, Bartels LJ: Rare tumors of the cerebellopontine angle. Otolaryng Head Neck Surg 88: 555-559, 1980.

Brackmann DE, Hitselberger WE: In neurological surgery of the ear, Vol II, Silverstein H and Norrel H. Edit Aesculapius Publ CO (Birmingham, Alabama) 173-177, 1979.

Brackmann DE: Acoustic neuroma surgery: Otologic medical group results. In neurological surgery of the ear, Vol II, Silverstein H and Morrel H Edit. Aesculapius Publ CO (Birmingham, Alabama) 248-259, 1979.

Brackmann DE: Trans-labyrinthine removal of acoustic neurinomas. In: Neurological surgery of the ear and skull base. Brackmann DE Edit. Raven Press Pub (New York): 235-241, 1982.

Brodersen BR, Barky N: Acoustic Tumor surgery: Anesthetic considerations. In: Acoustic tumors. Vol. II: Management. House WF, Luetje CM University Park Press publ: 3-14, 1979.

Burres S, Fisch U: The comparison of facial grading systems. Arch Otolaryngol Head Neck Surg 112: 755-758, 1986.

Chen JM, Fisch U: The transotic approach in acoustic neuroma surgery. J Otolaryngol 22:331-336, 1993.

Clark WC, Moretz WH, Acker JD, Gardner LG, Eggers F, Robertson JH: Nonsurgical management of small and intra-canalicular acoustic tumors. Neurosurgery 16: 801-803, 1985.

Clemis JD, Mastricola PG, Schuler I, Vogler M: Sudden hearing loss in the controlateral ear in post-operative acoustic tumor: three cases report. Laryngoscope 92/1: 76-79, 1982.

Clemis JD: Hearing conservation in acoustic tumor surgery: Pro's and con's. Otolaryng Head and Neck Surg 92/2: 156-161, 1984.

Cohen NH: Fluid management: In: Newfield P and Cottrell JE: Handbook of neuroanesthesia: Clinic and physiologic essentials. Little Brown Ed. 154-170, 1984.

Cohen NL: Acoustic neuroma surgery with emphasis on preservation of hearing. Laryngoscope 89: 886-896, 1979.

Conley JJ: Concept in head and neck surgery. Cancer of the ear. G Thieme Verlag Edit (Stuttgart): 69-79, 1970.

Conley JJ: Multiple paragangliomas in the head and neck. Ann Otol 65: 356-360, 1956.

Dany A, Vidal J, Dumas M, Ravon R, Bokor J: Les chondromes de l'angle ponto-cerebelleux. A propos d'une observation personnelle. Neurochirurgie 26: 355-357, 1980.

Djindjian R: Arteriographie superselective de la carotide interne et embolisation. Ann Med Int 26: 569-572, 1975.

Donaghy RMP, Numoto M, Wallman W, Flanagan ME: Pressure measurement beneath retractors for protection of delicate tissues. Am J Surg 123: 429-431, 1972.

Fisch U, Lanser MJ: Facial nerve grafting. Otolaryngol Clin North Am 24: 691-708,1991.

Fisch U, Mattox D: Microsurgery of the Skull Base. New York, Thieme Medical Publishers, 1988.

Fisch U, Nedzelski J, Wellauer J: Diagnostic value of meatocisternography. Arch Otolaryngol 101: 339-343, 1975.

Fisch U, Wegmuller A: Early diagnosis of acoustic neuromas. J. Oto Rhino Laryngol 36: 129-140, 1974.

Fisch U, Yasargil MG: Transtemporale, extrapyramidale eingriffe am inneren gehorgang. Pract Oto Rhino Laryngol 30: 377-379, 1968.

Fisch U: Facial nerve grafting. Otolaryngol Clin N Amer 7: 517-529, 1974.

Fisch U: Operations on the facial nerve in its labyrinthine and meatal course. In Miehlke A: Surgery of the Facial Nerve. Urban & Schwarzenberg, Munchen 1973.

Fisch U: Transtemporal extralabyrinthine operations on the internal auditory canal, the eighth and seventh cranial nerves. In Yasargil M.G: Microsurgery Applied to Neurosurgery. Thieme, Stuttgart 1969 (pp.195-210).

Fischer G, Bret Ph, Hor F, Pialat J, Massini B: Les kystes epidermoides de l'angle ponto-cerebelleux, 6 observations. Neurochirurgie 30: 365-372, 1984.

Fischer G, Constantini JL, Mercier P: Improvement of hearing after microsurgical removal of acoustic neurinoma. Neurosurgery 7/2: 154-159, 1980.

Friedmann J: Epidermoid cholesteatoma and cholesterol granuloma. Ann Otol Rhinol Laryngol 68: 57-79, 1959.

Gantz BJ, Fisch U: Modified transotic approach to the cerebellopontine angle. Arch Otolaryngol 109:252-56, 1983.

Garcia Ibanez E, Garcia Ibanez JL:Middle fossa vestibular neurectomy: a report of 373 cases. Otolaryngol Head Neck Surg 88: 486-490, 1980.

Gardner G, Robertson JH, et al: Transtemporal approaches to the cranial cavity. Am J Otol 7 (Suppl): 114-120, 1985.

Gardner G, Robertson JM, Clark WC: 105 patients operated for cerebello-pontine angle tumors. Experience using combined approach and C02 laser. Laryngoscope 93: 1049-1055, 1983.

German WJ: Acoustic neurinomas. A follow up. Chir Clin Neurosurg 7: 1-20, 1961.

Giannotta SL, Pulec JL, Goodkin R: Translabyrinthine removal of cerebello-pontine angle meningiomas. Neurosurgery 17-4: 620-625, 1985.

Glasscock ME, Hays JW, Jackson CG, Steenerson RL: A one stage combined approach for the management of large cerebello-pontine angle tumors. Laryngoscope 88/10: 1563-1576, 1978.

Glasscock ME, Hays JW, Miller GW, Drake FD, Kanok MM: Preservation of hearing in tumors of the internal auditory canal and cerebello-pontine angle. Laryngoscope 88/1: 43-55, 1978.

Glasscock ME, Hays JW, Murphy JP: Complications in acoustic neuromas surgery. Ann Otol Rhinol Laryngol 84: 530-540, 1975.

Glasscock ME, Kyeton JF, Jackson CG, Levine SC, McKennan KX: A systematic approach to the surgical management of acoustic neuroma. Laryngoscope 96: 1088-1094, 1986.

Graniek MS, Martuza RL, Parker SW, Ojemann RG, Montgomery WW: Cerebello-pontine angle meningiomas: clinical manifestations and diagnosis. Ann Otol Rhinol Laryngol 94: 34-38, 1985.

Granthil C, DuRot JC, Bouffier C, Latiere M, Colavolpe C: Place des epreuves fonctionnelles repiratoires dans l'-analyse du risque respiratoire en periode de sevrage post-operatoire. In: Mises au point en anesthesie reanimation. Kremlin Bicetre. Amene Edit 1: 89-98, 1986.

Granthil C, Lena P, Colavolpe C: Le sevrage de la ventilation artificielle en periode post-operatoire chez l'adulte. Ann Fr Anesth-Réanim 1: 617-628, 1982.

Hamer SG, Laws ER, Onofrio BM: Hearing preservation after removal of acoustic neurinoma. Laryngoscope 94: 1431-1434, 1984.

Harker LA, McNabe BF: Iowa results of acoustic neuroma operations. Laryngoscope 88: 1904-1911, 1978.

Hilding DA, Greenberg A: Surgery for large glomus iugular tumor. Arch Otolaryng 93: 227-231, 1971.

Hitselberger WE, Gardner G: Other tumors of the cerebello-pontine angle. In Monograph II. Acoustic neuroma, House WF. Edit Arch Otolaryng 88: 712-714, 1968

Hitselberger WE, House WF: Partial versus total removal of acoustic tumors. In acoustic tumors, Vol II: management House WF, Luetje CM. Edit University Park Press Baltimore 265-268, 1979.

Hitselberger WE, Hugues RL: Bilateral acoustic tumor and neurofibromatosis. In monograph II. Acoustic neuroma, House WF. Edit Arch Otolaryng 88: 700-711, 1968.

Hongo K, Kubayashi S, Yokon A, Sugita K: Monitoring retraction pressure on the brain. J Neurosurg 66: 270-275, 1987.

Horrax G, Poppen JL: Experiences with the total and intracapsular extirpation of acoustic neuromata. Ann Surg 110: 513-524, 1939.

House WF, Hitzelberger WE: The transcochlear approach to the skull base. Arch Otolaryngol Head Neck Surg 102: 334-342, 1976.

House WF, Luetje CM: Acoustic tumors: I Diagnosis. II Management. University Park Press Baltimore, 1979.

House WF: Acoustic neuroma. Monograph II. Arch Otolaryng 88: 575-715, 1968.

House WF: Cochlear effects. In acoustic tumors, Vol II. Management House WF, Luetje MC. Edit University Park Press Baltimore 209-211, 1979.

House WF: Evolution of trans-temporal bone removal of acoustic tumors. Arch Oto-Laryngol 80: 731-741, 1964.

Hughes GB, Sismanis A, Glasscock ME, Hays JW, Jakson CG: Management of bilateral acoustic tumors. Laryngoscope 92: 1351-1359, 1982.

Ishii S, Hayner R, Kelley WA, Evans JP: Studies of cerebellar swelling. II. Experimental cerebral swelling produced by supra-tentorial extra-dural compression. J Neurosurg 16: 152-166, 1959.

Jenkins HA, Fisch U: The transotic approach to resection of difficult acoustic tumor in the cerebello-pontine angle. Amer J Otol 70-76, 1980.

Kanzaki J, Ogawa K, et al: Postoperative complications in acoustic neuroma surgery by the extended middle cranial fossa approach. Acta Otolaryngol Suppl (Stockh) 487: 75-79, 1991.

Kanzaki J, Ogawa K, et al: Results of acoustic neuroma surgery by the extended middle cranial fossa approach. Acta Otolaryngol Suppl (Stockh) 487: 17-21, 1991.

Kasantikul V, Netsky MG, Glasscock ME, Hays JW: Acoustic neurilemmoma. Clinico anatomical study of 103 patients. J Neurosurg 52: 28-35, 1980.

King TT, Morrisson AW: Translabyrinthine and transtentorial removal of acoustic nerve tumors. J Neurosurg 52: 210-216, 1980.

Koos WT, Spetzler RF, Bock FW, Salah S: Microsurgery of cerebellopontine angle tumors. In clinical microsurgery. Koos WT, Bock FW, Spetzler RF. Edit G Thieme Publ Stuttgart 91-112, 1976

Laha RK, Dujovny M, Rao S, Barrionuevo PJ, Bunegin L, Hellstrom HR, Albin MS, Taylor FN: Cerebellar retraction: significance and sequellae. Surg Neurol 12: 209-215, 1979.

Le Corff G, Elias A, Bouvier JL, Serradimigni A: Prevention de la thrombose veineuse post-operatoire in: Journees Mediterranee d'Anesthesie-Reanimation, Marseille. Arnette Edit, 1986.

Lechat Ph, Guggiari M, Lascaut G, Fuschiardi M, Evans J, Drobinski G, Klimczac K, Grosgugeat Y: Detection par echographie de contraste d'un foramen ovale permeable avant neurochirurgie. Presse Med 30: 1409-1410, 1986.

Malis LI: Microsurgical treatment of acoustic neurinomas, in Microneurosurgery, Handa H. Edit Igaku Shoin Publ 105-120, 1975.

Mangez JF, Roux P, Alibert F, Colas G, Winckler C: Problemes per et post-operatoires poses par la chirurgie des neurinomes de l'acoustique. In: Resumes des communications. Forum de clubs d'anesthesie et reanimation chirurgicale. Cinquantenaire de la S.F.A.R. Septembre 1984. CHU Pitie Salpetriere Paris, 1984.

Mardllon M, Marcone C, Merot S, Blin F, Lereau L, Moisan L, Maestracci P: Le catheterisme de l'artere radiale en anesthesie-reanimation. Ann Fr Anesth-Reanim 5: 48-57, 1986.

Moret J, Delvert JC, Lasjaunias P: La vascularisation de l'appareil auditif. Normal, variantes, tumeurs glomiques. J Neuroradiol 9: 213-260, 1982.

Morrisson AW, King TT: Translabyrinthine removal of acoustic neuromas. In neurological surgery of the ear and skull base. Brackmann DE Edit. Raven Press. Publ 227-233, 1982.

Murata T, Akuba A, Okumura T, Mori K: Intra petrous neurinomas of the facial nerve. Report of three cases. Surg Neurol 23: 507-512, 1985.

Neely JG, Hough J: Histologic findings in two very small intracanalicular solitary schwannomas of the eight nerve. Ann Otol Rhinol Laryngol 95: 460-465, 1986.

Numoto M, Donaghy RMP: Effects of local pressure on conical vessels in the dog. J Neurosurg 33: 381-387, 1970.

Ojeman RG, Levine RA, Montgomery WM, Mc Gaffigan P: Use of intra operative auditory evoked potentials to preserve hearing in unilateral acoustic neuroma removal. J Neurosurg 61: 938-948, 1984.

Olivecrona H: Acoustic tumors. J Neurosurg 26: 6-13, 1967.

Paillas JE, Grisoli F, Farnarier Ph: Neurinomes du trijumeau. A propos de 8 cas. Neurochirurgie Paris 20: 41-54, 1973.

Palva T, Johnsson LG: Preservation of hearing after removal of the membranous canal with a cholesteatoma. Arch Otolaryngol, Head Neck Surg 112: 982-985, 1986.

Palva T, Troupp H, Jauhiainen T: Hearing preservation in acoustic neurinoma surgery. Acta Otolaryngol Stockholm 99: 1-7, 1985.

Panse R: Ein gliom des Akusticus. Arch Ohrenh 251-255, 1904.

Pech A, Cannoni M, Pellet W, Triglia JM, Zanaret M, Thomassin JM: Les tumeurs de l'angle ponto-cerebelleux a l'exception des neurinomes de l'acoustique. Ann Oto-Laryng Paris 103: 293-301, 1986.

Pellet W, Cannoni M, Lavielle J, Lehmann G, Vacherat S, Mouren P: Volumineuse tumeur du glomus jugulaire. Voie d'abord combinee Oto-Neuro-Chirurgicale. Neurochirurgie 19: 567-579, 1973.

Pellet W, Cannoni M, Pech A, Triglia JM: Le neurinome de l'acoustique. Approche oto-neuro-chirurgicale. Rev Neurol Paris 143: 614-619, 1987.

Pellet W, Cannoni M, Pech A: La collaboration oto-neurochirurgicale dans l'abord trans-labyrinthique des neurinomes de l'acoustique. Neurochirurgie 25: 84-90, 1979.

Pennybacker J, Cairns H: Results in 130 cases of acoustic neurinomas. J Neurol Neurosurg Psychiat 13: 272-277, 1950.

Pensak ML, Classcock ME, Gulya AJ, Hays JW, Smith HP, Dickens RE: Cerebellopontine angle lipomas. Arch Otolaryngol Head Neck Surg 112: 99-101, 1986.

Perlman H, Kimura R, Fernandez C: Experimentation on temporary obstruction of the internal auditory artery. Laryngoscope 69: 591-599, 1959.

Portmann M, Bebear JP, Lacaze JL: Neurectomie de la Vllleme paire cranienne par voie de la fosse cerebrale moyenne. Cahier O.R.L. (Montpellier) 7: 787-793, 1972.

Ricksten SE, Medegard A, Curelaru I, Gustavsson B, Linder LE: Estimation of central venous pressure by measurement of proximal axillary venous pressure using "halfway" catheter. Acta Anesthesiol Scand 30: 13-17, 1986.

Rosenbloom SB, Carson BS, Wang H, Rosenbaum AE, Uduarhelyi GB: Cerebello-pontine angle lipoma. Surg Neurol 23: 134-138, 1985

Rosenbloom Wl, El-Sabban F: Platelet aggregation and vasoconstriction in undamaged microvessels on cerebral surface adjacent to brain traumatized by a penetrating needle. Microvascular research 15: 299-307, 1978.

Roux FX, Cioloca E, Constans JP: Bases physiques et techniques de l'hemostase tumorale avec un laser CO2 en Neuro-Chirurgie 31: 412-415, 1985.

Roux FX, Oswald AM, Merienne L, Chodkiewicz JP: Neurochirurgie au Laser CO2. Bilan de 61 interventions. Neuro-chirurgie 31: 416-420, 1985.

Sceats DJ, Quislingr I, Rhoton AL, Ballinger WE, Ryan P: Primary leptomeningeal glioma mimicking an acoustic neuroma: case report with review of the literature. Neurosurgery 19: 649-654, 1986.

Scherpereel B, Rousseaux P, Bernard MH, Guyot JF: Le non rasage pre-operatoire en neurochirurgie. Neurochirurgie 25: 244-245, 1979.

Schuknecht HF: Pathology of vestibular schannoma acoustic neurinoma. In neurological surgery of the ear, Sylverstein H, Norrel HA, Vol 1. Aesculapius Publ 193- 197, 1977.

Schwartz HE, Morgan DE, Calcaterra TC: Recovery of eight nerve function after cerebello-pontine angle surgery. Arch Otolaryngol 104: 231-233, 1978.

Shapiro HM: Anesthesia effects upon cerebral blood flow, cerebral metabolism, electroencephalogram and evoked potentials. In: Miller RD Anesthesia. Vol 2. 2nd edition. Churchill Livingstone Edit 1249-1288, 1986.

Shea MC, Robertson JT: Acoustic neuroma. A comparative study of translabyrinthine and suboccipital approach. Amer J Otol 1: 94-99, 1979.

Sheptak PE, Jannetta PJ: The two stage excision of huge acoustic neurinomas. J Neurosurg 51: 37-41, 1979.

Silverstein H, Mc Daniel A, Norrel H, Wasen J: Conservative management of acoustic neuroma in the elderly patient. Laryngoscope 95: 766-770, 1985.

Spector GJ, Sobol S, Thawley SE, Maisel RH, Ogura JH: Patterns of invasion in the temporal bone. Laryngoscope 89: 1628-1639, 1979.

Steimle R, Pageaut G, Jacquet G, Bourghli A, Godard J, Bertaud M: Lipoma in the cerebello-pontine angle. Surg Neurol 24: 73-76, 1985.

Sterkers JM: Removal of bilateral and unilateral acoustic tumors with preservation of hearing, in neurological surgery of the ear. Silverstein H, Norrel NA Edits. Aesculapius Publi, Vol II. 269-277, 1979.

Sterkers JM, Batisse R, Gandon J, Cannoni M, Vaneecloo JM: Les voies d'abord du rocher. Librairie Arnette Publ Paris 1-195, 1984.

Sterkers JM, Desgeorges M, Sterkers O, Corlieu P, Viala P: Chirurgie du neurinome de l'acoustique et autres tumeurs du conduit auditif interne et de l'angle ponto-cerebelleux: a propos de 602 cas. Ann Oto-Laryng Paris 103: 487-492, 1986.

Sterkers JM, Hamann KF: Neurinomes de l'acoustique bilateraux a propos de 8 observations. Ann Otolaryng Paris 96: 623-635, 1979.

Sterkers JM: Microchirurgie du conduit auditif interne et des regions avoisinantes. Monographie de chirurgie O. R. L. et cervicofaciale. Arnette Edit. Paris, 1976.

Sterkers JM: Technique simplifiee de decouverte du conduit auditif interne par voie temporale. Ann Otol Laryngol (Paris) 90: 232-325, 1973.

Sterkers O, Viala P, Riviere F, Sterkers JM: Neurinomes du nerf facial intra-temporal. Classification anatomo-clinique de 12 cas. Ann Oto-Laryng Paris 103: 501-508, 1986.

Tarlov E: Total one stage suboccipital microsurgical removal of acoustic neuromas of all sizes. Surg Clinics North Amer 60: 565-591, 1980.

Tator CH, Medzelski JM: Preservation of hearing in patients undergoing excision of acoustic neuromas and others cerebellopontine angle tumors. J Neurosurg 63: 168-174, 1985.

Tos M, Thomsen J: The price of preservation of hearing in acoustic neuroma surgery. Ann Otol Rhinol Laryngol 91: 240-245, 1982.

Tran Ba Huy P, Levy C, Bensimon JL, Cophignon J: Cinq cas de kyste epidermoide ou cholesteatome primitif de la pyramide petreuse. Aspect clinique radiologique, pathogenique et therapeutique. Interet de la RMN dans le diagnostic et la surveillance post-opératoire. Ann Oto Laryng Paris 103: 363-371, 1968.

Uls C, Sehested P, Overgaard J: Intracranial Hypoglossal neurinoma: Diagnosis and post-operative care. Surg neurol 16:65-68, 1981.

Uziel A, Benezech J, Frerebeau Ph: Les possibilites de conservation de l'audition dans la chirurgie des neurinomes de l'acoustique. Ann Oto-Laryng Paris 103: 127-132, 1986.

Vaneecloo FM, Jomin M, Janssen B, Burny A, Lejeune E, Allouche F: Le traitement oto-neurochirurgical des tumeurs de l'angle ponto-cerebelleux a propos d'une serie de 93 cas. Ann Otol-Laryng Paris 102: 157-161, 1985.

Wade PJ, House WF: Hearing preservation in patients with acoustic neuromas via the middle fossa approach. Otolaryngol Head Neck Surg 92: 184-193, 1984.

Waters DC, Venes JL, Zis K: Case report: childhood cerebello pontine angle teratoma associated with congenital hydrocephalus. Neurosurgery 18: 784-786, 1986.

Whittaker CK, Leutje CM: Translabyrinthine removal of large acoustic neuromas. Am J Otol 7 (Suppl): 155-160, 1985.

Wigand ME, Haid T, et al: Extended middle cranial fossa approach for acoustic neuroma surgery. Skull Base Surg 1: 183-187, 1991.

Wigand ME, Rettinger G, Haid T, Berg M: Die Ausraumung von Octavus Neurinomen des Kleinhirnbruckenwinkels mit trans-temporalem Zugang uber die mittlere Schdelgrube. HNO. 33: 11-16, 1985.

Yasargil MG, Smith RD, Gasser JC: Microsurgical approach to acoustic neurinomas. Adv Technical Standard in Neurosurg, Krayenulh H, Edit, Vol 4. Springer Verlag Wien New-York 93-129, 1977.

Yliloski J, Palva T, Collan Y: Eight nerve in acoustic neuromas. Arch Oto-Laryngol 104: 532-537, 1978.

32

Middle cranial fossa approach

Patience and time accomplish more than force and anger.

STERKERS J.M.

The preservation of hearing is taking on an increasing greater importance in acoustic neuroma surgery, since these operations are reaching their primary objectives with increasing frequency, i.e. saving the patient's life, complete tumor removal, and preserving the facial nerve. It is natural, then, that surgery's next frontier is the preservation of hearing and that the use of middle fossa approach will increase. The improvements in diagnostic techniques enabling the surgeon to diagnose smaller and smaller tumors bring this objective to the fore. The importance of hearing preservation is underlined in treatment of type 2 neurofibromatosis (NF2) (see chapter 41).

INDICATIONS

The middle cranial fossa approach (supralabyrinthine transtemporal approach) is indicated for some pathologies:

- Removal of small intracanalicular neuromas or neuromas involving no more than 1 cm of the cerebellopontine angle, when attempting to preserve hearing.
- Exposure of the labyrinthine and tympanic parts of the facial nerve in idiopathic paralysis, and when the nerve is injured in the presence of longitudinal fractures of the temporal bone. This is the only method that provides access to the labyrinthine part of the facial nerve without compromising hearing.
- Removal of supralabyrinthine tumors, such as tumors of the facial nerve (neuromas and hemangiomas) and cholesteatomas.
- Vestibular neurectomy in patients with Mènière's disease, as an alternative to a vestibular nerve section with a retrolabyrinthine or retrosigmoid approach.
- Decompression of the internal auditory canal in patients with NF2.
- Treatment of extradural pathologies such as total facial nerve decompression, repair of a cerebro-spinal fluid leak in fractures of the petrosal bone, removal of pseudotumors such as cholesterol granulomas.
- With this technique, the internal auditory canal may be exposed from the fundus to the internal porus acusticus. A good view of the nerves in the IAC is obtained, and thus the cerebellum need not be compressed during surgery.
- We tend to select the middle fossa approach in the presence of usable hearing: generally for hearing loss up to 40 dB with at least 80% discrimination. If the tumor's development is predominantly in the CPA, with minimal IAC involvement (the tumor does not reach the fundus), the retrosigmoid approach is preferred. This is true even in cases of minimal residual hearing.
- Pre-operative clinical tests are valuable in predicting the possibility of preserving hearing, which depends not only on the tumor's size, but on its location as well. The closer the tumor is to the IAC fundus, the fewer are the chances of preserving hearing.

DISADVANTAGES OF THE MIDDLE FOSSA APPROACH

- In the middle fossa approach, the facial nerve lies beside and/or above the tumor, and is thus more easily damaged. In the translabyrinthine approach, on the other hand, the nerve's path is predominantly inferior to the tumor.
- Limited access to the posterior fossa is available in cases of hemorrhage.
- Symptoms of temporal lobe compression may be seen, especially in operations on the dominant hemisphere (e.g. left temporal lobe in right-handed patients).
- Patients over 60 suffer the greatest risk of intracranial complications due to the fragility of the dura. It is thinner, bleeds more copiously and is easily lacerated.
- In 5% of patients operated with a middle fossa approach from the left side, aphasia may ap-

pear, normalizing after 1-2 weeks (this applies to right-handed patients). In left-handed patients, the situation is reversed.

A rectangle is outlined with a plastic drape and disposable adhesive drapes. One side (approx. 12 cm) is tangent to the inferior part of the concha, another is tangent to the auricle (approx. 15 cm) and is crossed by a third approx. 7 cm over the apex of the elix.

PATIENT'S POSITION

Figures 6-23, 32-1

The electrodes of the facial nerve stimulator are positioned to monitor auditory evoked potentials.

ANESTHESIA

Hypotensive anesthesia with sodium nitroprusside is used to mantain the systolic pressure at or near 85 mm Hg.

To obtain brain relaxation, hyperventilation is performed to keep the PCO2 at 25 mm Hg. This is useful in all surgical procedures that expose the brain, as well as the intravenous infusion of Mannitol (0.5 mg/kg). Dexamethasone can be useful as well.

INCISION

The incision begins over the zygomatic root, anterior to the lowest point of the concha. It runs parallel to the helix, then curves slightly anteriorly for 8 cm, in proportion to its apex. The incision should not be prolonged beyond the zygomatic arch, and should be kept near the eye, at least initially. This is to avoid the frontal branches of the facial nerve and for esthetic purposes, since in this way the incision is kept within the hairline. The curvature of the incision makes it possible to spread the margins more amply, thus gaining space anteriorly.

The incision reaches the root of the zygomatic arch inferiorly and the fascia of the temporalis muscle underneath (Fig. 32-2).

If a frontal branch of the superficial temporal artery is encountered, it is tied with a silk thread to prevent delayed bleeding and a hematoma of the wound. The other vessels are coagulated.

ELEVATION OF THE MUSCLE FLAP

- The muscle flap is isolated from the subcutaneous planes with blunt instruments, such as the finger or the handle of the knife.
- The muscle is incised, creating a muscle flap based anteriorly. It is elevated and coagulated with the electric cautery on the bone.
- It is then anchored anteriorly, with silk sutures kept taut with Klemmer forceps. The flap thus created maintains its innervation and vascularization. In cases of persistent postoperative facial paralysis, it may be utilized by transposing the inferior hemiface.

ELEVATION OF THE BONE PLATE

- A craniotomy is performed with a 4 cm square bone plate (Fig. 32-3). This may be prepared under continuous aspiration-irrigation with a 4 mm cutting burr. When nearing the dura, a diamond burr is used instead. It is unnecessary to completely expose the dura underneath the sulcus of the burr. The craniotomy should be located two-thirds anterior to the external auditory canal.
- A Lempert periosteum dissector is then inserted between dura and bone, exerting an upward force, but without using the dura as a fulcrum.

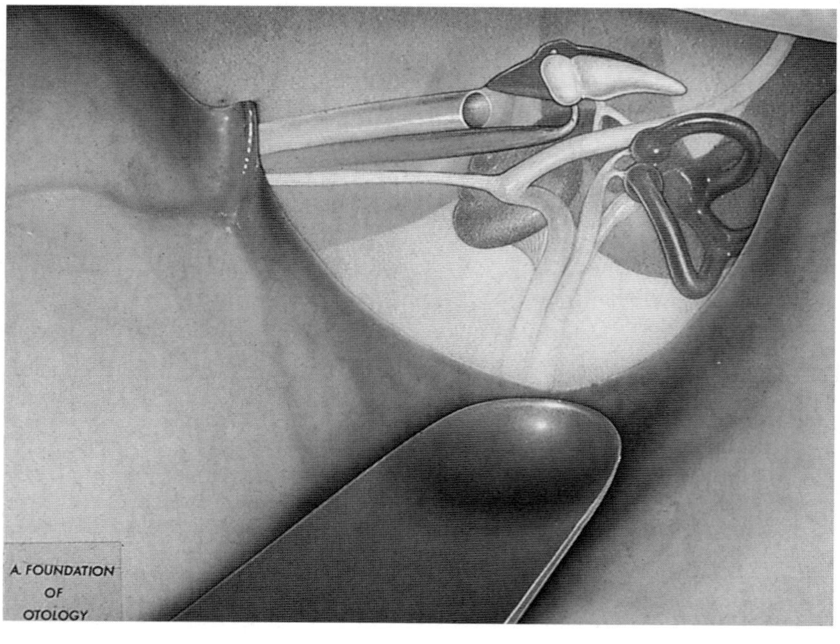

Fig. 32-1. The middle fossa approach. Surgical anatomy of the right temporal bone.

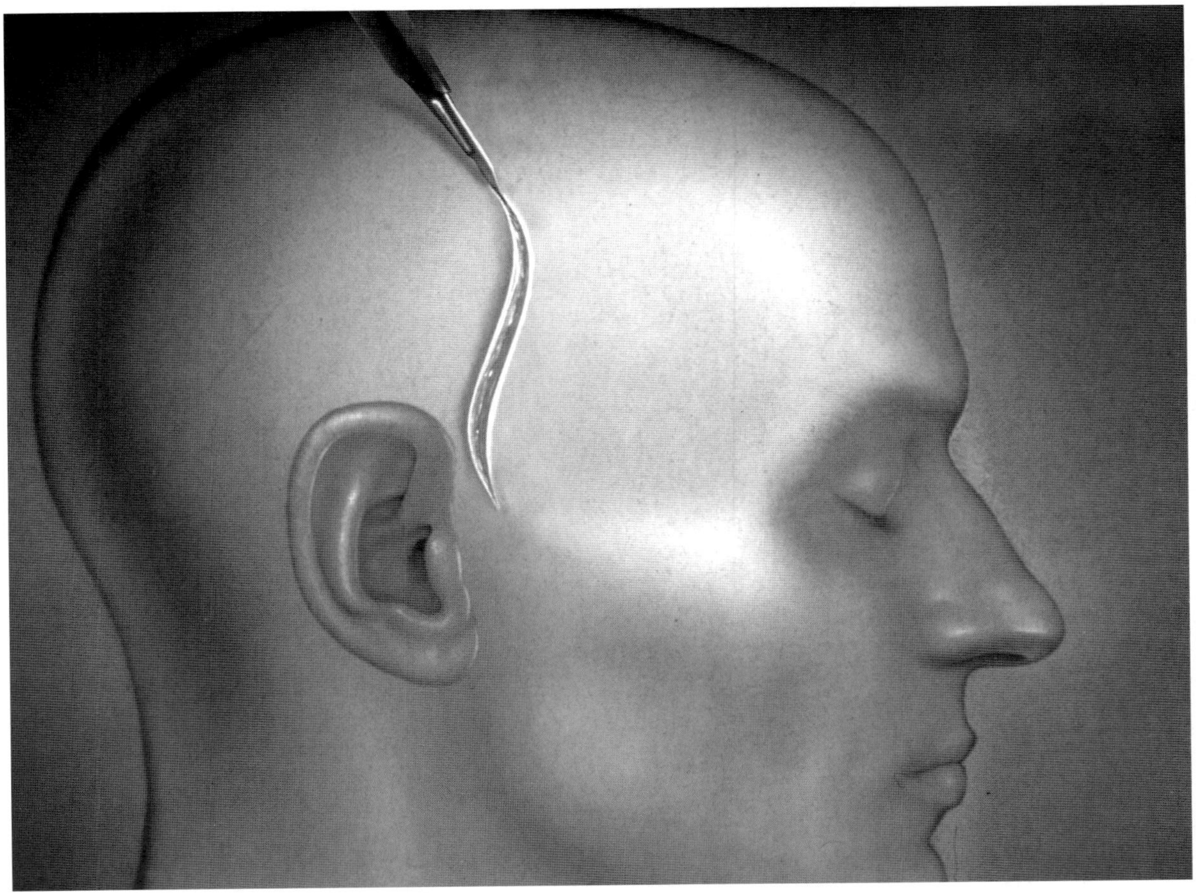

Fig. 32-2. Skin incision, beginning in the pretragal area.

Thus the bone plate is detached. This maneuver reduces the risk of lacerating the dura and herniating the temporal lobe.

- The bone margins are regularized with rongeurs.
- The inferior base of the bone plate must be as near as possible to the zygomatic root, to obtain the most favorable exposure of the internal auditory canal. It is possible to arrive no closer than 1 cm from the zygomatic root, since nearer, the squama of the temporal bone is too thick. The bone plate is removed and preserved in Ringer solution for later use.
- The anterior margins of the craniotomy may be enlarged as necessary with rongeurs and/or a diamond burr.
- There are often bleeding spots on the bone, which are sealed with bone wax.
- The margins of the craniotomy must be kept parallel, to facilitate the positioning of the self retaining retractor. The margins may be smoothed with a 5 mm diamond burr to prevent dural lacerations.
- If there is slight bleeding of the lateral margins of the craniotomy, it may be halted by placing strips of Surgicel at the margins, between the dura and bone.

DISSECTION OF THE DURA

- It is important to attempt to preserve the dural branches of the middle meningeal artery. If they bleed, they are coagulated with minimum intensity and continuous irrigation, to avoid dural lacerations and hernias of the temporal lobe later on. If dural lacerations do occur, they are repaired with silk sutures.
- The endocranial pressure is significantly reduced by the intraoperative administration of Mannitol and Dexamethazone.
- In rare instances dissection may be problematic, or the surgical view may be resistant, due to a high liquor pressure resistent to the preventative pharmacological measures. In this case a low point of the dura may be coagulated with the bipolar cautery. It is then opened by elevating the center of the coagulated zone with a hook and incising with the tip of the knife. The liquor will flow out and pressure will diminish.
- The dura is separated from the bone margins of the craniotomy with a dural elevator. This step is necessary to safely position the self retaining retractor.
- The claws of the retractor are placed against the two vertical sides of the bone plate (Fig. 32-4).

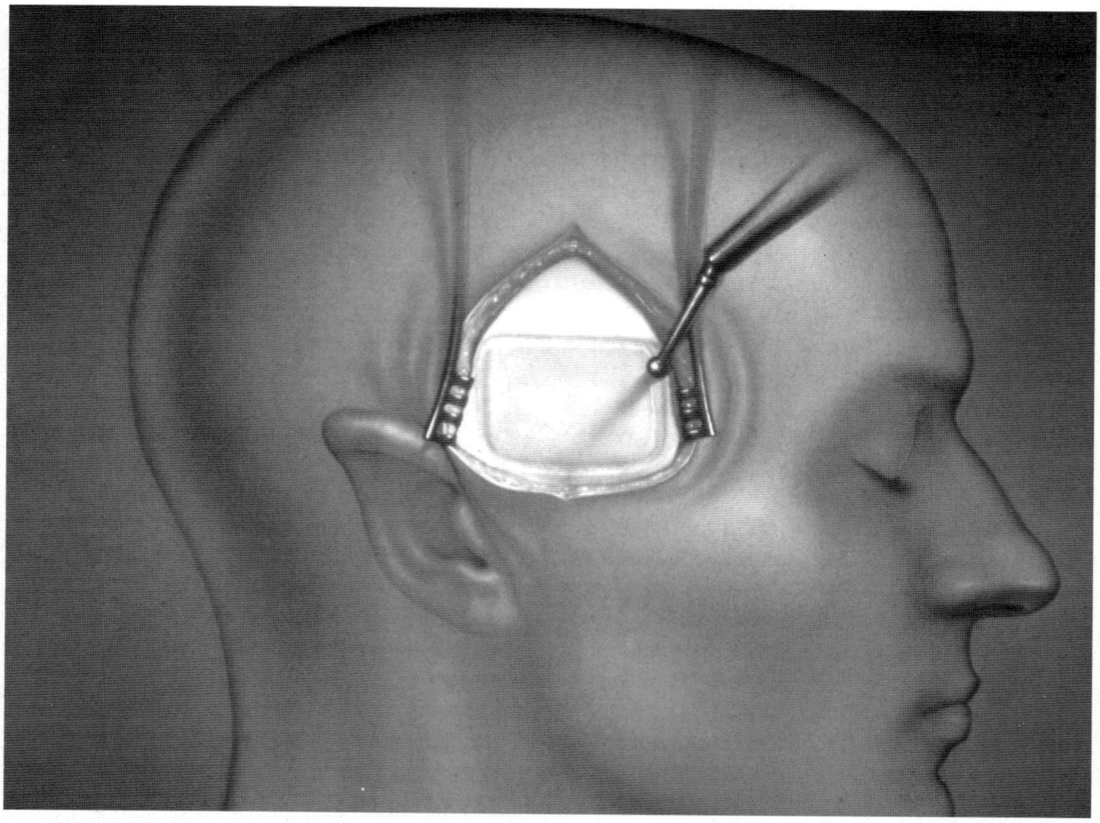

Fig. 32-3. Craniotomy

- With a suction-irrigator and a dural dissector, the dura of the anterior wall of the petrous ridge is divided. The anterior dissecting limit (and the most superficial) is the middle meningeal artery at its entrance into the foramen spinosum. Bleeding from the foramen spinosum is quite common, since the latter is rich in vascular junctions between bone and dura. The bleeding may be controlled by placing Surgicel in the foramen.
- The retractor is in situ, but the dura will be charged with the blade only after it has been completely dissected from the posterior floor of the middle fossa. This makes the procedure easier and quicker, and the intermittent pressure of the suction-irrigator proves less traumatic.
- The dura is carefully dissected from the bone, beginning posteriorly (postero-anterior direction). Posteriorly there are no important structures and adherences of dura to bone are rare.
- Dissection continues anteriorly working more on the dura than the bone, to avoid injuring the underlying structures. The greater superficial petrosal nerve is encountered, often protruding from its bone canal and the geniculate ganglion. Traction, but especially dissection of these structures, endangers the integrity of the facial nerve. Paresis or paralysis is the result. This part of the dissection must therefore be performed under microscopic control, to reduce the risks involved.
- The greater superficial petrosal nerve is found medial to the middle meningeal artery, and reaches the geniculate ganglion running parallel to the petrous apex.
- Superior to the geniculate ganglion is the tegmen tympani, thin and easily injured. Dissection must be very delicate in this phase, to prevent the spread of infection through a lesion of the tegmen, from the tube and the middle ear, through the internal auditory canal, and on to the endocranial spaces.

The bone overlying the internal carotid artery may also be very fragile and should not be touched, to avoid possible lesions to the artery.

EXPOSURE OF THE PLANE OF THE INTERNAL AUDITORY CANAL

- The dura has been completely dissected from the middle fossa floor, up to the petrous margin. Here we find the superior petrosal sinus, which must not be traumatized. If it does break, bleeding should be stopped with an extraluminal dressing with a large piece of Surgicel. Small pieces of Surgicel must not be used since they could go through the internal jugular vein

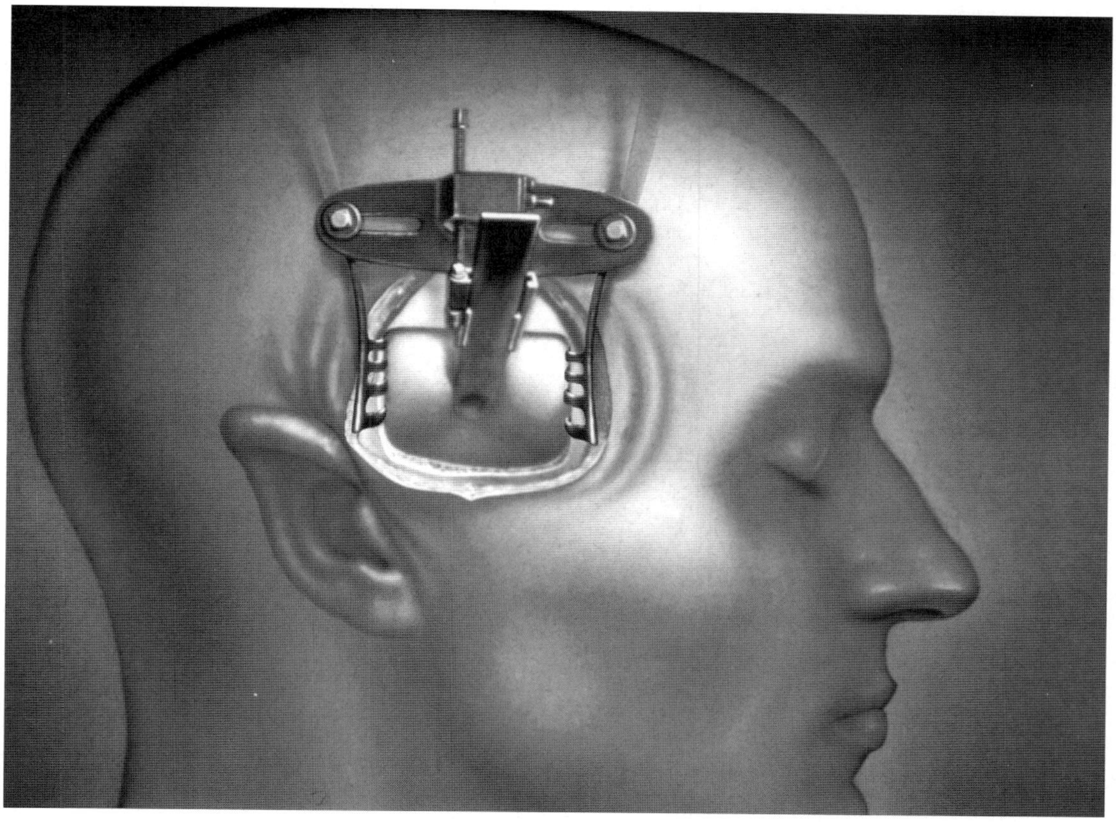

Fig. 32-4. The retractor is inserted inside the edges of the craniotomy.

and into the right side of the heart, and from there to the lungs, provoking an embolism.

- At the petrous margin (the inferior limit of the dissection), the blade of the self retaining retractor is put in place. It rests on the dura, projecting from the IAC, with its extremity just under the petrous margin, without twisting the petrosal sinus. The initial positioning of the retractor is performed without a microscope, to obtain a wider control of the operating field; at this point the operating table is placed in the anti-Trendelemburg position to improve visibility of the area underlying the retractor's blade. The final position of the retractor is reached with progressive advancements of the blade, which is later halted in the definitive position, under microscopic control (Fig. 32-5).
- No other maneuvers are performed before hemostasis is completed and a dry field is obtained. If there is an oozing of the dura, a bipolar cautery may be used to coagulate along a line, in a medial to lateral direction.
- The plane of the meatus lies before the arcuate eminence. The latter is a ridge corresponding to the superior semicircular canal. Its position is unpredictable. In this phase the largest diamond burr possible must be used, to avoid injury to the underlying structures.

Fisch's Technique

When identifying the IAC, the superior semicircular canal is first recognized with a blue line. A diamond burr is used on and posterior to the arcuate eminence, through the cells of the antrum and the attic. Continuous aspiration-irrigation is used to ensure working on a flat field, with no bony protruberances. The blue line must be recognized medial to the IAC rather than laterally. There is a risk of injury to the ampulla of the SSC, the cochlea, and the facial nerve. Once the blue line has been done (the membranous canal of the SSC visible through the thinned bone), the posterior dissection limit is reached. The drilling is within a 60° angle, the vertex of which is the SSC. The posterior side is the blue line of the SSC (Fig. 32-6).

The House technique calls for the identification of the greater superficial petrosal nerve, which is then followed to the hiatus of the facial nerve (see above).

Portmann & Garcia Ibanez Technique

The technique described by Portmann and diffused by Garcia Ibanez calls for the identification of the GSPN, beginning at the geniculate ganglion, to the identification of the superior semicircular canal. The internal auditory canal is ex-

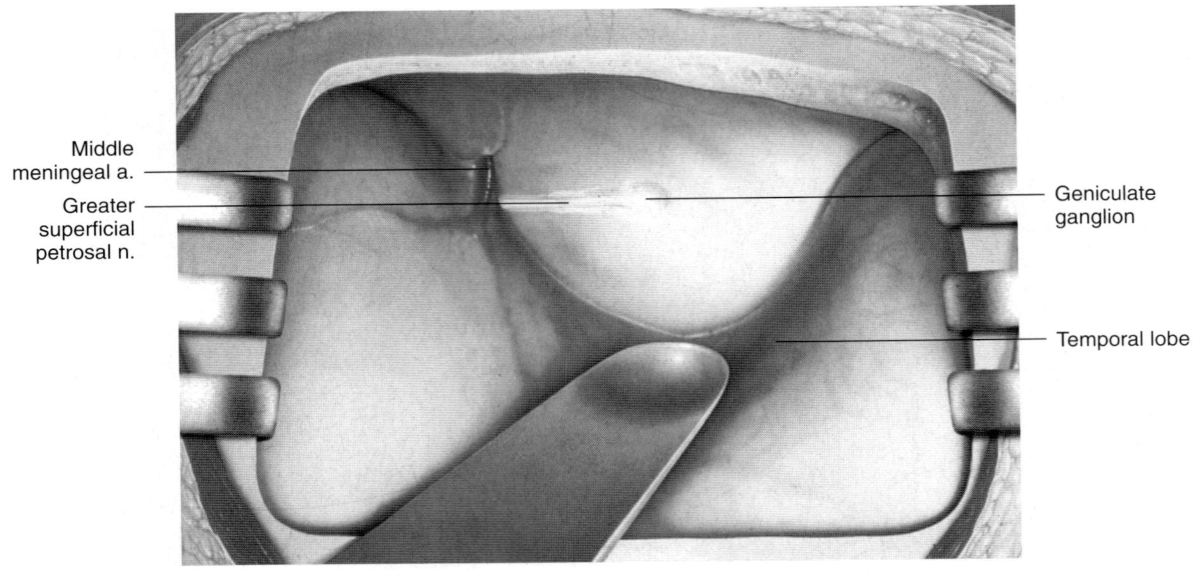

Fig. 32-5. Middle meningeal artery is identified. The greater superficial petrosal nerve is located medial to the MMA and followed backwards to the geniculate ganglion.

posed with the burr along the bisector of the angle formed by the GSPN and SSC.

Drilling proceeds medially in the temporal bone, so that only after having clearly exposed the internal auditory canal in a risk-free zone do we laterally approach the structures to be preserved (Fig. 32-7).

House Technique, adopted at the HEC before 1990

- The arcuate eminence and the greater superficial petrosal nerve are identified. The GSPN exits the foramen spinosum and runs diagonally in a posterior direction, becoming slightly more lateral.
- Following the nerve, we reach the facial nerve hiatus and then the geniculate ganglion. The ganglion is seen through a thin bone sheath, without having to completely expose it. This is often possible even without removing bone. A large diamond burr is used.
- The labyrinthine part of the facial nerve is followed from the geniculate ganglion to the internal auditory canal. The labyrinthine part of the

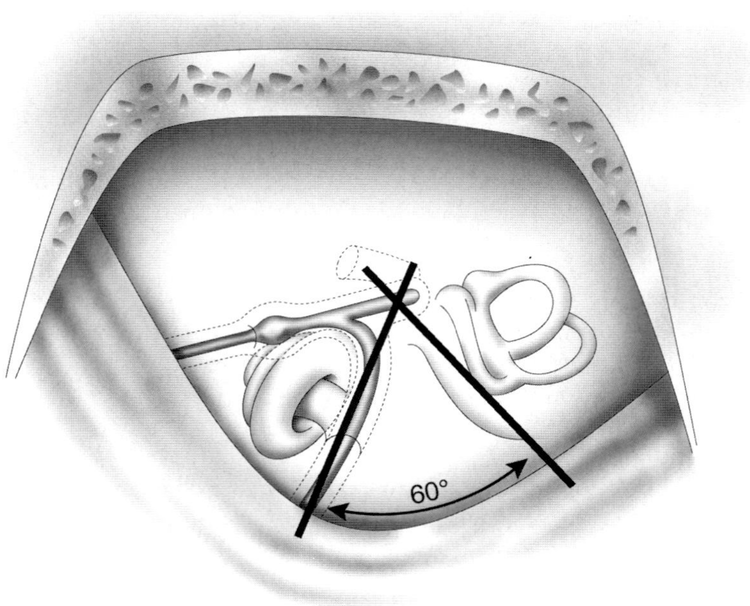

Fig. 32-6. The Fisch method for exposing the IAC.

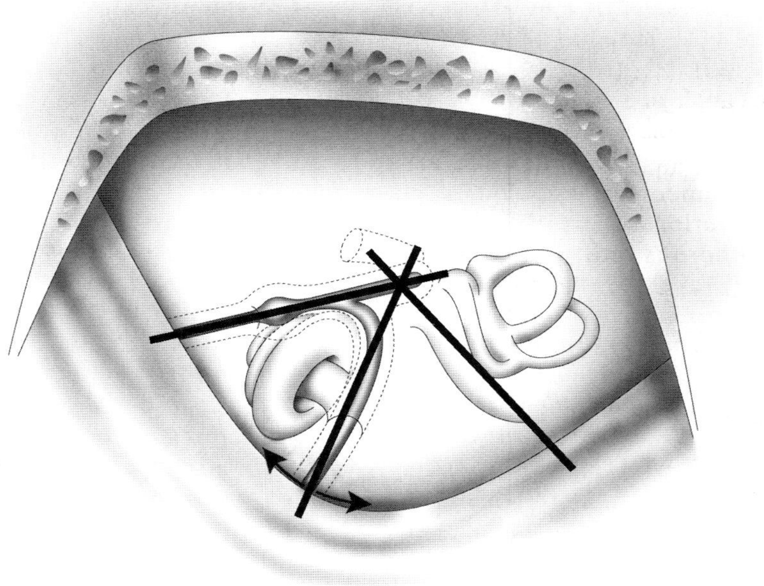

Fig. 32-7. The Portmann & Garcia-Ibanez method for exposing the IAC.

facial nerve runs parallel to the plane of the superior semicircular canal, which forms a 45-60° angle with the IAC (Fig. 32-8).

Modified House Technique

- The following technique is used currently at the House Ear Clinic. The arcuate eminence is identified, as well as the greater superficial petrosal nerve. Then, we drill along the bisector of the angle formed by these two structures.
- Drilling is begun near to the porus until the dura of the IAC is identified, and then we ascend medially following the landmark of the dura. In the medial part of the IAC, there are no vulnerable structures anteriorly or posteriorly, with the exception of the superior petrosal sinus running along the petrous bone margin. The cochlea is found in the lateral anterior position, whereas the superior semicircular canal is found in the lateral posterior position.

This technique reduces time in the operating room, as well as the risk of trauma to the facial nerve and the superior semicircular canal.

- It is preferable to begin by leaving a thin bony sheath on the internal auditory canal. A large-di-

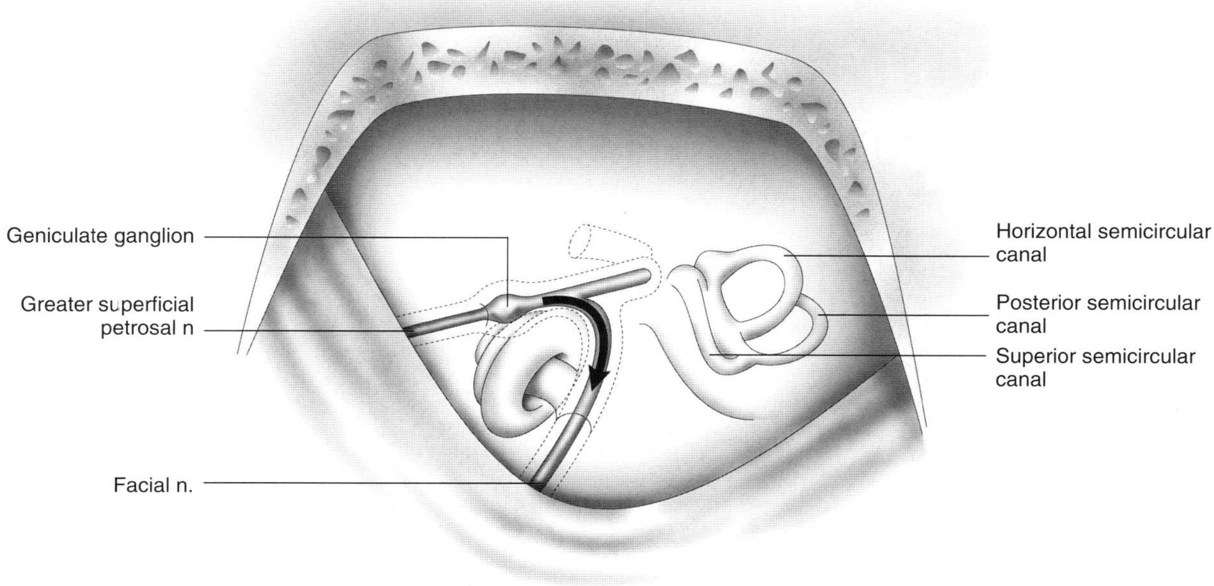

Fig. 32-8. The House method for exposing the IAC.

ameter diamond burr is used (3-4 mm). The internal auditory canal is skeletonized for approx. 270°, in its inferior two-thirds. The burr safely acts on the canal and at its anterior and posterior edges.

- The IAC is, in fact, the bisector of an acute angle with its vertex in the superior position, formed by the posterior semicircular canal and a line tangent to the posterior margin of the cochlea, anteriorly. Thus there is more space medially and is progressively restricted, laterally.
- The bone of the petrous margin is removed until the superior petrosal sinus within the dura has been completely exposed. Inferiorly there is a space free of structures, making identification of the IAC more difficult. Since we must overdrill, it is preferable to assume an anterior direction. This exposure is performed intentionally in the execution of the enlarged middle fossa technique (see the enlarged middle fossa chapter).
- The exposure of the superior third of the IAC requires more careful attention. Anteriorly, under the geniculate ganglion, is the cochlea. Its bony wall is in contact with the ganglion and the facial nerve, whereas posteriorly the ampulla of the superior semicircular canal is in contact with the top of the superior vestibular nerve.
- Thus the burr's diameter must be reduced (2mm diamond) and the superior part of the IAC is skeletonized staying on the canal, without proceeding laterally. A 1 mm diamond burr is then used. The lateral limits of the IAC are exposed as little as possible, proceeding in a lateral direction. At the lateral extremity only the superior part of the IAC is exposed, by approx. 90°. The presence of the cochlea and the ampulla of the superior canal make it impossible to expose the lateral part of the IAC.
- At the lateral extremity of the IAC, Bill's bar is identified. This is a thin bony sheath separating the facial nerve from the superior vestibular nerve. Following the infralabyrinthine part of the facial nerve from the geniculate ganglion, Bill's bar is posterior and medial to the IAC fundus.
- The entire IAC is now skeletonized and covered by a thin bony sheath which is removed with a House dissector.

Now that the phase of bone drilling has been completed and no bone remains on the petrous margin, it may be necessary to reposition the blade of the retractor.

The dura must be opened with a hook. Bill's bar is identified, followed by the facial nerve. The superior vestibular nerve is seen posterior to the facial nerve (Fig. 32-9).

TUMOR REMOVAL

- The superior vestibular nerve is cut laterally to the vertical crest. The nerve must be cut, with microscissors or with a sharp neurectomy scalpel. The use of a hook is not recommended, since it may take surrounding blood vessels with it. If an alteration of the internal ear vascularization does occur, the chances for postoperative hearing loss are greater.
- The superior vestibular nerve is reflected posteriorly. The inferior vestibular nerve is found medially with its two branches, the saccular nerve and the singularis nerve. The latter two nerves go frequently unrecognized due to their involvement with the tumor. The inferior vestibular nerve is incised at its lateral extremity with the method previously described.

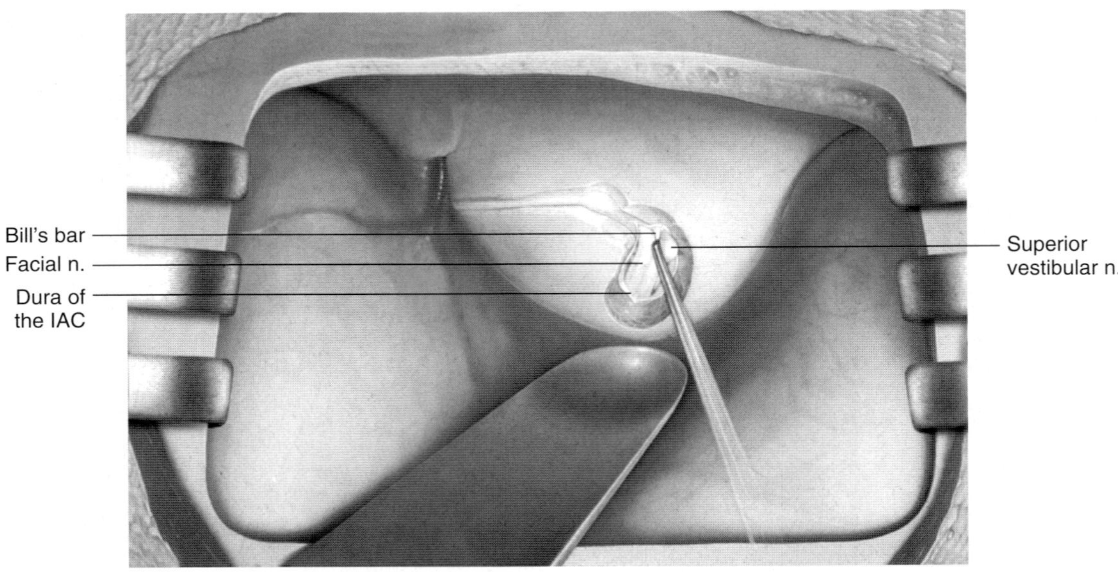

Fig. 32-9. The IAC is exposed. Bill's bar divides the facial nerve and the superior vestibular nerve.

- Both the vestibular nerves are sectioned. This prevents the postoperative instability likely to follow a partial section.
- The vestibulo-facial anastomoses are sectioned with a cutting instrument, in the attempt to avoid exerting traction on the facial nerve and altering the vascularization of the inner ear: cochlear artery, vestibular and vestibulo-cochlear-artery, which generally goes from the facial nerve to the cochlear nerve.
- This operation is selected when attempting to preserve hearing. Thus it is particularly important to try and exert as little traction as possible on the vascularization of the inner ear. Since the tumor must be removed, this is the most difficult objective to attain; much more so than the preservation of the cochlear and facial nerves. It is also difficult to detect an error in the making. Often the error is made evident only postoperatively, when hearing loss appears. In clinical practice, most of the tumors that extend into the cerebellopontine angle involve the vascularization of the cochlea. Thus they may not be removed without provoking irreversible ischaemic damage to the sensorineural epithelium. We thus underline the importance of the tumor's size in deciding whether to use a middle fossa approach.
- Preserving hearing is complicated by the dual function of the vessels originating in the anterior-inferior cerebellar artery (AICA): besides supplying blood to the tumor capsule, they may also serve the cochlea and the cochlear nerve. During removal of the tumor, the cochlear nerve may undergo irreversible trauma due to disturbances in the microcirculation of the endoneural vasa nervorum (Strauss). Other causes may be a vasospasm of the internal auditory canal, edema of the cochlear nerve, compressing action of the inner internal auditory meatus, or the growth of granulation tissue. Hearing may be damaged even by a cerebellar retraction or by the loss of cerebro-spinal liquor (Haid, Wigand). In some instances, hearing function may decrease compared to the unoperated ear even years after the operation (Shelton).
- The tumor is removed, separating it from the facial nerve. It is then removed from the posterior part of the IAC. This is why it is very important to remove as much bone as possible around the posterior margin of the IAC. Thus, even when following the IAC identification method recommended by William House for the facial nerve, a blue line of the SSC may be helpful, since it represents the posterior limit of the dissection.
- The tumor is moved posteriorly with a hook while the suction-irrigator's grasp is maintained. While working with the tumor, a fenestrated Brackmann aspirator should be used, since it reduces the suction exerted on the underlying structures.
- Irrigation is very useful: the field is cleared by the continuous rinsing and aspiration, and the flow of water acts as a delicate dissector. Thus the limits between nerves, vessels and tumor are outlined.
- The part of the tumor occupying the lateral extremity of the IAC is liberated.
- The tumor is reflected posteriorly and separated from the facial nerve and the cochlear nerve with a hook, or preferably by dissection (Figs. 32-10, 32-11, 32-12, 32-13). It is important not to lose this cleavage plane. The internal auditory

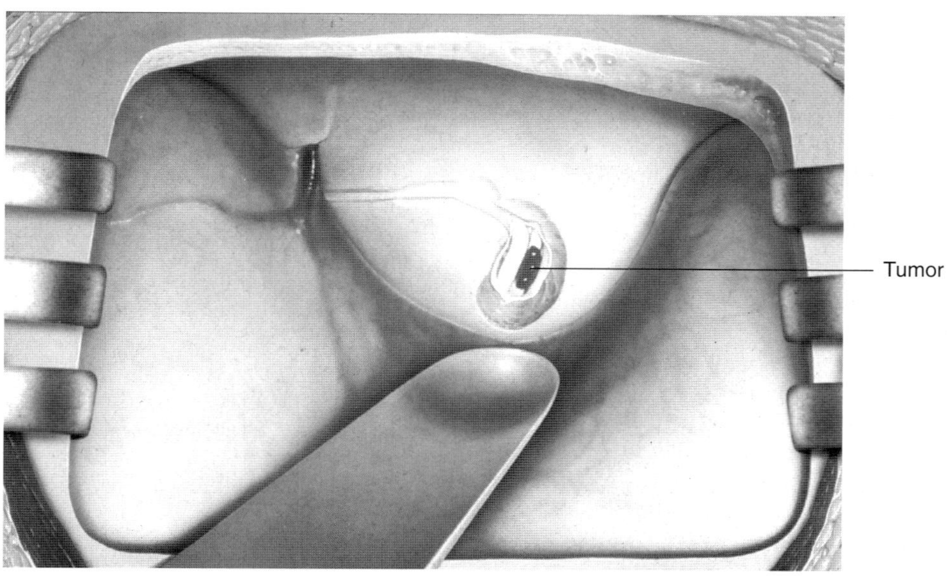

Fig. 32-10. Small tumor in the IAC.

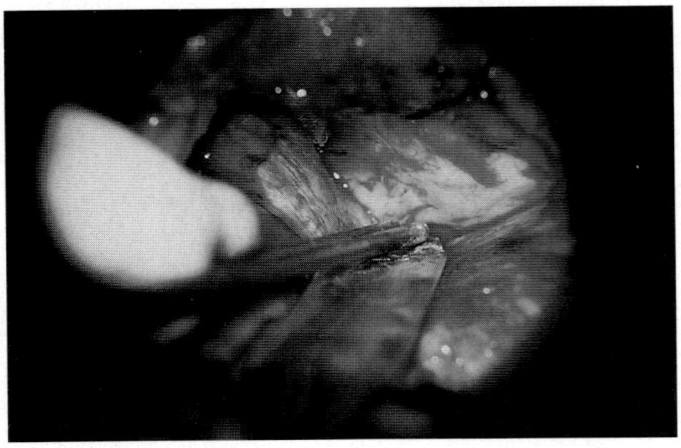

Fig. 32-11. The dura is elevated from the floor of the middle fossa with a blunt dural elevator and a suction irrigator. The House-Urban retractor is placed to gently support the temporal lobe.

artery is sought under the tumor and the cochlear nerve. The AICA may reach the cerebellopontine angle in its lateral-most part, at the fundus of the IAC, or in all the intermediate positions. It is important to detect it immediately, as if it occupied the lateral-most part of the IAC. Once the artery has been found, it is carefully separated from the surface of the tumor with a Rosen elevator.

Technique adopted at HEI until 1990
The tumor is progressively displaced posteriorly. If it does not reach the porus, and if the distal part of the vestibular nerves are easily seen at the medial extremity of the IAC, these are cut and the tumor is removed with forceps. If, on the other hand, the inferior limit is not very distinct, it is better to cut the tumor and remove the superior part first, to avoid exerting pressure on the facial nerve. The inferior part is then removed.

CURRENT TECHNIQUE
Intraoperative monitoring of the cochlear nerve has led us to concentrate on intraoperative injuries to the cochlear nerve and their causes, evaluated in realtime at their onset. Statistics (in terms of preserved hearing) are improved. The operative technique has been modified.

If the tumor originates in the superior vestibular nerve, the inferior vestibular nerve is preserved whenever possible to prevent vascular damage.

The cochlear nerve exits the multiple perforations of the habenula perforata of the cochlea with minuscule filaments that unite in one single trunk. These fibers are extremely delicate. Thus the dissection of the tumor from the facial nerve must not occur in a lateral-medial direction, which provokes a damaging traction on the cochlear nerve, but in a medial-to-lateral direction.

Intraoperative monitoring of the auditory evoked potentials is helpful in preserving the acoustic nerve, though the integrity of this nerve alone does not guarantee hearing preservation. Postoperative hearing may deteriorate or be lost immediately or at a later date, for various reasons:

- The preservation of the internal auditory artery alone does not guarantee vascular integrity. At times the vessels going from the AICA to the tumoral capsule may also supply the inner ear and the cochlear nerve.
- A mechanical trauma to the cochlear nerve during tumor removal may lead to disturbances in the microcircle of the endoneural vasa nervorum.
- Vasospasm of the internal auditory canal.
- Cochlear nerve edema.
- Internal IAC compression.
- Scar tissue growth.
- Cerebellar retraction; loss of cerebro-spinal liquor (both rare).
- Hearing in the operated ear may deteriorate over the years.

The tumor has now been completely removed. The surgical field is profusely irrigated with a suction-irrigator. The small bleeding vessels are observed, and generally stop bleeding spontaneously. If some vessels continue to bleed, hemostasis may be performed with a small piece of Surgicel placed at the end of the vessel and left in situ. The Surgicel must always be much smaller than the diameter of the IAC, since the former tends to enlarge and may exert damaging pressure on the facial and cochlear nerves. Hemostasis may also be performed with bipolar coagulation.

Closure of the field

- The IAC is closed with a free graft of temporalis muscle. If a lesion to the thin tegmen tym-

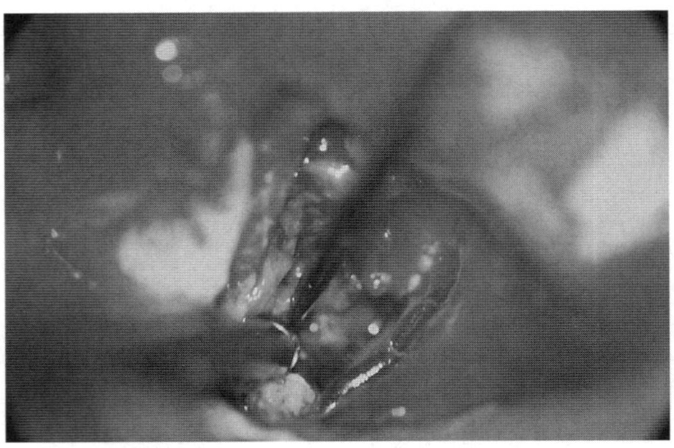

Fig. 32-12. Tumor is dissected away from the facial and cochlear nerves, rather then the nerves being retracted away from the tumor. The dissection along the VIII n. is done in a medial to lateral direction, in order to avoid tearing the filaments of the nerve that pass through the holes of the lamina cribrosa, at the fundus of the IAC.

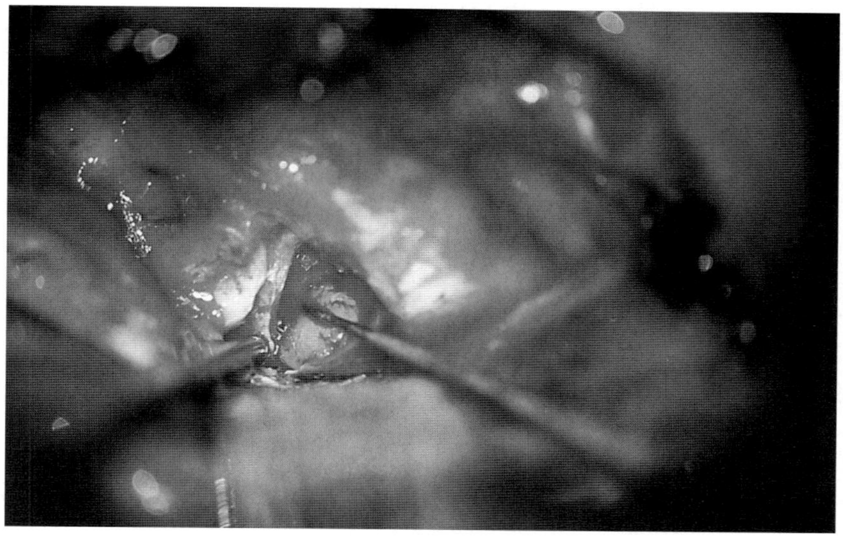

Fig. 32-13. Complete tumor removal. Facial nerve integrity is preserved.

pani has taken place, a fragment of bone from the craniotomy (from its thinnest margin) is shaped and put in place to close the gap, with the margins resting on intact bone. Kept in place with fibrin glue, it is later stabilized by the dural pressure. The blade of the dural retractor is retracted, the brain resumes position, and the dura recovers and fuses with the bone fragment. In this way the risks of infection and conductive hearing loss (from the pressure of the dura on the ossicles) are avoided.

- If a decompressive incision has been made on the dura, it is unnecessary to repair it. No permanent leak has ever been observed (Fisch).
- The plate of temporal bone is replaced. The temporalis muscle is replaced and sutured with 2-0 Vycril. If there is an excessive blood loss, a Penrose drain is put in place. The subcutaneous tissue is closed with 2-0 catgut and the skin is closed with 3-0 silk.

COMPLICATIONS

- One disadvantage of the middle fossa approach is the limited access available to the posterior fossa in the case of hemorrhage. If the AICA has undergone a lesion during the removal of the tumor, it may be necessary to drill the superior semicircular canal, to gain a more ample access to the IAC through the dura of the posterior cranial fossa. A clip is then positioned. If this is impossible, a translabyrinthine approach is performed. Otherwise, if the bleeding is in the cerebellopontine angle, a retrosigmoid approach is used.
- In cases of postoperative hemorrhage, the options are the same. In an emergency procedure, however, there is no time. This problem is not encountered with a translabyrinthine technique.
- An epidural hematoma, though rare, may occur shortly after surgery. A careful hemostasis and the use of a Penrose drain in the presence of blood ooze should prevent this from occurring. If the emergency does occur, the hematoma must immediately be evacuated, even in the Intensive Care Unit. Thus time is gained to safely move the patient into the operating room, perform general anesthesia, the sterile preparation of the field, and the subsequent thorough hemostasis.
- The rupture of the superior semicircular canal is a possible complication, when an SSC blue line is too aggressively performed.
- A similar complication is the opening of the basal turn of the cochlea during exposure of the IAC fundus.
- The perforation, in both cases, must be immediately closed with a fragment of fascia, upon which bone wax or bone paté is applied, followed by fibrin glue. In these instances, despite the rapid closure of the perforation, sensorineural hearing loss is common.
- If the superior petrosal sinus is cut, the temporal lobe may suffer.
- One possible complication to remember, common to every intracranial procedure, is meningitis.
- If the closure techniques are correct, no external CSF leaks are seen. A transitory rhynoliquorrhea may occur due to the flow of liquor through the tube.
- If care is used when working with the temporal lobe, rare but not impossible complications are avoided, such as hemiparesis and aphasia. Some patients (Haid: 5%) may show temporary cerebral disorientation or difficulty in speaking (anamnestic aphasia) for a few days (1-2 weeks), especially if they have been operated on on the left side: the left lobe is the dominant lobe in right-handed people, and vice versa.

Epileptic fits (temporal lobe epilepsy) may be present in approx. 2% of cases (Haid) and are prevented with antiepileptic therapy (Fenobarbital), beginning one week before the operation and terminating two months after surgery.

- Some patients may complain of dryness in the homolateral eye for some weeks after surgery. This is provoked by the stretching of the superior petrosal nerve.

TIPS AND PITFALLS

- All patients considering a middle fossa surgery undergo a thin cut CT exam, to identify the degree of bone pneumatization overlying the superior semicircular canal and the internal auditory canal.
- When the craniotomy is performed, the drilling may slip far forward, penetrating the antrum and the mastoid. This heightens the risk of CSF fistulas. It is advisable to maintain the superior margin of the zygomatic arch as the inferior margin of the craniotomy. If necessary, the craniotomy may later be safely enlarged.
- At times the surgeon may be left without a landmark, uncertain of the location of the IAC. In this case the tegmen tympani may be opened, to identify the malleus, the incus and the tympanic part of the facial nerve. Whether the tegmen has been opened intentionally or accidentally, the breach must be repaired at surgery's end.
- Anteriorly, approx. 1 cm under the cortical mastoid, the petro-squamous suture is found. This may attach to the dura with strong dural adherences. When the adherences are not resolved with a mere dissection (a rare occurrence), they must be coagulated and cut with microscissors near the bone.
- The vessels going from the bone to the dura and a vein going from the posterior bone to the superior petrosal sinus, when necessary, are coagulated and cut near the bone. The dural side of the vessel is thus longer and may be recoagulated as needed. The bony part of the vessels, if they bleed, may be closed with bone wax.
- It is important to keep in mind that there is almost always a blood ooze from the small vessels of the dura and the middle fossa floor. Surgery should continue, since this bleeding will spontaneously stop.
- The arcuate eminence is perpendicular to the petrous margin.
- The geniculate ganglion is approx. 1 cm lateral to the petrous margin and 2 cm medial to the cortical bone. The dimensions of the temporal bone may vary, but in general there is a one-to-two ratio. When approaching the geniculate ganglion in a lateral direction, the cochlea is near the IAC. This is similar to the ampulla of the SSC, which is nearer to the IAC than the SSC (Figs. 32-14, 32-15).
- The SSC describes an arch with superior convexity in the arcuate eminence. Thus it is more superficial at the vertex and deeper at the edges.
- Drilling is performed with continuous irrigation through a thin veil of water. The largest diamond burr possible is used (2-4 mm), while maintaining sufficient visual space between the tip of the burr and the structures at the sides.
- When the arcuate eminence is not very prominent, this means that the superior semicircular canal is near; care must be taken.
- As a general rule in cranial base surgery, the bone must be thinned and the underlying structures identified before removing the last bone layer. This is even more important in middle fossa surgery, where the operation is performed in restricted space.
- Bill's bar is slightly medial to the ampulla of the SSC (1 mm) and approx. 3 mm more medial than

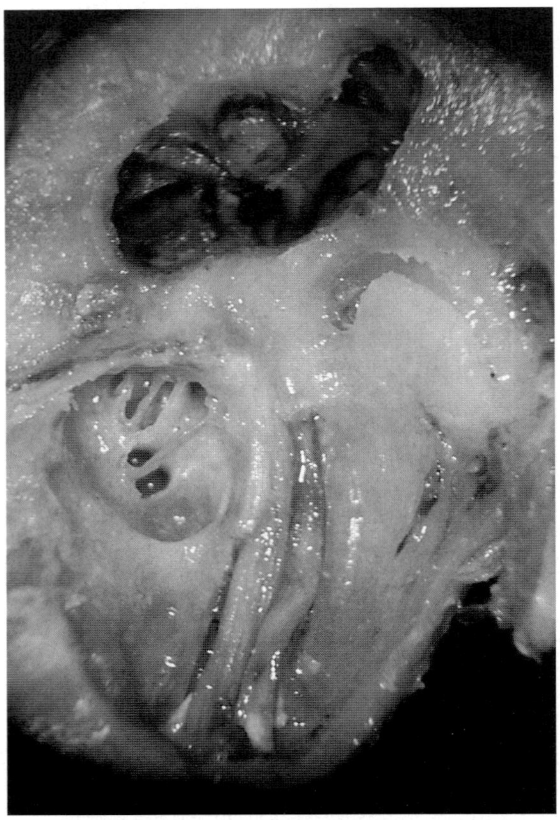

Fig. 32-14. Temporal bone dissection. Right ear. The internal auditory canal, the cochlea and the epitympanum are opened.

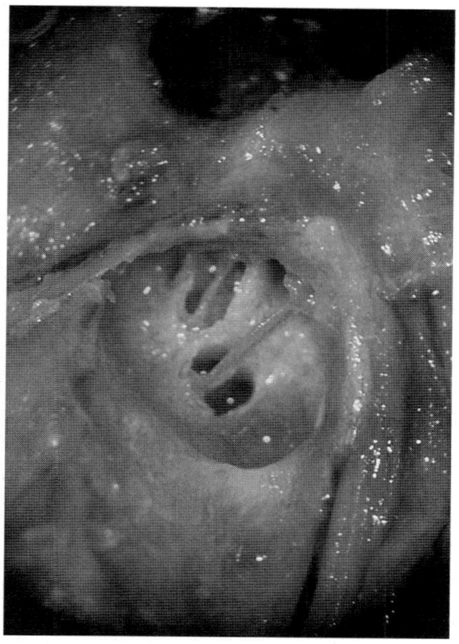

Fig. 32-15. Temporal bone dissection. The greater superficial petrosal n., the geniculate ganglion and the facial n. are exposed. The cochlea is opened for demonstration.

the geniculate ganglion. It divides the infralabyrinthine part of the facial nerve (2 mm) from the first part of the superior vestibular nerve.

- It is not advisable to expose the meatal foramen, since this is the narrowest portion of the fallopian canal, where the facial nerve is most delicate.
- It is the tumor which must be separated from the facial nerve, not vice versa. This reduces trauma to the nerve.
- A good landmark for the internal auditory canal is the external auditory canal. The two are perfectly aligned (Fig. 32-16).
- The labyrinthine part of the facial nerve lies parallel to the arcuate eminence.
- The subarcuate artery is found near the superior semicircular canal, lateral to the IAC.
- One way to identify Bill's bar without exposing the facial nerve is to follow the nerve backwards, from the geniculate ganglion to the IAC.
- After having exposed the IAC, it is helpful to penetrate between dura and bone with the House dissector, at both sides of the canal, to evaluate its size.
- Evoked potentials aid in predicting hearing preservation in intracanalicular tumors. The less they are altered, the greater the presence of a good preoperative conduction and the better the prognosis.
- Likewise, low electronystagmography test scores improve the prognosis for hearing preservation. This is because the ENG examines the function of the lateral semicircular canal. Part of the superior vestibular nerve fibers originates from its ampulla. A significant alteration in the reading hints at a SVN involvement. The tumors involving the SVN are more easily removed with the middle cranial fossa technique, since the SVN is lateral in the surgi-

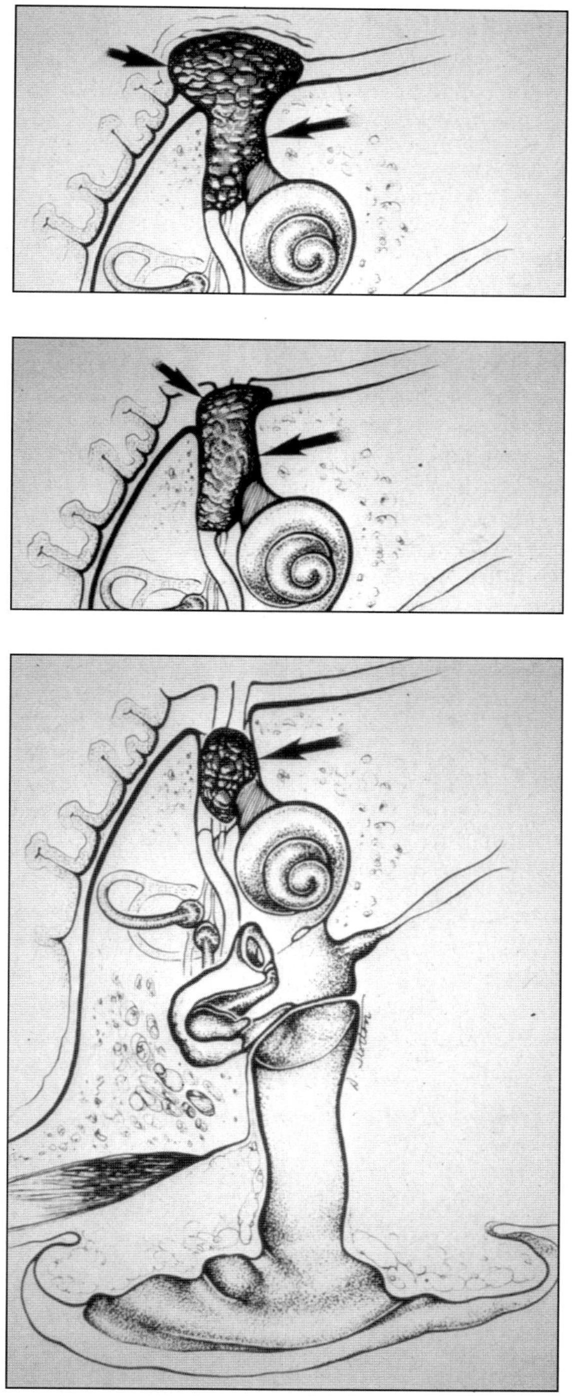

Fig. 32-16. Growing of the tumor from the IAC to the CPA.

cal perspective, whereas the IVN is medial to it. Their position means that they have less of a tendency to involve the cochlear nerve and they also tend to dislodge nerve VII anteriorly rather than infiltrating underneath it. In the HEI's data up to 1992, hearing was preserved in 48% of cases with a good EMG response, and in 64% of cases with a negative response.

- Since 1992, the percentage of hearing preservation has been improved by applying techniques of intraoperative acoustic nerve monitoring. Of 24 patients, 71% had unchanged hearing compared with preoperative levels. In 12% of cases some form of hearing was preserved, and in 17% of cases hearing was lost.
- When discussing the results of hearing preservation, it is important to keep in mind that in approx. 60% of patients, there is a deterioration in hearing of 20-30 dB 3-5 years after surgery. The cause is probably tied to the surgical alteration of the vascularization of the cochlea.
- If all vestibular nerve fibers are not removed with the tumor, postoperative instability is frequent due to a remaining labyrinthine function. A similar problem is seen in the retrosigmoid approach but not in the translabyrinthine approach, where vestibular function is destroyed. To prevent postoperative instability, the vestibular fibers must be completely sectioned. In any case, when we consider the advancements made in hearing preservation, temporary postoperative instability seems a fair and necessary price to pay.
- When the dura of the IAC is opened, the nerves are found on the surface of the fundus. They then proceed deeper in their path towards the porus, leaving more space for dissection. This general rule may naturally be altered by the tumor's development (Fig. 32-17).
- The middle fossa approach may be used for the closure of a hernia of the middle fossa dura in the mastoid bone, following a tympanoplasty. This approach avoids the risk of contamination in the mastoid bone (Sanna).
- *Antidromic stimulation of the GSPN.* Identification of the GSPN is not always easy. When working near the middle meningeal artery and the foramen ovale, bleeding is induced due to a nearby venous plexus. It is often useful to posteriorly identify the nerve which may be easily mistaken, in its diagonal path, with parallel lines of dura, or a small prominent petrous nerve. In these instances, electrical stimulation of the GSPN is helpful (Arriaga et al). What is believed to be the nerve is stimulated (Xomed Nerve Integrity Monitor), with an initial intensity of 1.0 mA, until an EMG activity is recorded. Then the intensity is lowered by degrees to 0.25, to receive confirmation of having effectively stimulated the great petrosal nerve and not a nearby structure. Once the GSPN has been identified, the usual steps are followed. The AA's experience has been that though some efferent visceral fibers do separate from the remaining facial nerve fibers, clinical practice shows that electrical stimulation of the GSPN is transmitted to facial nerve motor fibers, transversing the geniculate ganglion.

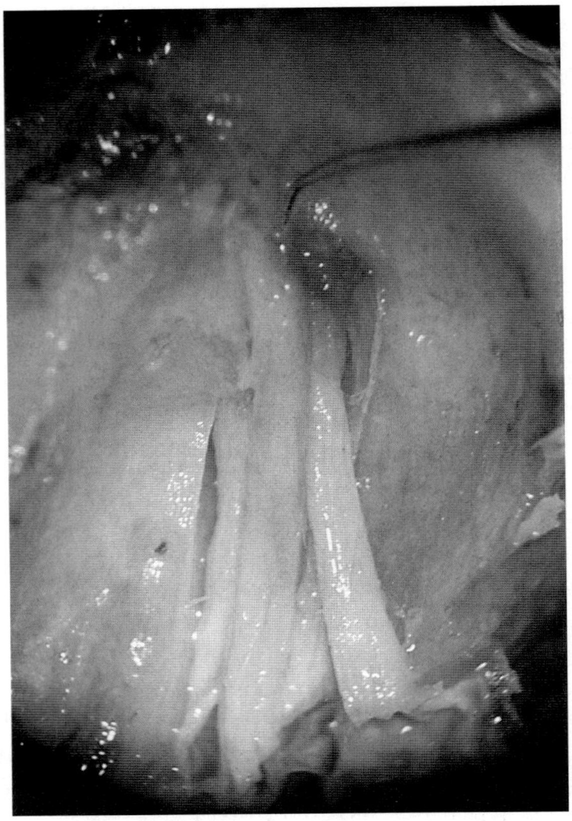

Fig. 32-17. The dura of the IAC is slit along the long axis of the canal at its posterior border, away from the facial nerve, which is anterior. The hook points out Bill's bar. Facial n. is on the left, vestibular n. is on the right.

THE ENLARGED MIDDLE FOSSA

Transpetrous approach through the middle fossa

This technique enlarges the scope of the middle fossa approach: it allows access to the posterior fossa, due to the removal of the petrous apex anteriorly to the IAC and medially to the carotid artery.

INDICATIONS

- Lesions of the cerebellopontine angle extended anteriorly into the cavernous sinus, along the prepontine region of the clivus, and even over the median line and superiorly through the tentorium and even over the anterior tentorial incisura (Arriaga, Brackmann, Hitselberger).
- Aneurisms of the basilar artery.

DISADVANTAGES

- Limited to lesions extended anteriorly to the IAC, since in these instances it is possible to preserve hearing. In lesions extending posterior to the IAC, the surgery may be combined with a suboccipital approach or with an extended retrolabyrinthine approach.
- Necessity of sectioning V3 to remove the bone from the tip of the petrous apex: torpidity of the cheek will result.
- Retraction of the temporal lobe. Greater problems are given by the retraction of the dominant lobe (the left in right-handed subjects). Temporary aphasia and/or epilepsy may occur. All patients should be treated with anticonvulsants beginning one week after surgery and continuing for 2 months.

SURGICAL TECHNIQUE

- The skin incision is the same as that of the middle fossa approach. The craniotomy is wider than normal: 5 cm along the zygomatic arch and 7 cm superior to it.
- The phases of IAC exposure are the same as those already described. An enlarged approach is used, however, giving access to the superior cerebellopontine angle at the clivus and the cavernous sinus (Fig. 32-18).
- Section of the middle meningeal artery at the foramen spinosum; the foramen is closed with bone wax. Section of the third branch of the trigeminal nerve at the foramen ovale. A greater retraction of the temporal lobe is thus possible for the anterior exposure.
- The petrous bone is drilled anterior to the IAC and anteromedial to the cochlea to the internal carotid artery at the foramen lacerum.
- Inferiorly we reach the superior petrosal sinus (SPS).
- Posteriorly the medial petrous bone is removed at the labyrinth.
- The temporal lobe is retracted with the self retaining retractor.
- Incision of the middle fossa dura, parallel and superior to the superior petrosal sinus, in the segment between the IAC and the V3.
- When necessary, the approach is amplified by sectioning the superior petrosal sinus between two clips and then incising the dura covering the posterior part of the petrous bone before bone removal.
- Incision of the tentorium in the gap opened by the incision of the SPS, posterior to the IVth cranial nerve, exposing nerves V, III, and VIII.

STRUCTURES TO PRESERVE

- The vein of Labbé, which enters the lateral sinus or the transverse sinus 2-3 mm behind the entrance of the superior petrosal sinus (SPS), should be preserved if possible. Sometimes it enters into the SPS. Given its variable point of confluence, it may be injured when sectioning the tentorium and the SPS. The lesion of the vein can lead to hemorrhagic necrotization of the temporal lobe.
- The IVth cranial nerve runs anterior and perforates the dura in the angle between the free margin and the attached margin of the tentorium in the posterior part of the triangle of the oculomotor nerve, and then enters the cavernous sinus.
- Nerve IV does not transverse the tentorium which is sectioned above the petrous apex. Its fragility and its length expose it to trauma when the dura is retracted anteriorly.
- Nerve V, more resistant and larger, is rarely damaged, but may be if inappropriate actions are taken.
- The IIIrd cranial nerve, before entering the cavernous sinus, is medial and anterior to IV. Following the superior petrosal sinus in an anterior direction, we reach its confluence in the cavernous sinus.

The bone to remove is found between the arcuate eminence posteriorly, the foramen spinosum superiorly, the trigeminal nerve anteriorly and the superior petrosal sinus inferiorly. In this quadrilateral, the cochlea is found (and preserved), as well as the GSPN nerve. The GSPN is sacrificed, to prevent traction on the facial nerve and to allow exposure of the internal carotid artery, which is parallel and medial to it.

The ICA is exposed in its horizontal intrapetrous tract from V3 to the posterior curve. It is important not to proceed posteriorly to the posterior curve because the basal turn of the cochlea lies approx. 1 mm from the artery.

Medial dissection extended to V3

The dissection may be medially extended to V3, after sectioning it. V3's section may be avoided by removing bone from the foramen ovale, found anteriorly and laterally, and moving the nerve towards the foramen.

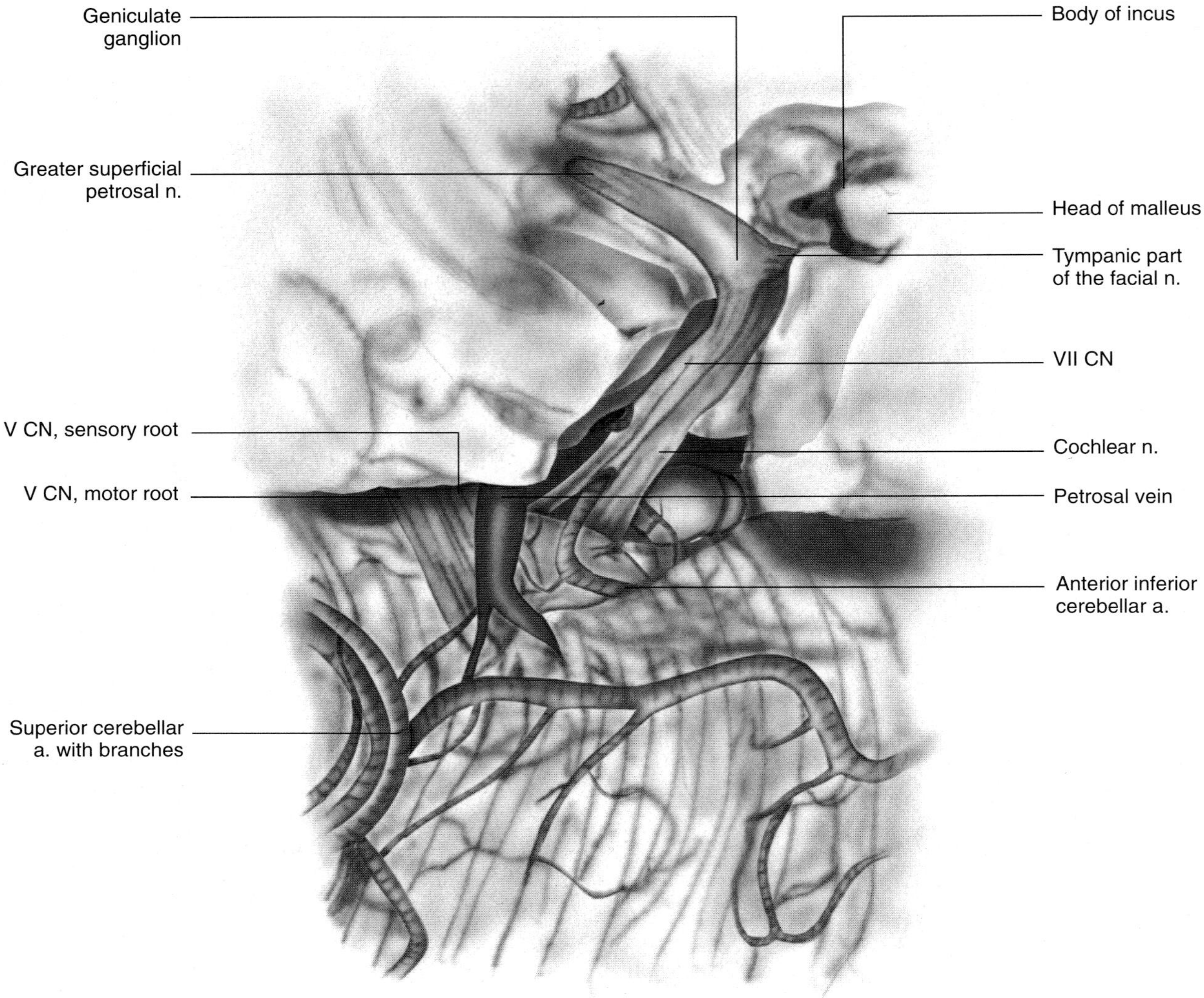

Fig. 32-18. Enlarged middle fossa approach. Exposure of the cerebellopontine angle.

Medial dissection extended to the SPS

- The bone between the superior petrosal sinus (sectioned to keep it out of the way) and the inferior petrosal sinus is removed. Here, maximal exposure of the posterior fossa dura has been obtained; from the IAC, to Meckel's cave, to the inferior petrosal sinus.
- The posterior fossa dura is safely exposed, because no structures transverse the dura from the IAC posteriorly to the petrosal apex anteriorly. Obviously, the IAC must be exposed before proceeding with the anterior and medial dissection.
- Once the dura has been opened, the CSF is aspirated. This helps to reduce endocranial pressure, along with hypotensive hyperventilation and the previous administration of Mannitol.
- The self retaining retractor may then be removed and the operation proceeds, using only the pressure of the dorsum of a Brackmann fenestrated suction-irrigator to move the temporal lobe. Thus the risk of complications due to excessive pressure on the temporal lobe is greatly reduced, since the pressure exerted by the aspirator is low and not continuous.

Closure

The dura is sutured under the temporal lobe. If zygomatic or mastoid cells have been opened, they are now closed with bone wax. Abdominal fat is positioned in the middle fossa floor, the bone plate is replaced, and the wound is closed in layers.

OTHER APPLICATIONS

The enlarged middle fossa approach is useful not only for neuroma removal, but also for other operations, such as neurovascular decompression in patients with hemifacial spasms, and/or vestibular neurectomy in patients with Mèniére's Disease. Extradural pathologies of the middle fossa can be treated in the following ways:

- Decompression or grafting of the facial nerve
- Repair of a CSF fistula due to fracture of the petrosal bone
- Removal of pseudotumors such as cholesterol granulomas, or penetrating cholesteatomas

This approach may be used to merely explore internal auditory canal structures and the cerebellopontine angle, though in these instances we prefer the retrosigmoid approach.

DECOMPRESSION OF THE INTERNAL AUDITORY CANAL

In patients with von Recklinghausen's Disease, -NF2-, tumors of the bilateral acoustic nerve are seen. If untreated, this pathology leads to total hearing loss. On the other hand, middle fossa tumor removal, even when performed in the initial stages, can rarely preserve hearing. This is because von Recklinghausen tumors are very aggressive and almost always involve the cochlear nerve, and frequently the cochlea itself. One compromise between the two therapeutic options is the decompression of the internal auditory canal.

- The IAC is identified with the methods described above. Care is taken to preserve the cochlea and the superior semicircular canal, which is preferably not blue lined. It is unnecessary to medially expose the IAC by 270°, since it is sufficient to free the superior part of the IAC -the roof- from the bone.
- The dura is incised along this structure. This gives the tumor an outlet for upward expansion. Thus the pressure exerted by the tumor in its growth on the cochlear nerve and the inner ear vascularization is diminished (Gadre).

The tumor's evolution is evaluated with an MRI 6 months after surgery, and then annually for 3-5 years.

Besides the technique above described, we treat NF-2 patients in the following way:

Surgery without hearing preservation

- Observation to make sure the patient's health is not at risk (i.e. brainstem compression, hydrocephalus); surgery if necessary, followed by auditory brainstem implant (ABI).

Surgery to preserve hearing

- Middle fossa surgery or transmeatal transigmoid approach. We do not perform partial surgery, because in this particular pathology, tumors grow very rapidly and hearing would deteriorate.
- If there is successful hearing preservation, another operation is performed after 6 months on the other ear.
- If the first operation is unsuccessful, the patient is observed periodically.

TOTAL DECOMPRESSION OF THE FACIAL NERVE

- In cases of idiopathic paralysis (Bell), decompressing surgery must be performed as soon as the summation potentials reach 10% or less than normal, within two weeks of the onset of the paralysis.
- In cases of Herpes zoster oticus, surgery must be performed when signs of inner ear suffering are seen, and in acute otitis media, when the summation potentials are reduced to 10% or less than the norm, even after medical therapy and/or miringotomy. (Fisch).

An S-shaped incision is made which includes the postauricular and temporal areas. The surgical technique is the same as in a middle cranial fossa, with the addition of the opening of the epitympanum (Figs. 32-19, 32-20, 32-21).

TREATMENT OF FACIAL NERVE TUMORS

The middle fossa approach can be used for the treatment of facial nerve tumors. It provides access to the facial nerve in the IAC. The tegmen bone is removed so that the geniculate ganglion and the horizontal facial nerve up to the midtympanic part are exposed. When additional exposure of the facial nerve is needed, this approach can be combined with a transmastoid approach, with opening of the facial recess. Facial nerve tumors can be hemangiomas, which are extraneural in origin and neuromas which are intraneural. Hemangiomas can be removed with sharp dissection, developing a plane between the nerve and the tumor, preserving the continuity of the facial nerve.

- The greater auricular nerve is a good donor for a nerve graft because of its similar diameter, adequate length and easy access in the surgical field.
- The nerve graft must be sutured with the facial nerve in a proximal to proximal and distal to distal fashion. In this way the larger part of the graft matches with the larger part of the nerve.
- The nerve is like a banana (Mark May). The excess fibrous tissue and epineurium must be removed from the nerve stumps. The ends of the graft are then trimmed sharply. The nerve stumps must not be cut with all the epineurium. The epineurium is like the sheath of a banana while the nerve is the banana. Cutting the sheath together with the banana places pressure on the fruit. Likewise, cutting the nerve with all the epineurium exposes the endoneurium to axonotmesis with a reduced recovery potential (see chapter 13).
- In the surgical manipulation, traction on the nerve must always be avoided, since it alters the nerve vascularity and subjects the nerve to internal disruption and scarring. It may be better to

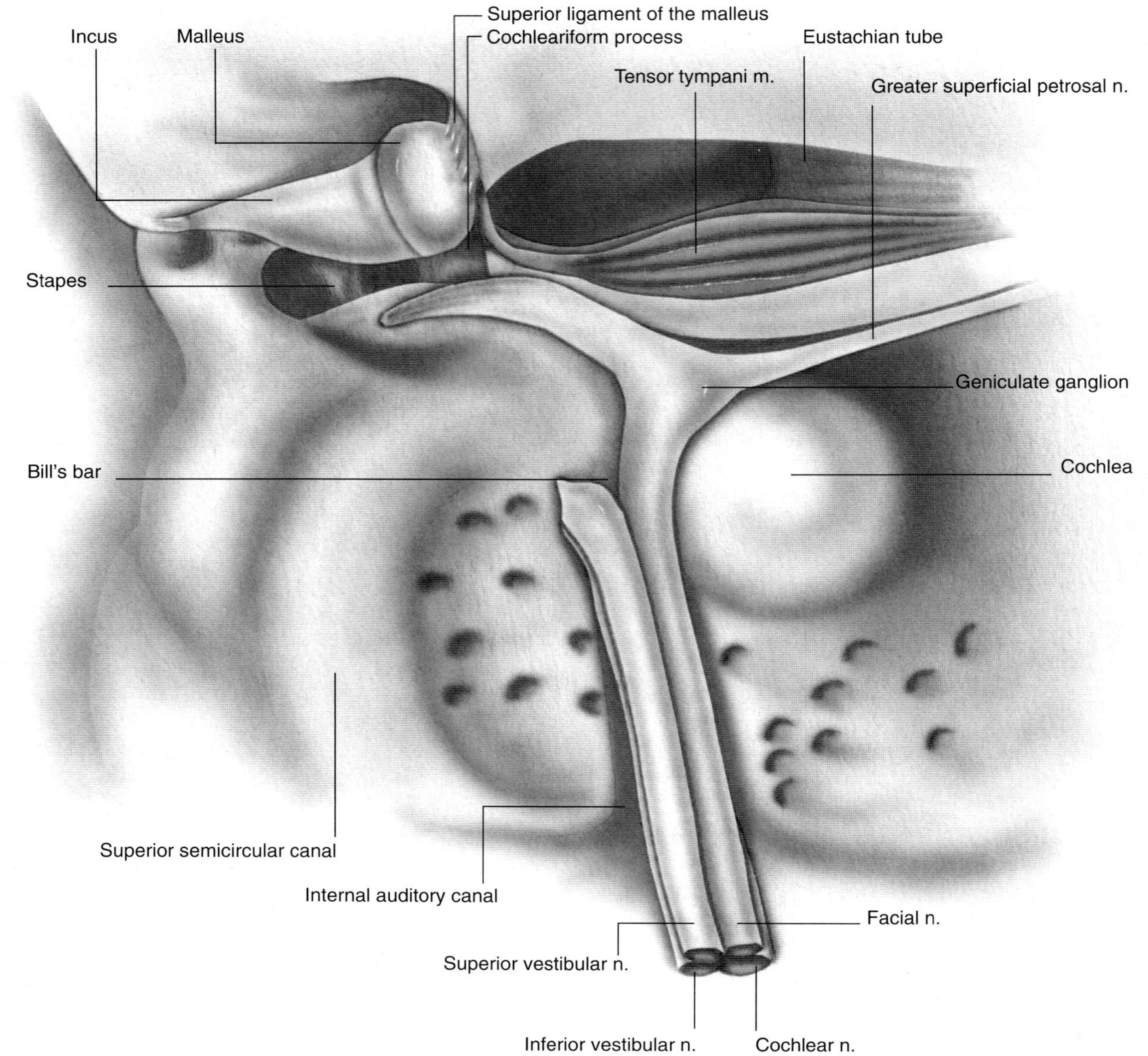

Fig. 32-19. Middle fossa approach. Left ear. The IAC has been opened and the nerves exposed. The epitympanum has been exposed to follow the facial nerve into the middle ear.

electively transect the nerve and successively graft it then to place aggressive traction on the nerve. Rerouting can be useful in CPA surgery, when lesions to n. VII occurr, since it gains additional nerve length and allows primary anastomosis.

- The nerve vascularization is altered by extensive nerve mobilization. It is important to prevent nerve dessication during surgery, by providing a moist environment. When a long nerve mobilization is required, the nerve should be positioned in a muscle flap at surgery's end (e.g. transferred temporalis muscle) to improve the nerve's revascularization.
- When sutures are used for grafting, the suture length is trimmed to 15 cm, to make it easier the control under the microscope.
- When dealing with tumors of the facial nerve, frozen sections of the nerve stump are necessary before grafting, to ensure complete tumor removal and to ensure that no residual tumor impedes axonal regrowth.

TOTAL FACIAL NERVE DECOMPRESSION AFTER LONGITUDINAL FRACTURES OF THE TEMPORAL BONE

- In cases of facial paralysis subsequent to fractures of the temporal bone, middle fossa surgery for the decompression and/or repair of the facial nerve must be performed in the following situations (May):
- Sudden and complete onset.
- Summation potentials reduce to 10% or less of the norm after 5 days.

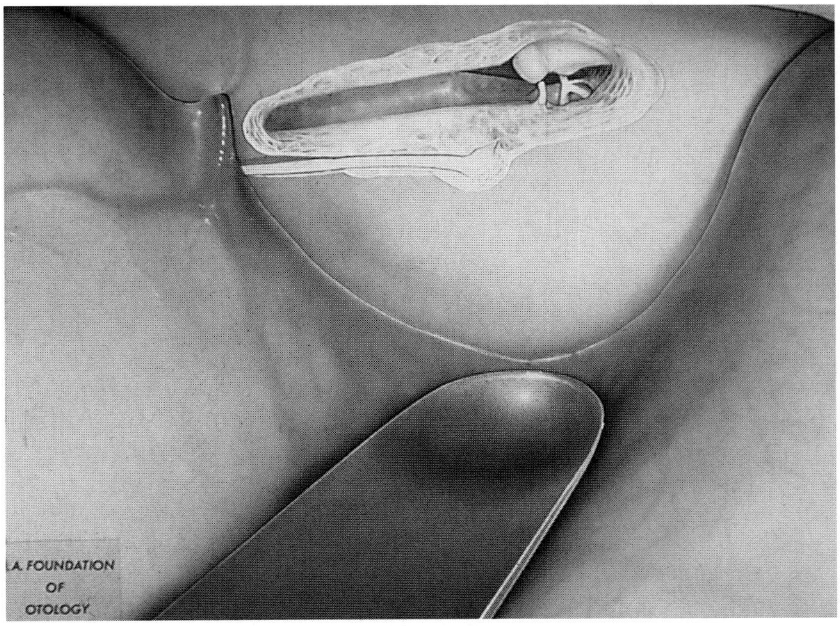

Fig. 32-20. The superior petrosal n. is located medial to the middle meningeal artery and is followed posteriorly up to the geniculate ganglion. The facial nerve can be followed laterally, posteriorly and inferiorly into the middle ear space. The canal of the tensor tympani muscle and the eustachian tube have been opened for demonstration.

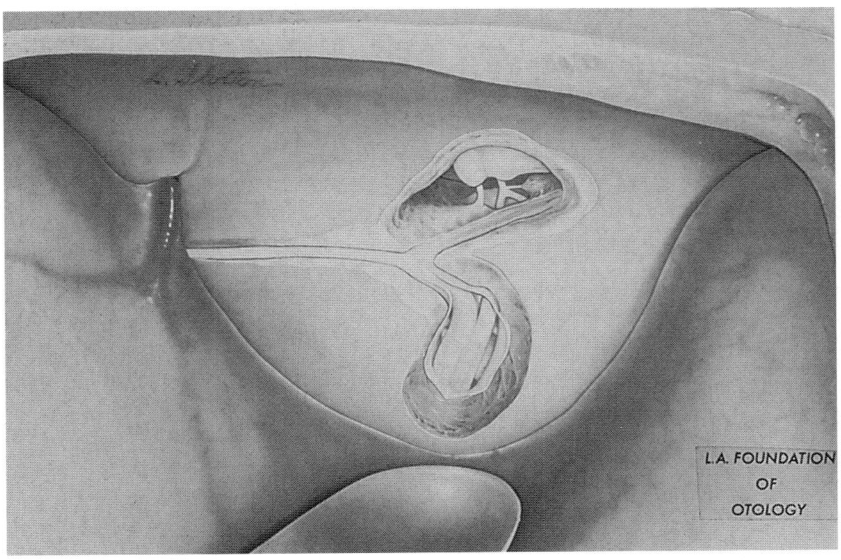

Fig. 32-21. The greater superficial petrosal n. is followed posteriorly to the geniculate ganglion and then medially and superiorly into the IAC.

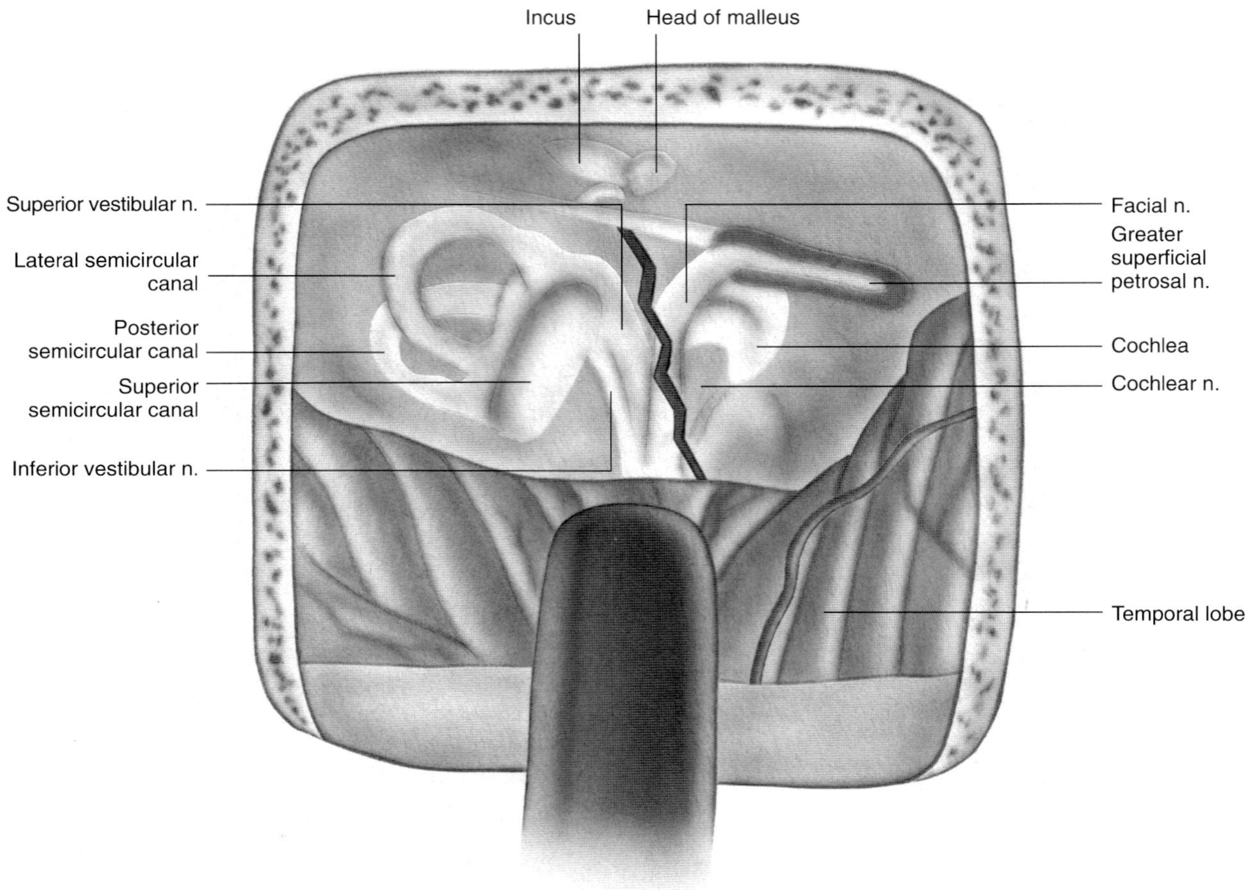

Fig. 32-22. Middle fossa approach can be used for temporal bone fractures involving the internal auditory canal and the facial nerve. Adapted from Miglets AW, Paparella MM, Saunders WH: Atlas of ear surgery, The C:V Mosby Company, 1986.

- CT shows damage to the fallopian canal; or, the fallopian canal is not damaged, but after 6 months facial function has not been recovered (Figs. 32-22, 32-23, 32-24, 32-25, 32-26).

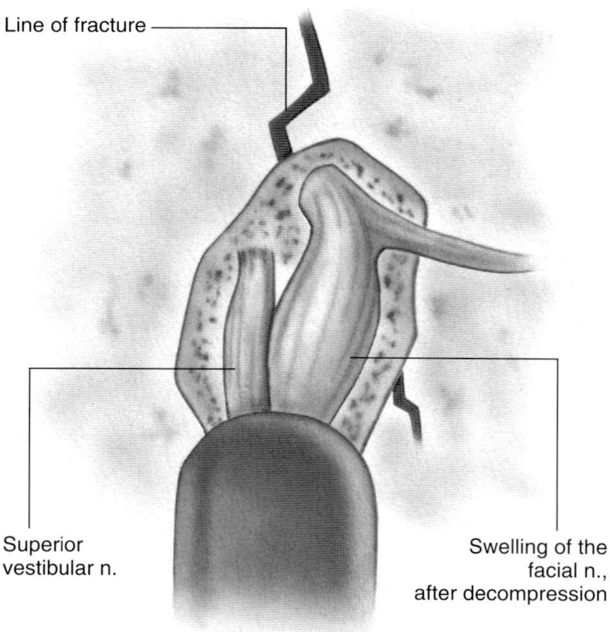

Fig. 32-23. Facial nerve, edematous, is decompressed up to the fundus of the IAC.

Fig. 32-24. Facial nerve is found lacerated. When laceration is >33% of the transversal extension of the nerve, we complete the transection and use a free graft (see chapter 11).

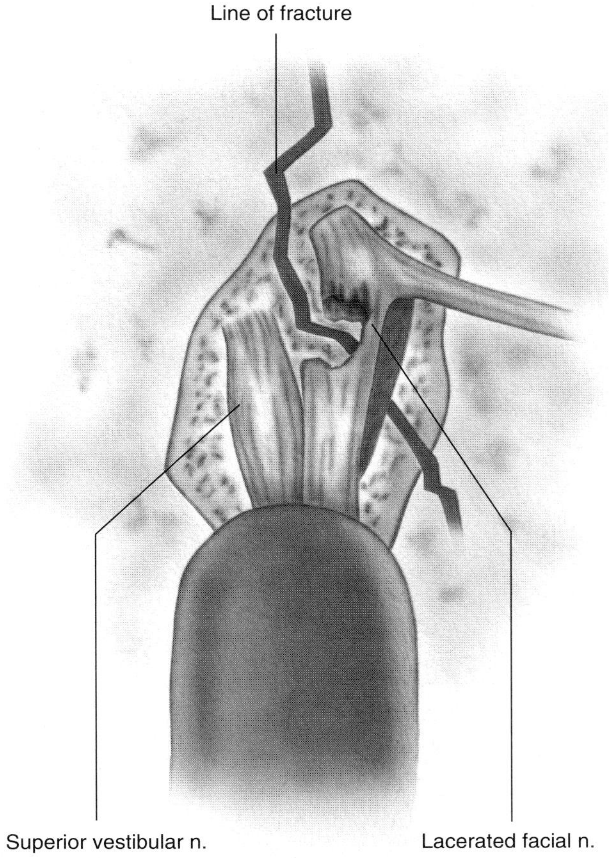

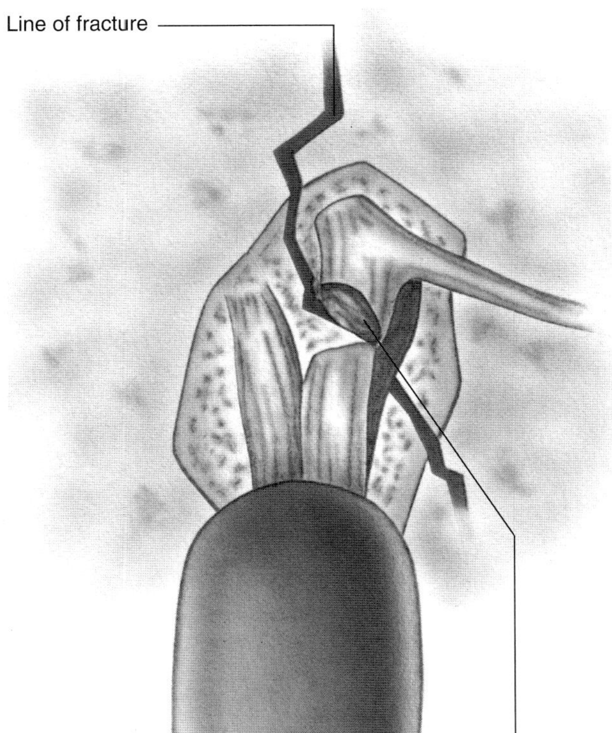

Fig. 32-25. Complete transection of the facial nerve.

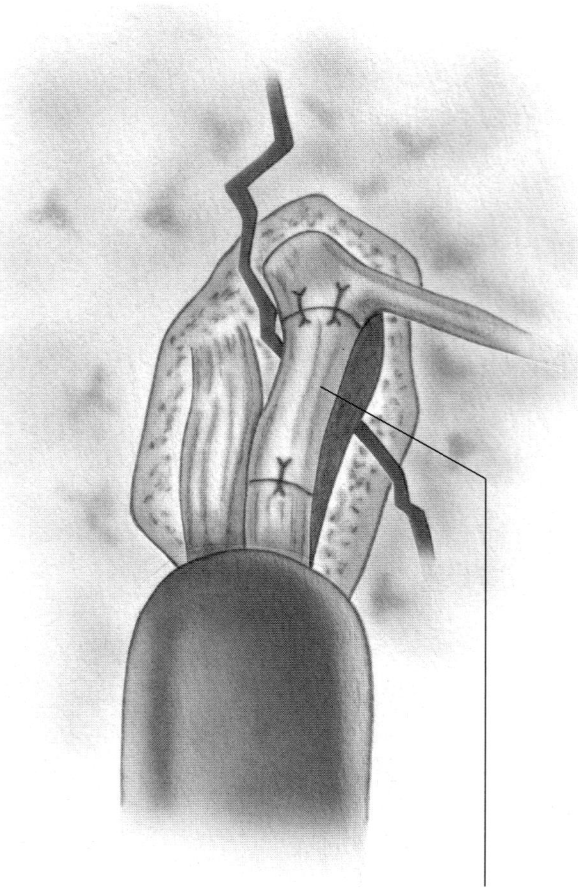

Fig. 32-26. When there is loss of substance and no termino-terminal suture can be used, the facial nerve is grafted with the greater auricular or sural nerve.

REFERENCES

Al-Mefty O, Fox JL, Smith RR: Petrosal approach for petroclival meningiomas. Neurosurgery 22: 510-517, 1988.

Andrews JC, Martin NA, Black K, Honrubia VF, Becker DP: Middle cranial fossa transtemporal approach to the intrapetrous internal carotid artery. Skull Base Surg 1:142-146, 1991.

Aristegui M, Cokkeser Y, Saleh E, Naguib M, Landolfi M, Taibah A, et al: Surgical anatomy of the extended middle cranial fossa approach. Skull Base Surg 4;188-95, 1994.

Arriaga MA, Brackmann DE, Hitselberger WE: Extended middle fossa resection of petroclival and cavernous sinus neoplasms. Laryngoscope 103:693-698, 1993.

Arriaga M, Haid MR, Masel D: Antidromic stimulation of the greater superficial petrosal nerve in middle fossa surgery. Laringoscope 105: 102-105, 1995.

Berliner KI, Shelton C, Hitselberger WE, Luxford WM: Acoustic tumors: Effect of surgical removal on tinnitus. Am J Otol 13:13, 1992.

Bochenek Z, Kukwa A: An extended approach through the middle cranial fossa to the internal auditory meatus and the cerebello-pontine angle. Acta Otolaryngol Stockh 80:410, 1975.

Brackmann DE: Middle cranial fossa approach. In House WF, Luetje CM eds: Acoustic Tumors, Vol 2: Management. Baltimore, University Park Press, 1979, p 15.

Bailey BJ, Johnson JT, Kohut RL, et al: Eds. J.B. Lippincott Co. Philadelphia. p. 1812, 1993.

Brackmann DE: Modifications of the middle fossa approach in acoustic neuroma surgery. Presentation to the Annual Meeting of the American Neurotology Society, Los Angeles, Calif, April 17. 1993.

Brackmann DE, Anderson RG: Cholesteatomas of the cerebellopontine angle. In Silverstein H, Norrell H eds: Neurological Surgery of the Ear. 1979, pp 340-344.

Cantu RC, Ojemann RG: Glucosteroid treatment of keratin meningitis following removal of a fourth ventricle epidermoid tumor. J Neurol Neurosurg Psychiatry 31: 75, 1968.

Dautheribes M, Migueis A, Vital JM, et al: Anatomical basis of the extended subtemporal approach to the cerebellopontine angle: Its value and limitations. Surg Radiol Anat 11:187, 1989.

De La Cruz A: The transcochlear approach to meningiomas and cholesteatomas of the cerebellopontine angle. In Brackmann DE ed: Neurological Surgery of the Ear and Skull Base. New York, Raven Press, 1982, pp 353-360.

De La Cruz A: Transcochlear approach to lesions of the cerebellopontine angle and clivus. Rev Laryngol Otol Rhinol Bord 1021-2: 33-36, 1981.

Eagleton WP: Unlocking the petrous pyramid for localized bulbar pontile meningitis secondary to suppuration of the petrous apex. Arch Otolaryngol Head Neck Surg 13: 386-422, 1931.

Fisch U, Kumar, A: Infratemporal surgery of the skull base. In Rand R: Microneurosurgery. Mosby, St. Louis 1985 pp.398-420.

Fisch U, Mattox D: Microsurgery of the Skull Base. New York, Thieme Medical Publishers, 1988.

Fisch U, Pillsbury HC: Infratemporal fossa approach to lesions in the temporal bone and base of the skull. Arch Otolaryngol Head Neck Surg 105: 99-107, 1979.

Fisch U, Pillsbury HC, Sasaki CT: Infratemporal approach to the skull base. In Sasaki CT, McCabe BF, Kirchner JA: Surgery of the Skull Base. Lippincott, Philadelphia 1984 pp. 141-160.

Fisch U, Pillsbury HC: Infratemporal fossa approach to lesions in the temporal bone and base of the skull. Arch. Otolaryngol 105: 99-107, 1979.

Fisch U: Current surgical treatment of intratemporal facial palsy. Clin Plast Surg 6: 377-388, 1979.

Fisch U: Diagnostic studies on idiopathic facial palsy. In Shambaugh GE, Shea JJ: Proceedings of the Shambaugh Fifth International Workshop on Middle Ear Microsurgery and Fluctuant Hearing Loss. Strode, Huntsville, Alabama 1977 pp.219-224.

Fisch U: Diagnostic studies on idiopathic facial palsy. In: Microsurgery and Fluctuating Hearing Loss. Strode, Huntsville, Alabama. Proeeedings of the Shambaugh Fifth International Workshop on Middle Ear Microsurgery and Fluctuant Hearing Loss, 219-224, 1976.

Fisch U: Excision of Scarpa's ganglion. Arch Oto-Laryngol 97: 147-149, 1973.

Fisch U: Facial nerve management in surgery of temporal bone and skull base. In Portmann, M: Facial Nerve. Masson, Paris 1985 pp.73-80.

Fisch U: Facial paralysis in fractures of the petrous bone. Laryngoscope 84: 2141-2154, 1974.

Fisch U: L'anatomie chirurgicale du systeme arteriel du conduit auditif interne chez l'homme. Rev Laryngol 89: 659-671, 1968.

Fisch U: Lateral infratemporal fossa approach to the skull base. In Chretien PB, Decker PC: Head and Neck Cancer, Vol.l. Mosby, St. Louis 1985 pp.251-262.

Fisch U: Management of intratemporal facial palsy. Advanc Tech Stand. Neurosurg.7: 215-238, 1980.

Fisch U: Maximal nerve excitability testing vs electroneuronography. Arch Otolaryngol 106: 352 357, 1980.

Fisch U: Operations on the facial nerve in its labyrinthine and meatal course. In Miehlke, A: Surgery of the Facial Nerve. Urban & Schwarzenberg, Munchen 1973 pp. 175-205.

Fisch U: Otochirurgische behandlung des akustikusneurinomes. In Plester D, Wende S, Nakayama N: Kleinhirn-Bruckenwinkel Tumoren. Springer, Berlin 1978 pp. 196-214.
Fisch U: Results of surgery versus conservative treatment in Bell's palsy and herpes zoster oticus. In Graham, MD, House, WF: Disorders of the Facial Nerve. Raven Press, New York 1982 pp.273-279.
Fisch U: Surgery for Bell's palsy. Arch. Otolaryngol 107: 1-11, 1981.
Fisch U: The surgical anatomy of the so-called internal auditory artery. X. Nobel Symposium. Almquist & Wiksell, Stockholm 1968 pp. 121-126.
Fisch U: The vestibular response following unilateral vestibular neurectomy. Acta Otolaryngol 76: 229-238,1973.
Fisch U: Total facial nerve decompression and electroneuronography. In Silverstein H, Norell H: Neurological Surgery of the Ear. Aesculapius, Birmingham 1977 pp.21-23.
Fisch U: Transtemporal extradural access to the internal auditory meatus. In Naumann, HH: Head and Neck Surgery, vol. III. Thieme, Stuttgart 1982 pp.465-507.
Fisch U: Transtemporal surgery of the internal auditory canal. Advanc Otolaryngol 17: 203-240, 1970.
Fisch U: Transtemporal Surgery of the Internal Auditory Canal: Report of 92 Cases. Adv Otorhinolaryngol, 17:202-240, 1970.
Fisch U: Vestibular and cochlear neurectomy. Trans Amer Acad Ophthalmol Otolaryngol 78: 252-255, 1974.
Fisch U: Vestibular nerve section. Amer J of Otology 5: 543-545, 1984.
Fisch U: Chirurgie im inneren gehorgang und an benaehbarten strukturen. In Naumann HH: Kopf- und Halsehirurgie: Ohrregion, vol. III. Thieme, Stuttgart 1976 pp.457-544.
Fisch U: Facial nerve grafting. Otolaryngol Clin N Amer 7: 517-529, 1974.
Fisch U: Meato-myosynangiosis. Acta Oto-Rhino-Laryngol Belg 30: 117, 1976.
Fisch U: Surgical treatment of vertigo. J Laryngol Otol 90: 75-86,1976.
Fisch U: The middle fossa approach to the internal auditory meatus. In Ballantyne, J: Operative Surgery. Ear. Butterworth, London 1976, pp. 179-192.
Fisch U: Transtemporaler, extraduraler zugang zum inneren gehorgang In Naumann, HH: Kopf- und Halsehirurgie, vol. III. Thieme, Stuttgart 1976 pp.457-499.
Fisch U: Lacrimation. In Fisch U: Facial Nerve Surgery. Aesculapius, Birmingham 1977 pp.147-153
Frerebeau PH, Benezech J, Uziel A, et al: Hearing preservation after acoustic neurinoma operation. Neurosurgery 21:197, 1987.
Gantz BJ, Parnes LS, Harker LA, et al: Middle cranial fossa acoustic neuroma excision: Results and complications. Ann Otol Rhinol Laryngol 95:454, 1986.
Garcia-Ibanez E, Garcia-Ibanez JL: Middle fossa vestibular neurectomy: A report of 373 cases. Otolaryngol Head Neck Surg 88:486, 1980.
Gardner G, Robertson JH: Hearing preservation in unilateral acoustic neuroma surgery. Ann Otol Rhinol Laryngol 97:55, 1988.
Glasscock M III, McKennan KX, Levine SC: Acoustic neuroma surgery: The results of hearing conservation surgery. Laryngoscope 97:785, 1987
Glasscock ME III, Hays JW, Josey AF, et al: Middle fossa approach for acoustic tumor removal and hearing preservation. In Brackmann DE ed: Neurological Surgery of the Ear and Skullbase. New York, Raven Press, 1982, p 223.
Glasscock ME III, Hays JW, Miller GW, et al: Preservation of hearing in tumors of the internal auditory canal and cerebellopontine angle. Laryngoscope 88:43, 1978.
Glasscock ME, Poe DS, Johnson GD: Hearing preservation in surgery of cerebellopontine angle tumors. In Fisch U, Valavanis A, Yasargil MG eds: Neurological Surgery of the Ear and Skull base. Amsterdam, Kugler & Ghedini, 1989, p 207.
Glasscock ME, Woods CI, Jackson CG, et al: Management of bilateral acoustic tumors. Laryngoscope 99:475, 1989.
Guidetti B, Gagliardi FM: Epidermoid and dermoid cysts. J Neurosurg 47: 12-18, 1977.
Haid T, Wigand ME: Advantages of the enlarged middle cranial fossa approach in acoustic neuroma surgery. Acta Otolaryngol: 112, 387-407, 1992.
Harker LA, McCabe BF: Iowa results of acoustic neuroma operations. Laryngoscope 88:1904, 1978.
Hitselberger WE, Horn KL, Hankinson HL, et al: The middle fossa transpetrous approach for petroclival meningiomas. Skull Base Surg 33:130-135, 1993.
Horn KL, Hankinson HL, Erasmus MD, et al: The modified transcochlear approach to the cerebellopontine angle. Otolaryngol Head Neck Surg 104: 37-41, 1991.
House F, Hitselberger WE: The middle fossa approach for removal of small acoustic tumors. Acta Otolaryngol Stockh 67:413, 1969.
House WF: Surgical exposure of the internal auditory canal and its contents through the middle cranial fossa. Laryngoscope, 71:1363-1385, 1961.
House WF, De La Cruz A: Transcochlear approach to the petrous apex and clivus. Trans Am Acad Ophthalmol Otolaryngol 84: 927-931, 1977.
House WF, Gardner Gl, Hughes RL: Middle cranial fossa approach to acoustic tumor surgery. Arch Otolaryngol Head Neck Surg 88:631, 1968.
House WF, Hitselberger WE, Horn KL: The middle fossa transpetrous approach to the anterior-superior cerebellopontine angle. Am J Otol 7: 1-4, 1986.
House WF, Hitselberger WE: The transcochlear approach to the skull base. Arch Otolaryngol Head Neck Surg 102: 334-342, 1976.
House WF: Middle cranial fossa approach to the petrous pyramid. Report of 50 cases. Arch Otolaryngol Head Neck Surg 78:460, 1963.
House WF: Middle cranial fossa approach to the petrous pyramid: A report of 50 cases. Arch Otolaryngol Head Neck Surg 78: 406-469, 1963.
House WF: Surgical exposure of the internal auditory canal and its contents through the middle cranial fossa. Laryngoscope 71: 1363-1385, 1961.
Fisch U: Analysis of surgical treatment for Mèniére's disease. In Vosteen, KH: Mèniére's Disease. Thieme, Stuttgart 1981 pp.215-219.
Josey AF, Glasscock ME, Jackson CG: Preservation of hearing in acoustic tumor surgery: Audiologic indicators. Ann Otol Rhinol Laryngol 97: 626, 1988.
Kanzaki J, Ogaura K, Shiobara R, et al: Hearing preservation in acoustic neuroma surgery and postoperative findings. Acta Otolaryngol Stockh 107:474, 1989.
Kanzaki J, Kunihiro T, Ouchi T, Ogawa K, Shiobara R, Toya S: Intracranial reconstruction of the facial nerve. Clinical observation. Acta Otolaryngol Suppl Stockh 487: 85-90, 1991.
Kanzaki J, Ogawa K, Ouchi T, Shiobara R, Toya S: Hearing preservation in acoustic neuroma surgery by the extended middle cranial fossa method. Acta Otolaryngol Suppl Stockh 487: 22-9, 1991.
Kanzaki J, Ogawa K, Tsuchihashi N, Inoue Y, Yamamoto M, Ikeda S: Postoperative complications in acoustic neuroma surgery by the extended middle cranial fossa approach. Acta Otolaryngol Suppl Stockh 487: 75-79, 1991.
Kanzaki J, Ogawa K, Yamamoto M, Ikeda T, Shiobara R, Toya S: Results of acoustic neuroma surgery by the extended middle cranial fossa approach. Acta Otolaryngol Suppl Stockh. 487: 17-21, 1991.

Kanzaki J, Shiobara R, Toya S: Classification of the extended middle cranial fossa approach. Acta Otolaryngol Suppl Stockh 487: 6-16, 1991.

Kartush JM, Kemink JL, Graham MD: The arcuate eminence: Topographic orientation in middle cranial fossa surgery. Ann Otol Rhinol Laryngol 94:25, 1985.

Kawase T, Toya S, Shiobara R, et al: Transpetrosal approach for aneurysms of the lower basilar artery. J Neurosurg 63: 857-861, 1985.

Kemink JL, LaRouere MJ, Kileny RP, et al: Hearing preservation following suboccipital removal of acoustic neuromas. Laryngoscope 100:597, 1990.

Kumar, A, Fisch U: The infratemporal fossa approach for lesions of the skull base. Advanc Tech Stand Neurosurg 10: 188-200, 1983.

Kurze T, Doyle IB Jr: Extra dural intracranial middle fossa approach to the internal auditory canal. J Neurosurg 19:1033, 1962.

Kwartler JA, Luxford WM, Atkins J, et al: Facial nerve monitoring in acoustic tumor surgery. Otolaryngol Head Neck Surg 104:814-817, 1991.

Landolfi M, Aristegui M, Taibah A, Russo A, Saleh E, Sanna M: Extended middle cranial fossa approach: a morphometric analysis. Acta Otorhinolaryngol Ital. Mar-Apr; 142: 127-134, 1994.

Lang J: Clinical Anatomy of the Posterior Cranial Fossa and Its Foramina. New York, Thieme Medical Publishers, 1988.

Leonetti JP, Smith PG, Linthicum FH: The petrous carotid artery: Anatomic relationships in skull base surgery. Otolarvngol Head Neck Surg 102: 3-12, 1990.

Mafee MF: MRI and CT in the evaluation of acquired and congenital cholesteatomas of the temporal bone. J Otolaryngol 224: 239-248, 1993.

Mangham CA, Skalabrin TA: Indications for hearing preservation in acoustic tumor surgery. Presented at the Annual Meeting of the American Neurotology Society, Kona, Hawaii, May 4, 1991.

Metson R: Facial nerve evoked potentials in the cat. Otolaryngol Head Neck Surg 98:130-132, 1988.

Miller E, Crockard HA: Transoral transclival removal of anteriorly placed meningiomas at the foramen magnum. Neurosurgery 20: 966-968, 1987.

Nadol JB Jr, Levine R, Ojemann RG, et al: Preservation of hearing in surgical removal of acoustic neuromas of the internal auditory canal and cerebellar pontine angle. Laryngoscope 97:1287, 1987.

Nager GT: Epidermoids involving the temporal bone: Clinical radiological, and pathological aspects. Laryngoscope 2Suppl 1-22, 1975.

Ogawa K, Inoue Y, Yamamoto M, Ikeda S, Kanzaki J: Surgical anatomy for the extended middle cranial fossa approach. Acta Otolaryngol Suppl Stockh 487: 41-47, 1991.

Ono M, Rhoton AL, et al: Microsurgical anatomy of the region of the tentorial incisura. J Neurosurg 60: 365-399, 1984.

Parisier SC: The middle cranial fossa approach to the internal auditory canal—an anatomical study stressing critical distances between surgical landmarks. Laryngoscope, 87Suppl. 4. Pt. 2: 1-20, 1977.

Paullus WS, Pait TG, Rhoton AL: Microsurgical exposure of the petrous portion of the carotid artery. J Neurosurg 47: 713-726, 1977.

Pensak ML, Lovern HV, Keith RW: Subtemporal transpetrosal approach to the petrous apex. Presented at the American Otological Society, 125th Meeting. Marriott Desert Springs Resort, Palm Desert, CA, April 12 and 13, 1992.

Rosomoff HL: The subtemporal transtentorial approach to the cerebellopontine angle. Laryngoscope 81:1448, 1971.

Ruenes R, De la Cruz A: Otologic Radiology, House Ear Institute and MacMillan Publishing Company, p. 1-183, 1986.

Sanna M, Zini C, Mazzoni A, et al: Hearing preservation in acoustic neuroma surgery. Middle fossa versus suboccipital approach. Am J Otol 8:500, 1987.

Sekhar LN, Schramm VL, Jones NF: Subtemporal-preauricular infratemporal fossa approach to large lateral and posterior cranial base neoplasms. J Neurosurg 67: 488-499, 1987.

Shelton C, Brackmann DE, House WF, et al: Acoustic tumor surgery: Prognostic factors in hearing conservation. Arch Otolaryngol Head Neck Surg 115:1213, 1989.

Shelton C, Hitselberger WE: The treatment of small acoustic tumors: Now or later? Laryngoscope 101:925, 1991.

Shelton MF, Brackmann DE, House WF, Hitselberger WE. Middle fossa acoustic tumor surgery: results in 106 cases. Laryngoscope 1989:99:405-408, 1972.

Shiobara R, Ohira T, Kanzaki J, Toya S: A modified extended middle cranial fossa approach for acoustic nerve tumors: Results of 125 operations. J Neurosurg 68: 358-365, 1988.

Spetzler RF, Daspit CP, Pappas CTE: Combined approach for lesions involving the cerebellopontine angle and skull base: Experience with 30 cases. Skull Base Surg 1: 226-234, 1991.

Strauss C, Fahlbusch R, Romstock J, Schramm J, Watanabe E, Taniguchi M, Berg M: Delayed hearing loss after surgery for acoustic neuromas: clinical and electrophysiological observations. Neurosurgery: 559, 28-30, 1991.

Velut SJ, Jan M: Anterior petrosectomy during approach to the petroclival area. In Schmidek HtI ed: Meningiomas and Their Surgical Management. Philadelphia, WB Saunders, 1991, pp 435-450.

Wade PJ, House WF: Hearing preservation in patients with acoustic neuromas via the middle fossa approach. Otolaryngol Head Neck Surg 92:184, 1984.

Wigand ME, Haid T, Berg M, et al: Extended middle cranial fossa approach for acoustic neuroma surgery. Skull Base Surg 1: 183-187, 1991.

Wigand ME, Haid T, Berg M, Rettinger G: The enlarged transtemporal approach to the cerebello-pontine angle: technique and indications. Acta Otorhinol Ital 2:571-82, 1982.

Wigand ME, Haid T, Berg M: The enlarged middle cranial fossa approach for surgery of the temporal bone and of the cerebellopontine angle. Arch Otorhinolaryngol 246:299, 1989.

Wigand ME, Haid T, Berg M: The enlarged middle cranial fossa approach for surgery of the temporal bone and of the cerebellopontine angle. Arch Otol Rhinol Laryngol 246: 299, 1989.

Yamakawa K, Shitara N, Genka S, et al: Clinical course and surgical prognosis of 33 cases of intracranial epidermoid tumors. Neurosurgery 244: 568-573, 1989.

Yasargil MG, Abernathy CD, Sarioglu AC: Microneurosurgical treatment of intracranial dermoid and epidermoid tumors. Neurosurgery 244: 561-567, 1989.

33

Lateral skull base surgery. Approaches centered on the temporal bone

It is essential to tailor the approach to the lesions. It means leaving the elementary stages behind and starting to control the lesions with your mind.

SANNA M.

The following approaches are centered on the temporal bone and used for lateral skull base surgery:

- Translabyrinthine approach (chapter 27).
- Retrolabyrinthine approach (chapter 18).
- Retrosigmoid approach (chapter 28).
- Infratemporal approach (chapter 15).
- Transtentorial retrolabyrinthine approach (chapter 33).
- Transsigmoid retrolabyrinthine approach (chapter 34).
- Petrosal approach (chapter 35).
- Transcochlear approach (chapter 36).
- Modified transcochlear approach (chapters 37, 38).

34

Transtentorial retrolabyrinthine approach

This approach was proposed by R.F. Canalis et al (1991) for the treatment of lesions to the petrous apex, the clivus, and the tentorium.
It is based on the combination of two operations already proposed: the retrolabyrinthine approach (Hitselberger and Pulec, 1972) and the transtentorial approach (Stiegliz 1899). It also resembles the suboccipital approach (Naffziger 1928) and the petrosal approach (Al-Mefty, 1988).
The patient is placed in a supine position, with his head turned 45 degrees.

ADVANTAGES

- Ample exposure of the petrous apex, the clivus, and the neurovascular structures, and treatment of specific pathologies: meningiomas, cholesteatomas, intradural petroclival chordomas, tentorial meningiomas, aneurisms of the basilar artery.
- Safe section of the tentorium with easy visualization of the superior petrosal sinus and the trochlear nerve.
- Only in rare instances is a retraction of the temporal lobe and the cerebellum necessary; in these cases, the retraction is minimal.

It is not necessary to section the sigmoid sinus.

DISADVANTAGES

- This technique is indicated only for chordomas with predominant lateral and intradural development.
- It is indicated only in the rare cases of cholesteatoma that do not involve the petrous part of the temporal bone. It is not indicated for petrous cholesteatomas or for cholesterol granulomas, since it does not permit the exteriorization of these lesions.

SURGICAL TECHNIQUE

Incision

An incision is made 4 cm behind the postauricular sulcus, and goes from the zygomatic arch superiorly to the mastoid tip inferiorly. The incision may be extended superiorly if the operation is combined with a middle fossa craniotomy, or posteriorly if a retrosigmoid approach is used (Fig. 34-1).

Bone removal. Extradural phase.

The same steps are used as in an enlarged retrolabyrinthine approach (see chapter 19):
Mastoidectomy "canal wall up".

- Exposure of the sigmoid sinus and the retrosigmoid dura. The sinus is exposed superiorly to approx. 1 cm beyond the exit of the superior petrosal sinus and inferiorly to the jugular bulb.
- Exposure of the third segment (vertical) of the facial nerve.
- Exposure of the lateral and posterior semicircular canal.
- Exposure of the dura of the posterior fossa, between the sigmoid sinus posteriorly and the lateral canal, the posterior canal and the facial nerve anteriorly (Fig. 34-2).
- The endolymphatic sac must be neither traumatized nor opened with the burr, since such occurrences would provoke the risk of an iatrogenic sensorineural hearing loss. Thus it is advisable to use the suction-irrigator placed flat, pressing the dura progressively in an anterior-medial direction, beginning with the sigmoid sinus. Along with the aspirator, a dural elevator is also used to separate the dural adherences from the bone. Thus part of the overlying bone is freed and it may be safely treated with a cutting burr. This procedure is repeated.
- Exposure of the dura underlying the tegmen of the middle fossa. The technique described above may also be used. If the extension of the pathology is in a cranial direction, a middle fossa craniotomy must be combined with the approach.
- A retrosigmoid craniectomy of approx. 3 x 3 cm is performed.
- At the end of the extradural phase, the dura of the middle fossa and the superior petrosal si-

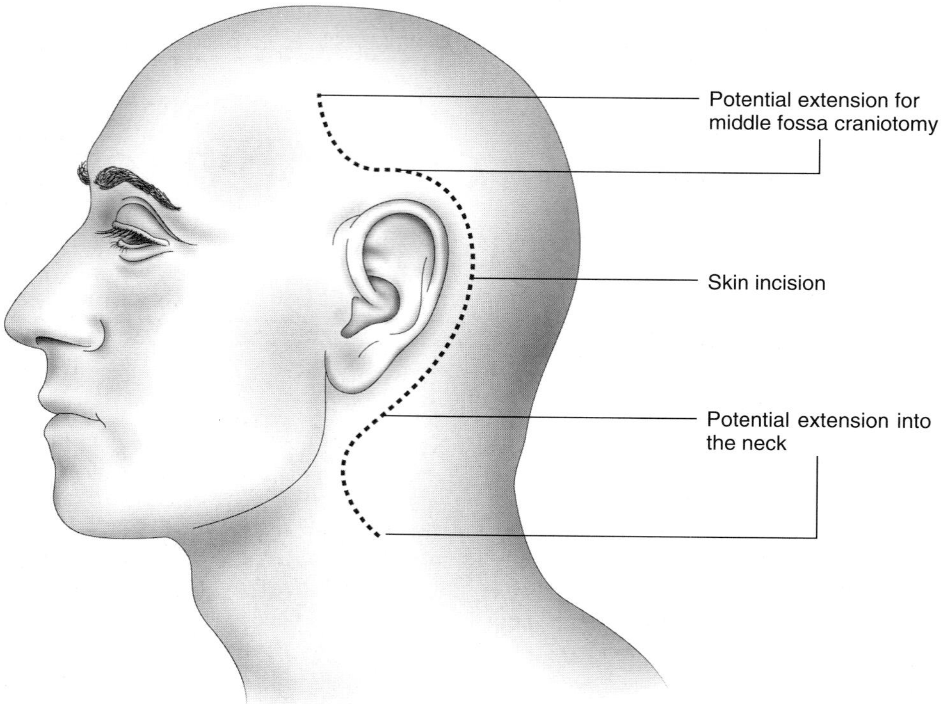

Fig. 34-1. Transtentorial retrolabyrinthine approach. Skin incision.

nus are exposed; the jugular bulb is exposed inferiorly; the dura of the retrosigmoid posterior fossa is exposed posteriorly, along with the sigmoid sinus, the presigmoid dura, and the endoymphatic sac; anteriorly, the lateral semicircular canal is exposed, as well as the posterior canal and the vertical tract of the facial nerve.

Intradural phase

- The dura is incised just posterior to the endolymphatic sac and is extended to the level of the superior petrosal sinus (Fig. 34-3). The petrosal sinus is closed with proximal and distal clips or with silk sutures, and is cut. The vein of Labbé is preserved. It goes from the middle cerebral vein or the superior sagittal sinus, passing over the temporal lobe to the transverse sinus a few mm behind the entrance of the superior petrosal sinus (see chapter 2). The aperture of the dura continues inferiorly to the jugular bulb. Superiorly, the incision is extended to the tentorium, which is divided along its insertion at the superior petrous margin; it is then prolonged medially to the "tentorial notch", taking care not to injure the trochlear nerve that runs infratentorially and parallel to the free edge, then proceeds through the tentorium to become supratentorial (see chapter 2) (Fig. 34-4).
- The dural flaps are anchored with silk sutures to spread the edges of the aperture (Fig. 34-5).
- Nerves V, VII, VIII, IX, X and XI are visible in a cranio-caudal direction.
- A lesion of nerve V may lead to corneal anesthesia. The consequences to the eye are more serious if there is also a lesion of VII, with paralysis of the eyelid and the blinking reflex, and thus serious risk of corneal trauma. Other possible complications are painful anesthesia, facial pain, and trigeminal neuralgia.
- The problems following lesions to the mixed nerves (IX, X, XI) may be dysphagia, vocal cord paralysis, depression of the coughing and vomiting reflexes, and the subsequent pulmonary complications.
- The slightest retraction of the cerebellum and/or temporal lobe, modifying the visual angle of the microscope, enables the surgeon to see the basilar artery system and the structures ventral to the pons.
- The operation is completed.
- All the residual mastoid cells are closed with bone wax.
- The dura is sutured. A small bone fragment drawn from the mastoid cavity is placed over the attic to separate the ossicles from the overlying fascia and thus prevent them from attaching to it. A flap of fascia lata is harvested and rests over the dural suture. Whenever possible, a second layer of fascia and fat are positioned.
- Suture of the skin-muscle flap and positioning of a pressurized dressing.

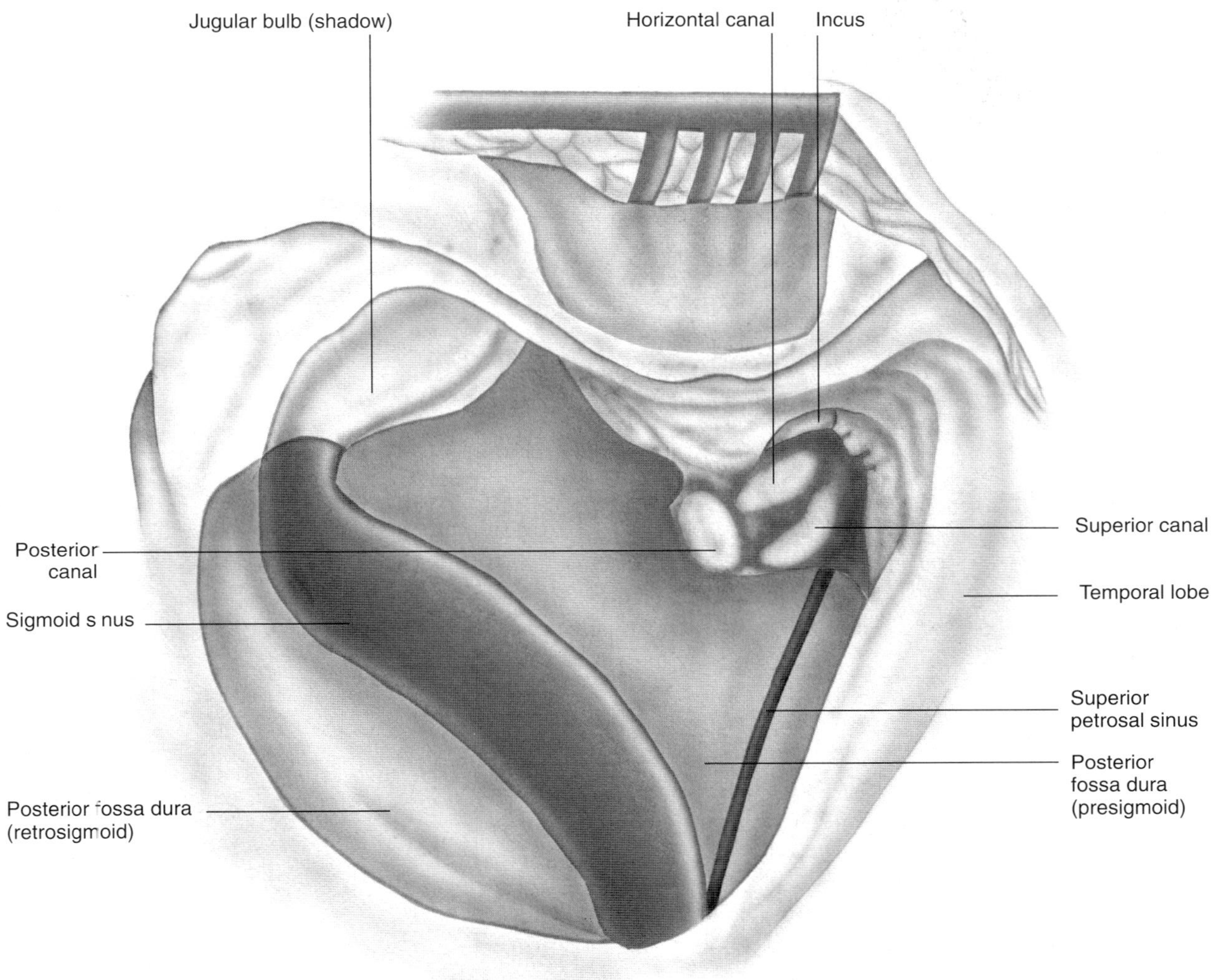

Fig. 34-2. Exposure of retrolabyrinthine fossa dura and retrosigmoid fossa dura.

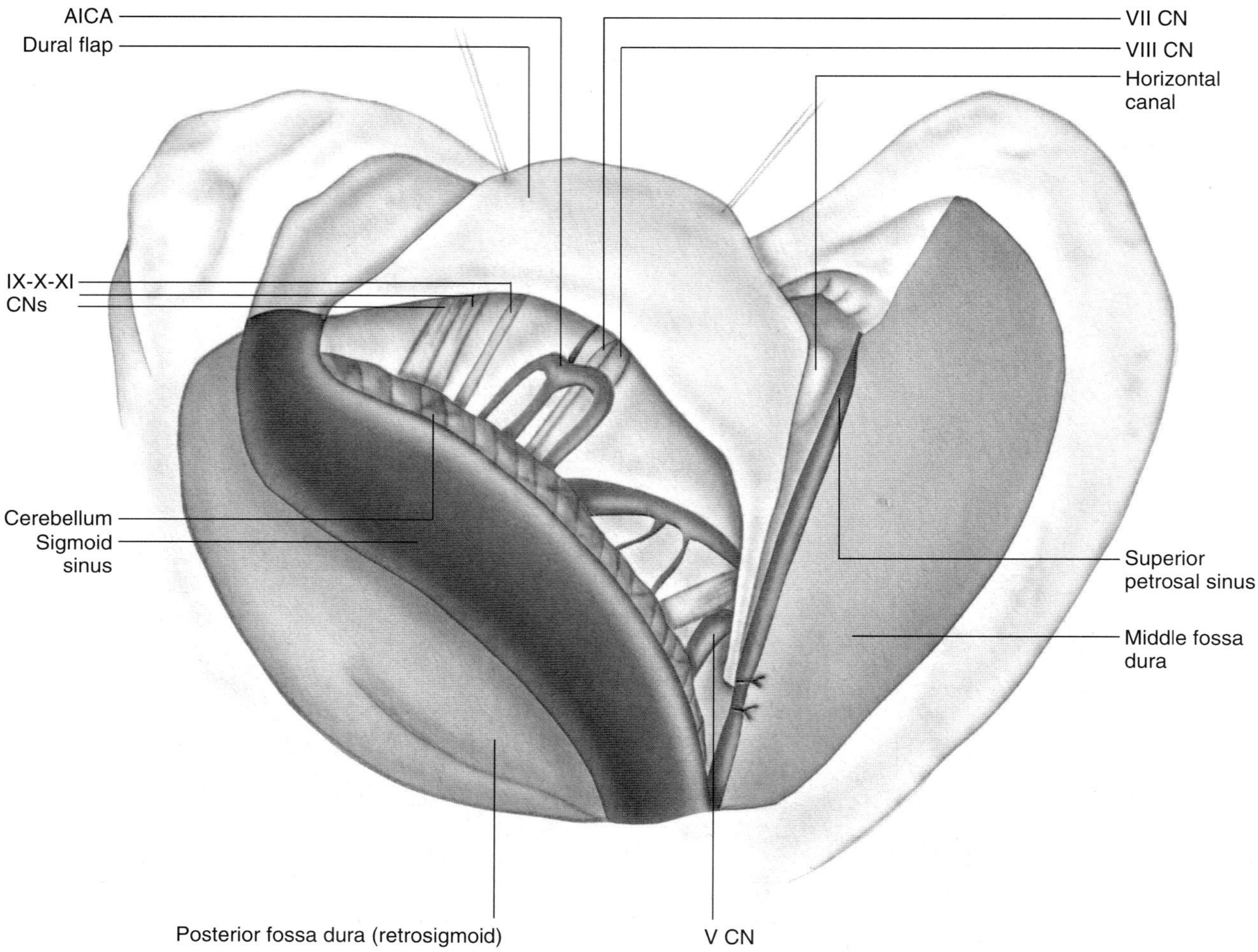

Fig. 34-3. Presigmoid dura is incised. The superior petrosal sinus is cut and the incision extended along the middle fossa dura.

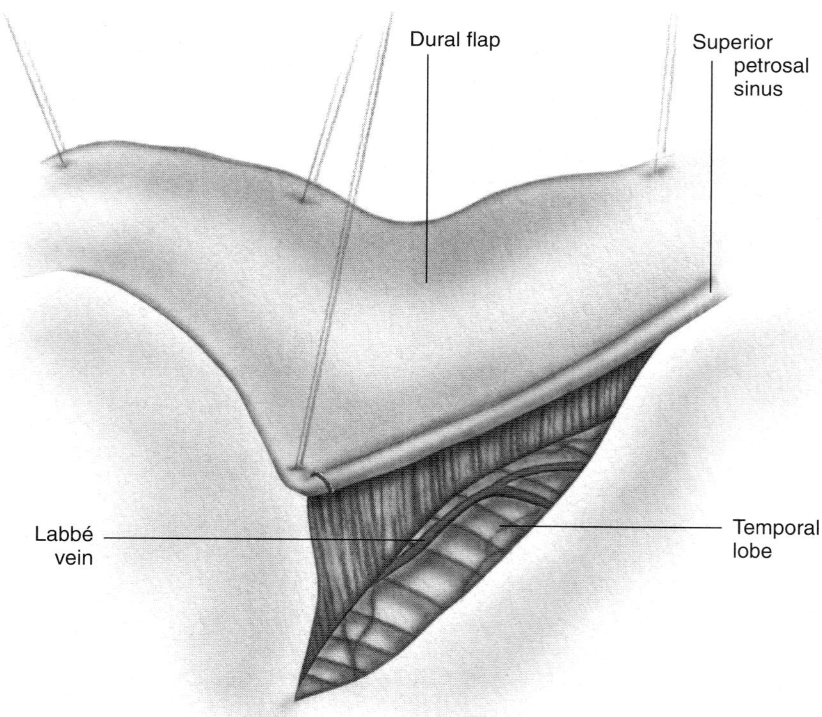

Fig. 34-4. The tentorium is divided along the superior petrosal ridge, taking care to avoid injury to the IV CN. Vein of Labbè is preserved.

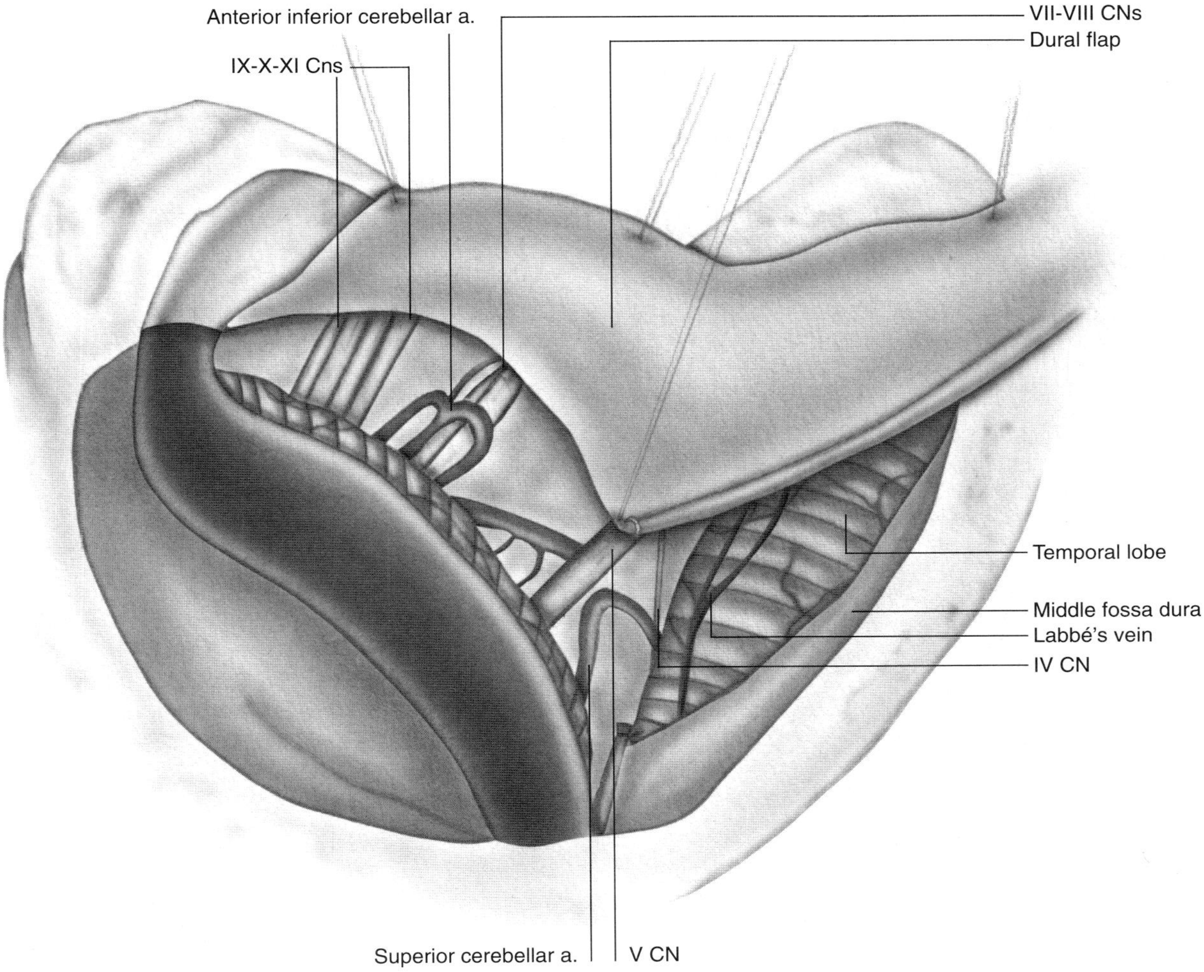

Fig. 34-5. Final exposure of the transtentorial retrolabyrinthine approach.

- Abdominal fat is harvested and positioned in small pieces over the fascia graft.
- A post-operative hydrocephalus may occur in rare instances. If its onset is rapid, it is caused by the increase in mass, reactive edema or hemorrhage; whereas if it is delayed, it is due to the poor reabsorption of CSF or to fibrosis of the basal cistern (Al-Mefty O).

In these cases, if the diagnosis is confirmed by the CT, a shunt is needed.

REFERENCES

Al-Mefty O, Fox JL, Smith RR: Petrosal approach for petroclival meningiomas. Neurosurgery, 22: 510-517, 1988.

Brackmann DE, Hitselberger WE: Retrolabyrinthine approach: Technique and newer indications. Laryngoscope, 88:286-297, 1978.

Canalis RF, Black K, Martin N et al: Extended retrolabyrinthine transtentorial approach to petroclival lesions. Laryngoscope 101, 6-13, 1991.

Cass SP, Sekhar LN, Pomeranz S, Hirsch BE, Snyderman CH: Excision of petroclival tumors by a total petrosectomy approach. Am J Otol 15:474-84, 1994.

Daspit CP, Spetzler RF, Pappas CTE: Combined approach for lesions involving the cerebellopontine angle and skull base: experience with 20 cases-preliminary report. Otolaryngol Head Neck Surg 105:788-796, 1991.

George B, Dematons C, Cophignon J: Lateral approach to the anterior foramen magnum. Surg Neurol 29:484-90, 1988.

Giannotta SL, Maceri DR: Retrolabyrinthine transigmoid approach to basilar trunk and vertebral basilar artery junction aneurysms. J Neurosurg, 69:461 466, 1988.

Hakuba A, Nishmura S, Tanaka K, et al: Clivus meningioma: Six cases of total removal. Neurol Med Chir (Tokyo), 17:63-77, 1977.

Hakuba A, Tsujimoto T: Transcondyle approach for foramen magnum meningiomas. In: Sekhar LN, Janecka IP, eds. Surgery of cranial base tumors. New York: Raven Press, 1993, 671-678.

Hakuba A, Nishimura S, Jang BJ: A combined retro-auricular and preauricular transpetrosal-transtentorial approach to clivus meningiomas. Surg Neurol 30:108-16, 1988.

Hitselberger WE, Gardner G Jr: Other tumors of the cerebellopontine angle. Arch Otolaryngol, 88:712-714, 1968.

Hitselberger WE, House WF: A combined approach to the cerebellopontine angle. Arch Otolaryngol, 84:267-285, 1966.

Hitselberger, WE and Pulec IL: Trigeminal nerve (posterior root) retrolabyrinthine selective section. Arch Otolaryngol, 96:412-415, 1972.

Jackler RK: Overview of surgical neuro-otology. In: Jackler RK, Brackmann DE, eds. Neuro-otology. Baltimore: Mosby, 651- 684, 1993.

Jackson CG, Glasscock ME, McKennan KX, et al: The surgical treatment of skull base tumors with intracranial extension. Otolaryngol Head Neck Surg 96:175, 1987.

Jackson CG: Surgery of skull base tumors. New York: Churchill Livingstone, 1991.

Kawase T, Toya S, Shiobara R, Mine S: Transpetrosal approach for aneurysms of the lower basilar artery. J Neurosurg 63:857-61, 1985.

Kinney SE, Hughes GB, Little JR: Retrolabyrinthine transtentorial approach to lesions of the anterior cerebellopontine angle. Am J Otol 13:426-30, 1992.

Malis LI: Surgical resection of tumors of the skull base. In: Neurosurgery Vol. 1. RH. Wilkins and S.S. Rongachary (Eds.). McGraw-Hill, New York, pp. 1011-1021, 1985.

Mann WJ, Amedee RG, Gilsbach J, Pemeczky A, Wolfensberger M: Transsigmoid approach for tumors of the jugular foramen. Skull Base Surg 1:137-41, 1991.

Naffziger HC: Brain surgery with special reference to exposure of the brain stem and posterior fossa; the principle of intracranial decompression, and the relief of impactions in the posterior fossa. Surg Gynecol Obstet, 46:241-248,1928.

Rosomoff HL: The subtemporal transtentorial approach to the cerebellopontine angle. Laryngoscope, 81:1448-1454, 1971.

Saleh E, Naguib M, Aristegui M, Cokkeser Y, Russo A, Sanna M: Surgical anatomy of the jugular foramen area. In: Mazzoni A, Sanna M, eds. Skull base surgery Update, 1. Amsterdam: Kugler, 1995 pp. 3-8.

Saleh E, Naguib M, Aristegui M, Cokkeser Y, Sanna M: The lower skull base: anatomical study with surgical implications. Ann Otol Rhinol Laryngol 104:57-61, 1995.

Saleh E, Taibah A, Achilli V, Aristegui M, Mazzoni M, Sanna A: Posterior fossa meningioma: surgical strategy. Skull Base Surg 4:209-219, 1994.

Samii M, Ammirati M: The combined supra-infratentorial presigmoid sinus avenue to the petro-clival region: surgical technique and clinical applications. Acta Neurochir 95:6-12, 1988.

Samii M, Draf W: Surgery of the skull base. Berlin: Springer, 1989.

Sasaki CT, Allen WE, Spencer D: Cerebral cortical veins in otologic surgery. Arch Otolaryngol, 103:730-734, 1977.

Sekhar LN, Estonillo R: Transtemporal approach to the skull base: an anatomical study. Neurosurgery 19:799-808, 1986.

Sekhar LN, Schramm VL, Jones NF: Subtemporal-preauricular infratemporal fossa approach to large lateral and posterior cranial base neoplasms. J Neurosurg 67:488-499, 1987.

Sen C, Sekhar LN: Extreme lateral transcondylar and transjugular approaches. In: Sekhar LN, Janecka I, eds. Surgery of cranial base tumors. NewYork: Raven Press, 389-412, 1993.

Sen C, Sekhar LN: An extreme lateral approach to intradural lesions of the cervical spine and foramen magnum. Neurosurgery 27:197-204, 1990.

Sen C, Sekhar LN: The subtemporal and preauricular infratemporal approach to intradural structures ventral to the brain stem. J Neurosurg 73:345-354, 1990.

Silverstein H, Norell H: Retrolabyrinthine surgery: A direct approach to the cerebellopontine angle. Otolaryngol Head Neck Surg, 88:462-469,1980.

Silverstein H, Norrell H: Retrolabyrinthine vestibular nerve section. Otolaryngol Head Neck Surg, 90:778-782, 1982.

Stieglitz, L, Gerster AG, Lilientual H: A study of three cases of tumor of the brain in which operation was performed—One recovery, two deaths. Am J Med Sci, III:509-531, 1886.

Thedinger BA, Glasscock ME, Cueva RA: Transcochlear transtentorial approach for removal of large cerebellopontine angle meningiomas. Am J Otol 13:408-415, 1992.

Velut S, Jan M: Anterior petrosectomy during approach to the petroclival area. In: Schmideck HE, ed. Meningiomas and their surgical management. Philadelphia: Saunders, 435-450, 1991.

Wiet RJ, Schramm DR, Kazan RP: The retrolabyrinthine approach and vascular loop. Laryngoscope, 99:1035-1039, 1989.

35

Transsigmoid retrolabyrinthine approach

This approach was proposed by Giannotta (1988) specifically for the treatment of aneurisms of the basilar artery and the vertebro-basilar arterial junction.

- A lumbar drain is inserted, and the patient is placed in a supine position, with his head inclined 45° and facing away from the surgeon. A Mayfield headrest may be used since it permits the attachment of a retractor, if necessary (e.g Yasargill blade).
- Postauricular incision (Fig. 35-1).
- A retrolabyrinthine approach is performed along with a retrosigmoid craniotomy, following the technique described above (Retrolabyrinthine transtentorial approach in this chapter, chapter 19, chapter 29) (Fig. 35-2).
- An incision is made above the retrosigmoid dura, which is then prolonged to the presigmoid zone beside the superior petrosal sinus. A similar incision is made in the retrosigmoid dura and then in the presigmoid dura, tangent to the jugular bulb.
- The sinus is tied above the junction with the transverse sinus and below the junction with the jugular bulb, and is divided. The flap of dura is reflected anteriorly, until the labyrinth is covered. In the underlying field, the following structures are visible: nerve V, the floccule with nerves VIII and VII at the center of the field, and the mixed nerves IX, X, and XI inferiorly (Fig. 35-3).
- The arachnoid of the prepontine and cerebellopontine cisterns is opened.
- The patient's position, the sloping position of the cerebellum and the brainstem, the CSF drain and the osmotic diuresis, all open the retroclival space wide. The basilar artery appears. The artery may be exposed from the zone adjacent to the confluence of the vertebral to the point in which the superior cerebellar artery originates. The brainstem detaches due to the weight of the clivus. Thus it becomes possible to treat even the aneurisms headed posteriorly in the basilar sulcus. Room for positioning is acquired, if necessary, by a clip on the proximal vertebral vessels.

Surgical side

The operation is characterized by the ample access and by the almost complete elimination of cerebellar retraction, as well as retraction of the temporal lobe and the brain; however, the section of the lateral sinus is required. This section may, though rarely, provoke serious complications (Sasaki).

It is thus advisable to follow a few indications:

- The dominant sigmoid sinus should be preserved. The dominant sinus is evident angiographically as the major drainage to the sagittal sinus. The non dominant sinus can be sacrificed if it's confluence is angiographically patent and the permeability of the contralateral sigmoid sinus is normal.

Spetzler and Daspit, who have had extensive experience with the petrosal approach, propose a simple technique.

- To be sure that the sigmoid sinus may be sacrificed, a No. 25 needle is inserted in the sinus and the pressure is recorded below the clip, before and after occlusion. In sinuses which result patent at the angiography, post-occlusion pressure does not rise more than 7 mm Hg. If pressure increase more than 10 mm Hg, the sinus is kept intact.
- The vein of Labbé enters the lateral sinus above the confluence of the superior petrosal sinus into the sigmoid sinus. Thus, when the sigmoid sinus is sacrificed, the ipsilateral vein of Labbé drains the blood in a contralateral direction.
- If the sinus is preserved, when the temporal lobe is elevated, the vein of Labbé may be damaged. Thus the sigmoid sinus and the tentorium should be elevated along with the temporal lobe, to avoid injury to the vein of Labbé (see chapter 2).

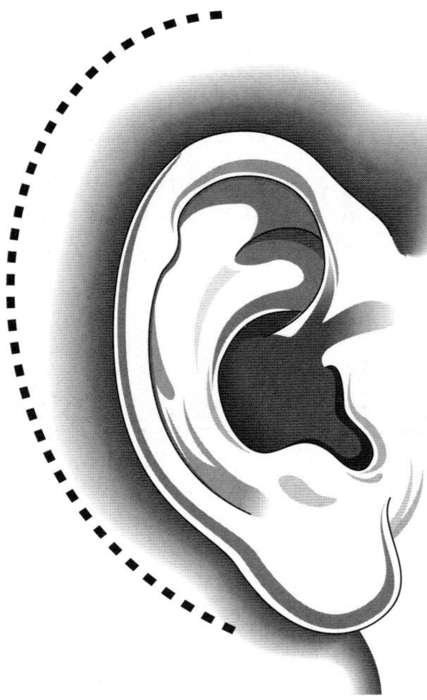

Fig. 35-1. Postauricular incision

- The approach must be beside the neck of the aneurism.
- If the aneurism has a superior or an inferior direction, and thus along the midline, the side where the sigmoid sinus is smaller is favored.
- It may be necessary to operate from the side of a very dominant sigmoid sinus. To avoid the risks associated with the ligation of the sinus, the sinus may be preserved, working anteriorly and posteriorly.
- A traditional suboccipital or subtemporal transtentorial approach may be used, or a transtentorial retrolabyrinthine approach, which does not require significant variations in technique.
- If hearing loss has already occurred, the posterior labyrinth (the semicircular canals) may be drilled with cutting burrs. The exposure of the bone must reach the third segment of the facial nerve, which represents the anterior boundary of dissection. To protect nerve VII, the anterior wall of the lateral semicircular canal is maintained, which makes up part of the fallopian canal. The posterior semicircular canal indicates that the facial nerve and its ampulla is in contact with the nerve. Medial to the ampulla of the superior semicircular canal is the origin of the superior vestibular nerve.

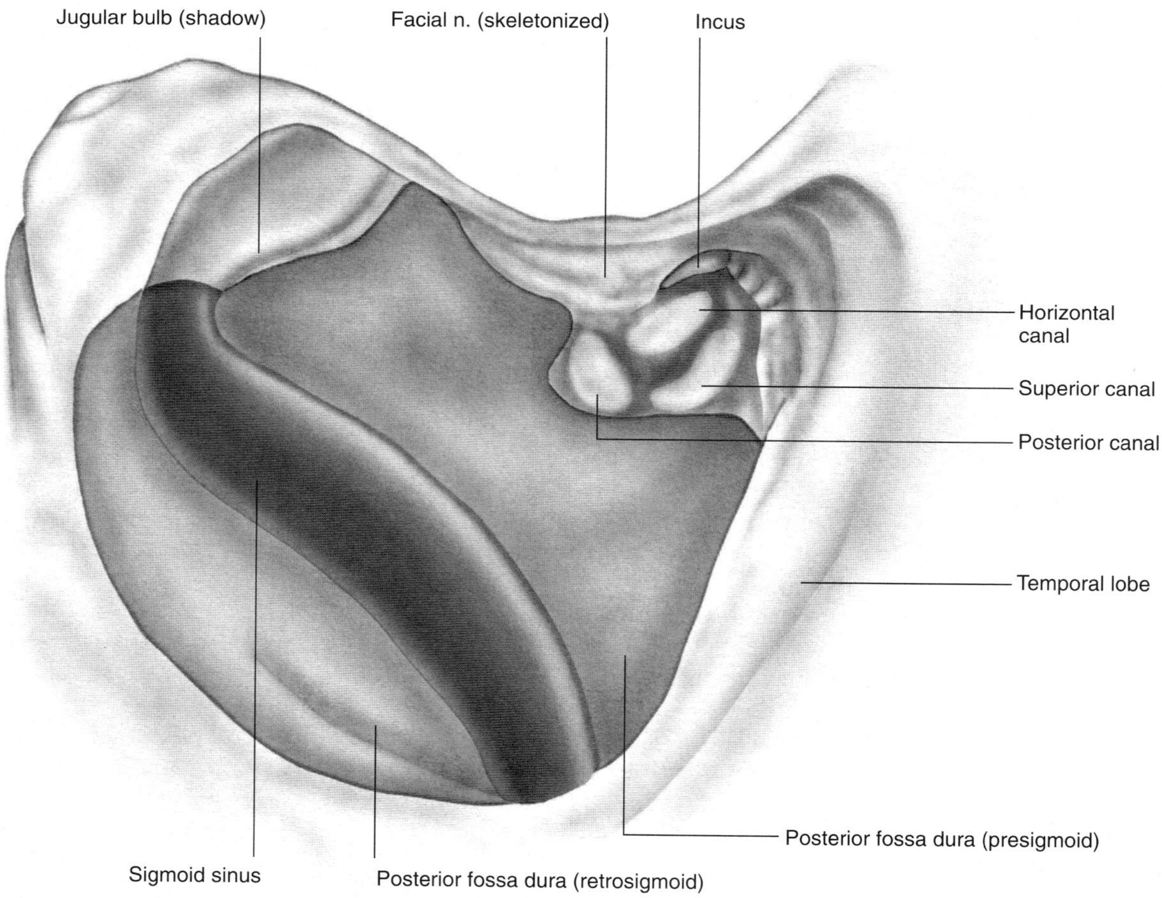

Fig. 35-2. Exposure of retrolabyrinthine fossa dura and retrosigmoid fossa dura.

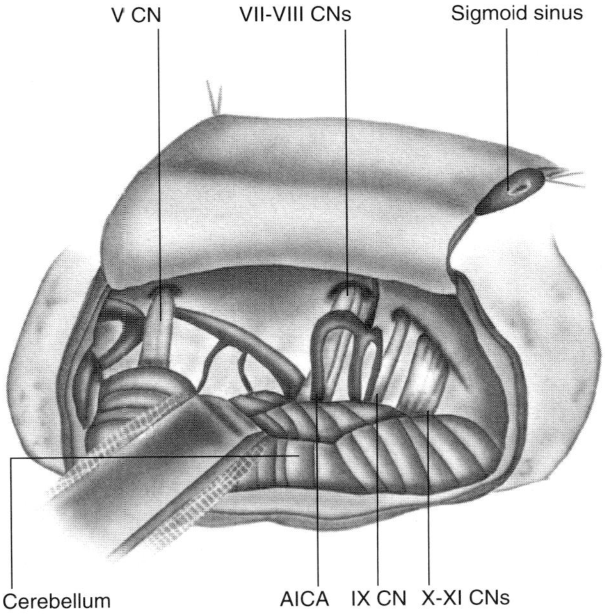

Fig. 35-3. The dura is opened on both sides of the sigmoid sinus. The sinus is ligated and divided. The dural flap is reflected anteriorly.

- The removal of the posterior labyrinth thus increases the anterior visual space and classifies the operation as translabyrinthine.
- Another alternative in cases of patients with hearing loss is the transcochlear approach (see chapter 37). The main disadvantage to this approach, which calls for the posterior transposition of the facial nerve, is related to the function of nerve VII. The nerve is moved from its bony mastoid canal and thus its vascularization is compromised. A paralysis is immediately seen, which will improve gradually. There is never a recovery superior to grade III (House-Brackmann scale, chapter 12). The complete loss of hearing is, of course, part of this disadvantage.

INDICATIONS

- The main advantage of this approach is in the absence of pressure on the temporal lobe and the cerebellum. The delicate pressure of the rod of a fenestrated suction is sufficient (Brackmann n. 5) resting on a cottonoid above the floccule. The suction pressure, unlike the self retaining retractors, is not continuous, and thus only rarely provokes effects of stasis.
- The approach is not very profound since it brings the entrance point through the dura near the clivus plane.
- The direction of penetration is along the shortest trajectory between the middle and inferior thirds of the clivus; thus the middle part of the basilar artery is exposed from the point where the superior cerebellar artery departs, to the area near the vertebro-basilar junction. Thus the required proximal and distal control are obtained for aneurisms of the basilar artery.

REFERENCES

Archer DJ, Young S, Uttley D: Basilar aneurysms: a new transclival approach via maxillotomy. J Neurosurg 67, 54-58, 1987.

Chou SN, Oniz-Suarez HJ: Surgical treatment of arterial aneurysms of the vertebrobasilar circulation. J Neurosurg 41:671-680, 1974.

Daspit CP, Spetzler RF, Pappas CTE: Combined approach for lesions involving the cerebellopontine angle and skull base: experience with 20 cases-preliminary report. Otolaryngol Head Neck Surg 105:788-796, 1991.

Drake CG: The surgical treatment of vertebral-basilar aneurysms. Clin Neurosurg 16:114-169, 1969.

Drake CG: The treatment of aneurysms of the posterior circulation. Clin Neurosurg 26:96-144, 1979.

Fox JL: Obliteration of midline vertebral artery aneurysm via basilar craniectomy. J Neurosurg 26:406-412, 1967.

George B, Dematons C, Cophignon J: Lateral approach to the anterior foramen magnum. Surg Neurol 29:484-90, 1988.

Giannotta SL, Maceri DR: Retrolabyrinthine transsigmoid approach to basilar trunk and vertebrobasilar artery junction aneurysm. J Neurosurg 69: 461-466, 1988.

Hakuba A, Tsujimoto T: Transcondyle approach for foramen magnum meningiomas. In: Sekhar LN. Janecka IP, eds. Surgery of cranial base tumors. New York: Raven Press, 1993: n-n.

Hakuba A, Nishimura S, Jang BJ: A combined retro-auricular and preauricular transpetrosal-transtentorial approach to clivus meningiomas. Surg Neurol 30:108-16, 1988.

Hammon WM, Kempe LG: The posterior fossa approach to aneurysms of the vertebral and basilar arteries. J Neurosurg 37:339-347, 1972.

Hayakawa T, Kamikawa K, Ohnishi T, et al: Prevention of postoperative complications after transoral transclival approach to basilar aneurysms. Technical note. J Neurosurg 54:699-703, 1981.

Heros RC: Lateral suboccipital approach for vertebral and vertebrobasilar artery lesions. J Neurosurg 64: 559-562, 1986.

House JW, Brackmann DE: Facial nerve grading system. Laryngoscope 93: n.2, 146-147, 1985.

Hook O, Norlen G, Guzman J: Saccular aneurysms of the vertebral-basilar arterial system. A report of 28 cases. Acta Neurol Scand 39:271-304, 1963.

Jackler RK: Overview of surgical neuro-otology. In: Jackler RK, Brackmann DE, eds. Neuro-otology. Baltimore: Mosby, 651-684, 1993.

Jackson CG, Glasscock ME, McKennan KX, et al: The surgical treatment of skull base tumors with intracranial extension. Otolaryngol Head Neck Surg 96:175, 1987.

Jackson CG: Surgery of skull base tumors. New York: Churchill Livingstone, 1991.

Jamieson KG: Aneurysms of the vertebrobasilar system. Surgical intervention in 19 cases. J Neurosurg 21: 781-797, 1964.

Kawase T, Toya S, Shiobara R, Mine S: Transpetrosal approach for aneurysms of the lower basilar artery. J Neurosurg 63:857-61, 1985.

Kinney SE, Hughes GB, Little JR: Retrolabyrinthine transtentorial approach to lesions of the anterior cerebellopontine angle. Am J Otol 13:426-30, 1992.

Mann WJ, Amedee RG, Gilsbach J, Pemeczky A, Wolfensberger M: Transsigmoid approach for tumors of the jugular foramen. Skull Base Surg 1:137-41, 1991.

Saleh E, Naguib M, Aristegui M, Cokkeser Y, Russo A, Sanna M: Surgical anatomy of the jugular foramen area. In: Mazzoni A, Sanna M, eds. Skull base surgery Update, 1. Amsterdam: Kugler, 1995 pp. 3-8.

Saleh E, Naguib M, Aristegui M, Cokkeser Y, Sanna M: The lower skull base: anatomical study with surgical implications. Ann Otol Rhinol Laryngol 104:57-61, 1995.

Saleh E, Taibah A, Achilli V, Aristegui M, Mazzoni M, Sanna A: Posterior fossa meningioma: surgical strategy. Skull Base Surg 4:209-219, 1994.

Samii M, Ammirati M: The combined supra-infratentorial presigmoid sinus avenue to the petro-clival region: surgical technique and clinical applications. Acta Neurochir 95:6-12, 1988.

Samii M, Draf W: Surgery of the skull base. Berlin: Springer, 1989.

Sasaki CT, Allen WE, Spencer D: Cerebral cortical veins in otologic surgery. Arch Otolaryngol, 103:730-734, 1977.

Sekhar LN, Estonillo R: Transtemporal approach to the skull base: an anatomical study. Neurosurgery 19:799-808, 1986.

Sekhar LN, Schramm VL, Jones NF: Subtemporal-preauricular infratemporal fossa approach to large lateral and posterior cranial base neoplasms. J Neurosurg 67:488-499, 1987.

Sen C, Sekhar LN: Extreme lateral transcondylar and transjugular approaches. In: Sekhar LN, Janecka I, eds. Surgery of cranial base tumors. New York: Raven Press, 389-412, 1993.

Sen C, Sekhar LN: An extreme lateral approach to intradural lesions of the cervical spine and foramen magnum. Neurosurgery 27:197-204, 1990.

Sen C, Sekhar LN: The subtemporal and preauricular infratemporal approach to intradural structures ventral to the brain stem. J Neurosurg 73:345-354, 1990.

Spetzler RF, Daspit CP, Pappas CTE: The combined supra- and infratentorial approach for lesions of the petrous and clival regions: Experience with 46 cases. J Neurosurg 76: 588-599, 1992.

Sugita K, Kobayashi S, Takemae T et al: Aneurysm of the basilar artery trunk. J Neurosurg 66: 500-505, 1987.

Thedinger BA, Glasscock ME, Cueva RA: Transcochlear transtentorial approach for removal of large cerebellopontine angle meningiomas. Am J Otol 13:408-415, 1992.

Velut S, Jan M: Anterior petrosectomy during approach to the petroclival area. In: Schmideck HE, ed. Meningiomas and their surgical management. Philadelphia: Saunders, 435-450, 1991.

36

Petrosal approach in petroclival tumors

Be prepared. Do not despair.

SEKHAR L.N.

The petrosal approach, centered on the petrous bone, was proposed by Al-Mefty, 1988. In Al-Mefty' s experience, several advantages are obtained:
- Minimal retraction of the cerebellum and the temporal lobe.
- Reduction by approx. 3 cm of the distance from the clivus.
- Direct view of the lesion and the anterior and lateral aspects of the brainstem.
- Preservation of the neuro-otologic structures and the anterior and posterior labyrinths.
- Preservation of the vascular structures: sigmoid sinus, transverse sinus, vein of Labbé, basal and occipital veins, and precocious identification of the vessels supplying the tumor (Fig. 36-1).
- This approach enables the surgeon to attack the tumor from various visual angles.

Indications
Petroclival meningiomas, trigeminal schwannomas, epidermoid tumors, neuromas over 4 cm in diameter.

SURGICAL TECHNIQUE

- The patient is placed in a supine position with his head turned 40-50° away from the side of the tumor.
- An incision is made going from the zygomatic root, along the temporal line, and then behind the ear to approx. 1 cm behind the mastoid tip.
- Three muscular flaps are made: the flap of temporalis muscle is retracted anteriorly, the sternomastoid muscle flap is retracted inferiorly, and a muscle-periosteum flap (see chapter 28) is retracted anteriorly.
- A temporo-parieto-occipital craniectomy is performed. Thus the transverse sinus and the sigmoid sinus are freed. It is important to take care to free the venous structures without injuring them, especially at the junction between the transverse and sigmoid sinuses. For this purpose, multifunction drills may be used. To reduce the extension of the bone plate, two separate parts may be distinguished: a temporal craniectomy and a craniectomy of the posterior cranial fossa.

Retrolabyrinthine mastoidectomy
A complete retrolabyrinthine mastoidectomy is performed from the tegmen to the middle fossa. Exposure is as follows:
- Superiorly, the dura of the middle cranial fossa is exposed, as well as the sinodural angle and the superior petrosal sinus.
- Posteriorly and inferiorly the sigmoid sinus is exposed to the jugular bulb.
- Anteriorly, the presigmoid dura is exposed to the posterior semicircular canal and the third segment of the facial nerve.

Dural incision
- An incision is made of the dura of the posterior cranial fossa (presigmoid) at approx. 3 mm from the margin of the lateral sinus, to the superior petrosal sinus. The incision of the dura near the sinus must always leave a safety margin, since the venous walls are never perfectly circular, but slope slightly at the boundaries. Thus this area may be injured by the scalpel.
- The dura of the temporal fossa is incised along its fundus. Ligation or clipping or coagulation are performed, as well as section of the superior petrosal sinus at approx. 1 cm from its confluence into the sigmoid sinus.
- The two incisions are joined.
- Along the floor of the temporal fossa, the incision of the tentorium is prolonged tangentially to the pyramid of the temporal bone.

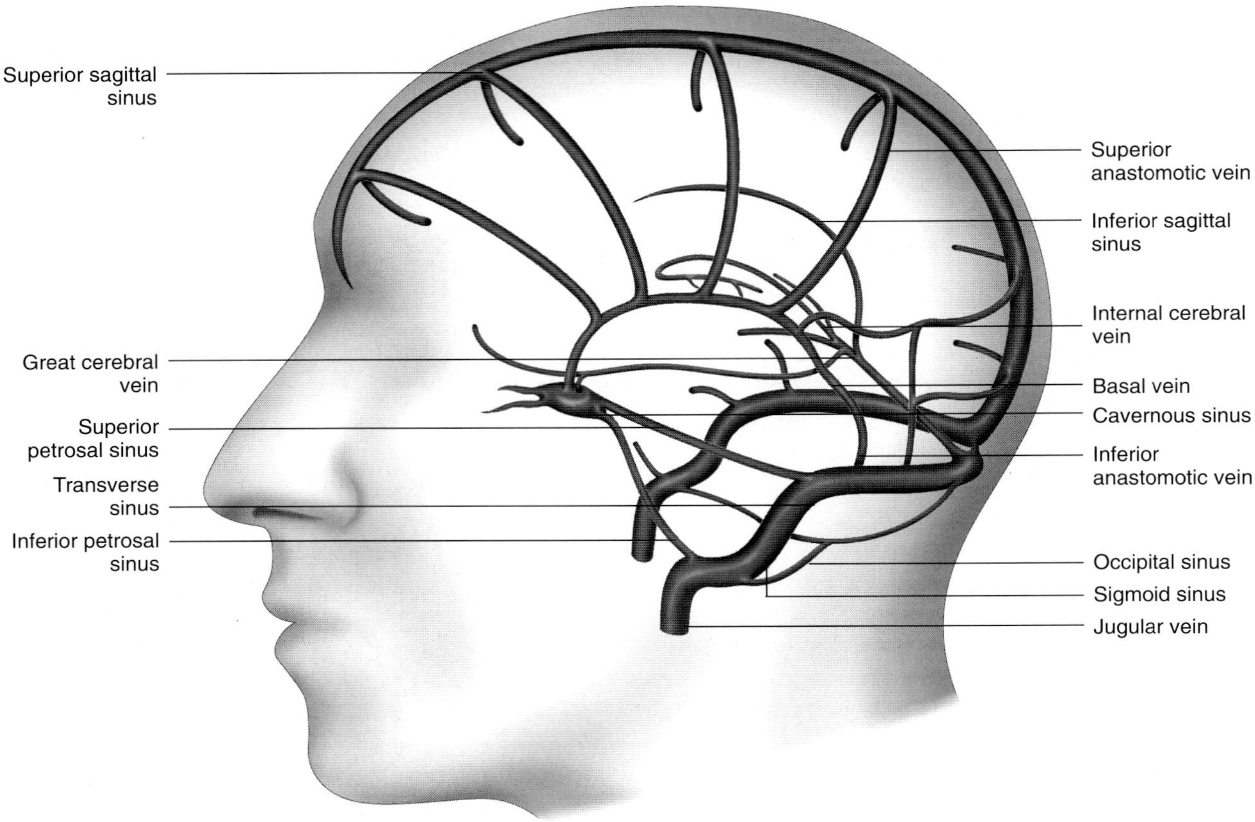

Fig. 36-1. Venous sinuses of the dura mater.

- To cut the tentorium, the temporal lobe must be moved superiorly. To avoid rupturing Labbé's vein with traction, the vein must be gently dissected from the surface of the temporal lobe. A lesion to this vein may lead to serious complications (see chapter 2).

Tumor removal
- The cerebellar-medullary cistern is opened to gain room to work. The small perforating arteries and the supratentorial vessels which supply the tumor are coagulated.
- The arachnoid plane is dissected and preserved and the underlying tumor is debulked.
- The vascular structures are preserved: the anterior-inferior cerebellar artery (AICA), the posterior-inferior cerebellar artery (PICA), the basilar artery, and its collateral branches.
- Tumor removal is performed with the same general indications as in the translabyrinthine approach to the neuroma.

Closure
- The presigmoid and temporal dura are sutured to be watertight. The temporalis muscle flap is repositioned on the mastoid and a flap of temporalis muscle is placed above it, made up of the anterior peduncle, which is sutured inferiorly at the sternocleidomastoid muscle.
- One variation in the technique to prevent liquor fistulas of the tube and/or the dural suture is to use fascia lata and completely cover the surgical area. To prevent the attachment of the malleus and the stapes, it is helpful to use a bone fragment as protection.
- A CSF fistula is treated as in the translabyrinthine and retrosigmoid approaches (see chapter 28-29).
- The presigmoid approach reduces the necessity of significant cerebellum retraction. For complications due to edema of the cerebellum, or post-operative hemorrhage of the posterior fossa, see chapter 28, on the treatment of surgical complications.

TIPS AND PITFALLS

- The nervous structures should be preserved. Depending on the size of the lesion, all the cranial nerves may be involved except for I and II. The facial nerve presents the same problems as in the translabyrinthine approach.
- Nerve III runs medial to nerve IV.
- While opening the tentorium, it is important to preserve the trochlear nerve by keeping the inci-

sion posterior to the spot where nerve IV transverses the tentorium. The trochlear nerve is in close relationship with the incisura. Nerve IV has a cisternal part, then passes through the tentorium and enters the posterior part of the cavernous sinus. The tentorium may be cut safely from V to IV. To proceed beyond the entrance point of IV, it is important to keep in mind that the trochlear nerve, once it crosses the tentorium, may reach the cavernous sinus with a straight or curved path, in a caudal direction.

- The roots of the trigeminal nerve must also be preserved. At times, pushed and stretched by the tumor, these roots are found just under the tentorium (see chapter 6).

- Nerve VI (see chapter 6).

- The criteria expressed for nerve VII-VIII preservation are the same as in the retrosigmoid approach.

- For lesions to the mixed nerves (see chapter 34-40).

- Nerve XII, when injured, increases the difficulty in swallowing, if concomitant with IX and X lesion. In this case, a VII-XII anastomosis is contraindicated.

- Thanks to the sigmoid sinus and the cut tentorium, the base of the temporal lobe, may be safely elevated without causing lesions to Labbé's vein (chapter 2).

Combined approach for skull base and CPA lesions (Daspit and Spetzler technique)

The aforementioned approach gives broad access to the midclivus and is indicated for those tumors which cross the medial petrosal margin and extend into the middle and posterior fossa, Meckel's cave, and the cavernous sinus.
It combines the subtemporal approach with the posterior fossa approach. The posterior fossa approach proposed is a subtemporal retrolabyrinthine (presigmoid) approach and is indicated for lesions posterior to the brain stem, without anterior extension and when the acoustic nerve must be preserved.

Daspit and Spetzler mantained the subtemporal part of the procedure, while extending the possibilities of posterior fossa approach utilizing three different variations: the aforementioned retrolabyrinthine approach, the translabyrinthine approach and the transcochlear approach.

- The translabyrinthine approach is used for any sized tumors of the CPA, when hearing preservation is not an objective.
- The transcochlear approach is used for CPA lesions with anterior extensions and clival lesions, when a wide exposure and a flat angle of approach to clivus is required.

In the transcochlear approach the entire tympanic part of the temporal bone is removed up to the temporomandibular joint. The jugular bulb is exposed. The bone occupying the space where the carotid turns anteriorly and the jugular turns posteriorly, called the crotch (jugulocarotid spine) is removed. Care must be taken not to injure the IX-X-XI cranial nerves, which pass through the jugular foramen.
The carotid artery is skeletonized anteriorly, leaving a thin shell of bone. The carotid artery can be exposed and if more exposure is needed, the mandibular condyle is displaced anteriorly and bone is removed around the ICA, exposing it by 270 degrees (see chapter 40).

Surgical resection of petrous bone tumors (Sekhar's Technique)

A technique of total petrous temporal bone resection has been proposed by Sekhar (see also chapter 10). This technique is applicable to tumors involving the petrous bone and surrounding structures: Benign lesions, low grade malignant lesions such as chordomas, chondrosarcomas, adenoid cystic carcinoma, pituitary adenoma and high grade malignant lesions such as carcinomas and osteogenic sarcoma.

- The skin incision is extended superiorly up to the frontal region and inferiorly, 5 cm below the mastoid tip, to expose the carotid artery, the jugular vein and the lower cranial nerves.
- Blind sac closure of the external auditory canal.
- Detachment of the splenius and semispinalis capitis muscles from the suboccipital bone.
- Exposure of the facial nerve from the stylomastoid foramen to the parotid gland. Section of the GSPN.
- Transection of the neck of the mandible and removal of the condyle.

- Exposure of the petrous and upper cervical ICA and anterior translocation. The eustachian tube is transected, packed and sutured.
- The extent of removal is dictated by the extension of the tumor. If the mastoid is not involved, the sigmoid sinus is skeletonized and a partial mastoidectomy is performed. If the tumor extends inferiorly and adequate cross-flow is present in the sigmoid sinus, the jugular vein is ligated, the sigmoid sinus is opened and packed with Surgicel, the jugular bulb is opened, and IX-X-XI nerves are dissected. When there is a good collateral drainage to the sylvian venous system, the vein of Labbé may be ligated and transected, in order to enlarge the surgical field.

The other surgical steps in benign and low-grade malignancy tumors are similar to those described in the petrosal approach, and the removal of the neoplasia can be accomplished piecemeal.

In high grade malignant tumors it is important to attempt to perform en bloc resection of petrous bone infiltrated by the tumor. The transverse sinus is ligated and transected and the dura of posterior and middle fossa is incised. The tentorium is incised from the transverse sinus to the tentorial notch to reach a middle fossa dural incision separating V3 and the trigeminal ganglion from the area of resection. The following structures are sacrificed:

- Tumor infiltrated dura and tentorium
- Petrosal vein
- Facial nerve
- Inferior petrosal sinus
- IX-XI CNs, when the jugular foramen is involved
- Bone of the petrous apex and clivus
- At the end of the procedure, the tumor-infiltrated petrous bone is completely resected
- The following surrounding structures, if tumor-infiltrated, are sacrificed:
- Occipital condyle
- Clivus
- Cavernous sinus
- ICA
- Tumor involved temporal lobe and/or cerebellum.

RECONSTRUCTION

- VII-XII CNs: Cable grafted (the greater auricular nerve and the sural nerve can be used).
- ICA: Reconstruction with a saphenous vein graft.
- Dural defect: Fascia lata is employed. Temporalis, sternocleidomastoid, semispinalis capitis and splenius capitis muscles are rotated to fill the defect. The posterior edge of the parotid is sewn to the muscles, as well as the temporal lobe dura. Sometimes a free rectus abdominis flap or another microvascular flap is used to close a residual defect.

Two closed system drains are positioned under the skin flap and mantained for 2-5 days after surgery. Lumbar drainage may be necessary.

When the ICA has been grafted or any minor surgical damage is suspected, angiography is performed the day after surgery. The surgical outcome is checked by means of a head CT.

COMPLICATIONS

Facial nerve injury is quite frequent as are IX and X cranial nerve palsy. When IX and X CNs are sacrificed and reconstructed, tracheostomy and gastrostomy are required and their removal may take several months.

Cranial nerve deficit in all series is more then 50% (Sekhar, Al Mefty, Mayberg's and Symon's, Daspit and Spetzler...). CSF leakage is quite frequent. Other complications are cerebral infarction, temporary hemiparesis, meningitis, abducens nerve paresis, aphasia, sepsis, pneumonia, hydrocephalus, wound dehiscences and flap hematoma. No intraoperative and perioperatively deaths have been reported in the major series.

The extensive temporal bone resection is made possible by several requirements:

- **Interdisciplinary collaboration**

  Radiologist

  Preoperative CT (axial and coronal) and MRI.

  Cerebral angiography. The dominance and connection between the sigmoid and transverse sinuses as well as the venous drainage and collateral flow of the temporal lobe are evaluated.

  Balloon occlusion test of the ICA and permanent balloon occlusion, if needed. Embolization of tumor feeder arteries.

  Anesthesiologist

  During surgery, for use of modern neurosurgical anesthesia without long-acting muscle paralysis, so as to allow neurophysiological monitoring.

  In the intensive care unit, for the postoperative care.

  Neurosurgeon, otolaryngologist, plastic surgeon, for surgical management.
- **Technical requirements**

  Bilateral somatosensory evoked response (SSER) preoperatively and postoperatively.

  Contralateral brain stem evoked response (BSER), preoperatively and intraoperatively, to detect brain stem compression.

  Intraoperative electroencephalograph monitoring.

  Facial and other cranial nerve monitoring.

CONCLUSION

- Surgery is the definitive choice for benign lesions involving the petrous bone.

- Surgery followed by radiotherapy is usually effective in low-grade malignant tumors.
- The surgical treatment of highly malignant petrous bone tumors is still a matter of controversy. In Sekhar's series, twenty-five percent of subjects are tumor free 2.5 years after surgery and adjuvant treatment and 10% have recurrent tumors. A mortality rate of 44% due to the primary disease has been observed within 1.5 years after surgery.

REFERENCES

Al-Mefty O, Fox JL, Smith RR: Petrosal approach for petroclival meningiomas. Neurosurgery 22: 510-517,1988.

Bochenek Z, Kukwa A: An extended approach through the middle cranial fossa to the internal auditory meatus and the cerebello-pontine angle. Acta Otolaryngol Stockh 80 410-414, 1975.

Brackmann DE: The facial nerve in the infratemporal approach. Otolaryngol Head Neck Surg 97: 15-17, 1987.

Daspit CP, Spetzler RF, Pappas CTE: Combined approach for lesions involving the cerebellopontine angle and skull base: experience with 20 cases-preliminary report. Otolaryngol Head Neck Surg 105:788-796, 1991.

Decker RE, Malis LI: Surgical approach to midline lesions at base of skull. J Mt Sinai Hosp 37: 84-102, 1970.

Fisch U: Infratemporal fossa approach for extensive tumors of the temporal bone and base of the skull. In Silverstein H, Norell H eds: Neurological Surgery of the Ear. Birmingham, AL, Aesculapius, 1977, pp 34-53.

Heros RC: Lateral suboccipital approach for vertebral and vertebrobasilar artery lesions. J Neurosurg 64: 559-562, 1986.

House WF, Hitselberger WE: The transcochlear approach to the skull base. Arch Otolaryngol Head Neck Surg 102: 334-342, 1976.

House WF: Translabyrinthine approach. In House WF, Luetje CM eds: Acoustic Tumors, Vol 2, Management. Baltimore, University Park Press, 1979, pp 43-87.

Jackler RK: Overview of surgical neuro-otology. In: Jackler RK, Brackmann DE, eds. Neuro-Otology. Baltimore: Mosby, 651 -84, 1993.

Jackson CG, Glasscock ME, McKennan KX, et al: The surgical treatment of skull base tumors with intracranial extension. Otolaryngol Head Neck Surg 96:175, 1987.

Jackson CG: Surgery of skull base tumors. New York: Churchill Livingstone, 1991.

Kawase T, Toya S, Shiobara R, Mine S: Transpetrosal approach for aneurysms of the lower basilar artery. J Neurosurg 63:857-861, 1985.

Malis LI: Surgical resection of tumors of the skull base. In Wilkins RH, Rengachary SS eds: Neurosurgery. New York, McGraw-Hill, 1985, pp 1011-1021.

Mann WJ, Amedee RG, Gilsbach J, Pemeczky A, Wolfensberger M: Transsigmoid approach for tumors of the jugular foramen. Skull Base Surg 1:137-141, 1991.

Mayberg MR, Symon L: Meningiomas of the clivus and apical petrous bone. Report of 35 cases. J Neurosurg 65: 160-167, 1986.

Morrison AW, King TT: Experiences with a translabyrinthine-transtentorial approach to the cerebello-pontine angle. Technical note. J Neurosurg 38: 382-390, 1973.

Pellet WT, Cannoni M, Pech A: The widened transcochlear approach to jugular foramen tumors. J Neurosurg 69: 887-894, 1988.

Saleh E, Naguib M, Aristegui M, Cokkeser Y, Russo A, Sanna M: Surgical anatomy of the jugular foramen area. In: Mazzoni A, Sanna M, eds. Skull base surgery Update, 1. Amsterdam: Kugler, 1995 pp. 3-8.

Saleh E, Naguib M, Aristegui M, Cokkeser Y, Sanna M: The lower skull base: anatomical study with surgical implications. Ann Otol Rhinol Laryngol 104:57-61, 1995.

Saleh E, Taibah A, Achilli V, Aristegui M, Mazzoni M, Sanna A: Posterior fossa meningioma: surgical strategy. Skull Base Surg 4:209-219, 1994.

Samii M, Ammirati M, Mahran A, et al: Surgery of petroclival meningiomas: Report of 24 cases. Neurosurgery 24: 12-17,1989.

Samii M, Ammirati M: The combined supra-infratentorial presigmoid sinus avenue to the petro-clival region: surgical technique and clinical applications. Acta Neurochir 95:6-12, 1988.

Samii M, Draf W: Surgery of the skull base. Berlin: Springer, 1989.

Sekhar LN, Estonillo R: Transtemporal approach to the skull base: an anatomical study. Neurosurgery 19:799-808, 1986.

Sekhar LN, Schramm VL, Jones NF: Subtemporal-preauricular infratemporal fossa approach to large lateral and posterior cranial base neoplasms. J Neurosurg 67:488-499, 1987.

Sekhar LN, Sen C, Jho HD: Saphenous vein graft bypass of the cavernous internal carotid artery. J Neurosurg 72: 35-41, 1990.

Sen C, Sekhar LN: Extreme lateral transcondylar and transjugular approaches. In: Sekhar LN, Janecka I, eds. Surgery of cranial base tumors. NewYork: RavenPress, 389-412, 1993.

Sen C, Sekhar LN: An extreme lateral approach to intradural lesions of the cervical spine and foramen magnum. Neurosurgery 27:197-204, 1990.

Sen C, Sekhar LN: The subtemporal and preauricular infratemporal approach to intradural structures ventral to the brain stem. J Neurosurg 73:345-354, 1990.

Spetzler RF, Daspit CP, Pappas CTE: The combined supra- and infratentorial approach for lesions of the petrous and clival regions: Experience with 46 cases. J Neurosurg 76: 588-599, 1992.

Spetzler RF, Fukishima T, Martin N, et al: Petrous carotid-to intradural carotid saphenous vein graft for intracavernous giant aneurysm, tumor, and occlusive cerebrovascular disease. J Neurosurg 73: 496-501,1990.

Spetzler RF, Grahm TW: The far-lateral approach to the inferior clivus and the upper cervical region: Technical note. Barrow Neurol Inst Q 64: 35-38,1990.

Spetzler RF: Two technical notes for microsurgery. Barrow Neurol Inst 42: 38-39,1988.

Thedinger BA, Glasscock ME, Cueva RA: Transcochlear transtentorial approach for removal of large cerebellopontine angle meningiomas. Am J Otol 13:408-415, 1992.

Velut S, Jan M: Anterior petrosectomy during approach to the petroclival area. In: Schmideck HE, ed. Meningiomas and their surgical management. Philadelphia: Saunders, 435-450, 1991.

37

Transcochlear approach to cerebellopontine angle lesions

We have to adapt the approach to the patient, not the patient to the approach. We have to choose the best approach for the patient, not the best patient for the approach.

The transcochlear approach is the most direct surgical route to midline intracranial lesions arising from the clivus, and to cerebellopontine angle masses arising anterior to the internal auditory canal. These lesions often extend around the basilovertebral artery and, since traditional surgical approaches were limited by the cerebellum and the brainstem, have been considered inoperable by many surgeons. The transcochlear approach does not have these limits and is designed primarily for:

Extradural lesions

- Large congenital petrous apex epidermoids.
- Primary intradural epidermoids anterior to the internal auditory canal.
- Recurrent neuromas with petrous bone extension.

Intradural lesions

- Meningiomas arising from the petroclinoid ridge.
- Intradural clivus lesions.
- Large acoustic tumors with complete facial nerve paralysis and anterior extension.
- Recurrent non acoustic CPA lesions with encasement of the vertebrobasilar artery and/or perforating arteries.

Transdural lesions

- Lesions that reach the endocranium from the clivus or petrous apex, such as chondrosarcomas, chordomas, and glomus tumors (Fig. 37-1).
- Lesions that reach the clivus or petrous apex from the endocranium, such as en plaque meningiomas.

The transcochlear approach evolved from the inability to excise the base of implantation and control the blood supply of these near-midline and midline tumors with other surgical approaches:

- *Suboccipital approach*: Total removal of these lesions is often impossible because of the interposition of the cerebellum and the brainstem.
- *Transpalatal-Transclival Approach*: this approach was attempted for these intradural midline lesions, with little or no success (House WF). The exposure is inadequate, the field is relatively far from the surgeon, the blood supply is lateral, away from the surgeon's view, and intracranial problems with oral contamination occur.
- *Retrolabyrinthine approach*: this approach is limited in its forward extension by the posterior semicircular canal.
- *Translabyrinthine approach*: tumor access is limited anteriorly by the facial nerve, which impedes removal of the tumor's base of implantation, which is anterior to the internal auditory canal, around the intrapetrous carotid artery, or anterior to the brainstem.
- *Anterior extended middle fossa approach*: The recent development of this approach enables complete removal of petroclinoid meningiomas and is used in patients with usable hearing. The primary limitation to this approach is that it cannot access tumors with inferior extension below the level of the inner ear (Shiobara, Wigand).

The transcochlear approach was developed by House and Hitselberger in the late 1960s and early 1970s as an anterior extension of the translabyrinthine approach. It involves complete rerouting of the facial nerve posteriorly and allows removal of the petrous bone, which exposes the intrapetrous internal carotid artery.

Surgical field

This approach affords wide exposure of the anterior cerebellopontine angle, cranial nerves V, VII, VIII, IX, X, and XI, both sixth cranial nerves, the clivus, and the basilar and vertebral arteries. The contralateral cranial nerves and the opposite cerebellopontine angle are also visible. It is the only approach during which the tumor base and

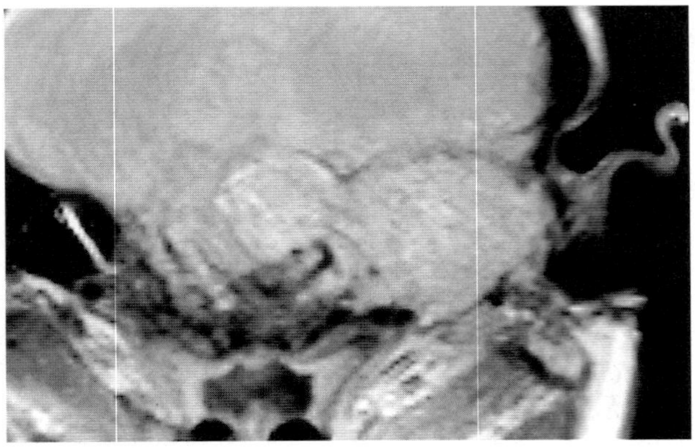

Fig. 37-1. MRI. Transdural left glomus jugularis tumor.

its arterial blood supply from the internal carotid artery are removed (Brackmann). The addition of excision and closure of the external auditory canal, recently advocated by Brackmann (Personal communication, 1993), further increases the anterior exposure.

ADVANTAGES OF THE TRANSCOCHLEAR APPROACH

- No cerebellar or temporal lobe retractors are required.
- Exposure and dissection of the petrous apex and clivus ensure complete removal of both the tumor and its blood supply. This is of particular importance in meningiomas.
- Careful handling and constant monitoring of the facial nerve during rerouting prevent injury to the intratemporal portion of the nerve. However, meningiomas often invade the nerve, and cholesteatomas tend to wrap themselves around it. If the facial nerve is lost during tumor removal, we recommend immediate repair using end-to-end anastomosis or nerve graft interposition.

DISADVANTAGES OF THE TRANSCOCHLEAR APPROACH

The main disadvantages of this approach are the sacrifice of residual hearing in the operated ear, and the risk of temporary facial palsy. This technique is used when no serviceable hearing exists in the involved ear, or when the tumor is too far inferior for the extended middle fossa craniotomy approach. With the use of continuous facial nerve monitoring, the incidence of permanent facial nerve palsy is low.

PATIENT EVALUATION AND PREOPERATIVE COUNSELING

Individuals with tumors that require transcochlear surgery may have minimal symptomatology, and the tumors are quite large at the time of diagnosis (De La Cruz, Brackmann).

SYMPTOMS

Petrous apex epidermoids

- Unilateral hearing loss and tinnitus are the presenting complaints in 80% of petrous apex epidermoids.
- Persistent otorrhea and facial twitch are common.
- Imbalance, ataxia, and parietal or vertex headache may be the only complaints in up to 20 per cent of patients (De La Cruz).

Meningiomas and intradural epidermoids

Patients may be nearly symptomless until they appear with fifth cranial nerve findings and signs of increased intracranial pressure. There is a relatively high rate of jugular foramen syndrome in patients with meningiomas. Seizures, dysarthria, and late signs of dementia from hydrocephalus were common presenting symptoms in the past (De La Cruz).

The evaluation proceeds with an examination of the cranial nerves and an audiometry. Hearing and vestibular function are frequently normal, and acoustic reflex decay or abnormal auditory brainstem response in the audiometric results may be the only anomalies (House WF).

Radiographic evaluation

High-resolution computed tomography (HRCT) with contrast enhancement and/or magnetic resonance imaging (MRI), are essential for diagnosis and surgical planning (Mafee).

- *HRCT.* Petrous apex and intradural epidermoids are expansile, spherical, or oval lesions, with scalloped bone edges. They are isointense with brain and CSF, with capsular enhancement.
- *MRI.* Petrous apex and intradural epidermoids are hypointense on T1 -and hyperintense on T2- weighted images; they do not enhance. Meningiomas enhance on CT and MRI.
- *Brain perfusion and flow studies.* Localization of the tumor may require angiography. In tumors surrounding or invading the intratemporal carotid artery, preoperative balloon occlusion, and/or embolization, are indicated (see Chapter 16).

Patient Counseling

Patients are counseled regarding the serious nature of their tumor. The natural history of petrous apex epidermoids is that they grow and may become superinfected. Treatment is difficult when such infections occur, and meningitis, sepsis, and death may result. Intracranial epidermoid tumors spread through the cisterns and subarachnoid planes to neighboring regions; petrous ridge meningiomas grow and are space-occupying lesions that increase intracranial pressure. Thus, surgical intervention is recommended. After surgery, intracranial pressure is reduced, and cranial nerve symptoms improve. Risks and complications in the immediate postoperative period include transient vertigo, complete hearing loss, and temporary facial nerve paresis, as well as infection, bleeding, cerebrovascular accidents, and death.

SURGICAL TECHNIQUE

Overview

- Complete mastoidectomy and labyrinthectomy, with exposure of the internal auditory canal.
- When first described by House and Hitselberger (1976), the tympanic ring was not removed and only the facial recess was opened to permit anterior exposure. Brackmann as well as Sanna have modified the approach by removing the entire tympanic ring, malleus, incus and stapes, and blind-sac closing the external auditory canal.
- Complete exposure of the facial nerve, with transection of the greater superficial petrosal and chorda tympani nerves. The facial nerve is rerouted posteriorly out of the fallopian canal.
- The cochlea is completely drilled out, and the internal carotid artery is identified.
- A large triangular window is created in the skull base. Its superior boundary is the superior petrosal sinus; inferiorly, it extends below and medially to the inferior petrosal sinus into the clivus. Anteriorly is the internal carotid artery, and the apex of the triangle is just beneath Meckel's cave.
- Tumor removal.
- The dura is reapproximated. Abdominal fat is used to fill the mastoidectomy defect and to cushion the facial nerve.

Setup

- General endotracheal anesthesia with arterial blood pressure monitoring is used, and a urinary catheter and a nasogastric tube are inserted. Long-acting muscle relaxants are avoided because they may produce false negative responses from the intraoperative facial nerve monitor, which is used in all cases. Anesthesia is kept light so that changes in blood pressure and pulse brought about by tumor manipulation are not masked.
- Prophylactic third-generation cephalosporin antibiotics and steroids are used routinely before the skin incision is made.
- Venous antiembolism compression boots are placed on the patient's legs before the procedure begins.
- The patient is placed supine on the operating table, with his head turned to the opposite side, and is maintained in a natural position without fixation. The surgeon sits by the side of the patient's head. This position avoids air embolization, minimizes surgeon fatigue, and allows stabilization of the surgeon's hands during the microsurgical procedure.

Incision

- A postauricular incision is made 3 cm. behind the postauricular fold, starting 1 cm above the ear and ending below the mastoid tip (Fig. 37-2).
- If the intracranial carotid artery and/or the lower cranial nerves are involved, the incision may be extended inferiorly into the neck to provide control of the large vessels and to obtain exposure of the lower cranial nerves. The superior limb of the incision extends to the level of the fascia temporalis.
- Inferiorly, the periosteum is incised above the linea temporalis from the level of the zygomatic root anteriorly to a point 1 cm posterior to the sigmoid sinus. The periosteal incision is carried inferiorly to the mastoid tip. The periosteal elevator is used to free the periosteum from the underlying cortex, to the sinodural angle posteriorly, and forward to the level of the external auditory canal.
- The skin of the external auditory canal is completely excised, including canal skin and tympanic membrane, and the meatus is closed in two layers.

Mastoidectomy

- An extended mastoidectomy is carried out with cutting and diamond burrs and continuous suction irrigation. Bone removal is begun along two lines, one along the linea temporalis, and another tangential to the external canal.
- The mastoid antrum is opened, and the lateral semicircular canal is identified. This canal is the most reliable landmark in the temporal bone and allows the dissection to proceed towards delineating the fallopian canal and the osseous labyrinth.
- The external opening of the mastoid cavity must be as large as possible and is extended posterior to the sigmoid sinus, exposing 1 to 2cm of suboccipital (posterior fossa) dura. The larger the tumor, the further back the posterior fossa dura is exposed, to a maximum of 2 to 3cm.
- The root of the zygomatic arch is drilled. This enhances the anterior visibility.
- Bone over the sigmoid sinus is removed with diamond burrs. An island of bone (Bill's island) may be left over the dome of the sinus, to avoid injury to the sinus from burr shafts. If bleeding occurs that cannot be controlled with preservation of the sigmoid sinus, it is reduced with a

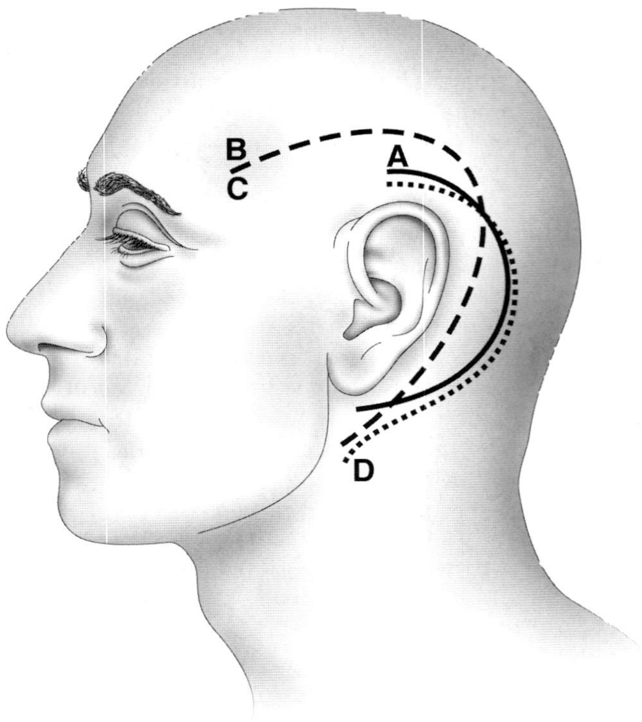

Fig. 37-2. Skin incision for transcochlear approach (A), type B and type C modified transcochlear approaches and modified type D transcochlear approach.

bipolar cautery, and the sinus is packed with a large piece of oxidized bovine cellulose (Surgicel), or ligated. No attempt is made to use small pieces of Surgicel, since they can reach the lung and cause a serious infarction. The mastoid emissary vein is dissected, and bleeding is controlled with bipolar cautery, a mixture of Surgicel and bone wax, or plain Surgicel packing.

- Bone is removed from the sinodural angle along the superior petrosal sinus. The mastoid air cells are exenterated from the sinodural angle, thereby skeletonizing the dura of the posterior fossa and the posterior 1 cm of middle fossa dura (Fig. 37-3).

Labyrinthectomy and Exposure of the Internal Auditory Canal

- After removal of all of the canal skin, the tympanic membrane and the ossicles, the bony external auditory canal is drilled out and excised circumferentially. This extension, together with the anterior dislocation of the mandibular condyle, gives a better control of the ICA, and opens the way to the mid-clivus (Sanna).

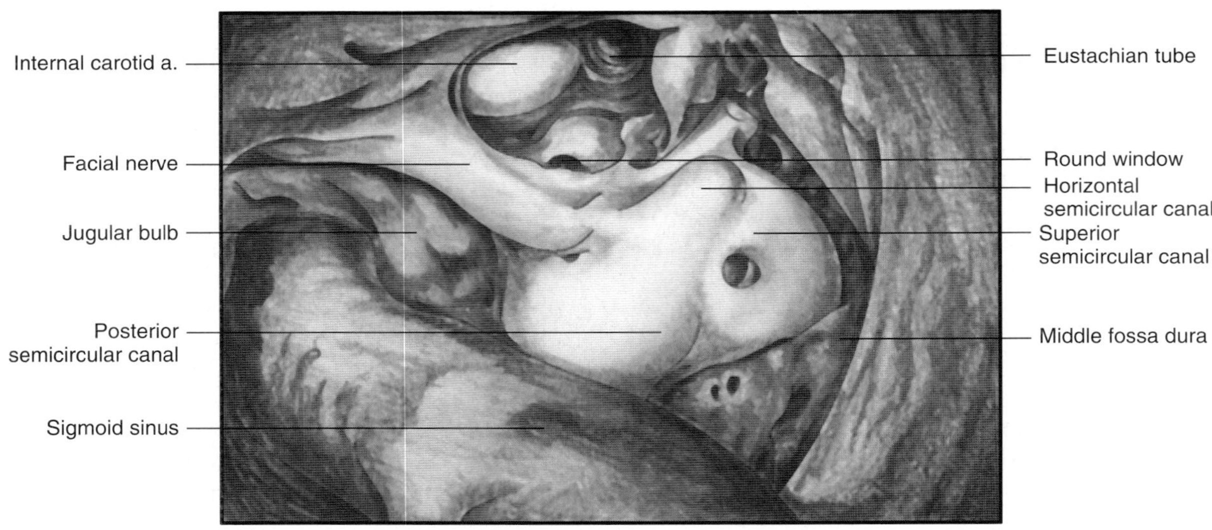

Fig. 37-3. Left ear. Complete mastoidectomy. Exposure of middle fossa dura, posterior fossa dura, sigmoid sinus, semicircular canals. The facial nerve is skeletonized.

- Dissection of the perilabyrinthine cells down to the lateral semicircular canal is completed. The facial nerve is identified between the nonampullated end of the lateral semicircular canal and the stylomastoid foramen. At this stage, exposing the perineurium of the nerve is not necessary, but it should be clearly and unmistakably identified in its vertical path.
- The labyrinthectomy is performed (see chapter 28). All three bony and membranous semicircular canals are removed, as well as the saccule and utricle in the vestibule (Figs. 37-4, 37-5).
- Dissection proceeds along the sinodural angle, and the dura of the posterior fossa is exposed anteriorly. The cells over the jugular bulb are removed, skeletonizing it. To obtain a better control of the lower cranial nerves and the vertebro-basilar junction, the jugular bulb is completely exposed and, if needed, lowered (see Chapter 28, Tips and Pitfalls).
- The internal auditory canal is identified, beginning inferiorly and then proceeding around to the porus acusticus, using the falciform (transverse) crest and vertical crest (Bill's bar) as identifying landmarks. The dissection and removal of the roof of the internal auditory canal is performed with diamond burr.

Facial Nerve Dissection

- Complete skeletonization of the facial nerve from the internal auditory canal to the stylomastoid foramen, including the geniculate ganglion and the beginning of the greater superficial petrosal nerve, is performed with diamond burrs.
- An extended facial recess opening may be created, but our current technique includes removal of the entyre tympanic bone, and ossicles and blind sac closure of the external auditory canal (Figs. 37-6, 37-7, 37-8).
- An area comprising 180% of the bony fallopian canal is exposed, removing the last shell of bone with a raspatory.

Care is taken to avoid placing traction on the nerve:

- The nerve is exposed up to the stylomastoid foramen, where the periosteum of the digastric muscle blends with the sheath of the VII nerve (Fig. 37-9). An uncomplete exposure of the VII up to this point would leave the VII nerve unrerouted. This would impede a complete control of the jugular bulb and limit the visualization of the tumor's lower pole.

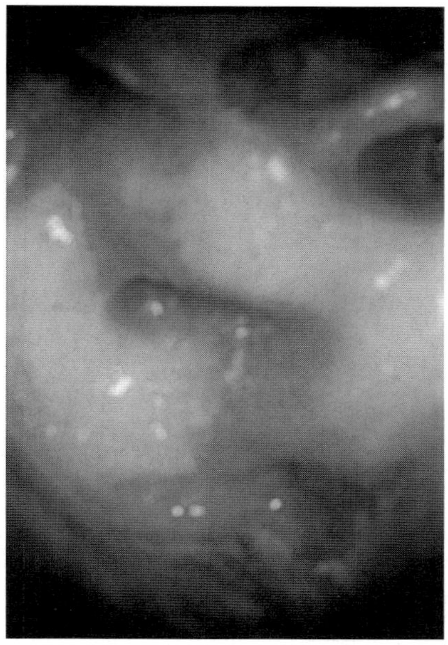

Fig. 37-4. The semicircular canals are exposed.

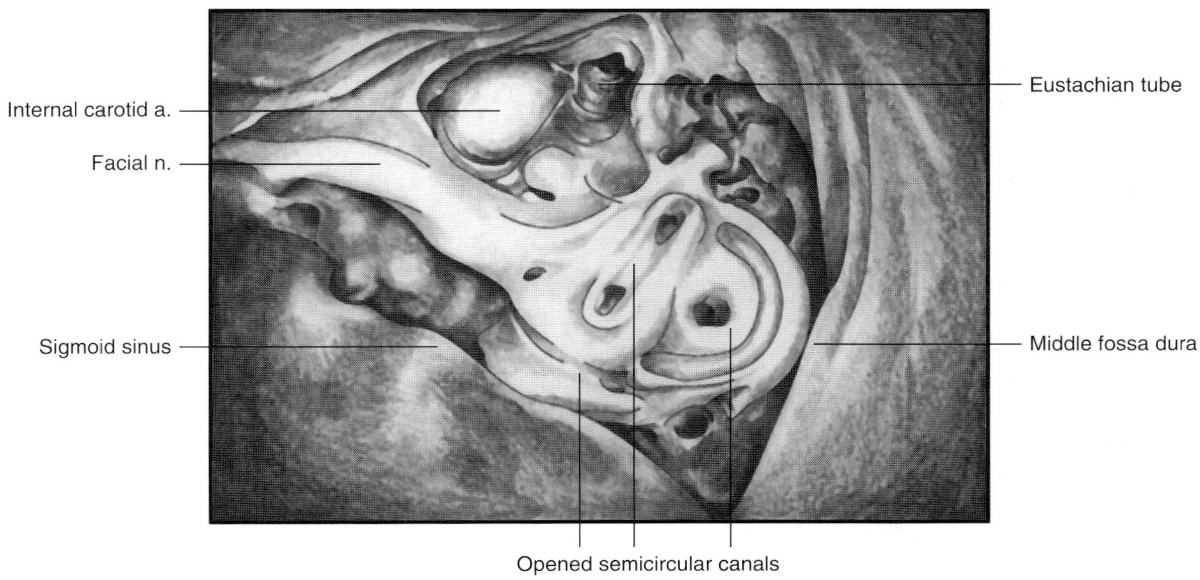

Fig. 37-5. Opening of the semicircular canals.

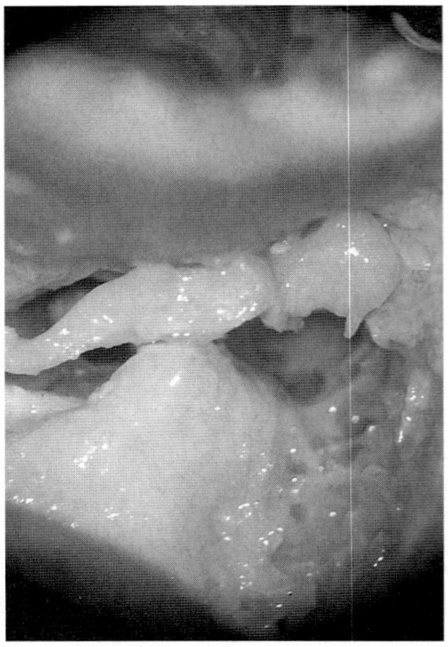

Fig. 37-6. Left ear. Transcochlear approach. Complete simple mastoidectomy. The ossicles are exposed through an extended facial recess opening. The incus is removed. When further anterior exposure is required, the malleus is removed and closure of the external auditory canal is included.

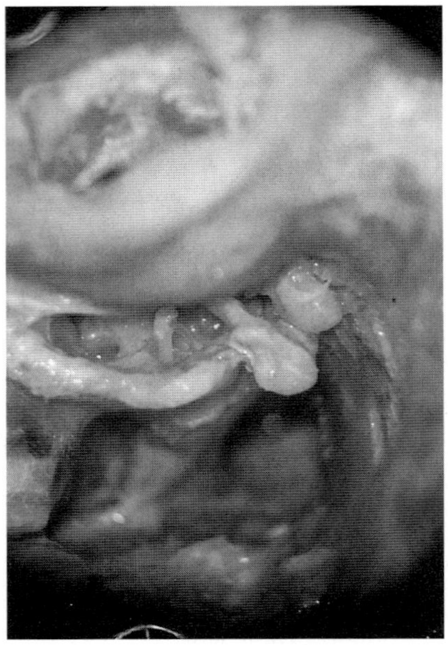

Fig. 37-8. The tympanic part and the mastoid part of the facial nerve are exposed, from the internal auditory canal to the stylomastoid foramen, including the geniculate ganglion. The internal auditory canal is exposed.

- Near the second genu, the nerve has adhesions to the fallopian canal and several branches of the stapedius muscle that must be cut with a sickle shaped knife. The trauma of a blunt dissection must be avoided.
- Special care is taken when working on the labyrinthine part of the nerve, near the geniculate ganglion. Here the nerve is reduced in size and forms an acute angle, therefore it is particularly liable to injury. It is important to completely expose this part, to avoid resistance of bony fragments when the nerve is rerouted. It is adivisable to completely expose the middle fossa dura, to depress it superiorly with a suction irrigator and to remove even the last shell of bone with diamond burr and dissectors.

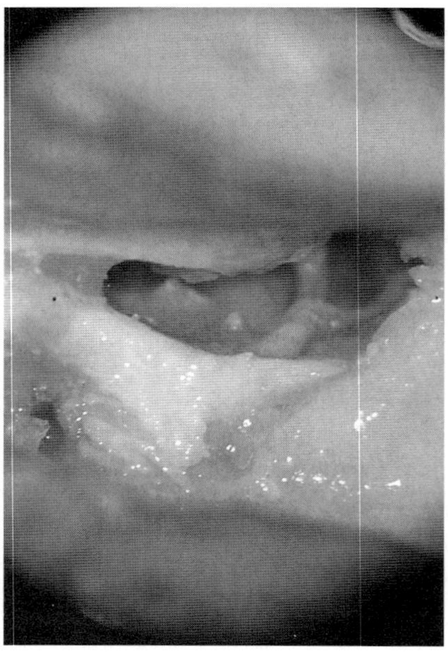

Fig. 37-7. An extended facial recess opening is created.

- The greater superficial petrosal nerve is cut from the geniculate ganglion at its origin with the incudostapedial joint knife. The nerve is then reflected posteriorly out of the bony fallopian canal with dental excavators (Figs. 37-10, 37-11).
- Since the geniculate ganglion and the labyrinthine facial nerve are the most fragile parts of the nerve, they are the first to be freed from the underlying bone. The tympanic segment and the mastoid segment follow.
- The internal auditory canal dura is preserved and the acousticofacial bundle, with all the protecting dura, is rerouted posteriorly. To this end, the anterior bony canal of the IAC is scraped with a dissector, carefully elevating the dura backwards.
- The nerve is moved out of the field, and fixed to the posterior fossa dura posteriorly with fibrin glue (Figs. 37-12, 37-13, 37-14).

Transcochlear Drill-Out

- The fallopian canal has been removed, the promontory has been exposed, and the ossicles have been removed.
- Starting with the basal coil, the cochlea is completely drilled. Bone removal is carried forward

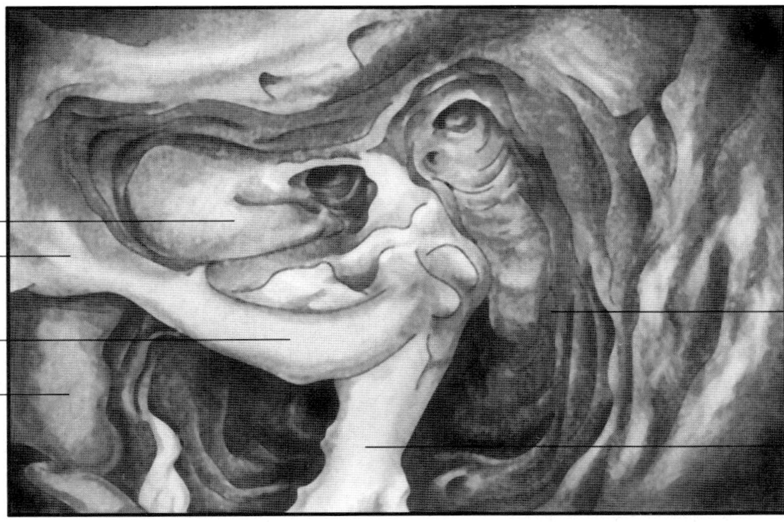

Fig. 37-9. The facial nerve is exposed, from the stylomastoid foramen to the IAC.

to the internal carotid artery with a diamond burr: no more then 1-2 mm of bone separates the ICA by the anterior part of the cochlea basal coil (Figs. 37-15, 37-16, 37-17, 37-18).

- The inferior limit of bone removal extends to the inferior petrosal sinus and jugular bulb. Superiorly the superior petrosal sinus is exposed to Meckels cave. Medially bone removal extends to the clivus. At this stage, a large window, covered by dura, has been created in the skull base. Its boundaries are superiorly the superior petrosal sinus; inferiorly, below and medial to the inferior petrosal sinus into the clivus; anteriorly the internal carotid artery; and medially the lateral clivus. The apex of the triangle is just beneath Meckel's cave (Figs. 37-19, 37-20).

Removal and closure of the external auditory canal is included (see Chapter 16 on glomus tumors).

- The mandibular condyle is anteriorly displaced with the Fisch infratemporal retractor.
- The petrous apex is drilled and the mid clivus is reached anteriorly. The differences between petrous and clival bone are easy to detect, the first being compact, the second cancellous.
- The posterior fossa dura is incised in front of the IAC, to avoid injury to the facial nerve. Care is also taken not to injure the VIth nerve, which runs underneath the dura, in the area between the IAC and the ICA (Fig. 37-21).
- In certain cases, the internal carotid artery must be sacrificed for complete tumor removal. Carotid resection affords greater anterior exposure, and the risks inherent to this procedure are minimized if the patient has tolerated the preoperative balloon occlusion of the artery.

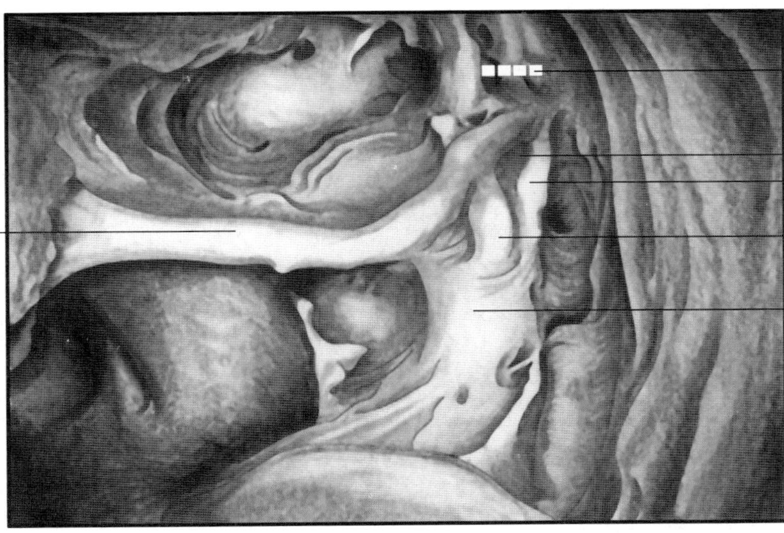

Fig. 37-10. The greater superficial petrosal nerve is cut.

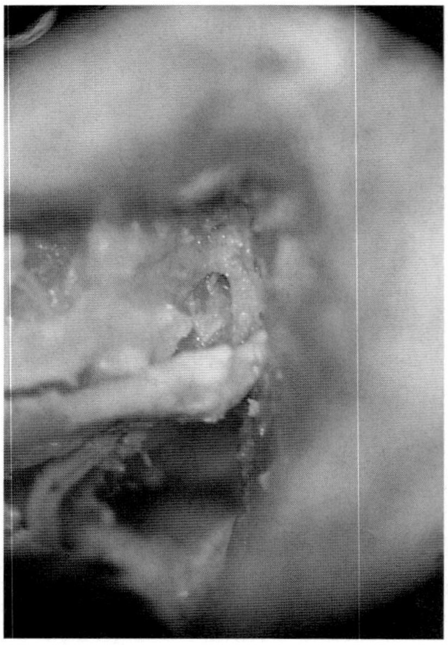

Fig. 37-11. The greater superficial petrosal nerve is cut at its origin from the geniculate ganglion with a hook or a sickle knife.

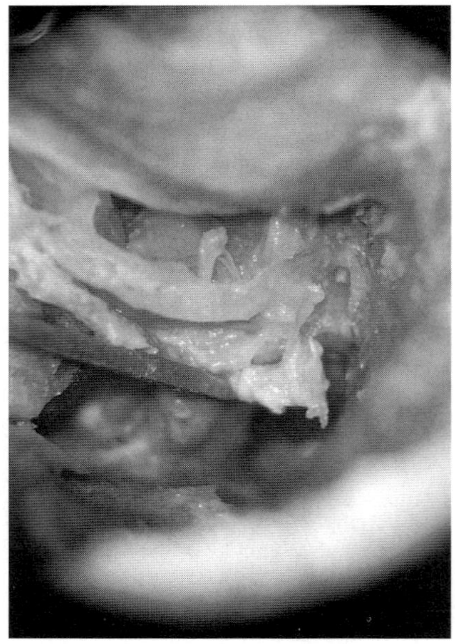

Fig. 37-13. The facial nerve is reflected posteriorly out of the bony fallopian canal, without exerting traction on it.

Tumor Removal

- In petrous ridge meningiomas, arterial feeder vessels from the internal carotid artery are encountered and eliminated at this stage. The diamond burr is used to excise these vessels and the base of implantation at the petrous tip. Using this approach, the surgeon removes the root of the tumor. The dura is opened as previously described and the opening is extended as far forward as is necessary for complete tumor exposure (Figs. 37-22, 37-23, 37-24, 37-25, 37-26).
- The facial nerve is seen on the posterior surface of the tumor. The junction of the intracranial portion of the facial nerve and the skeletonized intratemporal portion is now identified and the entire nerve is reflected posteriorly. The nerve

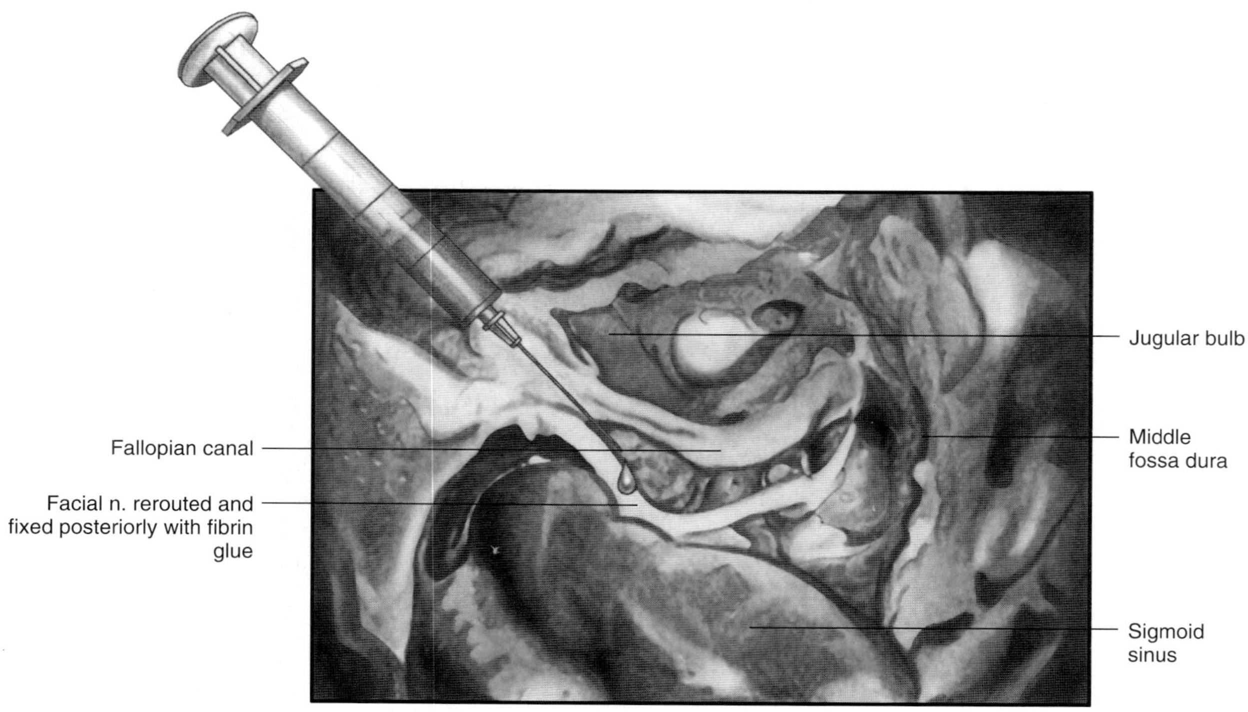

Fig. 37-12. The facial nerve is mobilized and rerouted posteriorly. It is fixed to the posterior fossa dura with fibrin glue.

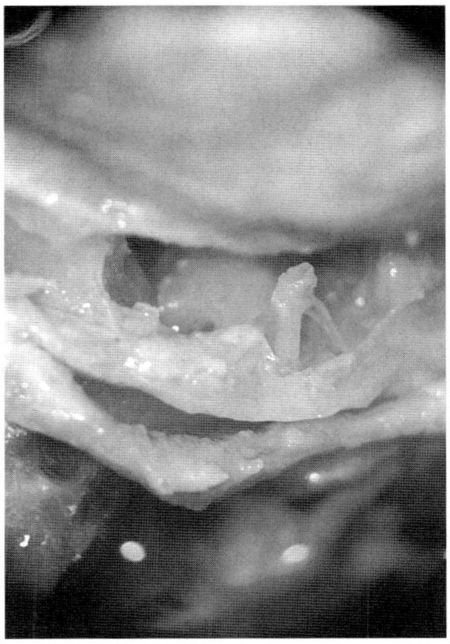

Fig. 37-14. The bony fallopian canal is drilled down. The stapedius muscle and the stapes are removed.

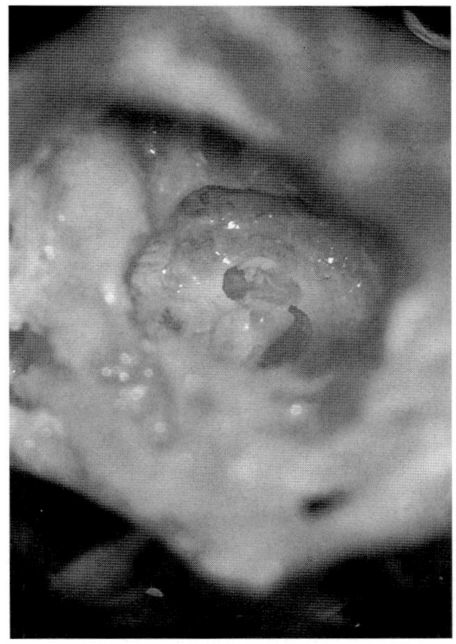

Fig. 37-16. Starting with the basal coil, the cochlea is completely drilled out. Approx. 1 mm. of bone separates anteriorly the basal coil of the cochlea from the petrous carotid artery.

is protected with a moist absorbable gelatine sponge (Gelfoam) pledget.

- The tumor capsule is opened, and the main mass of the tumor is removed. As the dissection proceeds forward and medially the basilar artery and sixth cranial nerves are identified anterosuperiorly. The vertebral arteries appear posteroinferiorly. The tumor capsule is removed from these vessels and their major tributaries under direct vision. In tumors extending across the midline, the basilar artery and its major branches can be dissected from the tumor capsule posteriorly. When the lesion is removed in this fashion, the cranial nerves and the internal auditory canal in the opposite cerebellopontine angle come into view.

Closure

- After the tumor has been removed, hemostasis is secured.

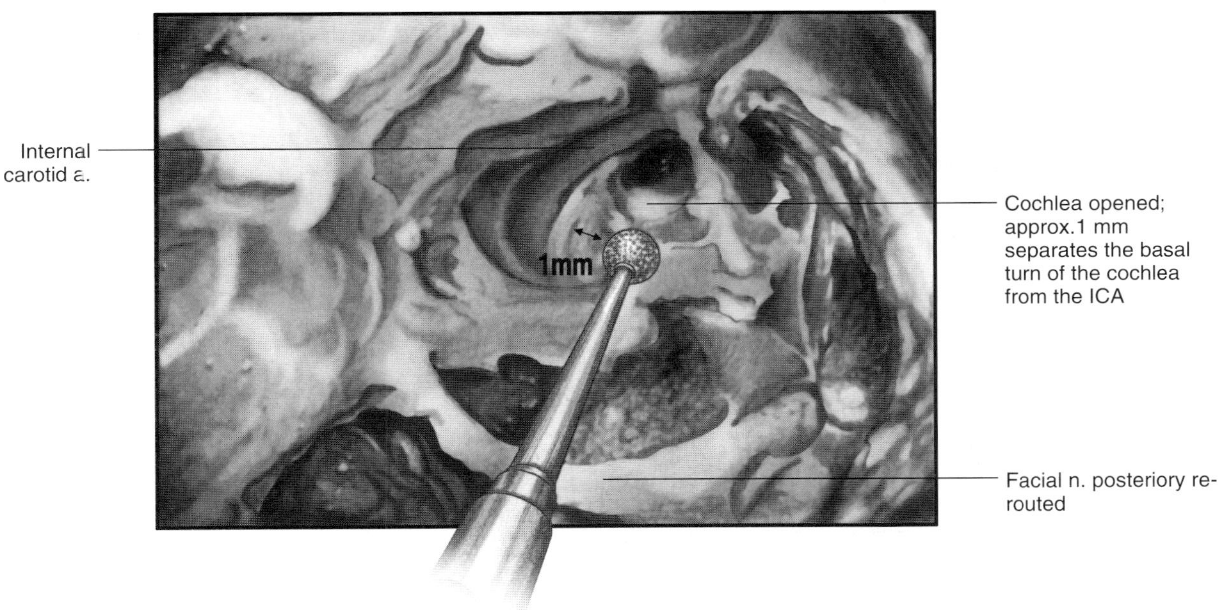

Fig. 37-15. The fallopian canal is drilled down. The cochlea is drilled down: only 1 mm separates the basal turn of the cochlea from the ICA.

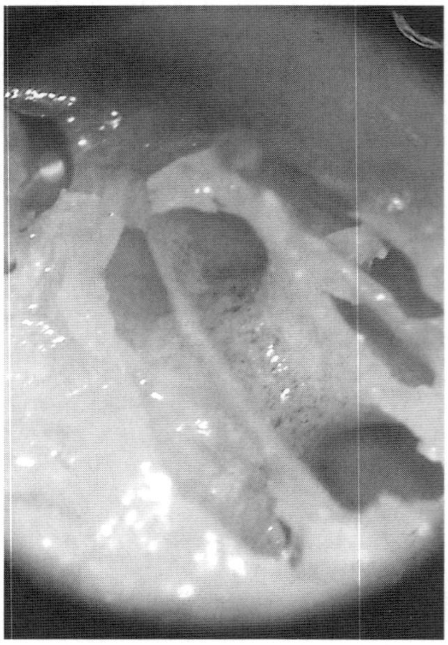

Fig. 37-17. Close-up view of the opened cochlea.

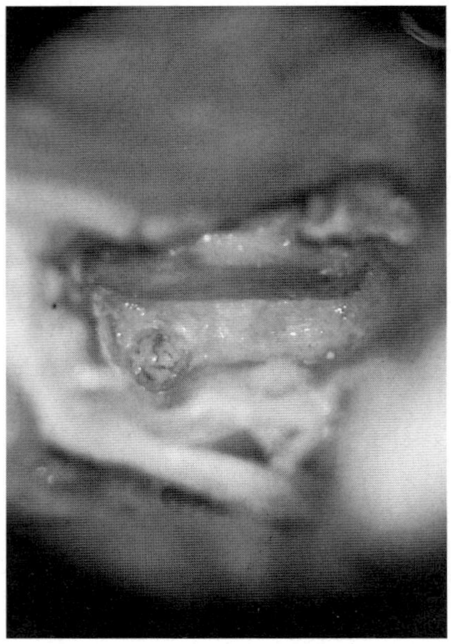

Fig. 37-18. Bone removal of the promontory is carried forward to the internal carotid artery while the inferior extent of bone removal extends to the inferior petrosal sinus and jugular bulb.

- The dura is reapproximated, and the facial nerve is freed and reflected forward. The eustachian tube orifice is plugged with Surgicel, bone wax, and bone paté.
- Abdominal fat is used to fill the mastoid and skull base defect, as well as to form a bed for the facial nerve.
- The postauricular incision is closed in three layers, and a compressive dressing is placed securely about the head.
- Lumbar drainage may be initiated and continued for 5 days.

POSTOPERATIVE CARE

The patient is observed in the intensive care unit for 48 hours after surgery, and remains in the hospital for 7 days. Steroids are continued for 48 hours, but antibiotics are not routinely continued after the perioperative period. Early mobilization and ambulation allow for the speedy return of balance, and prevents vascular complications.

RESULTS

In 1982, De La Cruz reviewed the results of 16 patients in whom the transcochlear approach was used. A combination transcochlear-middle fossa approach was used in the three cases involving dumbbell shaped tumors in both the posterior and middle cranial fossae. Total tumor removal was possible in

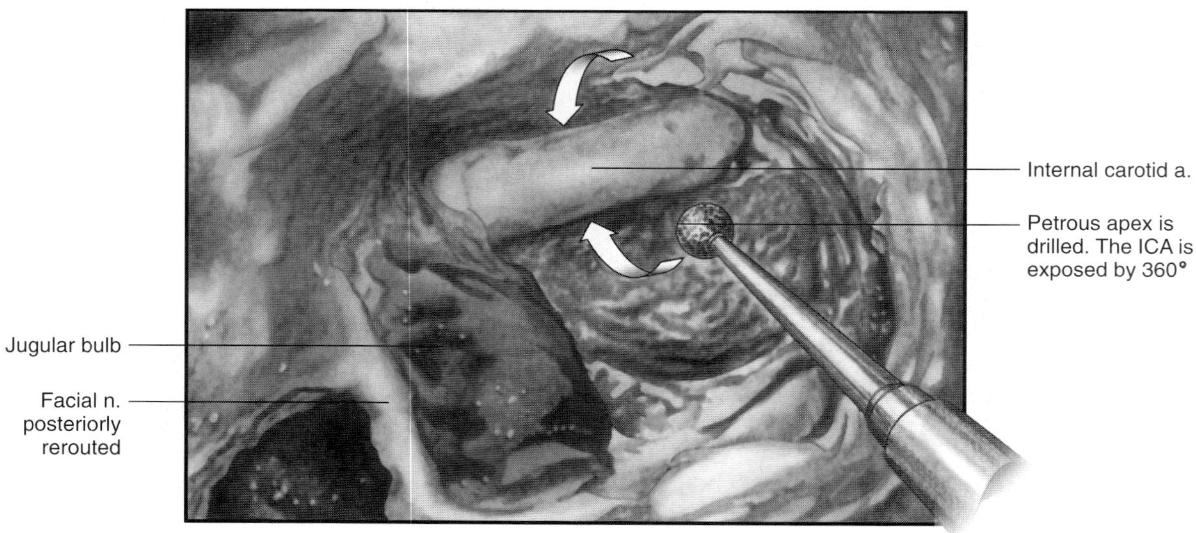

Fig. 37-19. The bone of the petrous apex is drilled. The ICA is exposed by 360 degrees. All the posterior fossa dura is exposed.

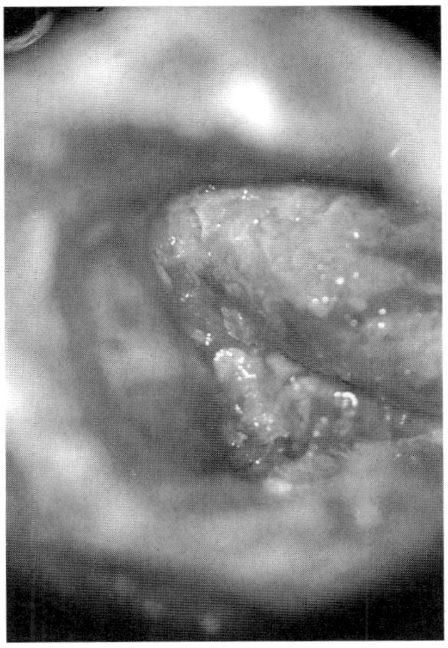

Fig. 37-20. The internal carotid artery and the jugular bone are exposed. The jugulocarotid bony spine (crotch) is drilled down.

13 of the 16 patients. Each of the other three patients had had surgery elsewhere and presented large recurrent meningiomas and extensive neurologic deficits preoperatively. During the transcoclear approach, scraps of tumor were left behind on the vertebral artery in two of these cases. None of these patients has had tumor recurrence.

Four patients had facial paresis or tics preoperatively; of the remaining 12, four had permanent facial paralysis due to tumor involvement of the nerve, and seven had temporary paresis with good-to-excellent recovery of facial function. This paresis was attributed primarily to the excessive manipulation necessary for total tumor removal, and these patients were operated on before facial nerve monitoring was available.

Two deaths occurred in this series. One individual experienced bleeding from the vertebral artery 1 week after surgery, and requiring clipping of the vessel, with subsequent infarction of the brainstem; the other was diabetic and succumbed 1 month postoperatively to gram-negative shock from pyelonephritis. This patient was reported as having a "permanent" facial paralysis. Autopsy revealed no evidence of residual tumor on the facial nerve or elsewhere.

In 1989 Yamakawa et al. published their results with the suboccipital approach, reporting subtotal tumor removal in 17 of 29 patients with intracranial epidermoids and tumor recurrence in seven patients. One of 14 patients with cerebellopontine angle tumors had postoperative seventh nerve paralysis, six had abducens palsy, four had dysphagia, and two had hearing loss.

The report by Yasargil et al. published in the same year analyzed results in 43 patients, 35 had epidermoid tumors while others had intracranial dermoid tumors. No recurrences were seen. Aseptic meningitis and transient cranial nerve palsies were the most common complications. Two deaths were reported.

COMPLICATIONS AND MANAGEMENT

- Temporary facial nerve paresis is the most common complication. If facial paresis occurs, prompt eye care is essential: adequate lubrication with drops, nighttime ointments, and a moisture shield prevents ocular complications. Unless the facial nerve has been severed, surgi-

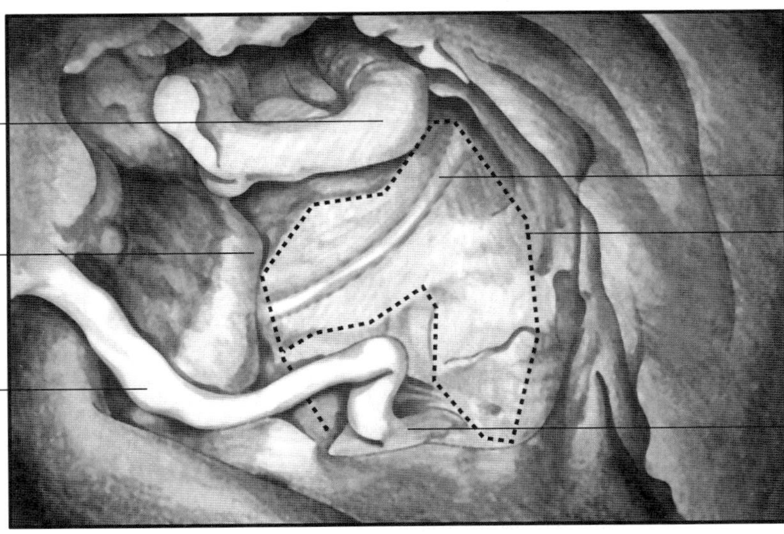

Fig. 37-21. Dural incision in front of the fundus of the IAC. Care is taken not to injure the underlying abducens nerve (Adapted from Sanna M).

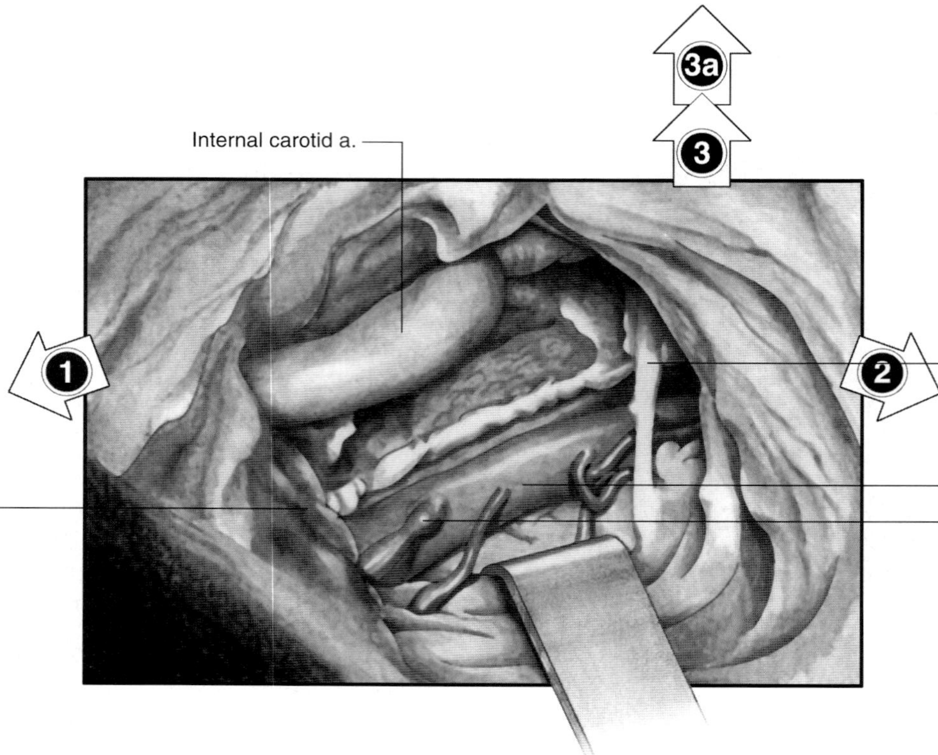

Fig. 37-22. Dura has been cut. The underlying structures can be seen. (Adapted from Sanna M).

cal intervention for facial reanimation is not indicated. The best approach in individuals with even complete facial paralysis after transcochlear surgery, if the facial nerve is anatomically intact, is eye care and "watchful waiting" because the great majority of these patients recover to an acceptable grade of facial function within the first year after surgery.

- Other cranial nerve palsies may occur and should be addressed individually. The neurotologist must attain a good working relationship not only with a neurosurgeon but also with an ophthalmologist and a laryngologist, to aid in the management of these cranial nerve deficits.
- Intracranial bleeding is controlled at the time of surgery. Close observation of the patient in the

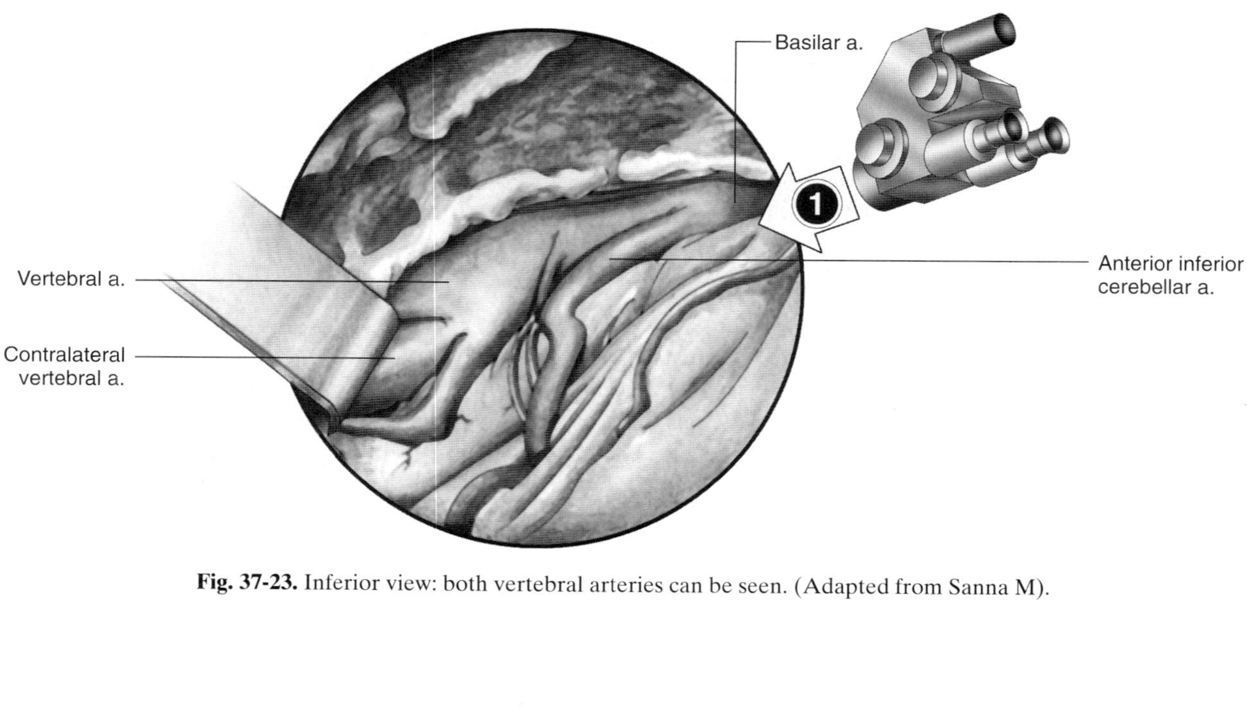

Fig. 37-23. Inferior view: both vertebral arteries can be seen. (Adapted from Sanna M).

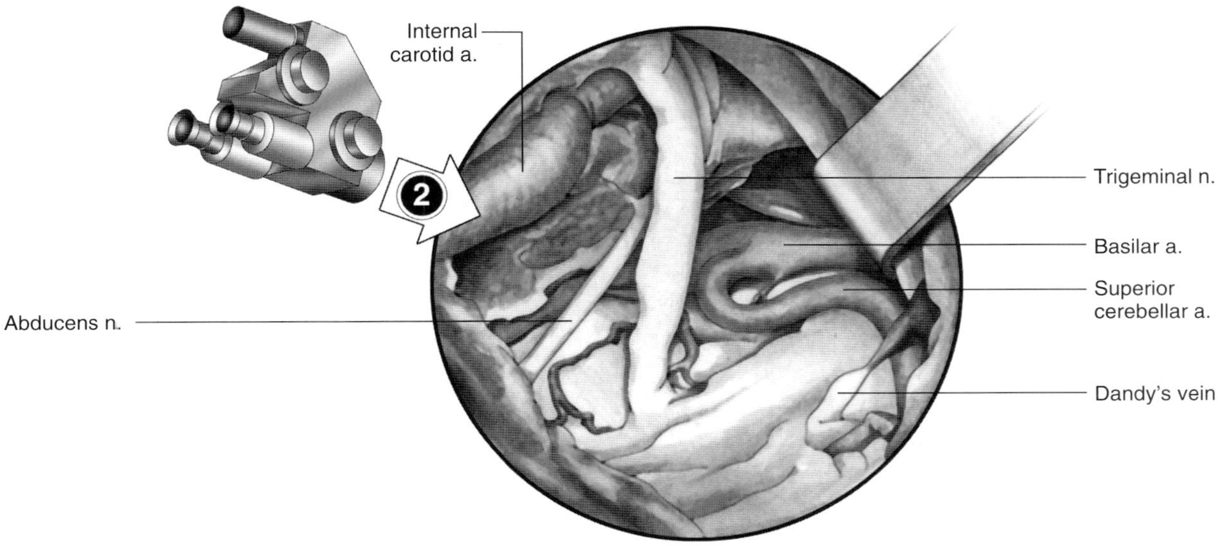

Fig. 37-24. Superior view. (Adapted from Sanna M).

intensive care unit for the initial 48 hours postoperatively allows early recognition of a delayed postoperative intracranial hemorrhage. In these cases, treatment consists of immediate reopening of the surgical wound and removal of the fat in the intensive care unit while the operating room is being prepared, followed by operative evacuation of the hematoma and control of the bleeding site(s).

- Meningitis is not unusual after complete excision of intracranial epidermoids (Cantu; Guidetti) and its incidence increases when the tumor capsule is left in place. If infectious, meningitis may be fatal, and it requires aggres-

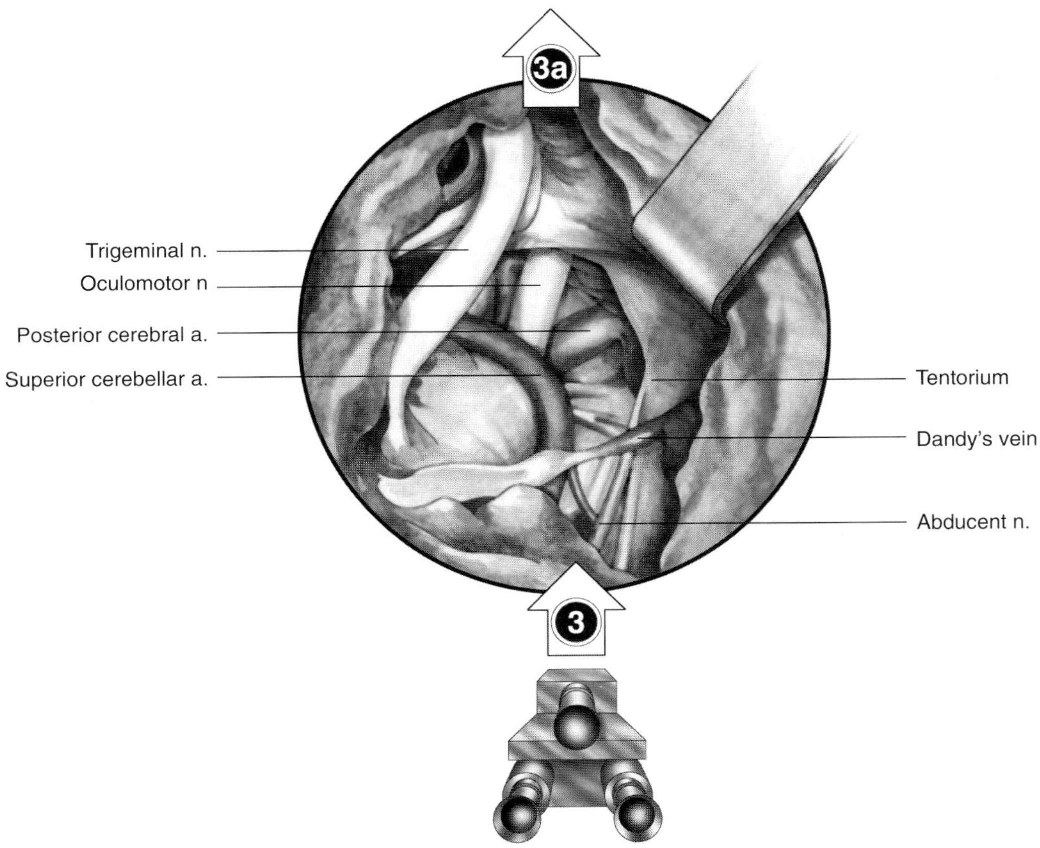

Fig. 37-25. Anterior view. Tentorium is retracted.

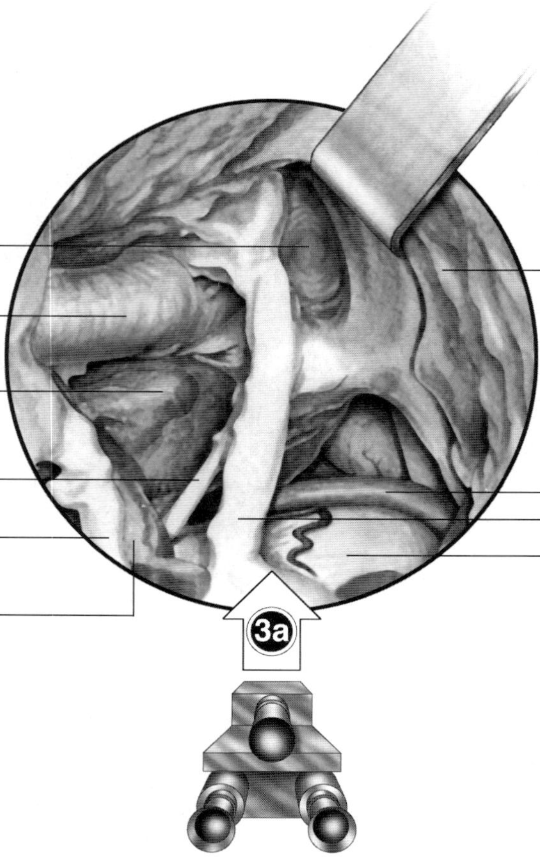

Fig. 37-26. More anterior view of the Fig. 37-25.

sive antibiotic therapy. More commonly, however, it is a chemical meningitis, and the patient is treated with dexamethasone.

- Normal-pressure hydrocephalus can occur and is treated with acetazolamide (Diamox). Postoperative pain is not as severe as that seen with the suboccipital approach, and it is handled with oral analgesics.

With this approach, tumor recurrence is rare if all of the visible tumor has been removed. Patients with recurrences do not present typically and may have vague complaints of unsteadiness or trigeminal neuropathy several years after the initial resection (De La Cruz). Biannual follow-up with gadolinium-enhanced MRI is necessary. In cases of suspected tumor regrowth or recurrence, a complete reevaluation is performed, and removal of the recurrent tumor is advised.

SUMMARY

Access to midline intracranial lesions, intradural clival tumors, and cerebellopontine angle tumors arising anterior to the internal auditory canal has traditionally been difficult. The transcochlear approach mobilizes the facial nerve, removes the cochlea, and dissects the internal carotid artery, allowing direct exposure of these lesions and of midline and contralateral structures. Total removal of the tumor and its base and blood supply is accomplished with this approach. The transcochlear approach is recommended for patients with poor or no hearing. Its safety and efficacy encourage its use.

REFERENCES

See Chapter 38.

38

Modified transcochlear approaches

Two principles of skull base surgery: Remove the bone; leave the brain undisturbed.

SANNA M.

Sanna and Mazzoni proposed these approaches which extend the indications of the basic transcochlear approach. Type A, B, C, D can be distinguished (Fig. 38-1).

TYPE A APPROACH

Essentially, it is that previously described, with removal of the posterior canal wall.

TYPE B

It is an anterior extension of the type A and follows the guidelines of Fisch infratemporal fossa approaches. It is indicated:

- In extradural lesions, such as clivus chordomas, involving the ICA.
- In intradural lesions, such as meningiomas, with limited extension beyond the midline.
- In transdural lesions, such as en plaque meningiomas or clivus chordomas extending to the parapharyngeal space. To avoid comunication between the endocranium and the parapharyngeal space, the operation is usually staged and the extracranial part is operated first. This reduces the rate of contamination and CSF leaks.

SURGICAL TECHNIQUE

Incision (Figs. 37-2, 38-1)

This approach incorporates all the techniques of the extended transcochlear approach. In addition:

- The glenoid fossa is drilled.
- When a wider exposure is needed, the zygomatic root is cut anteriorly and removed. It is repositioned and kept in place with silk passed through two burr holes, at the end of the operation (Fig. 38-2).
- The middle fossa bone is drilled with anterior direction, towards the petrous apex. The middle meningeal artery (MMA) coming from middle fossa dura is exposed, coagulated and transected. More anteriorly, V3 is exposed and, if needed, coagulated and transected. This provides better exposure of anterior and medial space (Fig. 38-3).
- Meckel's cave can be opened if it is involved by the tumor (Fig. 38-4).
- Sphenoid sinus can be opened, if it is involved by the tumor (Fig. 38-5). The mucosa is completely dissected from the cavity which is obliterated with fat. When the sphenoid sinus is opened by chance, the opening is closed with a muscle plug, to preserve the internal mucosal layer.

TYPE C

This approach is indicated for petroclival lesions, such as meningiomas, extended supratentorially.

SURGICAL TECHNIQUE

- Incision (Figs. 37-2, 38-1).
- The middle fossa dura is widely exposed and all the bone is drilled out. The middle fossa dura is opened 2-3 mm. above the superior petrosal sinus, on a parallel line. The superior petrosal sinus is coagulated and cut and Surgicel is used if needed.
- The tentorium comes into view below the junction between sigmoid sinus and superior petrosal sinus. It is cut from lateral to medial, up to the tentorial notch. The structures at risks are those close to the tentorium (see chapter 34) and must be preserved (Fig. 38-6).
- The field is bounded anteriorly by the ICA, inferiorly by the jugular bulb, posteriorly by the sigmoid sinus and superiorly by the oculomotor nerve and the posterior cerebral artery (PCA) (Fig. 38-7).
- With mild retraction of the temporal lobe, the field widens anteriorly up to the optic chiasm and the bifurcation of ICA into the middle cerebral and the anterior cerebral arteries comes into view.

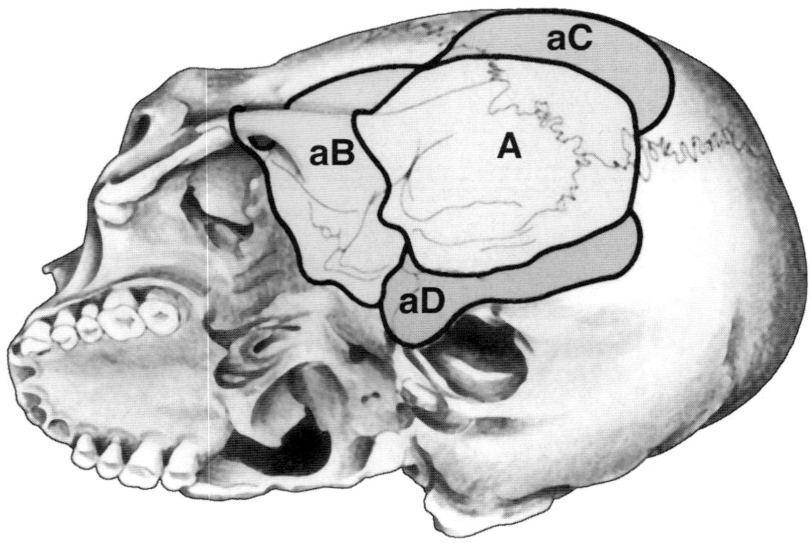

Fig. 38-1. Modified transcochlear approaches, as proposed by Sanna M and Mazzoni A. **A:** Type A. **aB:** Type B (anterior extension of type A). **aC:** Type C (anterior extension of type A). **aD:** Type D (inferior extension of type A).

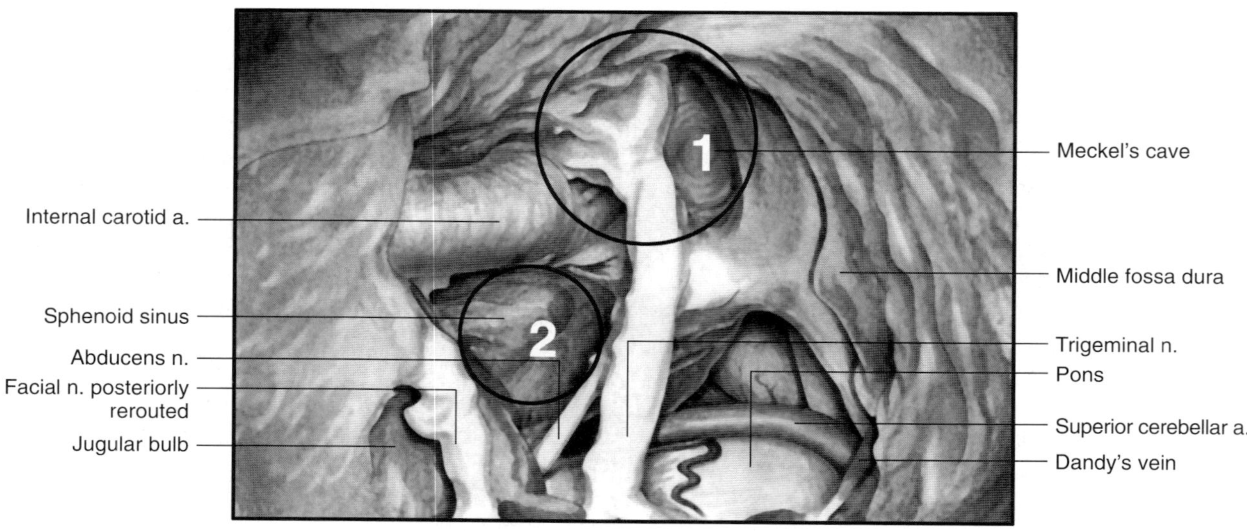

Fig. 38-2. Modified type B transcochlear approach: Meckel's cave and sphenoid sinus can be seen. 1): Meckel's cave. 2): Sphenoid sinus.

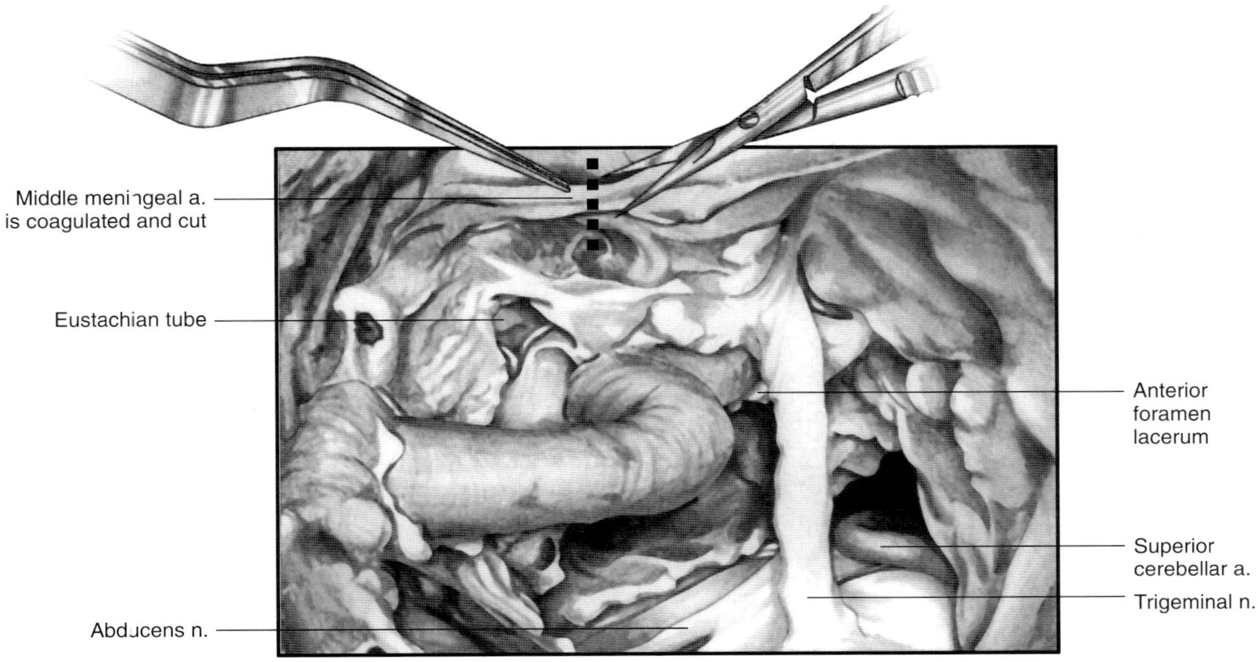

Fig. 38-3. Type B. To enlarge anterior extension, the glenoid fossa is drilled, while the middle meningeal artery is coagulated and cut. If more anterior extension is needed, V3 is cut, while the zygomatic arch is transected and later repositioned. (Adapted from Sanna M).

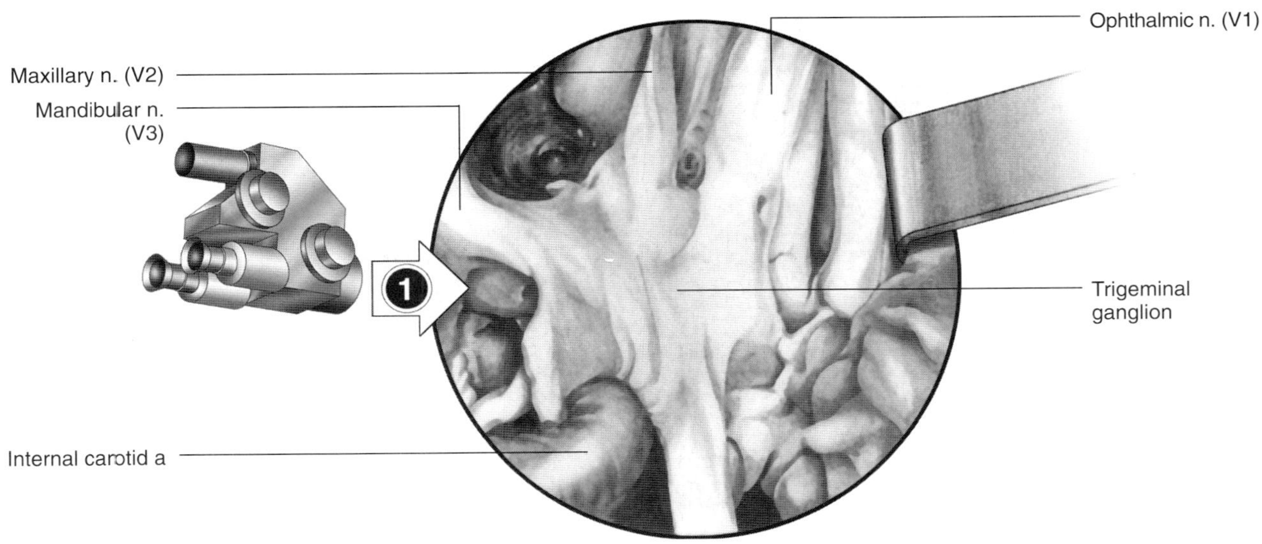

Fig. 38-4. Meckel's cave can be opened; the trigeminal ganglion can be seen.

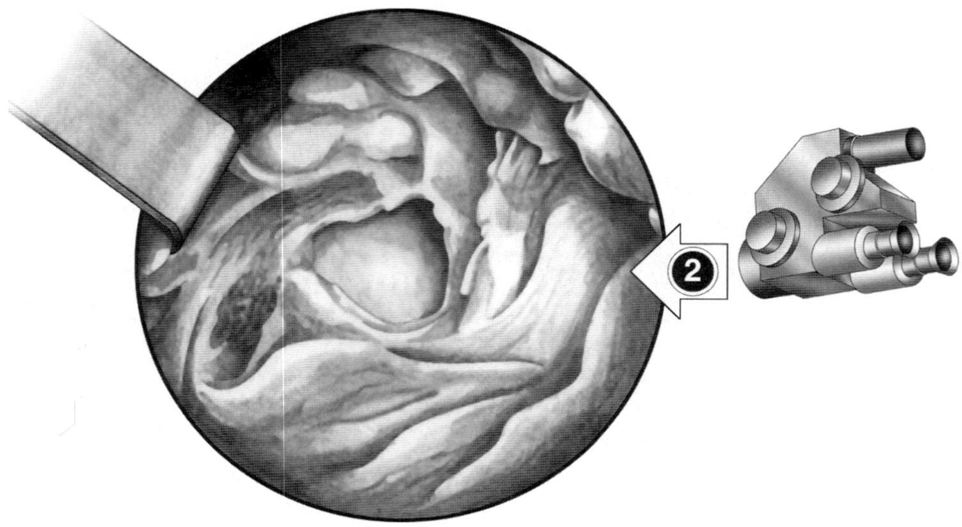

Fig. 38-5. Type B. Sphenoid sinus can be opened, when necessary.

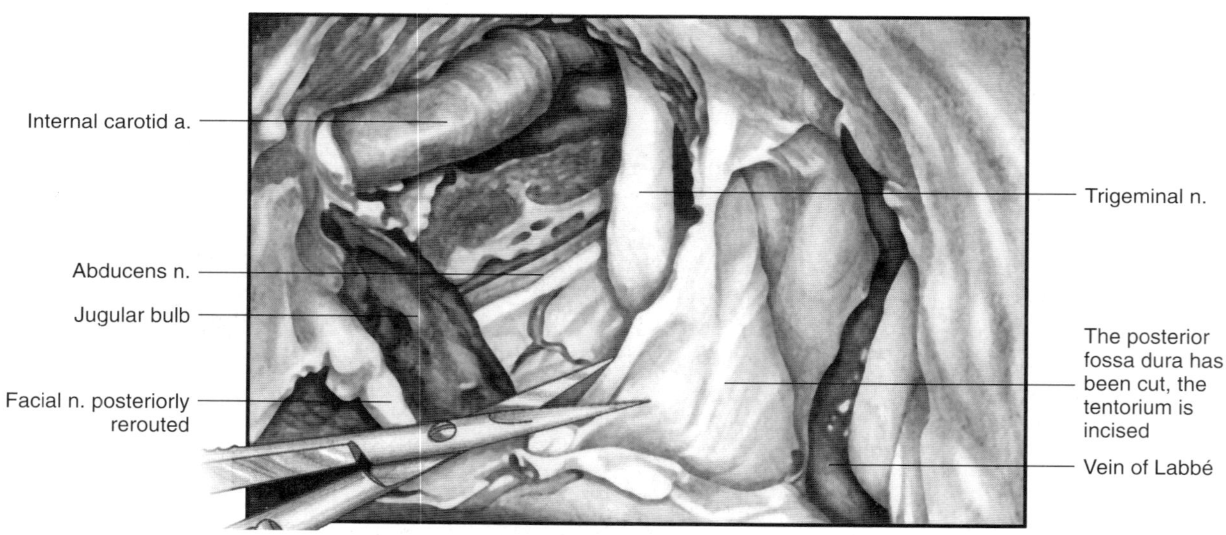

Fig. 38-6. Type C. Dura of the middle fossa has been opened.; vein of Labbé is preserved. Superior petrosal sinus is cut and packed with Surgicel. Tentorium is cut up to the tentorial notch. (Adapted from Sanna M).

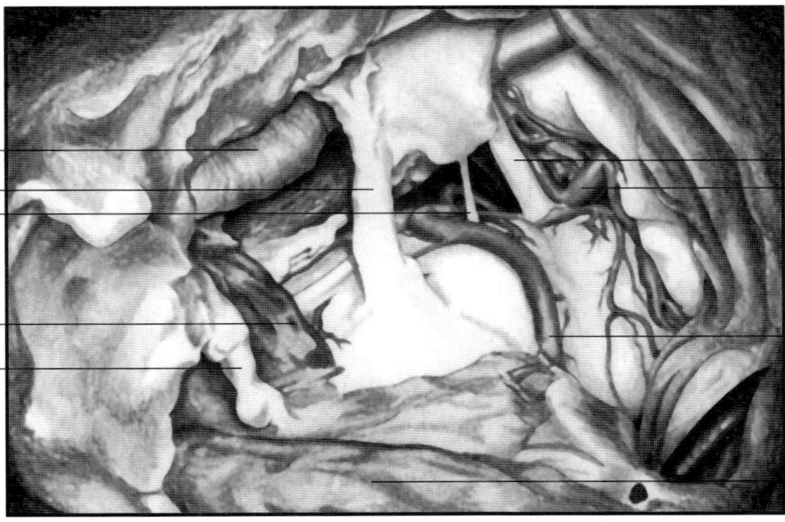

Fig. 38-7. Type C. The tentorium has been cut. Wide exposure has been obtained. (Adapted from Sanna M).

TYPE D

This approach is a combination of the type A with the petro-occipital transigmoid approach.
It is indicated for lesions of the middle and lower clivus, such as chordomas and petroclival meningiomas, that reach the foramen magnum.

SURGICAL TECHNIQUE

The same steps are performed as in Type A with the additional opening of the sigmoid sinus and jugular bulb.

- Incision (Figs. 37-2, 38-1).
- A periosteal flap, inferiorly based, is raised to be used at the end of the operation to reinforce the closure.
- Wide bone removal of the occipital bone, behind the sigmoid sinus, is performed.
- The sigmoid sinus is opened and packed intraluminally with large pieces of Surgicel or with sutures (see chapter 16, glomus tumors).
- The jugular vein is exposed in the neck, in front of the the transverse process of the atlas and ligated with two silk sutures.
- The dura is opened in the usual manner.
- The jugular bulb is opened. Bleeding from the inferior petrosal sinus is controlled with Surgicel (see chapter 16).
- The exposure is shown in Figure 38-8.

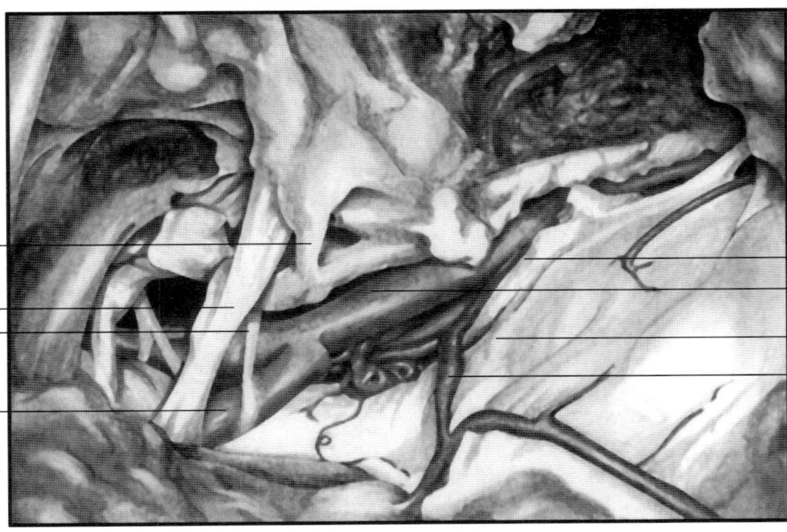

Fig. 38-8. The jugular bulb has been opened. Vertebral artery and IX-XII CNs can be seen. (Adapted from Sanna M).

REFERENCES

Brackmann DE, Anderson RG: Cholesteatomas of the cerebellopontine angle. In Silverstein H, Norrell H eds: Neurological Surgery of the Ear. 1979, pp 340-344.

Cantu RC, Ojemann RG: Glucosteroid treatment of keratin meningitis following removal of a fourth ventricle epidermoid tumor. J Neurol Neurosurg Psychiatry 31: 75, 1968.

Daspit CP, Spetzler RF, Pappas CTE: Combined approach for lesions involving the cerebellopontine angle and skull base: experience with 20 cases-preliminary report. Otolaryngol Head Neck Surg 105:788-796, 1991.

De La Cruz A: The transcochlear approach to meningiomas and cholesteatomas of the cerebellopontine angle. In Brackmann DE ed: Neurological Surgery of the Ear and Skull Base. New York, Raven Press, 1982, pp 353-360.

De La Cruz A: Transcochlear approach to lesions of the cerebellopontine angle and clivus. Rev Laryngol Otol Rhinol Bord 1021-1022: 33-36, 1981.

Guidetti B, Gagliardi FM: Epidermoid and dermoid cysts. J Neurosurg 47: 12-18, 1977.

Hitselberger WE, Horn KL, Hankinson H, et al: The middle fossa transpetrous approach for petroclival meningiomas. Skull Base Surg 33: 130-135, 1993.

Horn KL, Hankinson HL, Erasmus MD, Beauparalant PA: The modified transcochlear approach to the cerebellopontine angle. Otolaryngol Head Neck Surg 104:37-41, 1991.

House WF, De La Cruz A: Transcochlear approach to the petrous apex and clivus. Trans Am Acad Ophthalmol Otolaryngol 84: 927-931, 1977.

House WF, Hitselberger WE: The transcochlear approach to the skull base. Arch Otolaryngol Head Neck Surg 102: 334-342, 1976.

House WF, Luetje CM: Acoustic tumors: Vol II: management. University Park Press (Baltimore) 1: 239, 1979.

Mafee MF: MRI and CT in the evaluation of acquired and congenital cholesteatomas of the temporal bone. J Otolaryngol 224: 239-248, 1993.

Mazzoni A, Sanna M: The petro-occipital trans-sigmoid approach to the posterolateral skull base: results and indications [paper presented at the third Annual Meeting of the North American Skull Base Society, Acapulco, Mexico, 15-20 February 1992.

Mazzoni A: Jugulo-petrosectomy. Arch Ital Otol Rhinol Laryng 2:20-35, 1974.

Nager GT: Epidermoids involving the temporal bone: Clinical, radiological, and pathological aspects. Laryngoscope 2Suppl: 1-22, 1975.

Sanna M, Mazzoni A, Saleh E, Taibah A, Russo A: Lateral approaches to the median skull base through the petrous bone: the system of the modified transcochlear approach. J Laryngol Otol 108:1035-1043, 1994.

Sanna M, Mazzoni A, Taibah A, Saleh E, Russo A, Khashaba A: The modified transcochlear approaches to the skull base: results and indications. In: Mazzoni A, Sanna M eds. Skull base surgery update, 1. Amsterdam: Kugler, pp. 315-323, 1995.

Sanna M, Mazzoni A: The modified transcochlear approach to the tumors of the petroclival area and prepontine cistern [paper presented at the third Annual Meeting of the North American Skull Base Society, Acapulco, Mexico, 15-20 February 1992].

Sanna M, Saleh E, Russo A, Taibah A: Atlas of temporal bone and lateral skull base surgery. Thieme, 1-189, 1995.

Shiobara R, Ohira T, Kanzaki J, Toya S: A modified extended middle cranial fossa approach for acoustic nerve tumors: Results of 125 operations. J Neurosurg 68: 358-365, 1988.

Wygand ME, Haid T, Berg M: The enlarged middle cranial fossa approach for surgery of the temporal bone and of the cerebellopontine angle. Arch Otol Rhinol Laryngol 246: 299, 1989.

Yamakawa K, Shitara N, Genka S, et al: Clinical course and surgical prognosis of 33 cases of intracranial epidermoid tumors. Neurosurgery 244: 568-573, 1989.

Yasargil MG, Abernathy CD, Sarioglu AC: Microneurosurgical treatment of intracranial dermoid and epidermoid tumors. Neurosurgery 244: 561-567, 1989.

39

Surgery of meningiomas

Meningiomas of the posterior fossa require a surgical approach similar to that used for neuromas, and the problems involved are also similar.
The greatest problems in surgery are given by petroclival meningiomas. In these instances, the surgical approach must be different, since the translabyrinthine approach does not reach the anterior part of the petrous bone nor the prepontine cistern.

TECHNIQUE ACCORDING TO DESGEORGES

Meningiomas may be classified according to an anatomic-radiologic classification, based on the point of origin of the tumor.
The posterior skull base may be subdivided into four areas:

- Clivus area, medial to the trigeminal nerve.
- Posterior surface of the petrous bone, divided into three approximately equivalent areas:
- Anterior zone (zone A), located between the furrow of the trigeminal nerve and the anterior margin of the IAC
- Medial zone (zone M) which goes from the anterior margin of the IAC to a line just posterior to the labyrinthine block
- Posterior zone (zone P) which goes from the posterior line to the labyrinthine block up to the sigmoid sinus

The tumor's extension may involve one or more areas (AM; MP; AMP) (Fig. 39-1).
The primitive site of the meningiomas primarily involves the posterior surface of the petrous bone (97%).
In the posterior surface of the petrous bone, according to Desgeorge's statistics, there is a 20% involvement of zone A, 20% in zone M, 15% of zone P and a combined involvement of zone AM of 25%, MP of 12%, and 8% of zone AMP. A descending trend is noted in the location of the tumors of the anterior and exterior parts of the petrous bone.
Tumors of the clivus may extend into the petrous apex, the tentorium, and the cavernous sinus. Tumors of the posterior part of the petrous bone may extend to the clivus, Meckel's cave, the tentorium, and the foramen magnum.

Recommended approaches:

- Small tumors in zone A: subtemporal approach and reduced petrosectomy of the apex.
- Large tumors in zone A: enlarged translabyrinthine approach extended anteriorly with a transtentorial subtemporal approach.
- Small tumors in zone M: retrolabyrinthine approach.
- Large tumors in zone M: translabyrinthine approach.
- Tumors in zone P: retrolabyrinthine approach.

The choice of an approach

- In meningiomas, the choice of the approach is very important, since it must enable the surgeon to reach immediately the area of the tumor's primitive onset. This zone is defined preoperatively with CT, MRI, and reconstructions images.
- When the zone of primitive tumor onset is found on the dura, it is coagulated with a bipolar cautery or, better still, with a YAG laser. Thus the vascular pole is closed, the tumor decreases in volume, and bleeding diminishes.
- In the retrosigmoid approach, it is preferable to use a CO2 laser instead of the YAG. In this approach, the risk of spreading the electrocoagulation to the arachnoid membranes is present, since these retract and mask the view of the vasculo-nervous structures.
- When the site of primitive tumor onset is defined, the location of the vascular-nervous structures may also be predicted: e.g. a tumor in zone M of the clivus dislodges nerve III posteriorly, which is in turn dislodged anteriorly by a

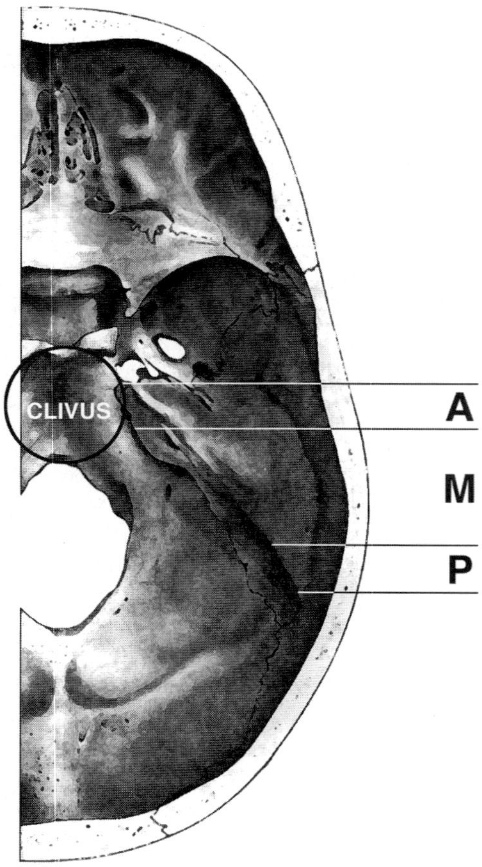

Fig. 39-1. The posterior side of the temporal bone and the clivus may be divided into four zones, according with Desgeorges M. **C**: Clivus zone. **A**: Anterior zone. **M:** Medial zone. **P**: Posterior zone.

tumor of zone A. A tumor in zone AM dislodges anteriorly the AICA while a tumor located in zone A dislodges it posteriorly.

VASCULAR COMPLICATIONS

The vascular complications are those already described in the translabyrinthine approach, but involve a greater number of structures, due to the wider extension of the approach.

Arterial complications.

The arterial structures involved are the antero-inferior, the postero-inferior, the superior cerebellar arteries and the perforating arteries.

Venous complications.

The venous structures involved are the sigmoid sinus, the vein of Labbé, and the petrosal vein (of Dandy).

- If the dominant sinus is closed, a venous infarction and/or hearing loss may be had due to venous hypertension. These complications do not occur when the jugular vein is tied in the neck, since it is below the superior petrosal sinus.
- The interruption of the transverse sinus risks lacerating the vein of Labbé coursing through the tentorium to the transverse sinus (see chapter 2 and chapter 34).

Post-operative hemorrhaging

To reduce the risk of bleeding, the following steps must be followed:

- Thorough hemostasis. Closure of the surgical field after hemostasis has been checked for at least 30 min.
- When in doubt, a small quantity of Avitene is placed in the endangered area.
- Keep in mind the greater chances for hemorrhage in older patients and/or cases of large tumors.
- Check the postoperative blood pressure.
- A hemorrhage may occur even 2-3 days after surgery.
- The portion of the dura involved in the meningioma must be removed. Mere coagulation is not sufficient and leads to relapses.

SUGGESTIONS

- When the vital structures are surrounded by the tumor, it is not always possible to completely remove it. In these cases it is preferable to leave small pieces of the tumor in place. The subsequent radiation treatment will aim at preventing their regrowth.

There are diverse possibilities for reducing postoperative liquorrhea, which may be utilized alone or in various combinations:

- Closure of the dura.
- Graft.
- Contrasting the endocranial pressure: bone reconstruction and/or fat packing.
- Reduction in CSF pressure.

Meningiomas are limited by capsules much thinner then those of neuromas. In neuromas the vascular-nervous structures are found preferentially between two arachnoid sheaths limiting the perimeter of the neoformation; hence the importance of preserving and dislodging the arachnoid from the tumor. As long as the gutting is intracapsular, no major neural or vascular structures are encountered. In meningiomas, the neurovascular structures are usually encased by the tumor, especially if the tumor is very large. Furthermore, tumors bleed more than neuromas. This makes the operation that much more difficult and delicate (Fig. 39-2). Thus, the removal of meningiomas requires different techniques then neuromas. The surgery is best performed with bipolar cauterization, which coagulates and shrinks the tumor and leaves a relatively dry surgical field. Removal is obtained by forceps and suction irrigation.

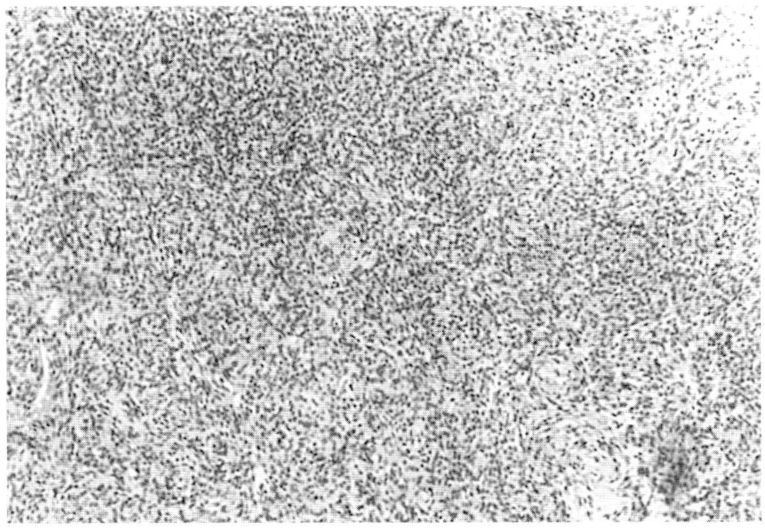

Fig. 39-2. Courtesy of Linthicum FH. Meningioma. ×115.

REFERENCES

Al-Mefty O, Fox JL, Smith RR: Petrosal approach for petroclival meningiomas. Neurosurgery 22:510-517, 1988.

Blom S, Ekbom KA: Early clinical signs of meningiomas of the foramen magnum. J Neurosurg 19:661-664, 1962.

Campbell E, Whitfield RD: Posterior fossa meningiomas. J Neurosurg 5:131-153, 1948.

Castellano F, Ruggiero G: Meningiomas of the posterior fossa. Acta Radiological, Suppl 104: 1-177, 1953.

Chennigton M, Schneck SA: Clivus meningiomas. Neurology 16:86-97, 1966.

Crockard HA, Sen C: The transoral approach for the management of intradural lesions at the craniovertebral junction: review of 7 cases. Neurosurgery 28:88-98, 1991.

Cushing HW, Eisenhardt L: Meningiomas. Their classification and regional behaviour. The history and surgical end results. Springfield, IL: Charles C. Thomas, 3-387, 1938.

Dodge HW Jr, Love JG, Gottlieb CM: Benign tumors at the foramen magnum: surgical considerations. J Neurosurg 13: 603-617, 1956.

Fujimoto K, Ikuno H, Hakuba A, Mishima Y, Kondou M, Maeno T: Foramen magnum neurinomas. Report of 5 cases. Central Jpn J Orthop Traumatic Surg 19: 1159-1163 in Japanese, 1976.

Guzowski J, Paparella MM, Rao KN, Hosmino T: Meningiomas of the temporal bone. Laryngoscope 86: 1141-1146, 1976.

Hakuba A, Nishimura S, Jang BJ: A combined retroauricular and preauricular transpetrosal-transtentorial approach to clivus meningiomas. Surg Neurol 30 108- 116, 1988.

Hakuba A, Nishimura S, Mishima Y, Kawano K: Foramen magnum tumors—report of 21 cases. Neuro Med Chir Tokyo 22:563-576, 1982.

Hakuba A: Foramen magnum meningiomas. Clin Neurosci 8:78-81 in Japanese, 1990.

Hakuba A: Total removal of cerebellopontine angle tumors with a combined transpetrosal-transtentorial approach. Neurol Surg 6:347-354 in Japanese, 1978.

House W, Hitselberger W: The transcochlear approach to the skull base. Arch Otolaryngol 102:334-342, 1976.

House WF, De la Cruz A, Hitselberger WE: Surgery of the skull base: transcochlear approach to the petrous apex and clivus. ORL J Otorhinolaryngol Relat Spec 86:770-779, 1978.

Howe JR, Taren JA: Foramen magnum tumors. Pitfalls in diagnosis. JAMA 225:1061-1066, 1973.

Komiyama M, Yagura H, Baba M, Yasui T, Hakuba A, Nishimura S, Inoue Y: MR imaging: possibility of tissue characterization of brain tumors using T1 and T2 values. A JNR 8:65-70, 1987.

Krayenbuhl H: Special clinical features of tumors of the foramen magnum. Schweiz Arch Neurol Neurochir Psychiatry 112: 205-218, 1973.

Long DM: Surgical approaches to tumors of skull base: an overview. In: Wilkins RH, Rengachary SS, eds. Neurosurgery update 1: diagnosis, operative technique. and neuro-oncology. New York: McGraw-Hill. 266-276, 1990.

Malis LI: Surgical resection of tumors of the skull base In: Wilkins RH, Rengachary SS, eds. Neurosurgery. Vol 1. New York: McGrawHill, 1011-1021, 1985.

Maniglia AJ: Intra and extra-cranial meningiomas involving the temporal bone. Laryngoscope Suppl 12: 88-89, 1978.

Mayberg MR, Symon L: Meningiomas of the clivus and apical petrous bone. Report of 35 cases. J Neurosurg 65:160-167, 1986.

Meyer FB, Ebersold MJ, Reese DF: Benign tumors of the foramen magnum. J Neurosurg 61:136-142, 1984.

Moller AR: Electrophysiological monitoring of cranial nerves in operations in the skull base. In Seckar LN, Schramm VL eds: Tumors of the cranial base: diagnosis and treatment. Mount Kisko, NY: Futura Publishing Company, 123-132, 1987.

Russel JR, Bucy PC: Meningiomas of the posterior fossa. Surg Gynec Obstet 96: 183-192, 1953.

Saleh E, Naguib M, Aristegui M, Cokkeser Y, Russo A, Sanna M: Surgical anatomy of the jugular foramen area. In: Mazzoni A, Sanna M, eds. Skull base surgery Update, 1. Amsterdam: Kugler, 1995 pp. 3-8.

Saleh E, Naguib M, Aristegui M, Cokkeser Y, Sanna M: The lower skull base: anatomical study with surgical implications. Ann Otol Rhinol Laryngol 104:57-61, 1995.

Saleh E, Taibah A, Achilli V, Aristegui M, Mazzoni M, Sanna A: Posterior fossa meningioma: surgical strategy. Skull Base Surg 4:209-219, 1994.

Samii M, Ammirati M, Mahran A, et al: Survey of petroclival meningiomas: report of 24 cases. Neurosurgery 24: 12-17, 1989.

Samii M, Ammirati M: The combined supra-infratentorial presigmoid sinus avenue to the petro-clival region: surgical technique and clinical applications. Acta Neurochir 95:6-12, 1988.

Samii M, Draf W: Surgery of the skull base. Berlin: Springer, 1989.

Sanna M, Saleh E, Russo A. Taibah A: Atlas of temporal bone and lateral skull base surgery. Thieme, 1-189, 1995.

Sekhar LN, Estonillo R: Transtemporal approach to the skull base: an anatomical study. Neurosurgery 19:799-808, 1986.
Sekhar LN, Jannetta PJ, Burkhart L, et al: Meningiomas involving the clivus: a six-year experience with 41 patients. Neurosurgery 27:764-781, 1990.
Sekhar LN, Jannetta PJ, Maroon JC: Tentorial meningiomas: surgical management and results. Neurosurgery 14:268-275, 1984.
Sekhar LN, Jannetta PJ: Petroclival and medial tentorial meningiomas. In: Sekhar LN, Schramm VL, eds. Tumors of the cranial base: diagnosis and treatment. Mount Kisco, NY: Futura Publishing Company, 623-640, 1987.
Sekhar LN, Schramm VL, Jones NF: Subtemporal-preauricular infratemporal fossa approach to large lateral and posterior cranial base neoplasms. J Neurosurg 67:488-499, 1987.
Sekhar LN, Sen C, Jho HD, Janecka IP: Surgical treatment of intracavernous neoplasms: a four-year experience. Neurosurgery 26: 18-30, 1989.
Sekhar LN, Sen C, Jho HD: Saphenous vein bypass of the cavernous internal carotid artery. J Neurosurg 72:35-41, 1990.
Sen C, Sekhar LN: An extreme lateral approach to intradural lesions of the cervical spine and foramen magnum. Neurosurgery 27: 197-204, 1990.
Stein BM, Leeds NE, Taveras JM, Pool JL: Meningiomas of the foramen magnum. J Neurosurg 20:741-750, 1963.
Takemoto K, Matsumura Y, Hashimoto H, et al: MR imaging of intraspinal tumors—capability in histological differentiation and compartimentalization of extramedullary tumors. Neuroradiology 30:303-309, 1988.
Velut S, Jan M: Anterior petrosectomy during approach to the petroclival area. In:Schmideck HE, ed. Meningiomas and their surgical management. Philadelphia: Saunders, 435-450, 1991.
Yagura H, Komiyama M, Fu Y, et al: Diagnosis of meningioma in magnetic resonance imaging. CT Kenkyu 8:675-682 in Japanese, 1986.
Yasargil MG, Mortara RW, Curcic M: Meningiomas of basal posterior cranial fossa. In: Krayenbuhl H, ed. Advances and technical standards in neurosurgery, vol. 7. Wien: Springer-Verlag. 1-115, 1980.

40

Petroclival tumors. Anterolateral approaches

A person who doesn't evolve is a dead person.

SEKHAR L.N.

The approaches described in this chapter have been proposed by L.N. Sekhar for the treatment of petroclival extradural benign lesions such as meningiomas, epidermoid cysts, glomus tumors, low grade malignant lesions such as chordomas, chondrosarcomas, adenoid cystic carcinoma, pituitary adenoma and high grade malignant lesions such as carcinomas, and osteogenic sarcoma (*see color plates*). Thanks to his efforts, there is now an array of surgical options for the treatment of lesions, some of which were previously considered inoperable. In highly malignant lesions, such as adenocarcinoma, squamous cell carcinoma, basal cell carcinoma, and osteogenic sarcoma, the primary problem is now metastasization. In the future, this problem will be addressed with new forms of adjuvant therapy.

- Extended frontal approach.
- Subtemporal, transcavernous, and transpetrous apex approach.
- Subtemporal and infratemporal approach.
- Extreme lateral, transcondyle, and transjugular approach.

EXTENDED FRONTAL APPROACH

The extended frontal approach was first proposed by Derome and was later modified by Sekhar.

INDICATIONS

- Midline tumors involving the upper, middle, and lower clivus from the dorsum of the sella to the foramen magnum.
- *Lateral limit.* The optic nerves, the cavernous and petrous internal carotids, and the hypoglossal nerves.
- *Inferior limit.* C1. The section may be extended to the margins of the foramen magnum.

DISADVANTAGES

- Complete anosmia for bilateral olfactory denervation.
- Changes in taste sensation.
- Possible damage to the frontal lobes and the optic and abducens nerves.

SURGICAL TECHNIQUE

- The patient is placed in a supine position, using a Mayfield head rest.
- The incision begins in front of one ear and ends at the other ear. The incision goes to the pericranium.
- The myocutaneous flap is reflected forward, to the nasofrontal suture medially, and the superior walls of the orbits laterally.
- The supraorbital foramina are exposed and the nerves and vessels are dissected.
- The periorbita is dissected at both sides up to the lacrimal sac.
- A frontal craniotomy is performed in two segments. Thus Sekhar reduces the risks of injury to the superior sagittal sinus.
- The subfrontal dura is separated from the floor of the anterior cranial fossa. It is almost impossible to avoid lacerating the dura during its dissection from the cribriform plates and the crista galli. The olfactory nerves are separated as close as possible to the cribriform plates. The dura is later repaired.
- The sequence of the incisions is outlined in Figure 40-1.
- Before beginning work on the temporal lobes, Mannitol is administered. The CSF pressure is reduced with a spinal drain and/or by opening the chiasmatic cisterns. By tilting the patient's head back, the force of gravity helps to dislodge

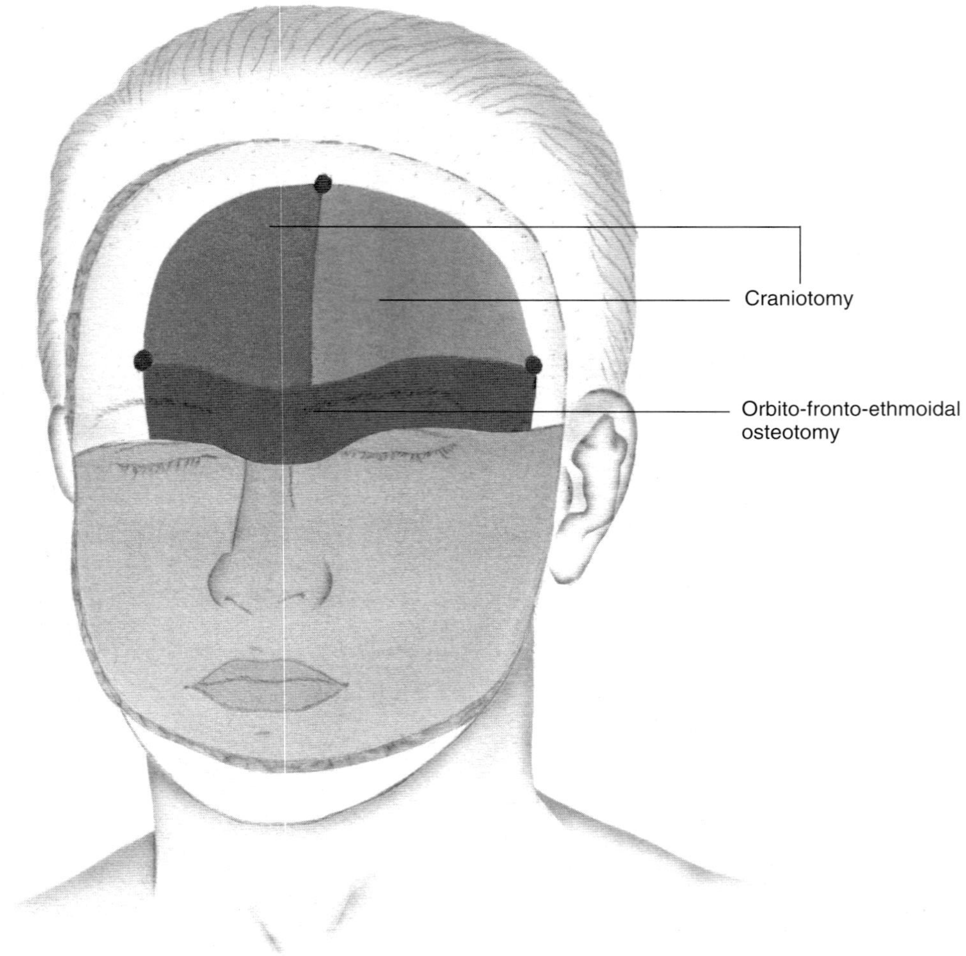

Fig. 40-1. Extended frontal approach. Bicoronal incision has been made. The underlying bone is exposed up to the superior orbital rims and the frontonasal suture. Two upper craniotomies are made, beyond the medial line, to avoid injury to the superior sagittal sinus. The lower craniotomy is the orbito-fronto-ethmoidal osteotomy. (Adapted from Seckar LN).

the temporal lobes from the floor of the anterior cranial fossa (Fig. 40-2).

- Orbito-fronto-ethmoidal osteotomies (Sekhar's technique) are performed.
- A slight midline retraction of the frontal lobes is performed.
- One or both optic nerves (depending on the extent of the lesion) are circumferentially unroofed. In this approach, a limited view is obtained of the anterior clinoid process; thus, the latter is only partially drilled.
- The sphenoid septum is reduced with the cutting burr and the mucosa is removed with a curette.

Tumor removal

- The clivus is exposed by resectioning the middle and posterior ethmoidal cells and opening the sphenoid (Fig. 40-3).
- The roof of the sphenoid sinus is dissected. The dura of the sella is exposed. The lateral wall of the sphenoid bone is sectioned in an anterior-posterior fashion, so that the cavernous ICA becomes visible posterior and inferior to the optic nerves.
- The dural layer is maintained on the lateral side of the sphenoid sinuses. This preserves the vascularity of the cavernous sinuses and very little bleeding is had. When the dura is invaded by the tumor, Surgicel is used to stop bleeding.
- The sphenoclival bone is removed from top to bottom until a safe area is reached.
- The clival bone is cancellous and is easily removed with a high-speed drill. Care is taken to avoid injuring the structures behind the dura. When the dura is infiltrated and must be sectioned, the basilar artery and the brainstem are carefully approached.
- The partial removal of the petrous apex is performed, unilaterally or bilaterally, as required. The ICA can be followed in the cavernous sinus to the petrous part, which is not visible with this approach. The abducens nerve entering Dorello's canal in the cavernous sinus must be preserved.

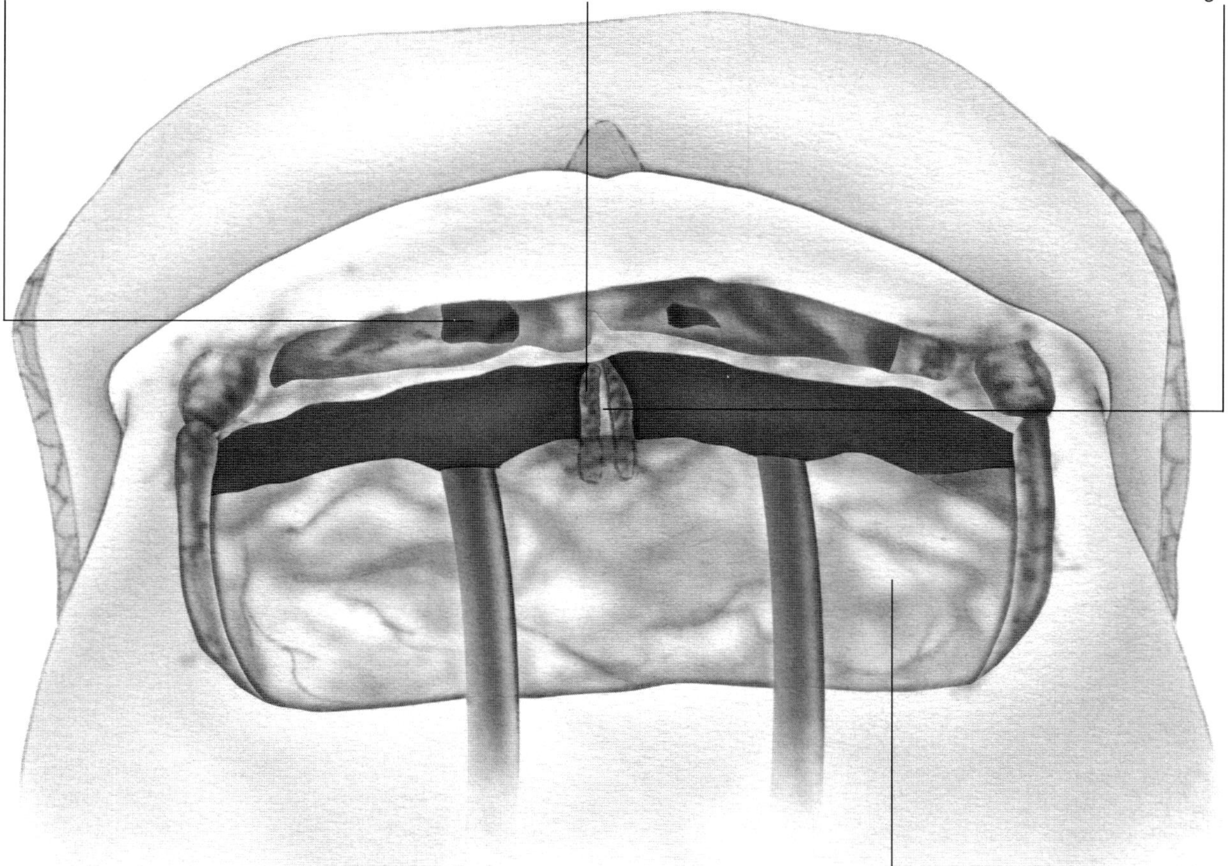

Fig. 40-2. The subfrontal dura is dissected from the orbital roofs and planum ethmoidalis.

- If the nasopharyngeal mucosa must be removed, the rhynopharyngeal mucosa may be damaged, provoking a fistula with a path of infection from the external to the internal cranium.

Closure
- The clivus opening, lacerations of the olfactory dura (a very common occurrence), and any other laceration in the dura are repaired with patches of fascia lata.
- Autologous fat is used to close any empty space in the sphenoidal and ethmoidal cavities. The fat must not compress the optic nerves. The operating site is closed with temporalis muscle and a galeo-pericranial flap.
- The bony fragments are replaced (first the orbito-frontal-ethmoidal and then the craniotomy fragments). To avoid necrotization of the muscular flap, excessive downward pressure by the bone should be avoided. The osseous rims can be reduced, if necessary. 2-0 Neurlon is used to anchor them.
- A gravity drain is put in place for 2-3 days.
- The spinal drain is removed before interrupting anesthesia.

TIPS AND PITFALLS
- The frontal approach can be combined with the subtemporal-infratemporal approach for the treatment of lesions involving the clivus and proceeding laterally. It is not necessary to separate V3 (Figs. 40-4, 40-5).

SUBTEMPORAL, TRANSCAVERNOUS AND TRANSPETROUS APEX APPROACH

This approach was first described by Kawase et al. and was modified by Sekhar et al.

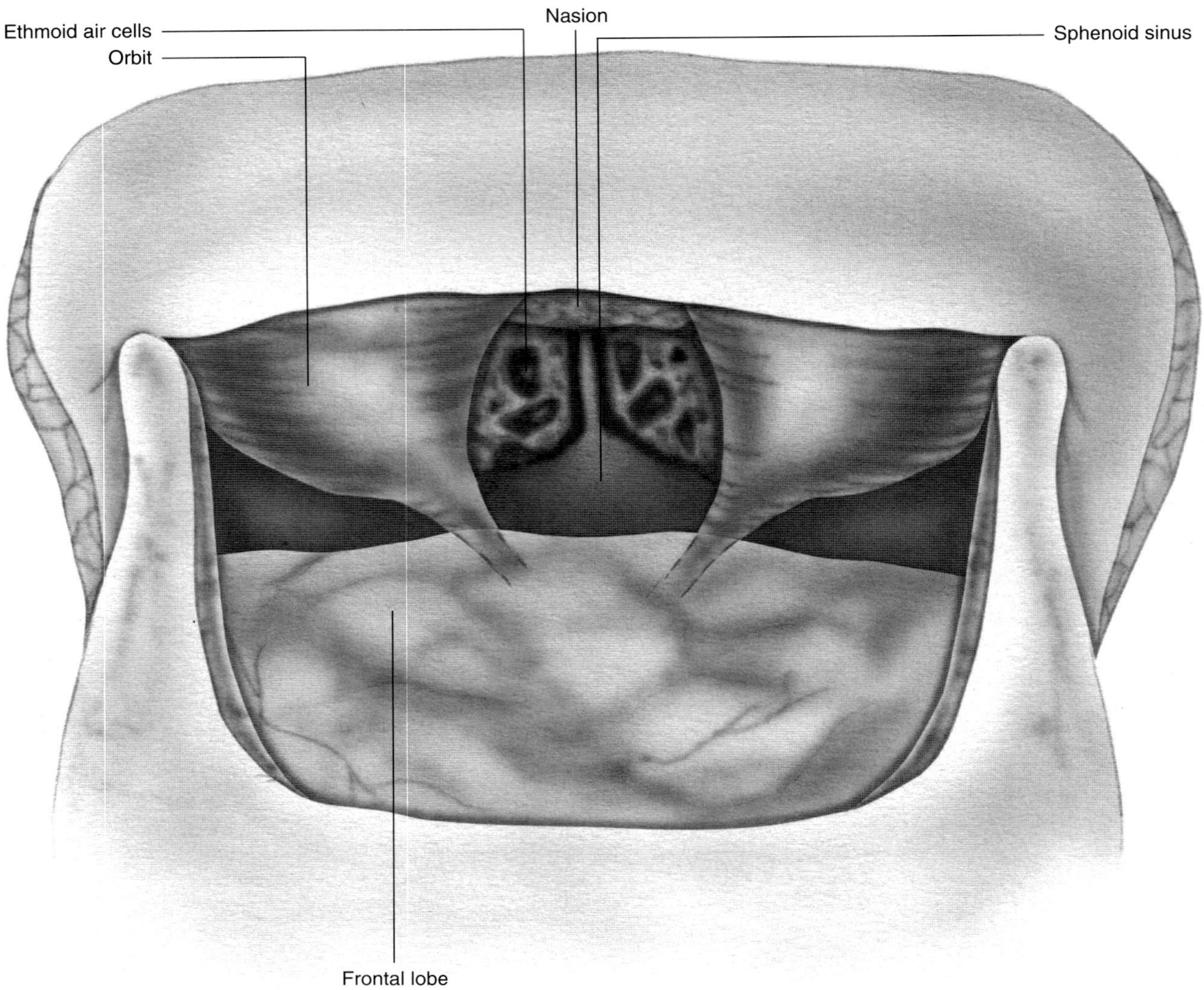

Fig. 40-3. Fronto-orbito-ethmoidal osteotomy is made. Resection of the ethmoidal cells open the way to the clivus. (Adapted from Sekhar LN).

Indications

- Lesions of the upper clivus and/or the petrous apex and/or the cavernous sinus on one side. In lesions with a lateral extension, the side involved is also the side of approach.
- For midline lesions, the side selected for the approach is on the nondominant hemisphere.

Position

The patient is supine, with his head on the Mayfield headrest and turned away from the surgeon at a 60° angle.

- Incision.
- The skin flap is elevated.
- The zygomatic arch is exposed and the periosteum is elevated.
- The temporalis muscle is elevated from above downwards.
- Temporal craniotomy.
- The capsule of the temporomandibular joint is opened. The meniscus is dissected and depressed.

Middle Fossa Extradural Dissection

- Typical landmarks in the middle fossa approach are the following: tegmen tympani, greater superficial petrosal nerve (GSPN), arcuate eminence, middle meningeal artery, V3, petrous internal carotid artery.
- The pressure exerted on the tegmen tympani must be very gentle, to avoid injuring this slight barrier between the operating field and the middle ear and the eustachian tube.
- The osseous external auditory canal is behind the temporomandibular joint, and must not be injured.

Intradural part

- Incision of the dura. Splitting of the sylvian fissure.

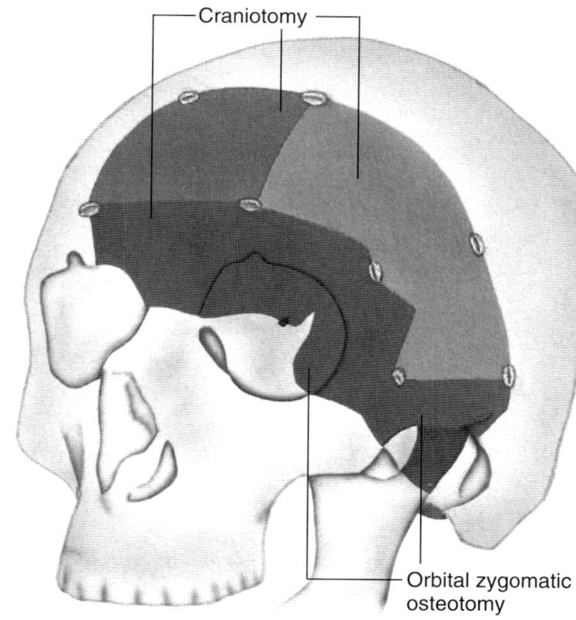

Fig. 40-4. For better exposure of clival tumors, the frontal approach can be combined with the subtemporal-infratemporal approach. Craniotomy and orbital-zygomatic osteotomy. (Adapted from Sekhar LN).

- Retraction of the temporal lobe.
- The superior cerebellar artery (SCA) and the posterior cerebral artery are preserved behind the arachnoid layer.
- The tentorium is divided by an incision beginning behind the IVth nerve and ending behind the superior petrosal sinus.
- The lateral wall of the cavernous sinus is exposed, using Surgicel as needed. The following structures are identified: the petrous ICA, petrous apex, clivus, homolateral and contralateral nerves VI, V, IV, homolateral and contralateral III, and the intradural portion of the ICA. The basilar artery and the cerebellum are posterior. The posterior clinoid and the pituitary gland are anterior.
- If the sphenoid sinus has been opened, the opening must be enlarged and packed with fat after removing the mucosa.

Closure

The dura is partially reconstructed and the residual openings are sealed with abdominal fat. The closure is reinforced with an overlying fascia lata graft.

SUBTEMPORAL AND INFRATEMPORAL APPROACH

This approach was first described by Sekhar et al in 1987 and represents a modification and an extension both of the middle fossa approach, de-

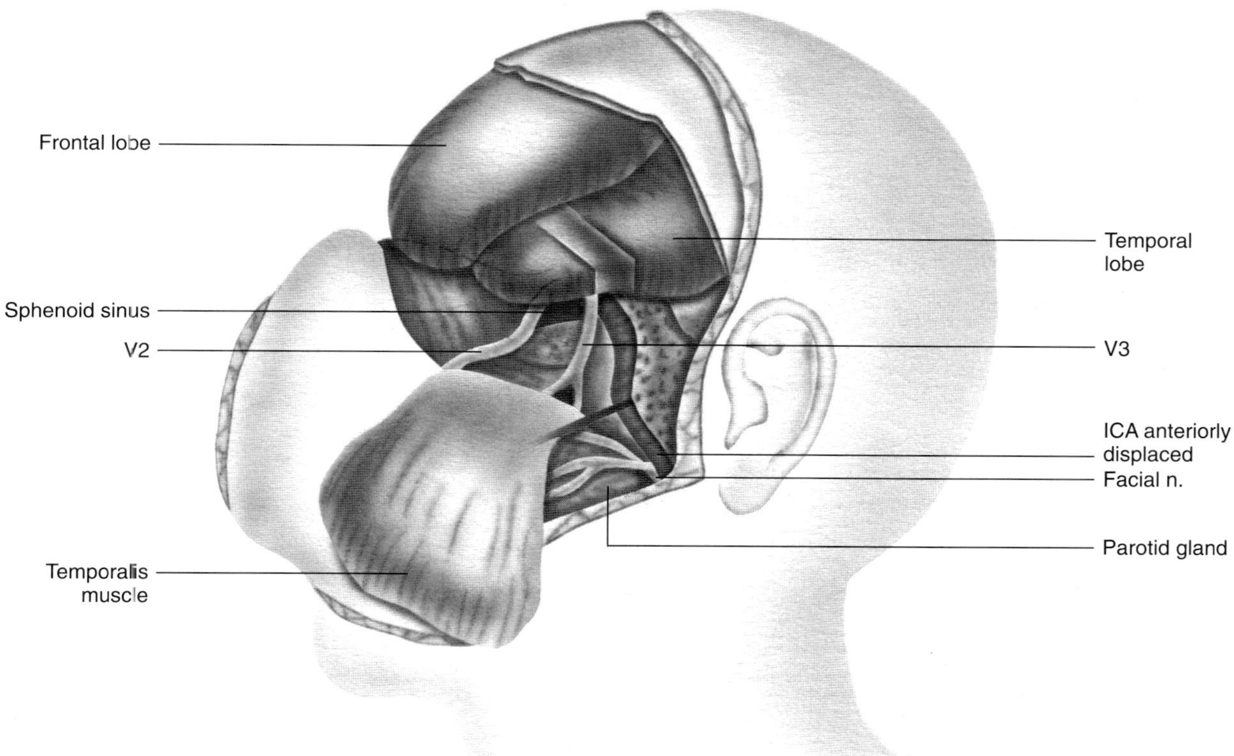

Fig. 40-5. Exposure of the combined anterior and lateral approach. (Adapted from Sekhar LN).

scribed by House in 1963 and of the infratemporal approach, described by Fisch in 1985.

Indications

- No V3 separation. Lesions that involve the petrous apex and the midclivus, inside the midline, with minimal invasion of the sphenoid sinus.
- With V3 separation. The indications are extended to lesions that involve the lower clivus, the lower cavernous sinus, the sphenoid, the infratemporal and pterygopalatine fossae, and lesions arising from the nasopharynx and extending to these structures.

Incision

- The periosteum is dissected from the zygomatic arch and the lateral orbital rim. When the incision is kept below the zygomatic arch, it is maintained superficial to the masseteric fascia up to the capsule of the temporomandibular joint. The flap is dissected anteriorly, while keeping in this plane, thus preserving the branches of the facial nerve found below (Figs. 40-6, 40-7, 40-8).
- The extratemporal facial nerve is exposed in the neck at the stylomastoid foramen (see glomus tumors...).
- Temporalis and masseter muscles are transposed, inferiorly, exposing the temporal fossa and the zygomatic arch.
- A temporal craniotomy is performed (Fig. 40-9). A zygomatic osteotomy is performed, extended to the condylar fossa, if more room is needed posteriorly.
- The capsule of the temporomandibular joint is opened. The meniscus is dissected and depressed.
- The mandibular condyle is freed from the pterygoid muscles. The condyle is divided with an oscillating saw and removed.
- The contents of the condylar fossa are removed.
- In the infratemporal fossa below, the styloid process is found. Medial to the styloid process is the stylomastoid process and the facial nerve.

Exposure of the Internal Carotid Artery

- The middle meningeal artery is coagulated and divided.
- The GSPN is identified; it may be useful in electrical stimulation of the nerve (NIM 2. Xomed-Treece, Jacksonville, Florida). Antidromic stimulation of the GSPN results in electrically recordable activity of the facial nerve.
- Medial to the GSPN are the tensor tympani muscle, the eustachian tube, and the horizontal segment of the intrapetrous ICA.
- The cartilaginous eustachian tube is packed with muscle and sutured.
- The petrous ICA runs medial to V2 and V3. Its superior border is proximal to the inferior margin of the gasserian ganglion.
- Once the petrous ICA has been identified, it is followed in its descending tract, drilling the overlying bone. A diamond burr may be used near the artery, leaving a thin shell of bone and taking care to preserve the periosteal layer of the carotid canal.

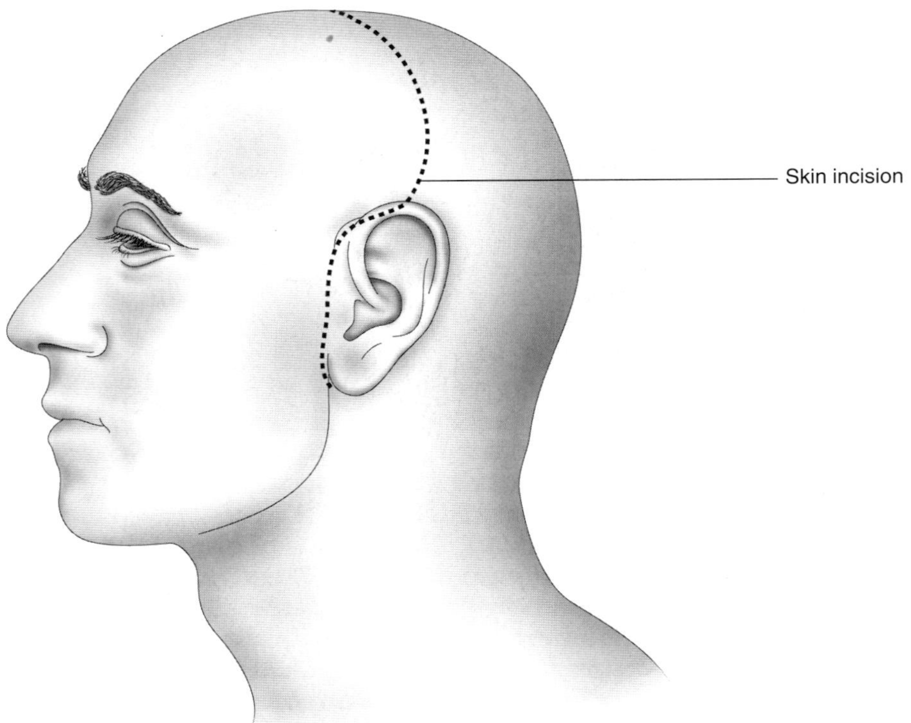

Fig. 40-6. Subtemporal-infratemporal approach. Skin incision.

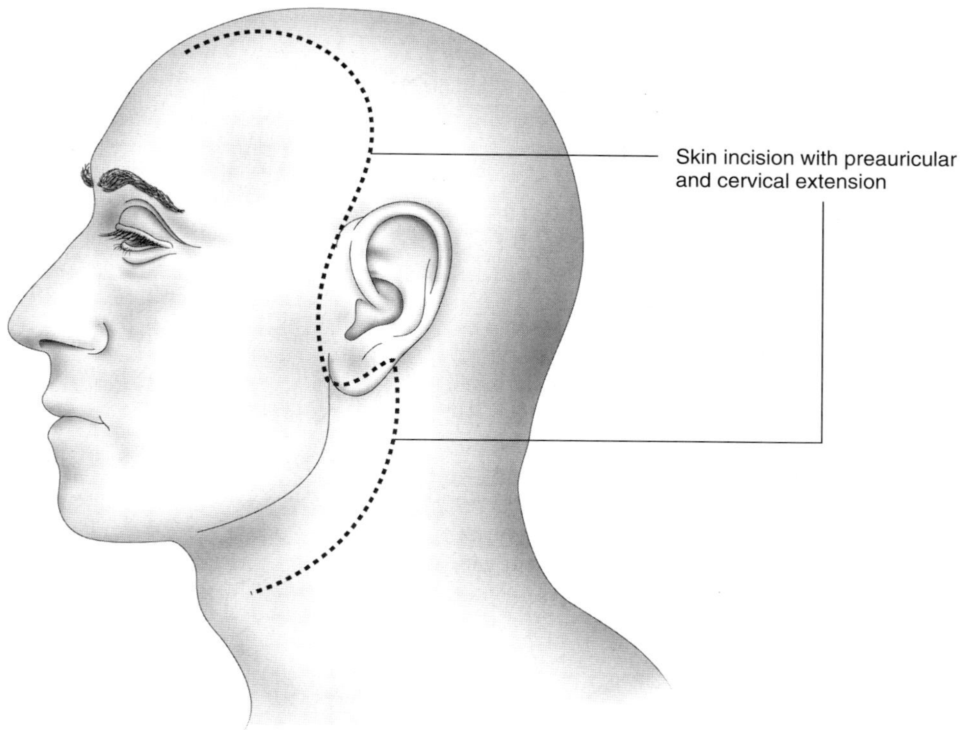

Fig. 40-7. Subtemporal-infratemporal approach. Skin incision when neck dissection or cervical ICA control is needed.

- The last shell of bone may be removed with a curette.
- The artery is followed to its entrance into the carotid canal.
- The carotid canal is medial to the styloid process; it contains a fibrocartilaginous ring that surrounds the ICA and must be opened to free the artery.

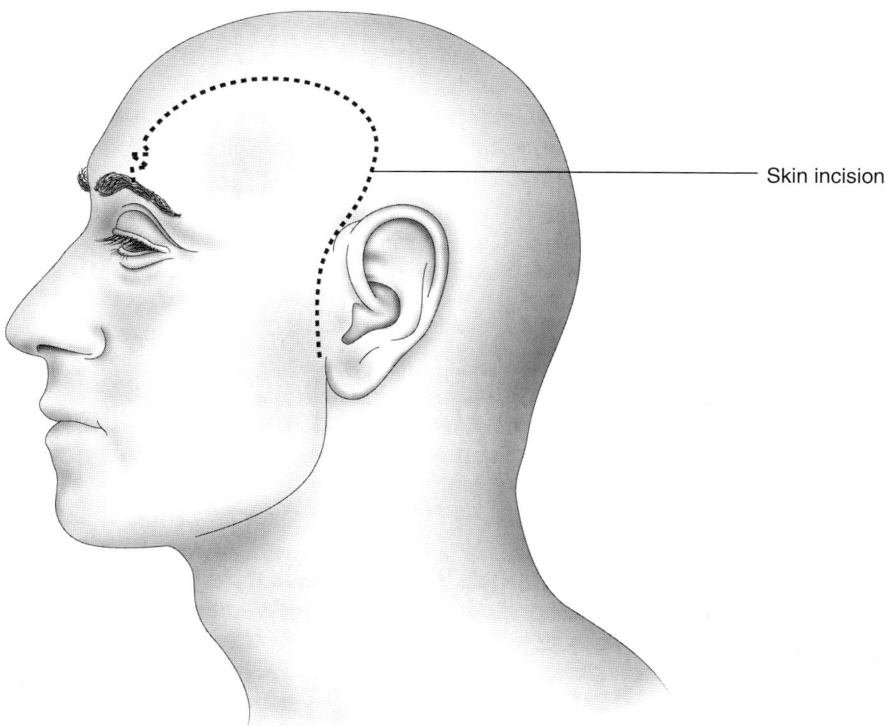

Fig. 40-8. Subtemporal-infratemporal approach. Skin incision when anterior extension is needed.

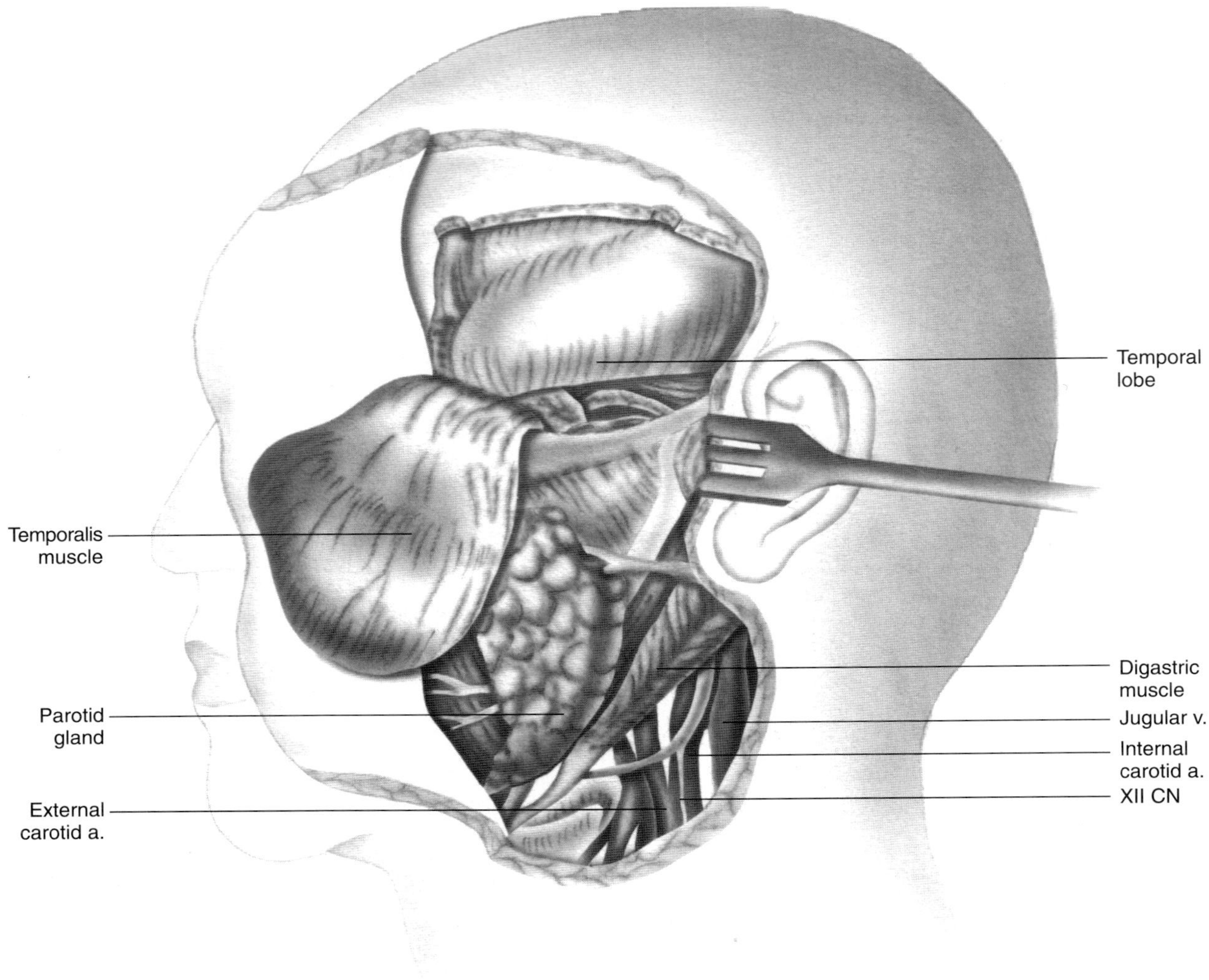

Fig. 40-9. Subtemporal-infratemporal approach combined with an upper cervical dissection. (Adapted from Sekhar LN).

- The carotid artery, the jugular vein, and nerves IX, X, and XI are exposed in the neck (Fig. 40-10).
- The ICA can be mobilized anteriorly to better expose the tumor.
- The petrous apex, free of structures, is drilled for approx. 1.5 cm.
- Tumor removal.
- To reach the central and inferior areas of the surgical field, the ICA must be mobilized in its petrous and cervical tract with an umbilical tape. The ICA cannot be moved from its path medial to V3 and V2, so that these two roots are not injured.
- If, however, V3 is divided at its exit through the foramen ovale, the ICA can be moved into this area. Greater control of the lesions extending into the cavernous sinus and the sphenoid sinus is thus achieved.
- An anterior extension of this approach enables us to reach the pterygoid fossa. up to the opposite petrous ICA.

Closure

- Fascia lata grafts to repair dural lacerations.
- Abdominal fat to fill the cavity.
- End-to-end anastomosis of V3 with epineural sutures.
- Splitting of the temporalis muscle and packing of the surgical cavity.
- If the temporalis muscle does not suffice to cover the surgical field or if the nasopharynx is open, the deficit must be covered with free flaps.

TIPS AND PITFALLS

- At the geniculate ganglion, the facial nerve heads medially in the IAC and laterally and posteriorly in the epitympanum.
- The bone forming the epitympanic wall—the tegmen antri bone—is very thin and must not be opened, to avoid communication of the skull base with the cavum tympani. If a breakage occurs, the breach must be repaired with a

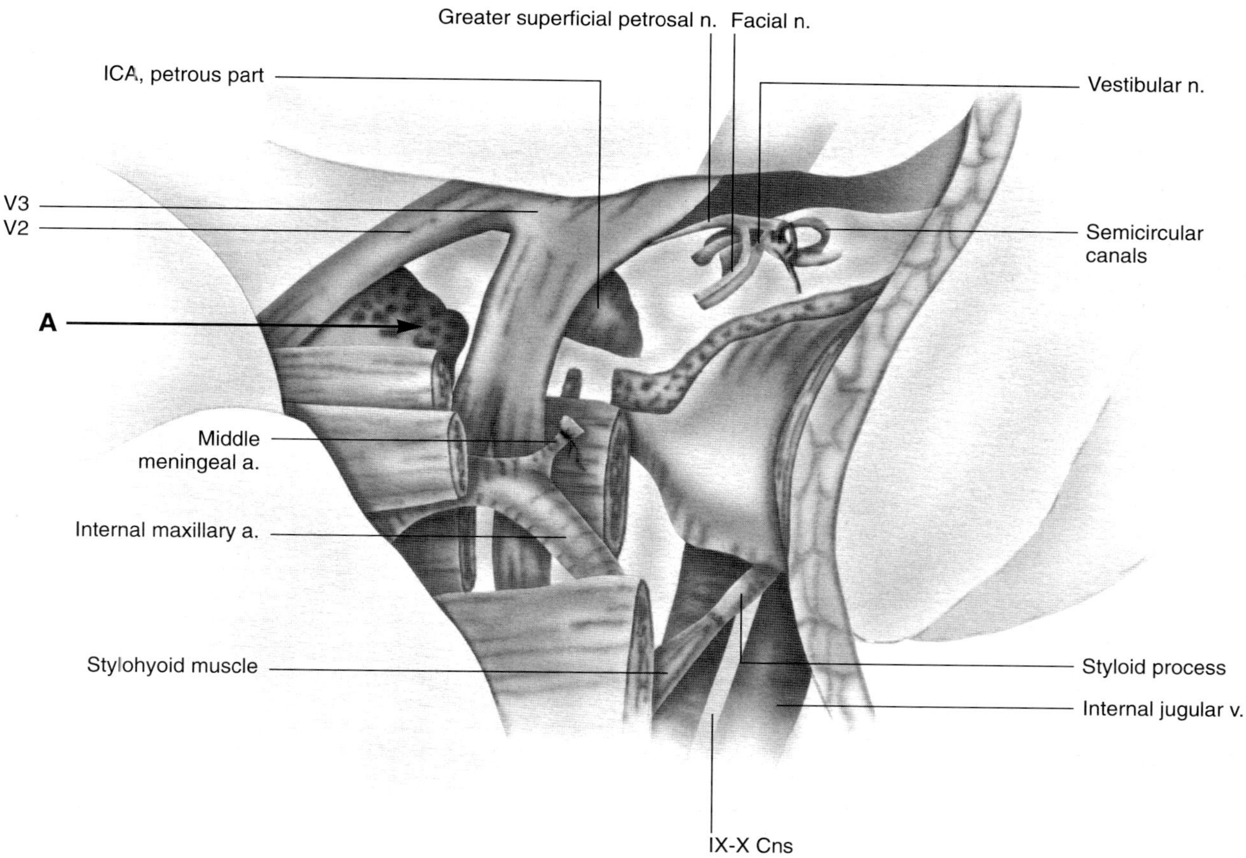

Fig. 40-10. The petrous carotid artery has been partially exposed. The position of the labyrinthine bone is shown (shadow). **A:** The sphenoid sinus can be reached passing between V2 and V3. When tumor extends into the jugular bulb, the jugular bulb can be opened posterior to the petrous ICA (**Fig. 3-3**). (Adapted from Sekhar LN).

bone fragment. This prevents the soft tissue from pressing on the ossicles and causing a transmissive hearing loss. A certain degree of transmissive hearing loss is always seen after the operation, due to the closure of the eustachian tube.

- The eustachian tube must be closed, to block communication between the nasopharynx and the skull base.
- Some instability in chewing will be had.
- Lacerations in the dura must be closed to prevent CSF leakage.

EXTREME LATERAL, TRANSCONDYLE, AND TRANSJUGULAR APPROACH

This approach was developed and has been used by Sekhar, Sen, et al, since 1985.

Indications

Extradural lesions of the inferior clivus, with possible extension to C1 and C2, to the jugular bulb and the occipital condyles.

Position

The patient is placed in a lateral position. The lower arm is positioned underneath the table, sustained by the horizontal bar of the Mayfield headrest.

Incision

- An inverted U-incision or a C-incision is performed.
- The sternocleidomastoid muscle is detached from the mastoid and reflected inferiorly.
- The lateral mass of C1 is palpated and used as a landmark for the vertebral artery.
- The jugular vein and the hypoglossal nerve are seen inferiorly.
- The splenius capitis is detached anteriorly and reflected posteriorly.
- The longissimus capitis muscle and part of the levator scapulae muscle are detached anteriorly and retracted posteriorly. The inferior oblique muscle is found under these muscles, and the extradural

segment of the vertebral artery (VA) runs tangent to its inferior margin (Figs. 40-11, 40-12).

- The C1 foramen transversarium is exposed posteriorly and laterally. The artery is exposed from the C1 foramen transversarium to the suboccipital membrane.

Bone removal

- *Predominantly cervical lesions which reach the foramen magnum*:
- It is sufficient to remove two-thirds of the articular facets and laminae.
- The vertebral artery courses anterior to the articular facets.
- *Cervical lesions reaching the foramen magnum from below*:
- The only bone to be removed is the anterior two-thirds of the articulated facet and the laminae. The vertebral artery is anterior to these structures.

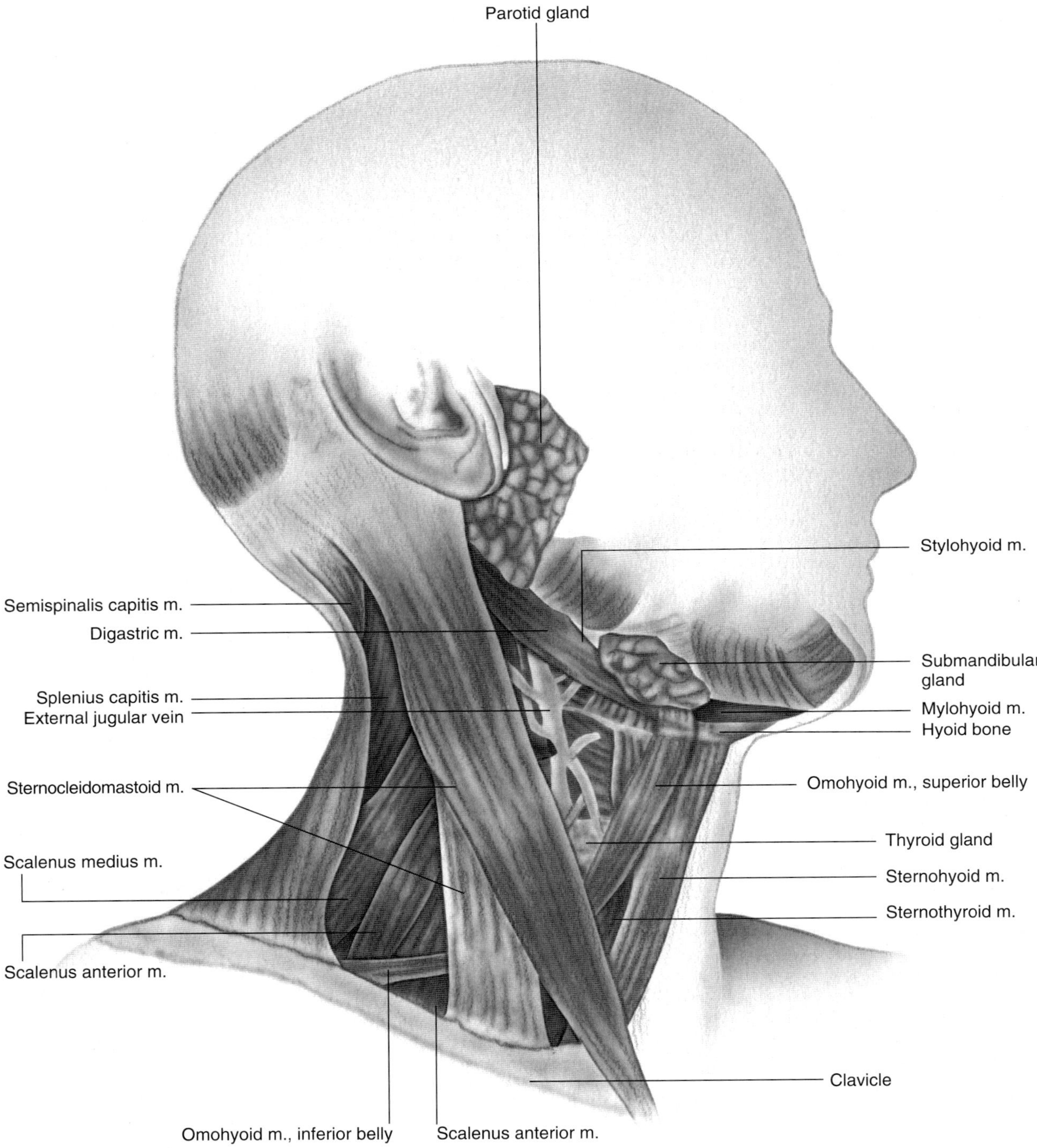

Fig. 40-11. Lateral aspect of the muscles of the neck.

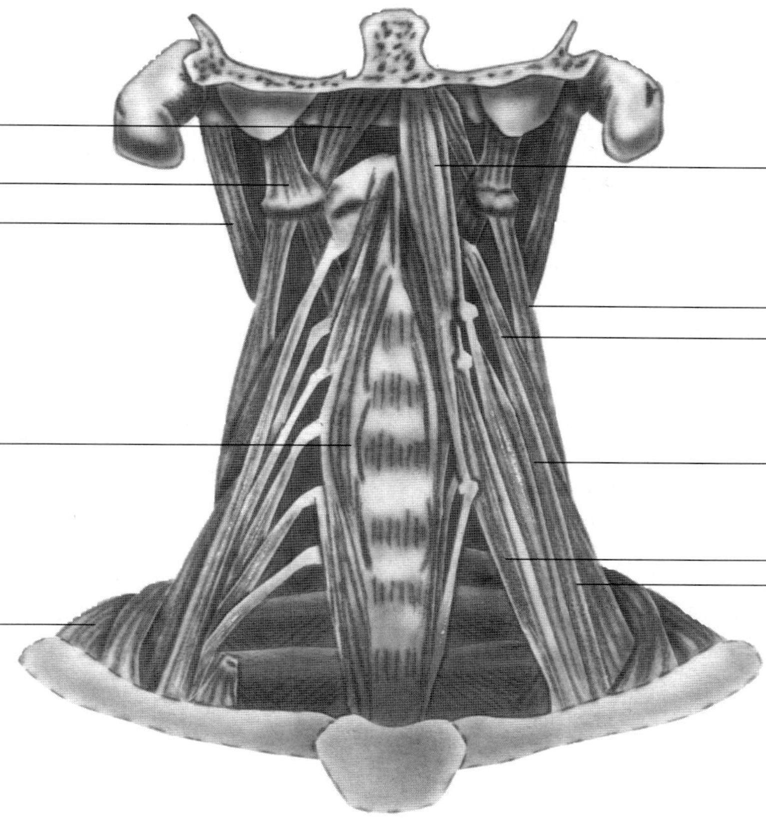

Fig. 40-12. Vertebral muscles. (Adapted from Gray's Anatomy).

- *Lesions going to the foramen magnum*:
- Mastoidectomy up to the mastoid tip. Skeletonization of the facial nerve helps in avoiding its injury. The middle ear is left untouched. Removal of the retrosigmoid bone and the posterior two-thirds of the occipital condyle.
- *Lesion touching the IAC*:
- The mastoidectomy can be extended to outline the semicircular canals.
- *Lesion involving the IAC*:
- The mastoidectomy can be extended into a translabyrinthine approach.

- The XI nerve, the VII nerve, and the jugular vein are exposed and preserved. The vertebral artery is followed to its entrance into the dura.
- The dura is cut from behind the sigmoid sinus up to and around the entrance of the VA into the dura, and is reflected anteriorly with all the sigmoid sinus. When the bulb is closed by the tumor, the sigmoid sinus is tied superiorly and the area of the bulb is opened, to better expose the underlying structures: the mixed nerves and the jugular foramen.
- When the lesion involves the lateral side of C1, the foramen transversarium is opened, the vertebral artery is dislodged, and the diseased bone is removed.
- In the area in which the artery surrounds the occipital condyle, surgical manipulations will provoke profuse venous bleeding, because of the venous plexus surrounding the artery.
- For the complete mobilization of the artery and the possibility of working in a 360° area, a partial removal of the condyle of the occipital bone is needed. The vertebral artery is often surrounded by the tumor and adheres to nerves IX, X, XI, and XII. The complete removal of the tumor from these structures is a very delicate and arduous task (Fig. 40-13).
- At the level of the brainstem, the dura is opened just posterior to the nerve roots.
- The tumor is removed under microscopic control with laser CO_2 and bipolar cautery. This lateral approach offers a good view of the brain stem interface, although there is a decreased visibility in the ventral facet of the medulla and the bulb. The midline and the area beyond it are seen with difficulty.
- The dural base, if infiltrated, is excised and then repaired with a dural graft.
- Up to two-thirds of the occipital condyle may be drilled without causing instability. If the entire condyle is treated, a titanium sheet must be used to steady it. After surgery, a rigid collar will have to be used.

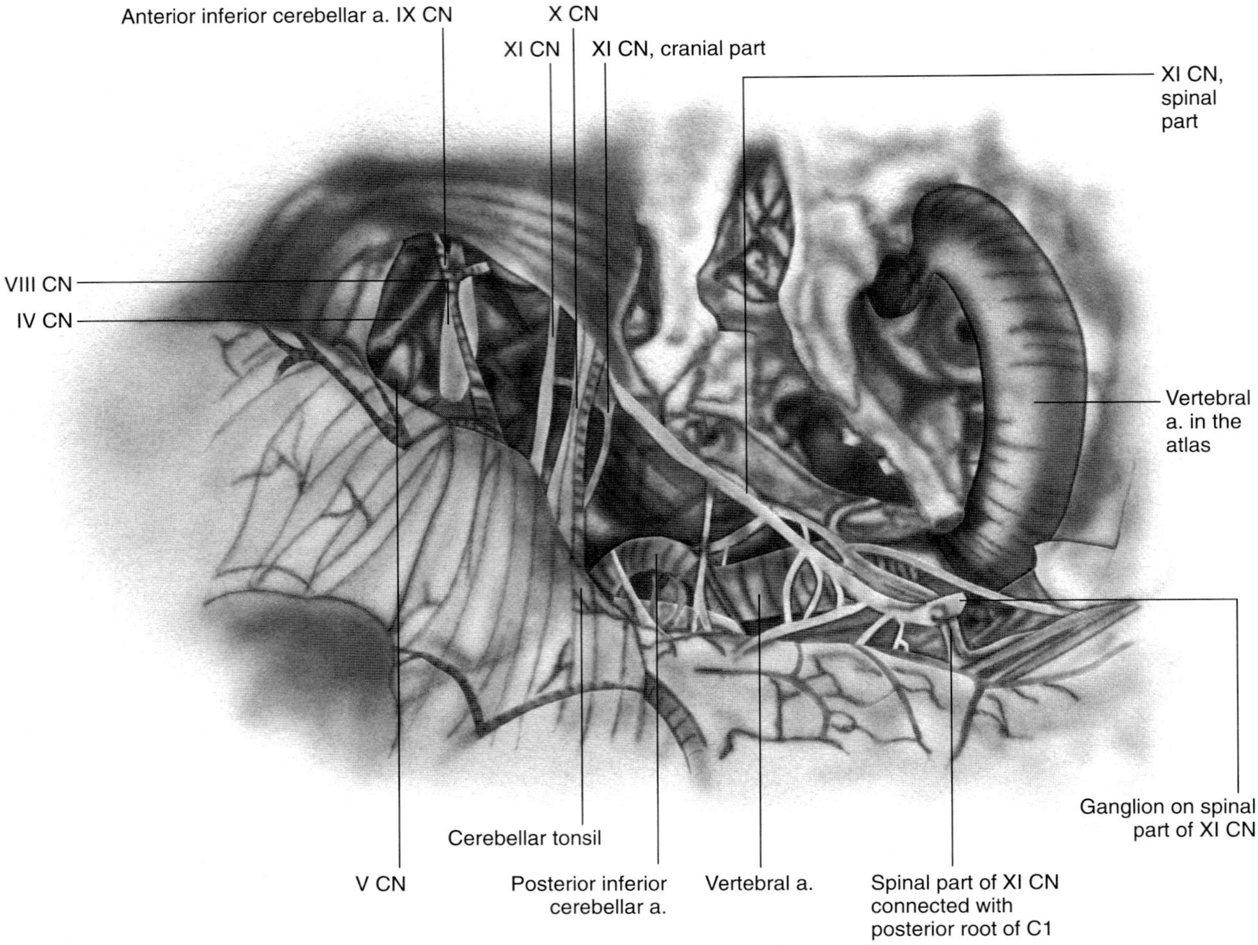

Fig. 40-13. Extreme lateral approach, right side. Dura has been opened, extradural vertebral artery has been exposed, the craniocervical junction and the CPA can be seen.

- At the operation's end, the dura is reconstructed. If the reconstruction does not hold, the lumbar drain is left in place for two days. The drain must not exceed 90 cc of liquor in 24 hours.
- If a postoperative lesion occurs to nerves IX, X, XI, and XII, it is important to prevent complications. The tracheotomy with insertion of a cuffed cannula prevents inhalation. Feeding is done with a nasogastric tube or a gastrostomy.
- When tumors of the mid and inferior clivus involve the petrous apexes, the approach may be combined with a subtemporal-infratemporal approach.

Caution
Before closing a sigmoid sinus, the demonstration of adequate venous drainage is necessary (see Chapter 35).

RESULTS

The approaches described above enable relatively complete tumor resection in most extradural petroclival tumors. In very extensive tumors, it may be necessary to perform the operation in stages.

- The rate of total removal (Sekhar series) is around 90% in benign lesions, such as meningiomas, glomus jugulare tumors, craniopharyngiomas, cholesterol granulomas, IX and X nerves neurilemomas, epidermoid cysts and benign teratomas.
- Apparently total excision is accomplished in almost 90% of high grade malignancies, such as squamous cell carcinomas, adenocarcinomas, basal cell carcinomas and osteogenic sarcomas. Partial excision is followed by radiation or chemotherapy.
- Apparently total excision is obtained in 50% of low grade malignancies, such as chordomas, chondrosarcomas, adenoid cystic carcinomas and invasive pituitary adenomas. Partial excision is followed by radiation therapy.

Paralysis of cranial nerves (III-XII) is generally temporary. Temporary palsy of the facial nerve (18%) usually follows the rerouting of its intratemporal part or its resection and grafting. Other, rarely observed, complications are those typical in skull base surgery: death, cerebral infarct, subdural hematoma, hydrocephalus, temporary hemiparesis, meningitis, and wound infection. CSF leakage is more frequent in patients with both intradural and extradural tumor.

Our capacity of achieving an apparently total tumor resection (based on postoperative CT and/or MRI studies) is improving steadily. However, the development of metastatic disease after surgery, expecially in highly malignant lesions, significantly reduces the success rate. Improvements in surgical technique and adjuvant therapy should provide positive results in the overall outcome in future, even in highly malignant lesions.

REFERENCES

Archer DJ, Young S, Uttley D: Basilar aneurysms: a new transclival approach via maxillotomy. J Neurosurg 67:54, 1987.

Cocke EW, Robertson JH, Robertson JT et al: The extended maxillotomy and subtotal maxillectomy for excision of skull base tumors. Arch Otolaryngol Head Neck Surg 11 6:92-104, 1990.

Crockard HA, Bradford R: Transoral transclival removal of a schwannoma anterior to the craniocervical junction. J Neurosurg 62:293, 1985.

Daspit CP, Spetzler RF, Pappas CTE: Combined approach for lesions involving the cerebellopontine angle and skull base: experience with 20 cases-preliminary report. Otolaryngol Head Neck Surg 105:788-796, 1991.

Derome PJ, Visot A, Monteil JP, Maestro JL: Management of cranial chordomas. In: Sekhar LN, Schramm VL Jr, eds. Tumors of the cranial base: diagnosis and treatment. Mount Kisco, NY: Futura, 607-622, 1987.

Fisch U, Kumar A: Infratemporal surgery of the skull base. In: Rand RW, ed. Microneurosurgery 3rd ed. St. Louis: Mosby, 398-420, 1985.

House WF, Hitselberger WE: The transcochlear approach to the skull base. Arch Otolaryngol 102:334, 1976.

House WF: Middle cranial fossa approach to the petrous pyramid. Report of 50 cases. Arch Otolaryngol 78:460-469, 1963.

Jackler RK: Overview of surgical neuro-otology. In: Jackler RK, Brackmann DE, eds. Neuro-otology. Baltimore: Mosby, 651-684, 1993.

Jackson CG, Glasscock ME, McKennan KX, et al: The surgical treatment of skull base tumors with intracranial extension. Otolaryngol Head Neck Surg 96:175, 1987.

Jackson CG: Surgery of skull base tumors. New York: Churchill Livingstone, 1991.

Jackson IT, Hide TH: A systematic approach to tumours of the base of the skull. J Maxillofac Surg 10:92-98, 1982.

Janecka IP, Sen C, Sekhar LN, Nuss D, Arriaga M: Facial translocation. A new approach to the cranial base. Otolaryngol Head Neck Surg 100:413-419, 1990.

Jones NF, Schramm VL, Sekhar LN: Reconstruction of the cranial base following tumour resection. Br J Plast Surg 40: 155-162, 1987.

Kawase T, Toya S, Shiobara R, et al: Transpetrosal approach for aneurysms of the lower basilar artery. J Neurosurg 63:857-861, 1985.

Lesoin F, Authricque A, Villette L, et al: Anteroexternal approach to the internal carotid artery at the base of the skull and intrapetrously. In: Proceedings of the International Symposium on Cavernous Sinus. Ljubljana, Yugoslavia: University Medical Centre. 265-274, 1986.

Mann WJ, Amedee RG, Gilsbach J, Pemeczky A, Wolfensberger M: Transsigmoid approach for tumors of the jugular foramen. Skull Base Surg 1:137-41, 1991.

Miller E, Crockard HA: Transoral transclival removal of anteriorly placed meningiomas at the foramen magnum. Neurosurgery 20:966, 1987.

Mullan S, Naunton R, Hekmat-Panah J, Vailati G: The use of an anterior approach to ventrally placed tumors in the foramen magnum and vertebral column. J Neurosurg 24:536, 1966.

Saleh E, Naguib M, Aristegui M, Cokkeser Y, Russo A, Sanna M: Surgical anatomy of the jugular foramen area. In: Mazzoni A, Sanna M, eds. Skull base surgery Update, 1. Amsterdam: Kugler, 1995 pp. 3-8.

Saleh E, Naguib M, Aristegui M, Cokkeser Y, Sanna M: The lower skull base: anatomical study with surgical implications. Ann Otol Rhinol Laryngol 104:57-61, 1995.

Saleh E, Taibah A, Achilli V, Aristegui M, Mazzoni M, Sanna A: Posterior fossa meningioma: surgical strategy. Skull Base Surg 4:209-219, 1994.

Samii M, Ammirati M: The combined supra-infratentorial presigmoid sinus avenue to the petro-clival region: surgical technique and clinical applications. Acta Neurochir 95:6-12, 1988.

Samii M, Draf W: Surgery of the skull base. Berlin: Springer, 1989.

Sanna M, Saleh E, Russo A, Taibah A: Atlas of temporal bone and lateral skull base surgery. Thieme, 1-189, 1995.

Sano K, Kinko M, Saito I: Vertebro-basilar aneurysms, with special reference to the transpharyngeal approach to the basilar artery aneurysms. Brain Nerve Tokyo 18: 1197, 1966.

Sekhar LN, Estonillo R: Transtemporal approach to the skull base: an anatomical study. Neurosurgery 19:799-808, 1986.

Sekhar LN, Janecka IP, Jones NF: Subtemporal-infratemporal and basal subfrontal approach to extensive cranial base tumors. Acta Neurochir Wien 92:83, 1988.

Sekhar LN, Schramm VL Jr, Jones NF, et al: Operative exposure and management of the petrous and upper cervical internal carotid artery. Neurosurgery 19:967, 1986.

Sekhar LN, Schramm VL Jr, Jones NF: Operative management of large neoplasms of the lateral and posterior cranial base. In: Sekhar LN, Schramm VL Jr, eds. Tumors of the cranial base: diagnosis and treatment. Mount Kisko, NY: Futura, 655-682, 1987.

Sekhar LN, Schramm VL Jr, Jones NF: Subtemporal-preauricular infratemporal fossa approach to large lateral and posterior cranial base neoplasms. J Neurosurg 67:488, 1987.

Sekhar LN, Schramm VL, Jones NF: Subtemporal-preauricular infratemporal fossa approach to large lateral and posterior cranial base neoplasms. J Neurosurg 67:488-499, 1987.

Sekhar LN, Sen C: Anterior and lateral basal approaches to the clivus. Contemp Neurosurg 11-18, 1989.

Sen C, Sekhar LN: Extreme lateral transcondylar and transjugular approaches. In: Sekhar LN, Janecka I, eds. Surgery of cranial base tumors. NewYork: Raven Press, 389-412, 1993.

Sen C, Sekhar LN, Schramm VL Jr, et al: Chordoma and chondrosarcoma of the cranial base: an 8-year experience. Neurosurgery 25:931-941, 1989.

Sen C, Sekhar LN: An extreme lateral approach to intradural lesions of the cervical spine and foramen magnum. Neurosurgery 27:197-204, 1990.

Sen C, Sekhar LN: The subtemporal and preauricular infratemporal approach to intradural structures ventral to the brain stem. J Neurosurg 73:345-354, 1990.

Snyderman CH, Janecka IP, Sekhar LN et al: Anterior cranial base reconstruction: role of galeal and pericranial flaps. Laryngoscope 100:49, 1990.

Stevenson GC, Stoney RJ, Perkins RK, et al: A transcervical transclival approach to the ventral surface of the brain stem for removal of a clivus chordoma. J Neurosurg 24:544, 1966.

Suzuki T, Tokuno H, Hakuba A: The orbito-zygomatic infratemporal approach: a new surgical technique. In: Proceedings of the International Symposium on Cavernous Sinus. Ljubljana Yugoslavia: University Medical Centre, 390-398, 1986.

Thedinger BA, Glasscock ME, Cueva RA: Transcochlear transtentorial approach for removal of large cerebellopontine angle meningiomas. Am J Otol 13:408-415, 1992.

Velut S, Jan M: Anterior petrosectomy during approach to the petroclival area. In: Schmideck HE, ed. Meningiomas and their surgical management. Philadelphia: Saunders, 435-450, 1991.

41

Auditory implants in the brainstem

The insane try to adapt reality to dreams. The sane try to adapt dreams to reality. Thus progress depends on the insane.

"The auditory brainstem implant permit bypassing both the cochlea and the cochlear nerve to directly stimulate the cochlear nuclei, giving the sensation of sound to an otherwise deaf patient". Hitselberger W.E. (Fig. 41-1).
Currently, patients who can receive a auditory brainstem implant are patients with bilateral acoustic neuromas and type 2 neurofibromatosis, according to a protocol monitored by the US Food and Drug Administration (Tables 41-1, 41-2).

Neurofibromatosis is a disease transmitted genetically, altering nerve cell growth.
Two types of neurofibromatosis can be distinguished. One has prevalent tropism for the peripheral system (NF-1), the other for the central system (NF-2).
The different modalities of presentation and the criteria for the differential diagnosis are expressed in Table 41-3.

Subjects with NF-2 have a greater risk of developing other tumors, such as schwannomas, meningiomas, gliomas, ependymomas, and plexiform neurofibromas.
Patients with NF-2 show an alteration of the acoustic nerve and thus no connection between the ganglion of Corti and the cochlear nuclei. A stimulus carried with a cochlear implant to the scala tympani would not in that case be transmitted to the Central Nervous System, due to the alteration in the acoustic nerve.

ANATOMY

- The structures having anatomic relationships with the lateral process of the fourth ventricle are the following: the foramen of Luschka, the choroid plexus, and the floccule (Fig. 41-2).
- The extremity of the lateral recess forms the foramen of Luschka, which is found at the edge of the bulbopontine sulcus. Just superior to the foramen is the root of nerves VII and VIII and inferior is the root of nerves IX and X.
- The choroid plexus is attached to the inner surface of the choroid tela and protrudes from the foramen of Luschka below entrance of nerves VII and VIII and slides to overlap the posterior part of nerves IX and X.
- The floccule is a cerebellar lobe which protrudes from the margin of the lateral recess and adheres to the rostral margin of the lateral recess and to the foramen of Luschka. The tenia passes across the roof of the lateral recess and outlines the area of the ventral cochlear nucleus (Fig. 41-3).

The stimulation should be carried to the ventral cochlear nerve, which is the most representative nucleus for the transmission of stimuli to the central auditory paths.
The further the electrode is inserted into the recess, the better is the result and the fewer are the side effects.

IMPLANTATION TECHNIQUE

- The translabyrinthine approach is the most common approach used at the House Ear Clinic for VIIIth nerve neuroma removal, but it is also the approach that gives the best surgical visibility for the positioning of a brainstem implant.
- The postauricular incision is able to produce a flap large enough to cover the implant with a margin with at least 1 cm of excess. The flap is more devascularized superiorly, while inferiorly it is more acute, since it must follow the mastoid tip. Thus cutting the soft tissue of the neck is to be avoided, since this results in unnecessary bleeding.
- Once the tumor has been removed, thorough hemostasis is performed. After positioning the implant, bipolar coagulation alone may be used, to avoid risking a shunt of current through the implant to the brainstem.
- The temporalis muscle is elevated with a self retaining retractor or with a Farabeuf retractor.

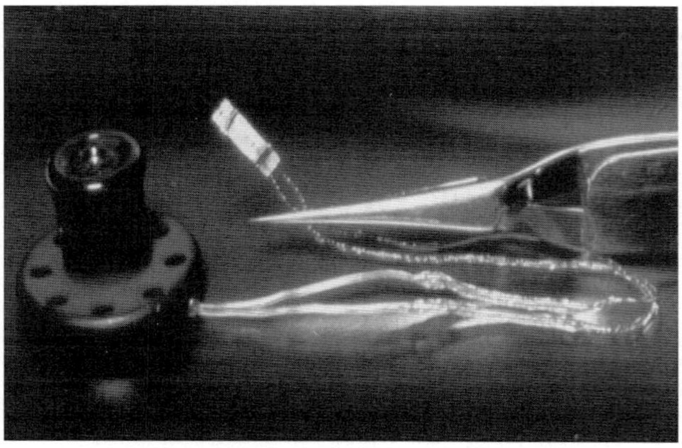

Fig. 41-1. Auditory brainstem implant: The electrode array for electrical stimulation.

Below the muscle, a butterfly burr or a cutting burr are used to prepare a niche in the squama of retromastoid bone, projecting from the sinodural angle, approx. 4-5 mm deep. A bone plate must be left in place medially to avoid exposing the dura. The correct amount of space to leave can be determined with a simulator. A dermographic pencil may also be used to draw the site of the correct position of the implant.

- Double points, connected, are drilled into the bone next to the niche. The coil of the niche is positioned in the niche and is anchored with nylon stitches across the lateral osseous holes. Once in place, the coil does not transmit oscillations to the electrodes during the delicate task of positioning.
- Identification of the lateral recess is based on the choroid plexus, which is generally preserved even after tumor removal. The choroid plexus protrudes laterally to the brainstem, and by following its posterior surface, the recess can be entered.
- If a large tumor has distorted the brainstem and it becomes difficult to find the usual landmarks, the stump of nerve VIII may be followed to the foramen of Luschka. The entrance point of nerve IX may also be followed by moving in a slightly superior direction.
- The location of the aditus of the lateral recess, once hypothesized, may be confirmed by the flow of liquor when the Valsalva maneuver is induced by the anesthesiologist.

Table. 41-1. FDA Criteria for Implantation.

- Presence of bilateral tumors of nerves VII/VIII involving the internal auditory canal or the cerebellopontine angle.
- Familiarity with the English language.
- Age at least 15.
- Good psychological state.
- Willingness to take part in research studies.
- Realistic expectations.

Table 41-2. FDA Criteria for the auditory brainstem implant in NF-2 patients.

- Secondary tumor in the only hearing ear.
- Any tumor larger than 1.5 cm in the hearing ear.
- Limited life expectancy due to other tumors, medical problems, or advanced age.
- Usable hearing with a tumor that does not demonstrate significant growth in MRI checks and stable hearing demonstrated in audiometric tests.
- Situations in which a tumor is observed in an ear with residual hearing of an NF-2 patient with bilateral neuromas, if the tumor does not endanger life nor significantly alter vital functions.

- The electrode holder is grasped carefully with delicate forceps, with the electrodes turned upwards, and inserted completely into the foramen of Luschka, to give the best yield. After insertion, the implant's function is evaluated in relation to its position and all of the electrodes are stimulated. The evoked potentials are sought, as well as any stimulation of nerves V, VII, and IX, and alterations in the vital signs (Fig. 41-4).
- The position of the electrode-holder is modified if necessary, in order to optimize the response of the evoked potentials and reduce side effects. Once a satisfactory position has been obtained, the electrode holder is held in place with a piece of fat in the meatus of the lateral recess and possibly with other fibrous tissue. The reference electrode is inserted into the temporalis muscle and the cable is positioned in the mastoid. The mastoid deficit is filled with adipose tissue.
- The subcutaneous closure is performed with Vycril and the cutaneous closure with silk (Fig. 41-5).

Evoked potential recording

The recording of evoked potentials in response to electrical stimulation of the cochlear nucleus through a brainstem implant is done with electrodes inserted under the skin at the vertex (Cz) of the head and of the neck (C7), with a grounded electrode on the neck near the hairline. The differential signal (Cz-C7) is amplified with a gain of 100,000 and filtered from 10 Hz to 10 KHz to avoid prolonging the stimulus artifact. 2000 stimuli are presented in 30 msec intervals. To eliminate the electrical connection with the patient, the stimulus is erogated through a pair of coils acting as a transformer. Biphasic voltage impulses are sent to the transmitting coil and the parameters are regulated to reduce the duration of the stimulus artifact to a minimum. The receiver coil is directly connected to the stimulating electrodes. The brainstem potentials revealed are fil-

Table. 41-3. Different modalities of presentation and criteria for the differential diagnosis between NF-1 and NF-2.

Definition
NF-1
Also called von Recklinghausen's disease or peripheral neurofibromatosis
NF-2
Also called bilateral hereditary syndrome of bilateral schwannomas.
Genetic
NF-1
Dominant autosomic disease. Transmitted to 50% of offspring. Gene located at band 17q on the long arm of chromosome 17, near the centromere.
NF-2
Dominant autosomic disease. Transmitted to 50% of offspring. Gene is located in the middle of chromosome 22's long arm.
Incidence
NF-1
1/40000
NF-2
1/40000
Age
NF-1
The skin spots appear mostly on the trunk within the first 4 years of life.
NF-2
Signs may manifest from 10 to 60 years, but in general later than those of NF-1.
Diagnosis
NF-1
At least 2 of the following signs:
- More than 5 coffee colored spots larger than 5 mm in children and 15 mm in adolescents and adults.
- Two or more neurofibromas or one plexiform neurofibroma.
- Freckles on the armpit or groin.
- Glioma of the optic nerve.
- Two or more raised melanocytic hamartomas, yellow or darker, on the surface of the iris.
- Specific osseous lesion, such as a displasia of the sphenoid or a thinning of the cortex of the long bones, with or without pseudoarthritis.
- Close relative with NF-1 defined with the aforementioned criteria.

NF-2
Subject has bilateral schwannomas of the vestibular nerve or a close relative with NF-2, or at least 2 of the following symptoms:
- Cutaneous or subcutaneous neurofibromas.
- Plexiform neurofibromas.
- Schwannomas.
- Gliomas.
- Posterior juvenile subcapsular cataract.

tered with filters that depend on the computer system utilized (Waring).

POSTOPERATIVE TREATMENT
According to FDA regulations, the implant must be positioned at the end of tumor-removal surgery. The postoperative treatment is thus similar to that of translabyrinthine surgery.
On the second day after surgery, patient's conditions permitting, a light pulsating signal may be administered, with progressively increasing intensity.

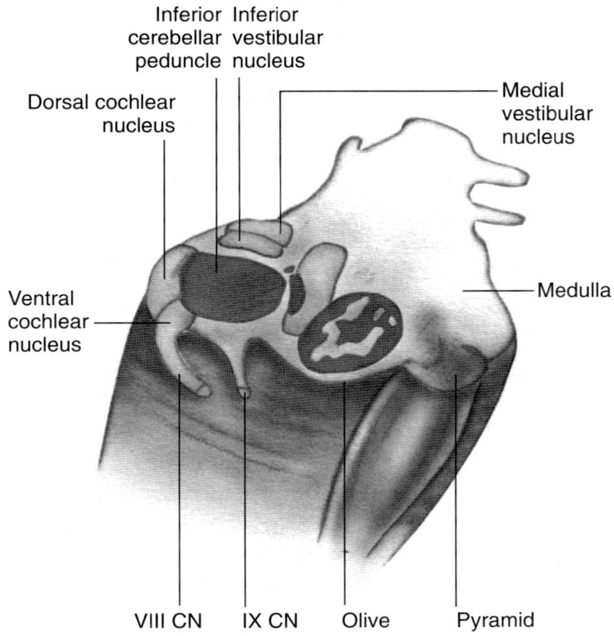

Fig- 41-2. The pons and the auditory nuclei. In humans the cochlear nuclear complex are covered by the cerebellar peduncle.

The best results and the fewest side effects have been obtained with a 300Hz sinusoid (Shannon).

SIDE EFFECTS
Among the side effects of electrical stimulation, symptoms of stimulation of the adjacent nervous structures may be seen:
- Nerve VII: Hemifacial movements.
- Vestibular part of nerve VIII: vertigo.
- Nerve IX: sensory alterations to the throat.
- Long brainstem pathways: tingling in the shoulder and arm.
- Cerebral floccule: vibratory and ocular sensations.

These side effects, if present, are eliminated or minimized by acting on the stimulation threshold of each electrode.

POSTOPERATIVE COMPLICATIONS
The most frequent postoperative complication is a cerebrospinal liquor fistula, which is more frequent than in the simple translabyrinthine operation, despite preventative measures. This is because the implant provides a path for liquor diffusion of the endocranial spaces to the internal coil and that of the external suture.
To prevent a liquor fistula
Care must be taken when closing the flap, following the aforementioned criteria (Chapter 28).
- Closure of the epitympanum is performed normally. In addition, it is advisable to open the fa-

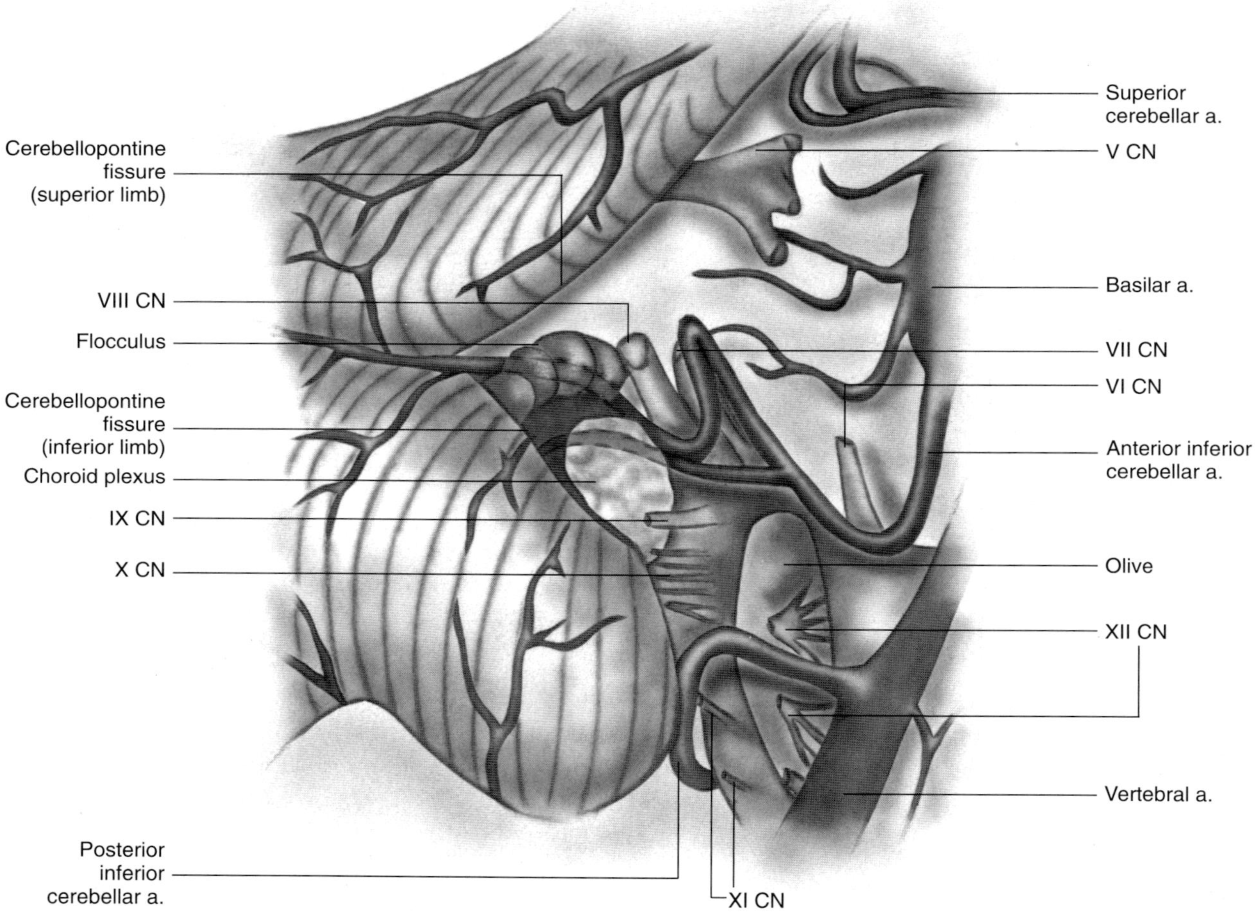

Fig. 41-3. The right CPA. Anterolateral view. Neurovascular relationship.

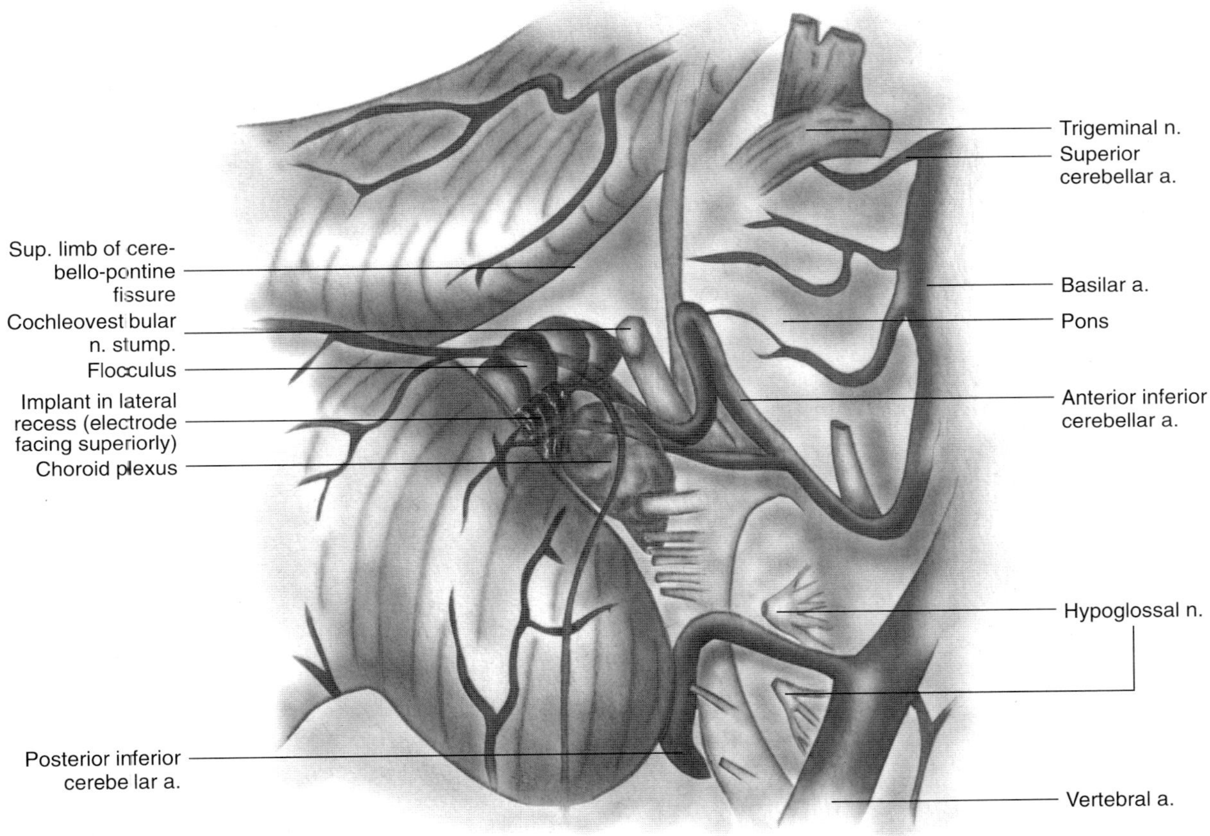

Fig. 41-4. The electrode array has been fully inserted into the lateral recess. The electrodes must face superiorly (Adapted from Hitselberger WE).

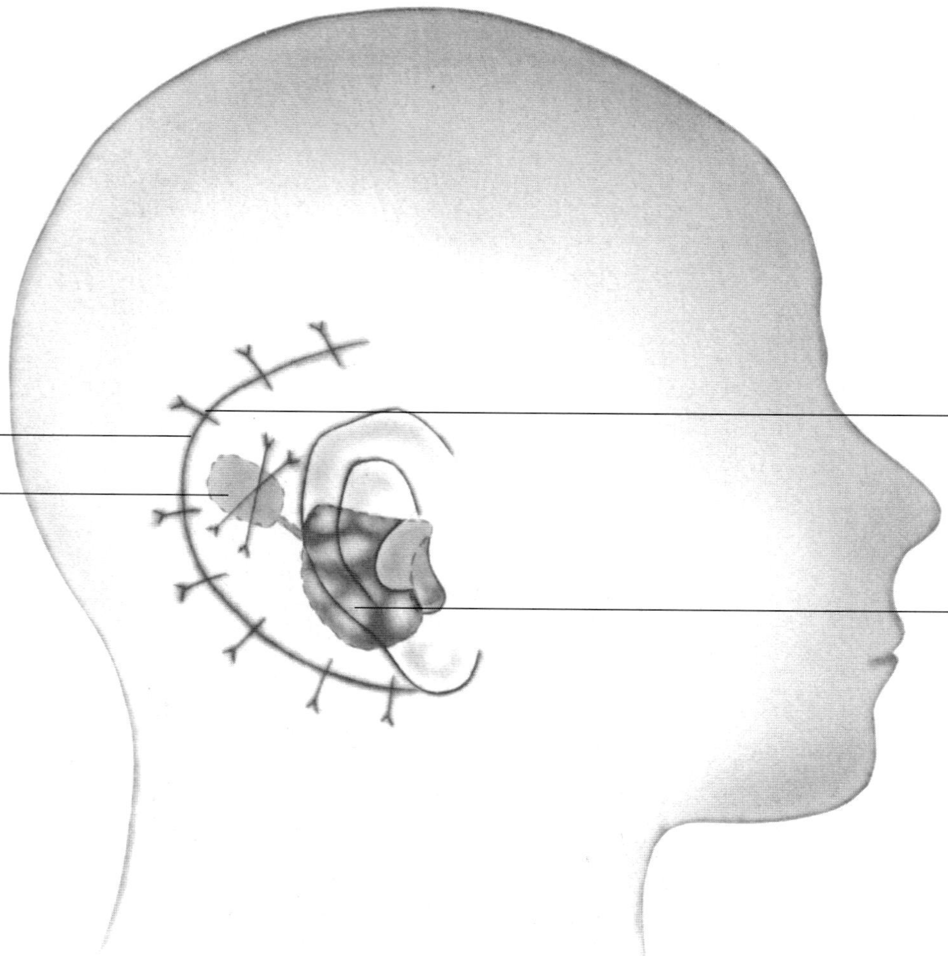

Fig. 41-5. Incision and positioning of the implant.

cial recess, close the tube with muscle and/or Surgicel and/or bone wax, and then reseal the facial recess with muscle.

- The dura is closed with 4-0 silk. It is impossible to attain a hermetic suture, but the technique of compressing abdominal fat in the ligation is helpful. The fat follows the paths of least resistance and goes to close the interstices in the suture. More abdominal fat is placed over the dura.
- If, despite these precautions, a fistula is seen, it is treated with the same procedure described for the therapy of translabyrinthine surgery complications (see chapter 28). The same procedure is followed for meningitis.

RECOVERY

Prophylactic medical treatment is initiated intravenously immediately after surgery and continued until the fifth day after surgery. The time needed for complete recovery of the operated area and for a stabilization of the implant, in the absence of complications, is 1 $^1/_2$ months.

RESULTS

Among 28 NF-2 patients implanted between 1979 and 1993, 19 have obtained auditory benefit, with no significant side effects,

Patients who have received an auditory brainstem implant report hearing a sound similar to that of a badly tuned radio station. Sounds are heard but not understood, but all users are aware of environmental sounds and show improved lip-reading scores.

REFERENCES

Brackmann DE, Hitselberger WE, Nelson RA, et al: Auditory Brainstem Implant: 1. Issues in Surgical Implantation. Otolaryngol Head Neck Surg 108:624-633, 1993.

Brackmann DE, Hitselberger WE, Nelson RA, Moore J, Waring MD, Portillo F, Shannon RV, Telischi FF: Auditory brainstem implant: I. Issues in surgical implantation [see comments]. Comment in: Otolaryngol Head Neck Surg , 1111:150-1, 1994.

El-Kashlan HK, Niparko JK, Altschuler RA, Miller JM: Direct electrical stimulation of the cochlear nucleus: surface vs. penetrating stimulation. Otolaryngol Head Neck Surg 105:533-543, 1991.

Hitselberger N, House WF, Edgerton BS, Whitaker S: Cochlear nucleus implant. Otolaryngol Head Neck Surg 92:52-54, 1984.

Luetje CM, Whittaker CK, Geier L, et al: Feasibility of multichannel human cochlear nucleus stimulation. Laryngoscope 1021, 23-25, 1992.

McCreery DB, Agnew WF, Yven TGM, Bullara I: Charge density and charge per phase as cofactors in neural injury induced by electrical stimulation. IEEE Trans Biomed Eng 37: 996-1001, 1990.

Monsell EM, McElveen JT, Hitselberger WE, House WF: Surgical approaches to the human cochlear nucleus complex. Am J Otol 85: 450-455, 1987.

Morest DK, Ostapoff EM, Potashner SJ, et al: The cellular basis for signal processing in the mammalian cochlear nuclei. In Merchan MA ed: The Mammalian Cochlear Nuclei: Organization and function. Europa Arts Graficas Salamanca, 1991.

Niparko JK, Altschuler RA, Xue XL, et al: Surgical implantation and biocompatibility of central nervous system auditory prostheses. Ann Otol Rhin Laryngol 98: 965-970, 1989.

Niparko JK, Kileny PR, Kemink JL, et al: Neurophysiologic intraoperative monitoring: II. Facial nerve function. Am J Otol 10: 55-61, 1989.

Ricardi VM: Neurofibromatosis. Neurol Clin 53: 337-349, 1987.

Shannon RV, Fayad J, Moore JK, et al: Auditory Brainstem Implant: II. Postsurgical issues and performance. Otolaryngol Head Neck Surg 108:634-642, 1993.

Shannon RV, Otto SR: Psychophysical measures from electrical stimulation of the human cochlear nucleus. Hear Res 47: 159-168, 1990.

Shannon RV: A model of safe levels for electrical stimulation. IEEE Trans Biomed Eng 39: 424-426, 1992.

Sinha VK, Terr LI, Galey FR, Linthicum FH: Computer aided three-dimensional reconstruction of the cochlear nerve root. Otolaryngol Head Neck Surg 113: 651-655, 1987.

Soussi T, Otto SR: Effects of electrical brainstem stimulation on tinnitus. Acta Otolaryngol Stockh. 1142: 135-40, 1994.

Terr LI, Edgerton BJ: Surface topography of the cochlear nuclei in humans: Two and three-dimensional. Hear Res 17: 51-59, 1985.

Waring MD: Electrically evoked auditory brainstem response monitoring of auditory brainstem implant integrity during facial nerve tumor surgery. Laryngoscope; 1021: 1293-1295, 1992.

42

Intraoperative neurophysiological monitoring

The following is the scale of priorities in the treatment of tumors of the skull base:
Preservation of the patient's life; complete tumor removal; preservation of cranial nerve integrity. Maintaining the cochlear nerve intact is important in operations attempting to preserve hearing. Nerve preservation is easier today thanks to intraoperative monitoring. This entails observing changes in evoked potentials during surgical manipulation, and modifying the stimulus accordingly, in time to prevent irreversible damage and/or its progression.

OPERATING ROOM SETUP

- All materials must be checked the evening before surgery, since an intraoperative malfunction may be irreparable.
- Before the first operation, the equipment must be checked in relation to the environment. Instruments which could provoke acoustic or electrical interference are identified and removed from the sensitive area. This procedure may be time-consuming the first time, but will henceforth be much more rapid.
- A preoperative evaluation of the BAEP's is performed. This makes it possible to compare the intraoperative and preoperative tracings. A preoperative evaluation is also done for the facial nerve.
- On the day of surgery, the electrodes are positioned on the sedated patient, before disinfection. Thus defective electrodes may be changed without contaminating the surgical field.
- Batteries must always be completely discharged after each operation to prevent a memory effect, and are recharged on the eve of surgery. This prolongs the life of the batteries and maintains their operative capacity.
- We use subdermic needle electrodes (Type E2, Grass Instrument Co., Quincy, MA), (Figs. 42-1, 42-2)

ANESTHESIA

When EMG modifications are to be recorded, no muscle relaxants should be used. An effective procedure requires:

- Intubation with rapid-action muscle relaxants for neuromuscular plate: Succinylcoline + D-tubocurarine (2-4 mg) or Atricurium.
- Maintenance with inhalants such as isoflurane or enflurane in a 2:1 solution with nitrogen and oxygen, or endovenous drugs, such as barbiturates or Propophol. Fentanyl or Morphine can be used to obtain an additional analgesic effect.

AUDITORY EVOKED POTENTIALS

BAEP's record electrical activity is induced in the nuclei and the fibers of the auditory channels by a sound stimulus.
The first five peaks (Wave I-V) are constant in most normal individuals (Table 42-1).

Selecting the most effective repetition frequency

Stimulation is performed with clicks. In clinical practice, a repetition frequency of approx. 11 clicks/sec is used. Lower frequencies improve response definition but increase the duration of the test. Thus we use a repetition of the stimuli at 35 clicks/sec intraoperatively. The weak point of the BAEP's is that a good tracing requires an average of 1000-2000 responses; thus too much time passes between the stimulus and the appearance of subsequent electrical modifications.
Sounds are produced with small auricular microphones, such as those used with portable radios.

Utilizing an adequate stimulus intensity

105 dB SPL (approx. 65 dB HL).

Filter adoption

We use digital filters, extended from 10 to 3000 Hz.

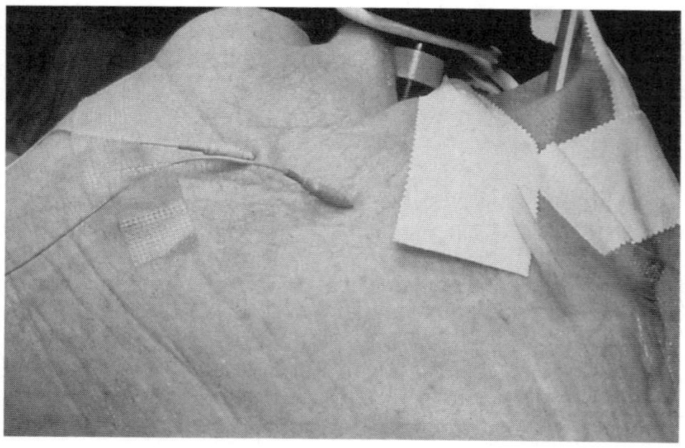

Fig. 42-1. Subdermal needle electrodes placed in the upper and lower face so that all facial muscles on one side can be monitored.

Table 42-1. Charateristics of evoked potential.

Denomination	Origin	Latency
AP	cochlea	1-6 msec
CM	nerve VIII	
SP		
ABR		
wave I	nerve VIII	1.5-1.8
II	cochlear nuclei	2.5-3.2
III	trapezoid body	3.5-4
IV	lateral lemniscus	4-5
V	inferior colliculus	5.1-6.7
VI	middle geniculate body	6.5-7.4
VII	thalamocortical acoustic radiation	7.5-8
FFR	brainstem	10-12
PAM	postauricular muscles	7-20
MLC	thalamus, auditory radiations, cortex I	10-50
SVR	cortex I, II	50-300
CNV P300	associational areas	300

Obtaining a base tracing

- A base tracing is recorded with an anesthetized patient, before the operation begins. The most evident BAEP wave, and thus the one most regarded in its intraoperative variations from the baseline, is wave V, followed by wave III. The most important parameter to consider is the decrease in peak size, followed by the decrease in latency.
- Wave III is generated mainly by the cochlear nuclei. A reduction in size and/or latency of wave III, followed by that of wave V, is thus a sign of acoustic nerve suffering.
- Wave V is generated by the inferior colliculi. The mere reduction of size and/or latency of wave V is thus a sign of alterations in the brainstem paths. Though there is no consensus in literature, a change in latency in wave V from 0.5 to 1.5 msec is considered significant by many authors.

Caution

During surgery, hypothermia or the irrigation of the electrode with a solution of a lower temperature than the body temperature will increase the latency values of the potentials.

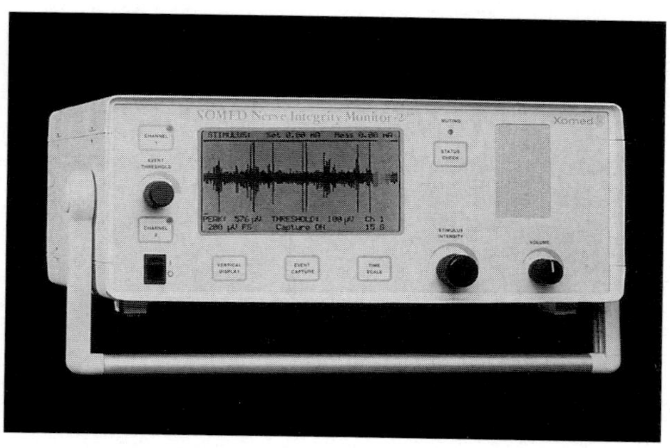

Fig. 42-2. The Xomed nerve integrity monitor.

Electrocochleography

The ECoG potentials are generated by the cochlea. They are recorded with a transtympanic electrode placed on the cochlea or in a non-invasive way with an electrode placed near the tympanic membrane (the potentials are slightly lower). These potentials are larger than those of the BAEP; they are thus more easily interpreted since few responses are needed for adequate tracings.
The benefits of auditory monitoring during acoustic neuroma surgery are limited, since only cochlear potentials are represented, and not, for example, those of the acoustic nerve. We do not utilize this method.

CAP MONITORING
(Compound Action Potentials)

Intraoperative monitoring of compound action potentials (CAP) is the most useful in intraoperative evaluation of the state of the acoustic nerve.

- Few responses are needed to generate the potential, so that the evaluation of possible nerve suffering is almost immediate, unlike in the BAEPs.
- A monopolar electrode is used, made of teflon-covered silver wire, with a tiny wad of cotton anchored to its non-teflon covered extremity. This extremity is placed on the acoustic nerve. This method is especially useful during vestibular nerve section in Mèniére's disease, or in the removal of small neuromas with the middle fossa approach.
- The BAEP's may be monitored simultaneously with the CAPs. The former are especially useful if

the electrode should become dislodged intraoperatively. The electrode should always be replaced, however, before continuing the operation.

A bipolar electrode may also be used, composed of two wires similar to those of the monopolar electrode. Its extremities are not isolated with cotton, so they must be placed on the nerve very cautiously.

CRANIAL NERVE MONITORING

Cranial nerve monitoring is based on the recording of EMG potentials from electrodes placed in the facial muscles.

FACIAL NERVE MONITORING

Facial nerves monitoring is useful in many surgical procedures; the removal of a tumor from the acoustic nerve, from the skull base, or a facial neuroma; the section of the vestibular nerve (vestibular neurectomy), microvascular decompression for hemifacial spasms, decompression of the facial nerve, the removal of parotid tumors, and facial trauma surgery.

The importance of the neurostimulator

- When the facial nerve is to be exposed, bursts of EMG activity are recorded before the nerve is reached. This has enhanced our understanding of the importance of continuous irrigation to avoid overheating of the nerve due to the burr's action. It has also facilitated the exposure of the nerve in the more difficult areas (blind spots), such as the second genu along the medial portion of the nerve, which is complicated by its proximity to the lateral semicircular canal.
- Awareness of the degree of nerve suffering during surgical maneuvers has led to modifications in technique. Along the descending part of the facial nerve, sharp dissection is preferable to blunt dissection, especially when the stapedial muscle anchors the nerve in the fallopian canal.
- In all surgical approaches to neuroma removal, it has been observed that separating the tumor from the facial nerve is less traumatic if performed with a disposable Beaver blade, rather than with a smooth dissection (Sterkers O).
- The identification of Bill's bar has become of secondary importance since it has become possible to use a probe to identify the nerve at its infralabyrinthine part and at the fundus of the IAC. Thus, the nerve's vulnerability to lesion is reduced.
- The discrimination of the facial nerve and the superior vestibular nerve at the IAC fundus is facilitated. The identification and the differentiation of the cochlear and facial nerves in the brainstem is also facilitated.
- The possibility of stimulating parts of the tumor and excluding the presence of nerve VII notably abbreviates time spent in surgery.
- When the nerve has been identified in skull base tumor operations, there is a tendency for the surgeon to relax psychologically and accelerate the tumor removal process, since the area is now reputed to be risk-free. Monitoring prevents the execution of maneuvers that can mechanically traumatize the nerve.

We use a Xomed Nim-2 facial nerve stimulator.

The facial nerve is primarily a motor nerve, with a lesser sensory component. The motor part innervates the stapedial muscle, the posterior belly of the digastric muscle, and the facial expression muscles: frontal, orbicular of the eye, anterior auricular, eyebrow arching muscles, zygomatic, orbicular of the mouth, lip depressor, elevator of the corners of the mouth, nasal, mental, platysma, buccinator, and risorius. Some of the facial expression muscles are typically utilized for intraoperative monitoring of the facial nerve. The most frequently used are the orbicular muscles of the eye and the mouth.

We use EEG needle electrodes, which are inserted under the skin covering the muscles to be monitored. One pair of electrodes is positioned to monitor the orbicular muscle of the eye, while the other pair is positioned to monitor the orbicular muscle of the mouth.

If desired, the same apparatus may be used to monitor another nerve, by positioning one pair of electrodes in one of the two muscles mentioned above, whereas the second pair of electrodes goes to monitor the second nerve.

The grounded electrode is positioned on the contralateral shoulder.

The electrodes are positioned as shown in Figure 42-1 and kept in place with tape.

Stimulation

We use a monopolar stimulating electrode to stimulate the nerve (Prass Monopolar Stimulator Probe). It is best to use a current with a semiconstant voltage. Thus the risk of shunting is avoided, which would alter the signal by modifying the field conditions (for example, cerebrospinal liquor or intraoperative irrigation).

The use of a bipolar stimulating electrode is not advised, since stimulation is affected by the placement of the stimulator. In very long and complex operations, the stimulation procedure must be as simple as possible, since it must be repeated many times during surgery.

Stimulus intensity

The stimulus intensity required to record an adequate response depends on various factors, among

them: the state of the nerve, the type of stimulating probe (monopolar or bipolar), the duration of the stimulus, the distance from the electrode to the nerve, and the presence of cerebrospinal liquor. The general rule is to utilize the lowest intensity possible. In general a stimulus of 0.05 (the minimum) to 0.3 mA is sufficient. The stimulus is kept at a low intensity at the beginning, when the nerve is known to be intact, until a response is recorded. If nerve suffering is manifested as surgery progresses, no response will be elicited with the previous stimulus intensity, and it must be progressively increased to obtain a response.
It is preferable that the surgeon know in real time any significant modification in the EMG potentials intraoperatively, to understand the motivations and modify his technique, before causing irreversible damage.

Recognizing artifacts
EMG responses may be obtained independent of the electrical stimulus, for many reasons. The most frequent is due to mechanical stimulation of the nerve, due to surgical manipulation. Thermal stimulation, e.g. with water at below body temperature, is manifested with a chain of repetitive stimuli. During electrical stimulation, the stimuli are quieted by the apparatus, but an electrical loss may be verified by the thermocautery. Another signal artifact is when the surgeon uses two metal instruments together in the surgical field, e.g. an aspirator with a dissector. This signal, and others like it, are typically monophasic, with a sudden beginning and end. They appear on the screen as acute-peak responses, in a single direction.

Conclusion of surgery
Before closing the field, the functional integrity of the nerve must again be evaluated, by stimulating as far as possible medially and distally inside the surgical field.
Monitoring must be continued until the incision has been closed. It may be that too much fat, compressed by the skin flap, will damage the nerve. If a repetitive electrical activity is seen, the wound must be reopened (in general, nerve suffering will be noted at the first 2-3 sutures) and the dressing loosened.

CRANIAL NERVE MONITORING III-IV-V-VI

OCULOMOTOR NERVE (III)

The oculomotor nerve enters the orbit through the superior orbitary fissure, where it divides into a superior and an inferior branch which innervate the ocular muscles. The superior branch innervates the levator palpebrae superioris and the superior rectus muscle. The inferior branch innervates the medial rectus, the inferior rectus and the oblique inferior muscles. The parasympathetic fibers from the Edinger Westphal nucleus innervate the pupillary constrictor muscle and the ciliary muscle, which enables the lens to dilate and vary its thickness in the process of accommodation.
To monitor the oculomotor nerve, EMG activity is generally recorded from the inferior rectus.
An EEG needle electrode or a simple hook electrode may be positioned in or near the inferior rectus muscle percutaneously. The electrode must merely be near the muscle, since EMG activity needs not be intramuscular.
The electrode must be inserted with the point of the needle pointed away from the eye, to avoid injuring it.
A second electrode is positioned on the opposite shoulder. This electrode serves as a point of reference for the recording electrode.
To be able to monitor nerves III and IV and/or VI, a grounded electrode must be used, located on the patient's forehead.

TROCHLEAR NERVE (IV)

The trochlear nerve enters the orbit through the superior orbitary fissure and terminates in the superior oblique muscle.
The electrode is placed in or near the superior oblique muscle, percutaneously, and pointed away from the eye.
The reference electrode and the grounded electrode are positioned as described above.

TRIGEMINAL NERVE (V)

Monitoring of the trigeminal nerve alone is less frequent than monitoring of other cranial nerves. The surgical procedures in which the trigeminal nerve may be monitored alone are during microvascular decompression for trigeminal neuralgia (Moller, 1988), and during the section of the nerve for intractable pain.
The trigeminal nerve is more often monitored along with the facial nerve during surgery for the removal of large tumors from the posterior fossa, such as neuromas of the acoustic nerve or meningiomas.
The motor part of the trigeminal nerve innervates the chewing muscles: the internal and external pterygoid muscles, the temporalis muscle, the masseter and mylohyoid muscles, and the anterior belly of the digastric muscle.
EMG activity is generally recorded from the masseter and/or temporalis muscles when monitoring the trigeminal nerve.
To monitor nerve V, bipolar electrodes are used, such as the "double hookwire" or a pair of sub-

dermal EEG electrodes, placed 1-2 mm apart. If "hookwire" electrodes are used, they must be inserted intramuscularly in the appropriate muscle. If EEG needle electrodes are used, they must be inserted in a subdermal position in the area overlying the specific muscle, without touching.

In general, a pair of electrodes is positioned to monitor the masseter muscle. If another pair of electrodes is used, they are positioned to monitor the temporalis muscle.

The grounded electrode is positioned on the patient's forehead.

ABDUCENS NERVE (VI)

The abducens nerve enters the orbit through the superior orbitary fissure and terminates in the lateral rectus muscle which abduces or deviates the eye laterally.

The electrode is positioned in or near the lateral rectus muscle, percutaneously, pointing away from the eye.

The reference electrode and the grounded electrode are positioned as described above.

IMPROVEMENT

- Facial nerve monitoring makes it possible to improve the prognosis of facial nerve preservation. Time in surgery is abbreviated, since identification of the nerve is easier and thus tumor removal is also more rapid in other areas. The postoperative function of the nerve can be predicted by the intraoperative stimulation.
- Intraoperative BAEP registration has not led to statistically significant improvements in hearing preservation, since much of the credit for better results may be attributed to improvements in surgical technique. At any rate, improvements in surgical technique have been aided by the monitoring of electrophysiological modifications, and the understanding of their relationships by means of surgical manipulation.

REFERENCES

Babin RM, Jai HR, McCabe BF: Bipolar localization of the facial nerve in the internal auditory canal. In Graham MD, House WF eds: Disorders of the Facial Nerve: Anatomy, Diagnosis, and Management. New York, Raven Press, 1982, pp 35.

Belal A, Lynthicum FH, House WF: Acoustic tumor surgery with preservation of hearing. Histopathologic report. The Amer J Otology 4/1: 9-16, 1982.

Benecke JE, Calder HB, Chadwick G: Facial nerve monitoring during acoustic neuroma removal. Laryngoscope 97: 697-700, 1987.

Bennett MH, Bunegin L, Albin MS, Dujovny M, Hellstrom HR, Jannetta PJ: Evoked potential correlates of graded brain retraction pressure. Stroke 8: 487-492, 1977.

Campbell KCM, Abbas PJ: The effect of stimulus repetition rate on auditory brainstem response in tumor and nontumor patients. J Speech Hear Res 30: 494-502, 1987.

Coats AC: Human auditory nerve action potentials and brainstem evoked responses latency intensity functions in detection of cochlear and retrocochlear pathology. Arch Otolaryngol Head Neck Surg 104: 709-717, 1978.

Coats AC: The summating potential and Mèniére's disease. I. Summating potential amplitude in Mèniére and non Mèniére ears. Arch Otolaryngol Head Neck Surg 107: 199-208, 1981.

Daube JR, Harper CM: Surgical monitoring of cranial and peripheral nerves. In Desmedt JE ed: Neuromonitoring in Surgery. Amsterdam, Elsevier Science Publishers, 1989, pp 115-138.

Daube JR: Intraoperative monitoring of cranial motor nerves. In Schramm J, Moller AR eds: Intraoperative Neurophysiologic Monitoring in Neurosurgery. Heidelberg, Springer-Verlag, 1991, pp 246-267.

Davis H, Hirsh SK: A slow brain stem response for low frequency audiometry. Audiology 18: 445-461, 1979.

Delgado TE, Buchheit WA, Rosenholtz HR, Chrissian S: Intraoperative monitoring of facial muscle evoked responses obtained by intracranial stimulation of the facial nerve: a more occurate technique for facial nerve dissection. Neurosurg 4: 418-421, 1979.

Dickins JRE, Graham SS: A comparison of facial nerve monitoring systems in cerebellopontine angle surgery. Am J Otol 12: 16, 1991.

Doyle DJ, Hyde ML: Analogue and digital filtering of auditory brainstem responses. Scand Audiol 10: 81-89, 1981.

Duncan PG, Sanders RA, McCullough DW: Preservation of auditory brainstem responses in anesthetized children. Can J Anaesth 26: 492-495, 1979.

Eggermont JJ: Electrocochleography. In Keidel WD, Neff WD eds: Handbook of Sensory Physiology, Vol 3, New York, Springer-Verlag, 1976, pp 625-705.

Ferraro JA, Best LG, Arenberg IK: The use of electrocochleography in the diagnosis, assessment, and monitoring of endolymphatic hydrops. Otolaryngol Clin North Am 16: 69-82, 1983.

Ferraro JA, Murphy GB, Ruth RA: A comparative study of primary electrodes used in extratympanic electrocochleography. Semin Hear 7: 279-287,1986.

Fischer C, Ibanez V, Mauguiere F: Monitorage per-operatoire des potentiels evoques auditifs precoces. Presse Med (Paris): 14-37, 1914-1918, 1985.

Grundy BL, Jannena PJ, Procopio PT, Lina A, Boston JR, Doyle E: Intraoperative monitoring of brain stem auditory evoked potentials. J Neurosurg 57: 674-681, 1982.

Grundy BL: Evoked potentials monitoring. In Blitt CD ed: Monitoring in Anesthesia and Critical Care Medicine. New York, Churchil Livingstone, 1985, pp 345-411.

Grundy BL: Intraoperative monitoring of sensory evoked potentials. Anesthesiology 58: 72-87, 1983.

Halner SG, Daube JR, Beatty CW, Ebersold MJ: Intraoperative monitoring of the facial nerve. Laryngoscope 98: 209-212, 1988.

Hardy RW Jr, Kinney SE, Lueders H, Lesser RP: Preservation of cochlear nerve function with aid of brain stem auditory evoked potentials. Neurosurgery 11: 16-18, 1982.

Harner SG, Daube JR, Ebersold MJ, Beatty CW: Improved preservation of facial nerve functions with use of electrical monitoring during removal of acoustic neuromas. Mayo Clin Proc 62: 92-102, 1987.

Hashimoto I, Ishiyama Y, Yoshimoto T, Nemoto S: Brainstem auditory evoked potentials recorded directly from human brainstem and thalamus. Brain 104: 841-859, 1981.

House JW, Brackmann DE: Facial nerve grading system. Otolaryngol Head Neck Surg 93: 146-167, 1985.

Jannetta PJ, Moller AR, Moller MB: Technique of hearing preservation of small acoustic neuromas. Ann Surg 200: 513-523, 1984.

Kanzaki J, Ouchi T, Yokobbori H, Ino T: Electrocochleographic study of summating potentials in Mènièrе's disease. Audiology 21: 409-424, 1982.

Kartush JM, Bouchard KR: Intraoperative facial monitoring. Otology, Neurotology, and Skull base surgery. In Kartush JM, Bouchard KR eds: Neuromonitoring in Otology and Head and Neck Surgery. New York, Raven Press, 1992, pp 99-120.

Lambert PR, Ruth RA: Simultaneous recording of noninvasive ECoG and ABR for use in intraoperative monitoring. Otolaryngol Head Neck Surg 98: 575-580, 1988.

Lang J: Clinical Anatomy of the Head, Neurocranium, Orbit, and Craniocervical Region. New York, Springer Verlag, 1983.

Lanser MJ, Jackler RK, Yingling CD: Regional monitoring of the lower ninth through twelfth cranial nerves. ln Kartush J, Bouchard K eds: Intraoperative Monitoring in Otology and Head and Neck Surgery. New York, Raven Press, 1992, pp 131-150.

Lazorthes G, Lacomme Y, Gaubert J, Planel H: La constitution du nerf auditif. Presse Med 69: 1067-1068, 1961.

Legatt AD, Arezzo JC, Vaughn HG: Short latency auditory evoked potentials in the monkey. II. Intracranial generators. Electroencephalogr Clin Neurophysiol 64: 53-73, 1986.

Leonetti JP, Brackmann DE, Prass RL: Improved preservation of facial nerve function in the infratemporal approach to the skull base. Otolaryngol Head Neck Surg 101: 747-748, 1989.

Levine RA, Ojemann RG, Montgomery WW, McGaffigan PM: Monitoring auditory evoked potentials during acoustic neuroma surgery. Insights into the mechanism of the hearing loss. Ann Otol Rhinol Laryngol 93: 1161-1123, 1984.

Levine RA: Monitoring auditory evoked potentials during acoustic neuroma surgery. In: Neurological of the ear. Silverstein H, Norrel H Edit Aesculapius Publ (Birmingham alab) 2: 285-293, 1980.

Linden RD, Tator CH, Benedict C, et al: Electrophysiological monitoring during acoustic neuroma and other posterior fossa surgery. J Sci Neurol 15: 73-81,1988.

Lorente del No R: Analysis of the distribution of action currents of nerve in volume conductors. Stud Rockefeller Inst Med Res 132: 384-482, 1947.

Markand ON, Lee BI, Warren C, et al: Effects of hypothermia on brainstem auditory evoked potentials in humans. Ann Neurol 22: 507-513, 1987.

Moller AR, Burgess JE: Neural generators of the brainstem auditory evoked potentials BAEPs in the rhesus monkey. Electroencephalogr Clin Neurophysiol 65: 361-372, 1986.

Moller AR, Jannetta PJ, Moller MB: Neural generators of brainstem evoked potentials. Results from human intracranial recordings. Ann Otol Rhinol Laryngol 90: 591-596, 1981.

Moller AR, Jannetta PJ: Auditory evoked potentials recorded intracranially from the brainstem in man. Exp Neurol 78: 144-157, 1982a.

Moller AR, Jannetta PJ: Evoked potentials from the inferior colliculus in man. Electroencephalogr Clin Neurophysiol 53: 612-620, 1982b.

Moller AR, Jannetta PJ: Monitoring auditory functions during cranial nerve micro vascular decompression operations by direct recording from the eighth nerve. J Neurosurg 59: 493-499, 1983.

Moller AR, Jannetta PJ: Monitoring of facial function during removal of acoustic tumor. Am J Otol Suppl: 27-29, 1985.

Moller AR, Jannetta PJ: Neural generators of the auditory brainstem response. In Jacobson JT ed: The Auditory Brainstem Response. San Diego, College Hill Press, 1984b, pp 13-31.

Moller AR, Jannetta PJ: Preservation of facial function during removal of acoustic neuromas: Use of monopolar constant voltage stimulation and EMG. J Neurosurg 61: 757-760, 1984a.

Moller AR, Moller MB, Jannetta PJ, Jho HD: Auditory nerve compound action potentials and brain stem auditory evoked potentials in patients with various degrees of hearing loss. Ann Otol Rhinol Laryngol 100: 488-495, 1991a.

Moller AR, Moller MB, Jannetta PJ, Jho HD: Compound action potentials recorded from the exposed eighth nerve in patients with intractable tinnitus. Laryngoscope 102: 187-197, l991b.

Moller AR, Moller MB: Does intraoperative monitoring of auditory evoked potentials reduce incidence of hearing loss as a complication of microvascular decompression of cranial nerves? Neurosurgery; 24: 257-263, 1989.

Moller AR: A digital filter for brain stem evoked responses. Am J Otolaryngol 1: 372-377, 1980.

Moller AR: Electrophysiological monitoring of cranial nerves in operations in the skull base. In Sekhar LN, Schramm V eds: Tumors of the Cranial Base: Diagnosis and Treatment. Mt Ki sco, NYs Futura Publishers, 1987, pp 123-132.

Moller AR: Evoked Potentials in Intraoperative Monitoring Baltimore, Williams & Wilkins, 1988a.

Moller AR: Intraoperative monitoring of evoked potentials: An update. In Wilkins RH, Rengachary SS eds: Neurosurgery Update I. Diagnosis, Operative Technique, and Neuroncology. New York, McGrawHill, 1990, pp 169-176.

Moller AR: Neural generators of auditory evoked potentials BAEP. In Jacobson JT ed: Principles and Applications in Auditory Evoked Potentials. San Diego, Allyn & Bacon, 1994, pp 23-46.

Moller AR: Neuromonitoring in operations in the skull base. Keio J Med 40: 151-159, 1991.

Moller AR: Use of zerophase digital filters to enhance brainstem auditory evoked potentials BAEPs. Electroencephalogr Clin Neurophysiol 71: 226-232, 1988b.

O'Hara DA, Derbyshire GJ, Overdyk FJ, et al: Closed look infusion of atracurium with four different anesthetic techniques. Anesthesiology 74: 258-263, 1991.

Ojemann RG, Levine RA, Montgomery WM, McGaffigan PM: Use of intraoperative auditory evoked potentials to preserve hearing in unilateral acoustic neuroma removal. J Neurosurg 61: 938-948, 1984.

Prass R, Lueders H: Acoustic loudspeaker facial electromyographic monitoring. Part I. Neurosurgery 19: 392-400, 1986.

Prass RL, Luders H: Acoustic (Loudspeaker) facial electromyographic monitoring: Part 1: evoked electromyographic activity during acoustic neuroma resection. Neurosurgery 19: 392-400, 1986.

Prass RL, Kinney SE, Hardy RW, et al: Acoustic loudspeaker facial electromyographic monitoring: Part II. Use of evoked EMG activity during acoustic neuroma resection. Otolaryngol Head Neck Surg 97: 541-551, 1987.

Prass RL, Lueders H: Constant current versus constant voltage stimulation. J Neurosurg 62: 622-623, 1985.

Radtke RA, Erwin W, Wilkins RH: Intraoperative brainstem auditory evoked potentials: Significant decrease in postoperative morbidity. Neurology 39: 187-191, 1989.

Rand RW, Kurze TL: Facial nerve preservation by posterior fossa transmeatal microdissection in total removal of acoustic tumours. J Neurol Neurosurg Psychiatry 28: 311-316, 1965.

Raudzens PA, Shener AG: Intraoperative monitoring of brainstem auditory evoked potentials. J Neurosurg 57: 341-348, 1982.

Raudzens PA: Intraoperative monitoring of evoked potentials. Aml N Y Acad Sci 388: 308-326, 1982.

Richmond IL, Mahla M: Use of antidromic recording to monitor facial nerve function intraoperatively. Neurosurgery 16: 435-462, 1985.

Sabin HI, Bentivoglio P, Symon L, et al: Intraoperative electrocochleography to monitor cochlear potentials during acoustic neuroma excision. Acta Neurochir Wien 85: 110-116, 1987.

Sanders RA, Duncan PG, McCullough DW: Clinical experience with brain stem audiometry performed under general anesthesia. J Otolaryngol 8: 24-32, 1979.

Schwartz DM, Rosenberg SI: Facial nerve monitoring during parotidectomy. In Kartush J, Bouchard K eds: Intraoperative Monitoring in Otology and Head and Neck Surgery, New York, Raven Press, 1992, pp 121-130.

Sekhar LN, Moller AR: Operative management of tumors involving the cavernous sinus. J Neurosurg 64: 879-889, 1986.

Sekiya T, Hatayama T, Iwabuchi T, Maeda SH: A ring electrode to record extraocular muscle activities during skull base surgery. Acta Neurochir Wien 117: 66-69, 1992.

Sekiya T, Hatayama T, Iwabuchi T, Takiguchi M: Thermal effect of irrigation in the cerebellopontine angle on brainstem auditory evoked potentials: Experimental and clinical study. Clin Thermometry 12: 72-79, 1992. [Abstract]

Sekiya T, Iwabuchi T, Suzuki S, et al: Recordings of evoked electromyographic response from the extraocular muscle to monitor the oculomotor, trochlear, and abducens nerve function during skull base and orbital surgery. No Shinkei Geka 18: 447-451, 1990.

Sekiya T, Iwabushi T, Kamata S, lshida T: Deterioration of auditory evoked potentials during cerebellopontine angle manipulations. J Neurosurg 63: 598-607, 1985.

Silverstein H, Norrell H, Hyman S: Simultaneous use of C02 laser with continuous monitoring of eighth cranial nerve action potential during acoustic neuroma surgery. Otolaryngol Head Neck Surg 92: 80-84, 1984.

Silverstein H, Smouha E, Jones R: Routine identification of facial nerve using electrical stimulation during otological and neurotological surgey. Laryngoscope 98: 726-730, 1988.

Smith DI, Mills JH: Anesthesia effects: Auditory brain stem response. Electroencephalogr Clin Neurophysiol 72: 422-428, 1989.

Sohmer H, Gold S, Cahani M, Attias J: Effects of hypothermia on auditory brainstem and somatosensory evoked response. A model of a synaptic and axonal lesion. Electroencephalogr Clin Neurophysiol 74: 50-57, 1989.

Soulier MJ, Fraysse B, Lazorthes Y, Da Mona M: Potentiels evoques auditifs per-operatoires dans la chirurgie de la fosse posterieure: Neuro-chirurgie 31: 519-526, 1985.

Spoendlin H, Schrott A: Analysis of the human auditory nerve. Hear Res 43: 25-38, 1989.

Sugita K, Kobayashi S: Technical and instrumental improvements in the surgical treatment of acoustic neurinomas. J Neurosurg 57: 747-752, 1982.

Wigand ME, Rettinger G, Haid T, Berg M: Die ausraumung von oktavusneurinomen des kleinhirnbruckenwinkels mit transtemporalem zugang ber die mittlere schadelgrube. HNO 33: 11-16, 1985.

43

The informed consent

The following are informed consent forms used in common clinical practice at the House Ear Clinic.

MYRINGOTOMY AND INSERTION OF VENTILATION TUBES

(Incision of eardrum membrane and insertion of plastic tube)

ADENOIDECTOMY
(AND/OR TONSILLECTOMY)
(Removal of adenoids and/or tonsils).

Infection
Ear infection may develop following ventilation tube insertion. It is easily controlled with antibiotics in most cases.

Hearing Loss
It is very rare to develop permanent hearing loss following ventilation tube insertion .

Eardrum Perforation
Ventilation tube insertion is performed to produce a temporary eardrum perforation. On rare occasions, when the tube is dislodged or removed, the eardrum fails to heal. Should this happen the perforation can be repaired surgically at a later time.

Hemorrhage
Hemorrhage is the major risk in adenoidectomy or tonsillectomy. Although not common, should this occur. blood transfusions might be necessary and hospitalization could be prolonged. Hemorrhage may occur in the immediate postoperative period or be delayed, occurring approximately one week after surgery. Death from hemorrhage is an extremely rare complication.

General Anesthesia Complications
Anesthetic complications are very rare, but can be serious. You may discuss these with the anesthesiologist if desired.

I have read, and I understand, and have considered and accept the risks and complications of this surgery as stated above. Alternative methods of treatment have been discussed with me.

Signature:.................................

STAPEDECTOMY. TIMPANOTOMY AND STAPES EXPLORATORY TYPE OF OPERATION

(Operation of the middle ear performed through the ear canal)

Dizziness
Some unsteadiness is common during the first few postoperative days; dizziness on sudden head motion may persist for several weeks. On rare occasions dizziness is prolonged.

Taste Disturbance
Taste disturbance and mouth dryness is not uncommon for a few weeks following surgery. In some patients this disturbance is prolonged.

Loss of Hearing
Further hearing loss develops in 2% of patients due to some complications in the healing process. In 1% this hearing loss is very severe and may prevent the use of an aid in the operated ear.

Tinnitus
Should the hearing be worse following stapedectomy, tinnitus (head noise) likewise may be more pronounced.

Eardrum Perforation
A perforation (hole) in the eardrum membrane develops in less than 1% and usually is due to an infection. Fortunately, the membrane may heal spontaneously. If healing does not occur, surgical repair (myringoplasty) may be required.

Weakness of the Face
A very rare complication of stapedectomy is temporary weakness of the face. This may occur as the result of an abnormality or swelling of the facial nerve.

I have read, and I understand, and have considered and accept the risks and complications of this surgery as stated above. Alternative methods of treatment have been discussed with me.

Signature:.................................

MYRINGOPLASTY. TYMPANOPLASTY. MASTOID SURGERY AND OTHER OPERATIONS FOR CORRECTION OF CHRONIC EAR INFECTION

(Operations to eliminate middle ear and/or mastoid infection, to repair the eardrum and/or to repair the sound transmission mechanism)

Ear Infection
Ear infection, with drainage, swelling and pain, may persist following surgery or, on rare occasions, may develop following surgery due to poor healing of the ear tissue. Were this to be the case, additional surgery might be necessary to control the infection.

Loss of Hearing
Further permanent impairment of hearing develops in 3% of patients due to problems in the healing process. In 2% this loss of hearing may be severe or total in the operated ear. Nothing further can be done in these instances.
When a two-stage operation is necessary the hearing is usually worse after the first operation.

Tinnitus
Should the hearing be worse following surgery, tinnitus (head noises) likewise may be more pronounced.

Dizziness
Dizziness may occur immediately following surgery due to irritation of the inner ear structures. Some unsteadiness may persist for a week postoperatively. Prolonged dizziness is rare unless there was dizziness prior to surgery .

Taste Disturbance and Mouth Dryness
Taste disturbance and mouth dryness is not uncommon for a few weeks following surgery. In some patients this disturbance is prolonged.

Facial Paralysis
A rare postoperative complication of ear surgery is temporary paralysis of one side of the face. This may occur as a result of an abnormality or a swelling of the nerve and usually subsides spontaneously.
On very rare occasions the nerve may be injured at the time of surgery or it may be necessary to excise it in order to eradicate infection. When this happens a skin sensation nerve is removed from the upper part of the neck to replace the facial nerve. Paralysis of the face under these circumstances lasts six months to a year and there would be a permanent residual weakness. Eye complications, requiring treatment by a specialist could develop.

Hematoma
A hematoma (collection of blood) develops in a small percentage of cases, prolonging healing. Reoperation to remove the clot may be necessary if this complication occurs.

General Anesthesia Complications
Anesthetic complications are very rare, but can be serious. You may discuss these with the anesthesiologist if desired.

Complications Related to Mastoid Surgery
A cerebrospinal fluid leak (leak of fluid surrounding the brain) is a very rare complication. Reoperation may be necessary to stop the leak. Intracranial (brain) complications such as meningitis or brain abscess, even paralysis, were common in cases of chronic otitis media prior to the antibiotic era. Fortunately these now are extremely rare complications.

I have read, and I understand, and have considered and accept the risks and complications of this surgery as stated above. Alternative methods of treatment have been discussed with me.

Signature:.................................

INFRALABYRINTHINE DRAINAGE OF PETROUS APEX CHOLESTEROL GRANULOMA

(Drainage of inner ear bone cyst through an incision behind the ear)

Hearing Loss
Total loss of hearing occurs in up to 10% of patients. Partial loss of hearing may occur in others.

Tinnitus
Should the hearing be worse following this surgery, tinnitus (head noise) usually accompanies the hearing loss.

Dizziness
Dizziness is common following surgery and, at times, may be severe for days to weeks. It may be followed by prolonged unsteadiness on head motion.

Facial Weakness
Weakness of the face from swelling of the nerve is a rare complication of surgery. Permanent paralysis is extremely uncommon.

Spinal Fluid Leak
This operation may result in a temporary leak of cerebrospinal fluid (fluid surrounding the brain). This leak is always closed prior to the completion of surgery. On occasion, however, this leak reopens and further surgery may be necessary to close it.

Infection
Infection may occur following surgery. Should it develop, it could lead to meningitis, an infection in the fluid and tissues surrounding the brain, and this would require prolonged hospital treatment.

Hematoma
A hematoma (collection of blood) develops in a small percentage of cases, prolonging hospitalization and healing. Reoperation to remove the clot may be necessary if this complication occurs.

Recurrence of Cyst
Most of the time a permanent drainage tube is placed into the cyst to prevent it from redeveloping. This tube may become blocked with recurrence of the cyst. Should this occur, a revision operation may be required.

General anesthesia complications
Anesthetic complications are very rare, but can be serious. You may discuss these with the anesthesiologist if desired.

I have read, and I understand, and have considered and accept the risks and complications of this surgery as stated above. Alternative methods of treatment have been discussed with me.

Signature:.................................

MASTOID EXPLORATION & DECOMPRESSION OF THE FACIAL NERVE

(Uncovering the facial nerve in the mastoid through an incision behind the ear)

Hearing Loss
All patients notice some hearing impairment in the operated ear immediately following surgery. In an occasional case scar tissue forms and results in a permanent hearing impairment. It is rare to develop a severe impairment.

Tinnitus
Tinnitus (head noise) may develop following surgery. In a rare case this may persist.

Dizziness
Dizziness is uncommon following surgery but may develop due to irritation of the inner ear structures. Some unsteadiness may persist for a few days. On rare occasions dizziness is prolonged.

Hematoma
A hematoma (collection of blood) develops in a small percentage of cases, prolonging hospitalization and healing. Reoperation to remove the clot may be necessary if this complication occurs.

Spinal Fluid Leak
Spinal fluid leak (leak of fluid surrounding the brain) is a rare complication. Reoperation may be necessary to stop the leak.

Infection
Infection is a rare occurrence following facial nerve surgery. Should it develop, however, it

could lead to meningitis, an infection in the fluid and tissue surrounding the brain, and would require prolonged hospital treatment. Fortunately, this complication is very rare.

General Anesthesia Complications
Anesthetic complications are very rare, but can be serious. You may discuss these with the anesthesiologist if desired.

I have read, and I understand, and have considered and accept the risks and complications of this surgery as stated above. Alternative methods of treatment have been discussed with me.

Signature:.................................

TRANSMASTOID FACIAL NERVE DECOMPRESSION

(Uncovering the facial nerve in the mastoid through an incision behind the ear)

Hearing Loss
All patients notice some hearing impairment in the operated ear immediately following surgery. In an occasional case scar tissue forms and results in a permanent hearing impairment. It is rare to develop a severe impairment.

Tinnitus
Tinnitus (head noise) may develop following surgery. In a rare case this may persist.

Dizziness
Dizziness is uncommon following surgery but may develop due to irritation of the inner ear structures. Some unsteadiness may persist for a few days. On rare occasions dizziness is prolonged.

Hematoma
A hematoma (collection of blood) develops in a small percentage of cases, prolonging hospitalization and healing. Reoperation to remove the clot may be necessary if this complication occurs.

Spinal Fluid Leak
Spinal fluid leak (leak of fluid surrounding the brain) is a rare complication. Reoperation may be necessary to stop the leak.

Infection
Infection is a rare occurrence following facial nerve surgery. Should it develop, however, it could lead to meningitis, an infection in the fluid and tissue surrounding the brain, and would require prolonged hospital treatment. Fortunately, this complication is very rare.

General Anesthesia Complications
Anesthetic complications are very rare, but can be serious. You may discuss these with the anesthesiologist if desired.

I have read, and I understand, and have considered and accept the risks and complications of this surgery as stated above. Alternative methods of treatment have been discussed with me.

Signature:.................................

ENDOLYMPHATIC SHUNT OPERATION

(Drainage of excess inner ear fluid)

Hearing Loss
Further permanent hearing loss occurs in 5% of cases. Total loss of hearing occurs in 1%.

Dizziness
Dizziness is common immediately following surgery due to swelling of the ear and irritation of the inner ear structures. In approximately one-third of patients, dizziness is not improved following this surgery.

Tinnitus
Should the hearing be worse following surgery, tinnitus (head noise) may likewise be more pronounced.

Weakness of the Face
Temporary weakness of one side of the face is a rare postoperative complication of ear surgery. It may occur as the result of an abnormality or a swelling of the nerve. Permanent paralysis is extremely rare. Eye complications, requiring treatment by a specialist, could develop.

Spinal Fluid Leak
This operation may result in a temporary leak of spinal fluid. This leak is always closed prior to the completion of surgery. On occasion, however, the leak reopens and further surgery may be necessary to stop it.

Infection
Infection is a rare occurrence following surgery. Should it develop, however, it could lead to meningitis, an infection in the fluid and tissues surrounding the brain, and would require prolonged hospital treatment. Fortunately this complication is very rare.

Hematoma
A hematoma (collection of blood) develops in a small percentage of cases, prolonging hospitalization and healing. Reoperation to remove the clot may be necessary if this complication occurs.

General Anesthesia Complications
Anesthetic complications are very rare, but can be serious. You may discuss these with the anesthesiologist if desired.

I have read, and I understand, and have considered and accept the risks and complications of this surgery as stated above. Alternative methods of treatment have been discussed with me.

Signature:................................

SACCULOTOMY OR TRANSCANAL LABIRINTHECTOMY

(Puncture or removal of inner ear balance mechanism through the ear canal)

POSTAURICULAR LABIRINTHECTOMY

(Removal of balance mechanism through an incision behind the ear)

Hearing Loss
Labyrinthectomy results in total loss of hearing in the operated ear. Sacculotomy results in total loss of hearing in the operated ear in 80% of the cases.

Dizziness
Dizziness is common following this surgery and may be severe for a few weeks. Imbalance or unsteadiness on head motion is prolonged in some patients.

Tinnitus
Tinnitus (head noise) may be worse following surgery.

Taste Disturbance and Mouth Dryness
Taste disturbance and mouth dryness is not uncommon for a few weeks following surgery. In some patients this disturbance is prolonged.

Facial Paralysis
Temporary weakness of one side of the face is a rare postoperative complication. It may occur as the result of an abnormality or a swelling of the nerve, or nerve damage, and may require further surgery. Eye complications, requiring treatment by a specialist, could develop.

General Anesthesia Complications
Anesthetic complications are very rare, but can be serious. You may discuss these with the anesthesiologist if desired.

Complications related to Postauricular Labyrinthectomy
A hematoma (collection of blood) develops in a small percentage of cases, prolonging healing. Reoperation to remove the clot may be necessary if this complication occurs.
A cerebral spinal fluid leak (leak of fluid surrounding the brain) is a rare complication. Reoperation may be necessary to stop the leak.

I have read, and I understand, and have considered and accept the risks and complications of this surgery as stated above. Alternative methods of treatment have been discussed with me.

Signature:................................

RETROLABYRINTHINE OR RETROSIGMOID FIFTH NERVE SECTION

(Cutting the sensation nerve to the face through an incision behind the ear)

RETROLABYRINTHINE RETROSIGMOID VESTIBULAR NERVE SECTION

(Cutting the balance nerve through an incision behind the ear)

Hearing Loss
Hearing loss in the operated ear is an uncommon complication. When it occurs, however, it may be severe and permanent.

Tinnitus
Should the hearing be worse following this surgery, tinnitus (head noise) usually accompanies the hearing loss.

Dizziness
Dizziness is common immediately following surgery due to irritation of the inner ear structures. It is uncommon for permanent dizziness to result.

Facial Weakness
The facial nerve is in close relationship to the fifth cranial nerve. Weakness of the face from swelling of the facial nerve is a rare complication of surgery. Permanent paralysis is extremely uncommon.

Eye Complications
The nerve responsible for eye movement lie in close proximity to the fifth cranial nerve. A rare complication of this surgery is paralysis of one or more of the eye muscles. In this case, double vision results and treatment is necessary.
Numbness of the cornea is a rare complication of this surgery. If this occurs it may result in irritation of the eye and, rarely, ulceration of the cornea. In this case, treatment by an eye specialist would be necessary.

Numbness of the Face
Partial numbness of the face occurs frequently following surgery. Some permanent loss of skin sensation of that side of the face is common.

Spinal Fluid Leak
This operation results in a temporary leak of cerebrospinal fluid (fluid surrounding the brain). This leak is always closed prior to the completion of surgery. On occasion, however, this leak reopens and further surgery may be necessary to close it.

Infection
Infection may occur following surgery. Should it develop it could lead to meningitis, an infection in the fluid and tissues surrounding the brain, and this would require prolonged hospital treatment.

Hematoma
A hematoma (collection of blood) develops in a small percentage of cases, prolonging hospitalization and healing. Reoperation to remove the clot may be necessary if this complication occurs.

Transfusion Reaction
It is very uncommon to administer blood transfusions during fifth nerve section surgery. Fortunately, immediate adverse reactions to transfusion are rare. A potential late complication of a blood transfusion would be a viral infection such as hepatitis. When this complication occurs, medical treatment and possibly hospitalization would be necessary. It is possible for patients to donate their own blood for use during their own surgery. This should be discussed with your surgeon well in advance of your surgery.

General Anesthesia Complications
Anesthetic complications are very rare, but can be serious. You may discuss these with the anesthesiologist if desired.

I have read, and I understand, and have considered and accept the risks and complications of this surgery as stated above. Alternative methods of treatment have been discussed with me.

Signature:.................................

TRANSLABYRINTHINE LABYRINTHECTOMY AND EIGHTH NERVE SECTION

(Removal of balance canals and cutting of the balance and hearing nerves)

Hearing Loss
This operation results in total loss of hearing in the operated ear.

Tinnitus
Tinnitus (head noise) may be worse following surgery.

Taste Disturbance and Mouth Dryness
Taste disturbance and mouth dryness is not uncommon for a few weeks following surgery. In some patients this disturbance is prolonged.

Dizziness
Dizziness is common following surgery and may be severe for days to a few weeks. Fortunately, severe attacks of dizziness are eliminated in nearly every instance. Imbalance, or unsteadiness on head motion, is prolonged in some patients.

Facial Paralysis
Temporary weakness of one side of the face is a rare postoperative complication. It may occur as

the result of an abnormality or a swelling of the nerve, or nerve damage, and may require further surgery. Eye complications, requiring treatment by a specialist, could develop.

Spinal Fluid Leak
This operation results in a temporary leak of cerebrospinal fluid (fluid surrounding the brain). This leak is always closed prior to the completion of surgery. On occasion, however, the leak reopens and further surgery may be necessary to stop it.

Infection
Infection is a rare occurrence following this surgery. Should it develop, however, it could lead to meningitis, an infection in the fluid and tissues surrounding the brain, and this would require prolonged hospital treatment.

Hematoma
A hematoma (collection of blood) develops in a small percentage of cases, prolonging hospitalization and healing. Reoperation to remove the clot may be necessary if this complication occurs.

General Anesthesia Complications
Anesthetic complications are very rare, but can be serious. You may discuss these with the anesthesiologist if desired.

I have read, and I understand, and have considered and accept the risks and complications of this surgery as stated above. Alternative methods of treatment have been discussed with me.

Signature:................................

MIDDLE FOSSA SURGERY

(Surgery on the upper portion of the inner ear through an incision above the ear)

Hearing Loss
Up to 10% of patients may develop a severe hearing impairment in the operated ear.

Tinnitus
Tinnitus (head noise) usually remains the same as before surgery. If the hearing is worse following surgery, tinnitus may likewise be more noticeable.

Dizziness
Dizziness may occur following surgery and, at times, may be severe for days to weeks. It may be followed by prolonged unsteadiness on head motion.

Weakness of the Face
Temporary weakness of one side of the face is an uncommon postoperative complication of ear surgery. It may occur as the result of an abnormality or a swelling of the nerve, or nerve damage, and could require further surgery. Eye complications, requiring treatment by a specialist, could develop.

Spinal Fluid Leak
This operation results in a temporary leak of cerebrospinal fluid (fluid surrounding the brain). This leak is always closed prior to the completion of surgery. On occasion, however, the leak reopens and further surgery may be necessary to stop it.

Infection
Infection is a rare occurrence following surgery. Should it develop, however, it could lead to meningitis, an infection in the fluid and tissues surrounding the brain, and would require prolonged hospital treatment.

Hematoma
A hematoma (collection of blood) develops in a small percentage of cases, prolonging hospitalization and healing. Reoperation to remove the clot may be necessary if this complication occurs.

Brain Complications
Temporary paralysis of half the body has occurred following a middle fossa operation due to brain swelling. This complication is, however, extremely rare.

Transfusion Reaction
It is sometimes necessary to administer blood transfusions during middle fossa surgery. Fortunately, immediate adverse reactions to transfusion are rare. A potential late complication of a blood transfusion would be a viral infection such as hepatitis. When this complication occurs, medical treatment and possibly hospitalization would be necessary. It is possible for patients to donate their own blood for use during their own surgery. This should be discussed with your surgeon well in advance of your surgery.

General Anesthesia Complications
Anesthetic complications are very rare, but can be serious. You may discuss these with the anesthesiologist if desired.

I have read, and I understand, and have considered and accept the risks and complications of this surgery as stated above. Alternative methods of treatment have been discussed with me.

Signature:................................

MIDDLE FOSSA ACOUSTIC TUMOR REMOVAL

(Acoustic tumor removal through an incision above the ear)

Hearing Loss
60% of patients develop a total hearing loss in the operated ear.

Tinnitus
Tinnitus (head noise) usually remains the same as before surgery. If the hearing is worse following surgery, tinnitus may likewise be more noticeable.

Taste Disturbance and Mouth Dryness
Taste disturbance and mouth dryness is not uncommon for a few weeks following surgery. In some patients this disturbance is prolonged.

Weakness of the Face
Acoustic tumors are in intimate contact with the facial nerve. Temporary weakness of the face commonly occurs as a result of nerve swelling. This weakness may persist for six months to a year and there may be permanent residual weakness. In 5% of the cases it is necessary to remove all or a portion of the facial nerve in order to remove the tumor. In some cases it is possible to reconnect the facial nerve at the time of surgery or to remove a skin sensation nerve from the upper part of the neck to replace the missing portion of the facial nerve. In this case paralysis of the face lasts from six months to a year and there would be a permanent residual weakness. When it is not possible to repair the facial nerve immediately, further surgery may be necessary to substitute another nerve.

Eye Complications
Should facial paralysis develop, the eye may become dry and unprotected. It might be necessary to apply artificial tears or to tape the eye shut. In some cases surgery on the eyelid is necessary.

Dizziness
Dizziness is common following removal of acoustic tumors. It is often severe for a few days to weeks. Rarely there is permanent imbalance.

Spinal Fluid Leak
This operation results in a temporary leak of cerebrospinal fluid (fluid surrounding the brain). This leak is always closed prior to the completion of surgery. On occasion, however, the leak reopens and further surgery may be necessary to close it.

Infection
Infection occurs in less than 10% of the patients following surgery. Should this develop in your case, it could lead to meningitis, an infection of the fluid and tissue surrounding the brain, and would require prolonged hospital treatment. A rare complication are bladder and lung infection.

Hematoma
A hematoma (collection of blood) develops in a small percentage of cases, prolonging hospitalization and healing. Reoperation to remove the clot may be necessary if this complication occurs.

Brain Complications
Temporary paralysis of half the body due to brain swelling has occurred following middle fossa surgery. This complication is, however, extremely rare. Permanent paralysis has not occurred but is possible.

Transfusion Reaction
It is sometimes necessary to administer blood transfusions during acoustic tumor surgery. Fortunately, immediate adverse reactions to transfusion are rare. A potential late complication of a blood transfusion would be a viral infection such as hepatitis. When this complication occurs, medical treatment and possibly hospitalization would be necessary. It is possible for patients to donate their own blood for use during their own surgery. This should be discussed with your surgeon well in advance of your surgery.

General Anesthesia Complications
Anesthetic complications are very rare, but can be serious. You may discuss these with the anesthesiologist if desired.

I have read, and I understand, and have considered and accept the risks and complications of this surgery as stated above. Alternative methods of treatment have been discussed with me.

Signature:................................

MIDDLE FOSSA FACIAL NERVE DECOMPRESSION

(Uncovering the facial nerve through an incision above the ear)

Hearing Loss
All patients notice some hearing impairment in the operated ear immediately following surgery.

In an occasional case scar tissue forms and results in a permanent hearing impairment. It is rare to develop a severe impairment.

Tinnitus
Tinnitus (head noise) may develop following surgery. On occasions this persists.

Dizziness
Dizziness may occur following surgery and, at times, may be severe for days to weeks. It may be followed by prolonged unsteadiness on head motion.

Hematoma
A hematoma (collection of blood) develops in a small percentage of cases, prolonging hospitalization and healing. Reoperation to remove the clot may be necessary if this complication occurs.

Spinal Fluid Leak
A cerebrospinal fluid leak (leak of fluids surrounding the brain) develops in an occasional case. Reoperation may be necessary to stop the leak.

Infection
Infection is a rare occurrence following facial nerve surgery. Should it develop, however, it could lead to meningitis, an infection in the fluid and tissues surrounding the brain, and this would require prolonged hospital treatment. Fortunately, this complication is very rare.

Paralysis
Temporary paralysis of half the body has occurred following a middle fossa operation, due to brain swelling. This complication is, however, extremely rare.

Transfusion Reaction
It is sometimes necessary to administer blood transfusions during middle fossa surgery. Fortunately, immediate adverse reactions to transfusion are rare. A potential late complication of a blood transfusion would be a viral infection such as hepatitis. When this complication occurs, medical treatment and possibly hospitalization would be necessary. It is possible for patients to donate their own blood for use during their own surgery. This should be discussed with your surgeon well in advance of your surgery.

General Anesthesia Complications
Anesthetic complications are very rare, but can be serious. You may discuss these with the anesthesiologist if desired.

I have read, and I understand, and have considered and accept the risks and complications of this surgery as stated above. Alternative methods of treatment have been discussed with me.

Signature:...................................

TOTAL (MASTOID AND MIDDLE FOSSA) FACIAL NERVE DECOMPRESSION

(Uncovering the facial nerve through an incision above the ear and an incision behind the ear)

Hearing Loss
All patients notice some hearing impairment in the operated ear immediately following surgery. In an occasional case scar tissue forms and results in a permanent hearing impairment. It is rare to develop a severe impairment.

Tinnitus
Tinnitus (head noise) may develop following surgery. On occasions this persists.

Dizziness
Dizziness is common immediately following surgery due to irritation of the inner ear structures. Some unsteadiness may persist for a few days postoperatively. On rare occasions dizziness is prolonged.

Hematoma
A hematoma (collection of blood) develops in a small percentage of cases, prolonging hospitalization and healing. Reoperation to remove the clot may be necessary if this complication occurs.

Spinal Fluid Leak
A cerebrospinal fluid leak (leak of fluids surrounding the brain) develops in an occasional case. Reoperation may be necessary to stop the leak.

Infection
Infection is a rare occurrence following facial nerve surgery. Should it develop, however, it could lead to meningitis, an infection in the fluid and tissues surrounding the brain, and this would require prolonged hospital treatment. Fortunately, this complication is very rare.

Paralysis
Temporary paralysis of half the body has occurred following a middle fossa operation, due to brain swelling. This complication is, however, extremely rare.

Transfusion Reaction
It is sometimes necessary to administer blood transfusions during facial nerve decompression

surgery. Fortunately, immediate adverse reactions to transfusion are rare. A potential late complication of a blood transfusion would be a viral infection such as hepatitis. When this complication occurs, medical treatment and possibly hospitalization would be necessary. It is possible for patients to donate their own blood for use during their own surgery. This should be discussed with your surgeon well in advance of your surgery.

General Anesthesia Complications
Anesthetic complications are very rare, but can be serious. You may discuss these with the anesthesiologist if desired.

I have read, and I understand, and have considered and accept the risks and complications of this surgery as stated above. Alternative methods of treatment have been discussed with me.

Signature:.................................

INFRATEMPORAL FOSSA REMOVAL OF TUMOR

(Removal of tumor involving the middle ear or inner ear or mastoid or petrous apex or all of these structures)

Type of Tumor:...

Hearing Loss
The larger the tumor the more likely one is to experience further loss of hearing following surgery. On occasion, there is a total loss of hearing in the operated ear.

Tinnitus
Should the hearing be worse following surgery, tinnitus (head noise) will usually be more pronounced and of a different character.

Taste Disturbance and Mouth Dryness
Taste disturbance and mouth dryness may occur following surgery. In some cases these disturbances may be prolonged.

Dizziness
Dizziness is common immediately following surgery due to irritation of the inner ear structures. In some cases it is necessary to remove the inner ear structures, in which case the dizziness may be severe and some permanent balance disturbance may result.

Facial Paralysis
At times it is necessary to move the facial nerve from its canal, in which case a temporary paralysis is common. Rarely the tumor involves the facial nerve and it may be necessary to excise a portion of the nerve in order to remove the tumor. In this case, a skin sensation nerve is removed from the upper part of the neck to replace the facial nerve. Paralysis of the face under these circumstances lasts from six months to a year and there would be a permanent residual weakness. Eye complications, requiring treatment by a specialist, could develop.

Other Cranial Nerve Weaknesses
These tumors may involve other nerves of the head and neck. In order to remove the tumor, temporary or permanent injury to these nerves might result. In this case there could be decreased sensation in the throat, weakness of the voice and shoulder, paralysis of muscles of the tongue on the side of surgery, and difficulty in swallowing.

Brain Complications
Rarely, in the large tumor case, it is necessary to ligate (tie) the major artery to the brain on the side of the tumor (carotid artery). Were this necessary, paralysis of the opposite side of the body (arm and leg) would be expected to occur in over 50% of the cases, and the paralysis would be permanent. Difficulties in speaking may also occur and would be permanent.

Spinal Fluid Leak
At times this operation results in a temporary leak of cerebrospinal fluid (fluid surrounding the brain). When this occurs, the leak is always closed prior to the completion of surgery. On occasion, however, the leak reopens and further surgery may be necessary to stop it.

Infection
Infection is uncommon following surgery. Should it develop, however, it could lead to meningitis, an infection in the fluid and tissues surrounding the brain, and would require prolonged hospital treatment.

Hematoma
A hematoma (collection of blood) develops in a small percentage of cases, prolonging hospitalization and healing. Reoperation to remove the clot may be necessary if this complication occurs.

Transfusion Reaction
It is sometimes necessary to administer blood transfusions during tumor surgery. Fortunately, immediate adverse reactions to transfusion are rare. A potential late complication of a blood transfusion would be a viral infection such as hepatitis. When this complication occurs, medical treatment and possibly hospitalization would be necessary. It is possible for patients to donate their own blood for use during their own surgery. This should be discussed with your surgeon well in advance of your surgery.

Arterial Line Monitoring
In large tumors it may be necessary to monitor the patient's general status by inserting a small tube into an artery in the arm or leg. When this is necessary there may be pain in the hand or foot following surgery . Occasionally a blood clot forms in the artery following surgery. Should this complication occur further surgery may be necessary to remove the clot.
A very rare complication of this arterial line monitoring is the loss of a finger, toe, or even a hand or a foot.

General Anesthesia Complications
Anesthetic complications are very rare, but can be serious. You may discuss these with the anesthesiologist if desired.

I have read, and I understand, and have considered and accept the risks and complications of this surgery as stated above. Alternative methods of treatment have been discussed with me.

Signature: ....

TRANSLABYRINTHINE ACOUSTIC TUMOR REMOVAL

(Acoustic tumor removal through an incision behind the ear with removal of inner ear structures)

Hearing Loss
All patients have a total permanent loss of hearing in the operated ear following translabyrinthine acoustic tumor removal.

Dizziness
Dizziness is common following acoustic tumor removal and may be severe for days or a few weeks. Imbalance, or unsteadiness on head motion, is prolonged in some patients .

Tinnitus
Tinnitus (head noise) remains the same as before surgery in most patients. In some patients the tinnitus may be more noticeable.

Taste Disturbance and Mouth Dryness
Taste disturbance and mouth dryness is not uncommon for a few weeks following surgery. In some patients this disturbance is prolonged.

Weakness of the Face
Acoustic tumors are in intimate contact with the facial nerve. Temporary weakness of the face commonly occurs as a result of nerve swelling. This weakness may persist for six months to a year and there may be permanent residual weakness. In 5% of the cases it is necessary to remove all or a portion of the facial nerve in order to remove the tumor. In some cases it is possible to reconnect the facial nerve at the time of surgery or to remove a skin sensation nerve from the upper part of the neck to replace the missing portion of the facial nerve. In this case paralysis of the face lasts from six months to a year and there would be a permanent residual weakness. When it is not possible to repair the facial nerve immediately, further surgery may be necessary to substitute another nerve.

Eye Complications
Should facial paralysis develop the eye may become dry and unprotected. It might be necessary to apply artificial tears or to tape the eye shut. In some cases surgery on the eyelid is necessary.

Other Complications
Acoustic tumors often contact the nerves (glossopharyngeal, vagus, hypoglossal, spinal nerves) which supply the eye muscles, the face, the mouth, the throat, the muscles of the shoulder. Following surgery there could be decreased sensation in the throat, weakness of the voice and shoulder, paralysis of muscles of the tongue on the side of surgery, and difficulty in swallowing. These problems may be permanent.

Respiratory and Circulatory Complications
Acoustic tumors are located adjacent to the vital centers of the brain responsible for control of breathing, heart rate and blood pressure. During the course of removal of these tumors the brain itself, or the blood vessels supplying this area of the brain, may be injured. These serious complications are rare but a patient may have injury to these vital structures, in which case death could occur.

Spinal Fluid Leak
This operation results in a temporary leak of cerebrospinal fluid (fluid surrounding the brain). This leak is always closed prior to the completion of surgery. On occasion, however, this leak reopens and further surgery may be necessary to close it.

Infection
Infection occurs in less than 10% of the patients following surgery. Should this develop in your case it could lead to meningitis, an infection of the fluid and tissue surrounding the brain, and would require prolonged hospital treatment. A rare complication are bladder and lung infections.

Hematoma
Hematoma (collection of blood) develops in a small percentage of cases, prolonging hospitalization and healing. Reoperation to remove the clot may be necessary if this complication occurs.

Brain Complications
Temporary paralysis of the arms and legs may occur following acoustic tumor surgery. Permanent paralysis is rare. At times it is necessary to remove a portion of the brain responsible for balance. In this case persistent unsteadiness may occur.

Transfusion Reaction
It is sometimes necessary to administer blood transfusions during acoustic tumor surgery. Fortunately, immediate adverse reactions to transfusion are rare. A potential late complication of a blood transfusion would be a viral infection such as hepatitis. When this complication occurs, medical treatment and possibly hospitalization would be necessary. It is possible for patients to donate their own blood for use during their own surgery. This should be discussed with your surgeon well in advance of your surgery.

Arterial Line Monitoring
In large tumors it is often necessary to monitor the patient's general status by inserting a small tube into an artery in the arm or leg. When this is necessary there may be pain in the hand or foot following surgery. Occasionally a blood clot forms in the artery following surgery. Should this complication occur, further surgery may be necessary to remove the clot.
A very rare complication of this arterial line monitoring is the loss of a finger, toe or even a hand or a foot.

General Anesthesia Complications
Anesthetic complications are very rare, but can be serious. You may discuss these with the anesthesiologist if desired.

I have read, and I understand, and have considered and accept the risks and complications of this surgery as stated above. Alternative methods of treatment have been discussed with me.

Signature:................................

FACIAL-HYPOGLOSSAL NERVE ANASTOMOSIS

(Connecting the facial nerve and the nerve which moves the tongue through incisions behind the ear and in the upper portion of the neck)

Hearing Loss
Many patients requiring this surgery have a total loss of hearing in the operated ear. If the hearing is normal, it is unusual for hearing loss to result from this surgery.

Tinnitus
Should the hearing be worse following surgery, tinnitus (head noise) may develop or be more pronounced.

Dizziness
Dizziness is uncommon following this type of surgery. If it does occur, it is rarely prolonged.

Tongue Weakness
The nerve controlling the muscles of one side of the tongue is cut and sutured to the facial nerve. The result is loss of muscle control on one side of the tongue. This may produce some speech disability and difficulty in swallowing and chewing. Over a period of time the muscles of one side of the tongue atrophy (shrink).

Voice Weakness
A very rare complication of this surgery is weakness of the voice due to injury of the nerve to the vocal cord.

Prolonged Facial Paralysis
A period of several months to a year or more is necessary for the tongue nerve to grow into the facial muscles. When movement does occur it will not be normal. There will be persistent weakness of the face. On moving the face, all of the muscles tend to contract at once, and some face motion may occur when speaking.

Spinal Fluid Leak
At times this operation results in a temporary leak of cerebrospinal fluid (fluid surrounding the

brain). If this occurs, the leak is always closed prior to the completion of surgery. On occasion, however, the leak reopens, and further surgery may be necessary to close it.

Infection
Infection is uncommon following surgery. Should it develop, however, it could lead to meningitis, an infection in the fluid and tissues surrounding the brain, and this would require prolonged hospital treatment.

Hematoma
A hematoma (collection of blood) develops in a small percentage of cases, prolonging hospitalization and healing. Reoperation to remove the clot may be necessary if this complication occurs.

Transfusion Reaction
It is sometimes necessary to administer blood transfusions during facial-hypoglossal nerve anastomosis surgery. Fortunately, immediate adverse reactions to transfusion are rare. A potential late complication of a blood transfusion would be a viral infection such as hepatitis. When this complication occurs, medical treatment and possibly hospitalization would be necessary. It is possible for patients to donate their own blood for use during their own surgery. This should be discussed with your surgeon well in advance of your surgery.

General Anesthesia Complications
Anesthetic complications are very rare, but can be serious. You may discuss these with the anesthesiologist if desired.

I have read, and I understand, and have considered and accept the risks and complications of this surgery as stated above. Alternative methods of treatment have been discussed with me.

Signature:.................................

Color plates

CHAPTER 7

Surgical treatment of congenital malformations of the temporal bone

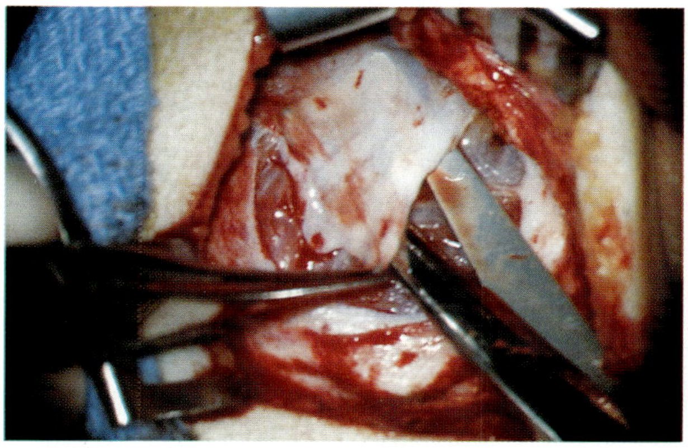

Fig. 7-49. Congenital aural atresia. Temporalis fascia is harvested and placed to dry.

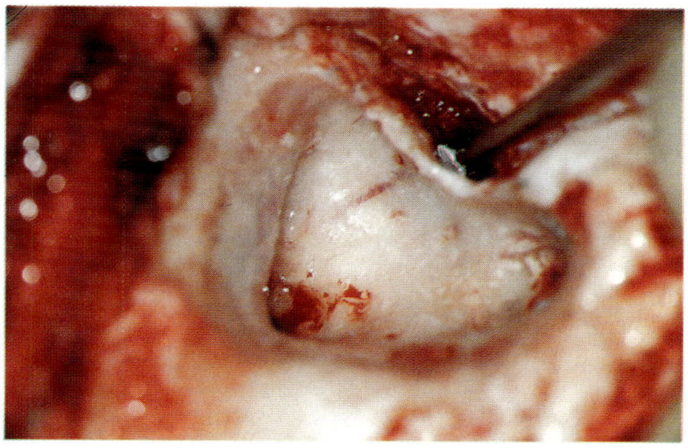

Fig. 7-50. Right ear. The temporomandibular joint space is anteriorly dissected.

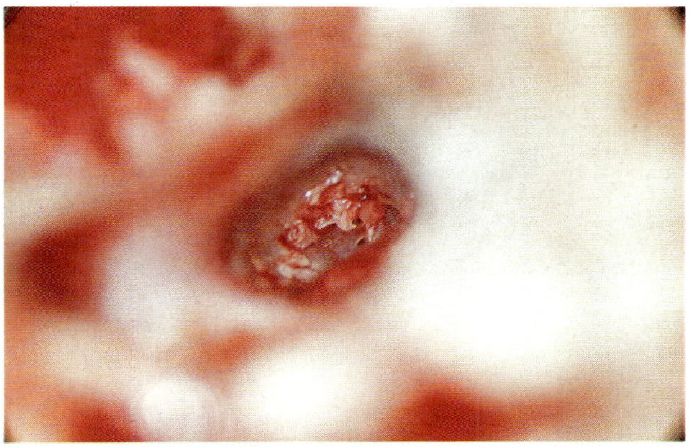

Fig. 7-51. Left ear. Initial removing of the atresia plate.

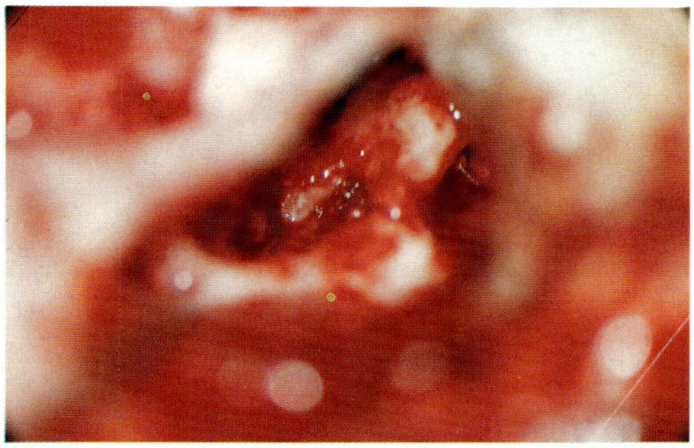

Fig. 7-52. Left ear. The ossicles are exposed. The facial nerve canal can be seen.

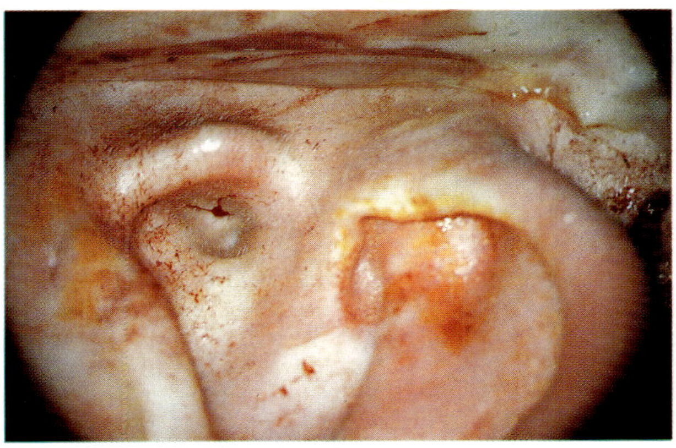

Fig. 7-53. Left ear. Stenosis of the external ear meatus.

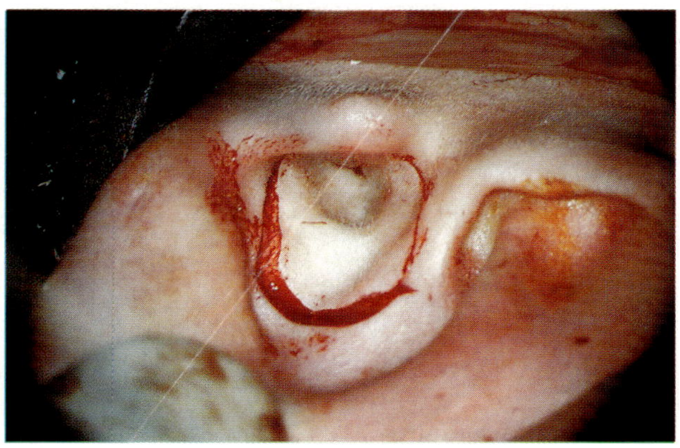

Fig. 7-54. Left ear. Skin, subcutaneous tissue and cartilage are removed in a 1.4 cm diameter core over the new meatus.

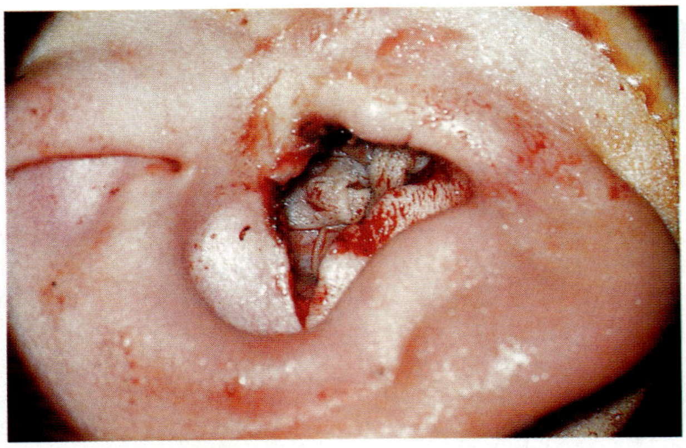

Fig. 7-55. Right ear. Meatoplasty is completed.

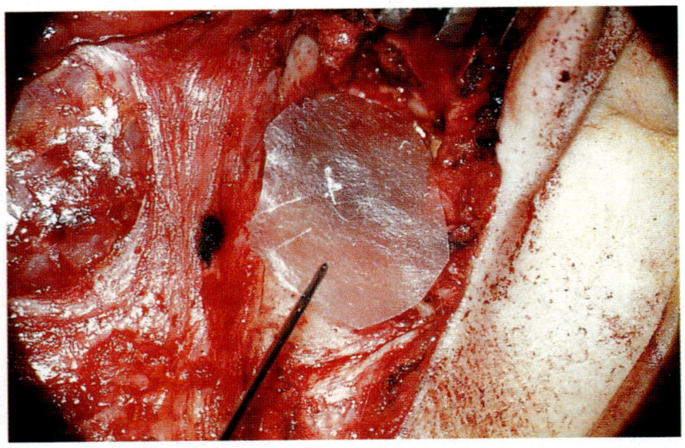

Fig. 7-56. Temporalis fascia trimmed to adequate size. Tabs are cut to prevent lateralization of the tympanic membrane graft.

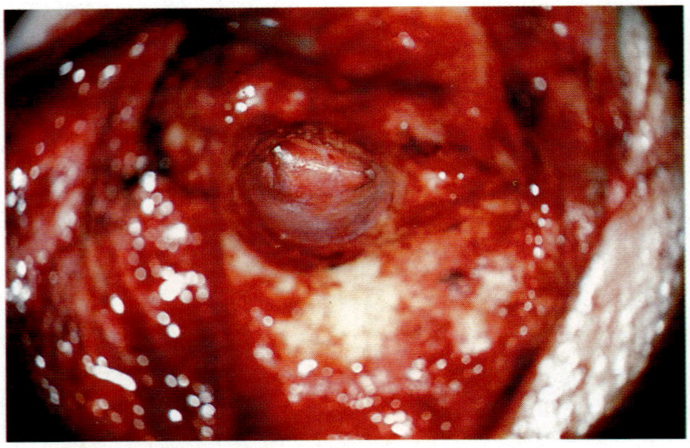

Fig. 7-57. Fascia is placed in site.

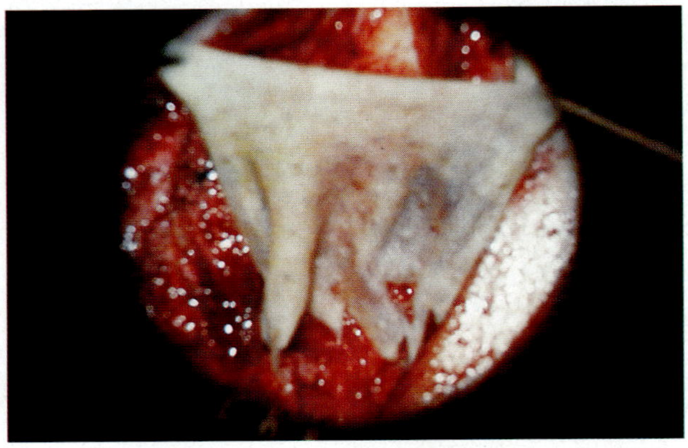

Fig. 7-58. A 0.012-inch thick, 6 cm × 6 cm split-thickness graft is harvested.

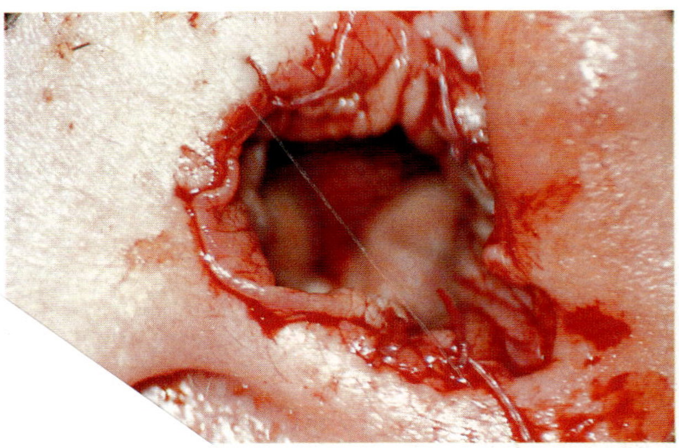

-es of 5-0 Ti-Cron attach the lateral
·mferentially to the meatal skin.
.ıst absorbing plain gut) is used
. each Ti-Cron suture.

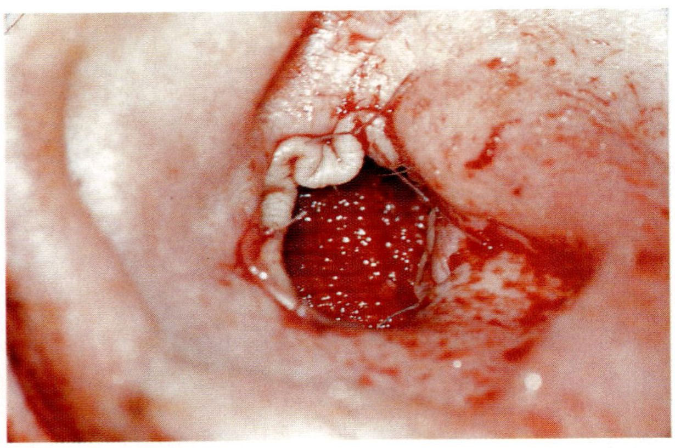

Fig. 7-60. The lateral portion of the EAC and the meatus are packed.

CHAPTER 8

Cochlear implant surgery

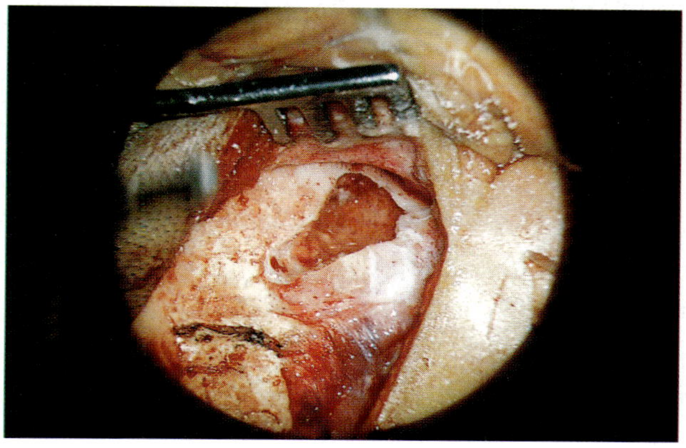

Fig. 8-33. Surgery for cochlear implantation. Left ear. Beginning of the transmastoid, facial recess approach.

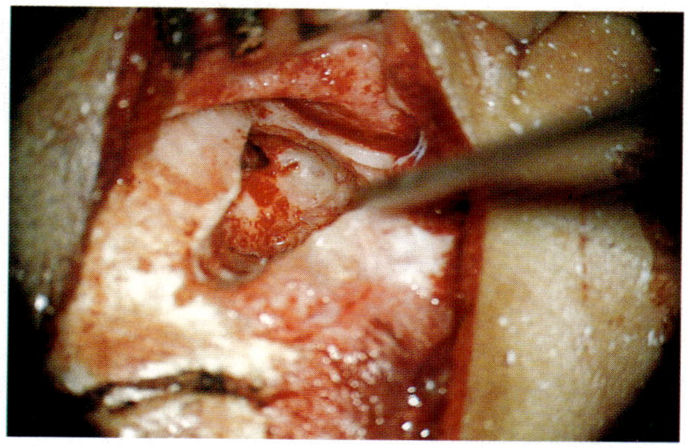

Fig. 8-34. Beginning of mastoidectomy: the antrum is opened.

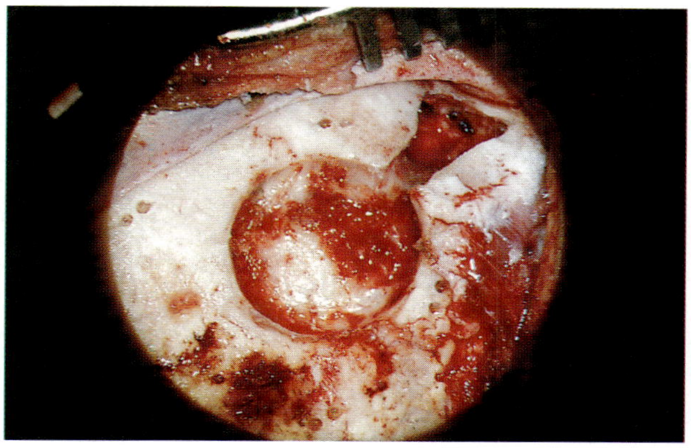

Fig. 8-35. The site for the internal receiver with the suture tunnel holes is completed.

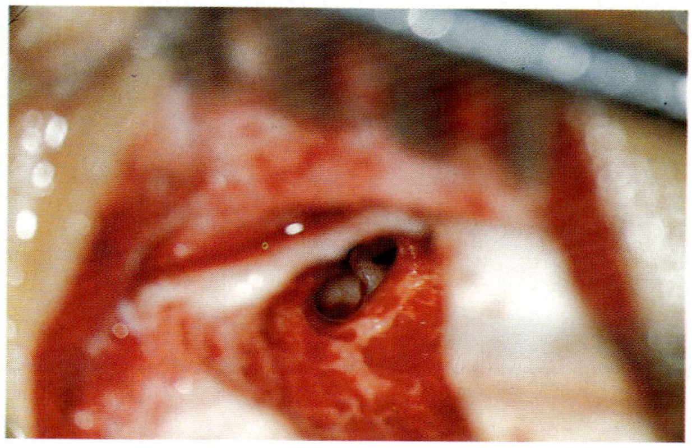

Fig. 8-36. The round window is opened.

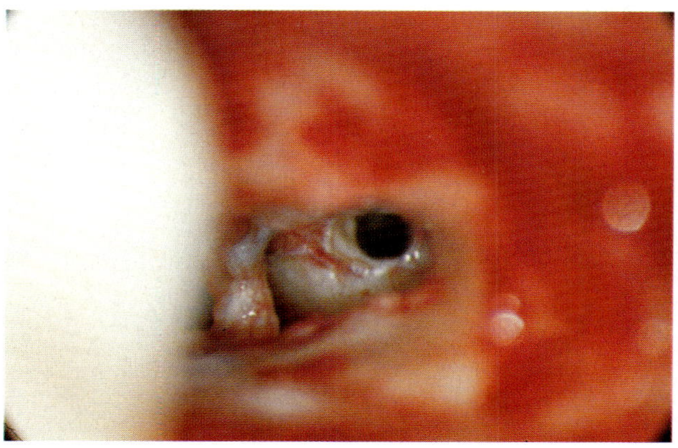

Fig. 8-37. Close-up view of fig. 8-36.

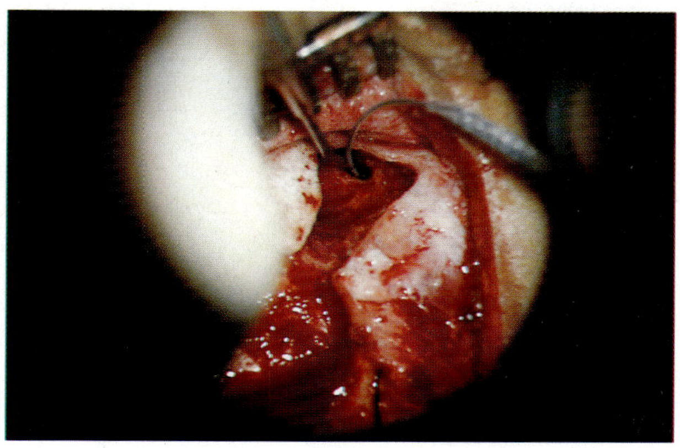

Fig. 8-38. Claw forceps is used to direct the electrode tip into the scala tympani.

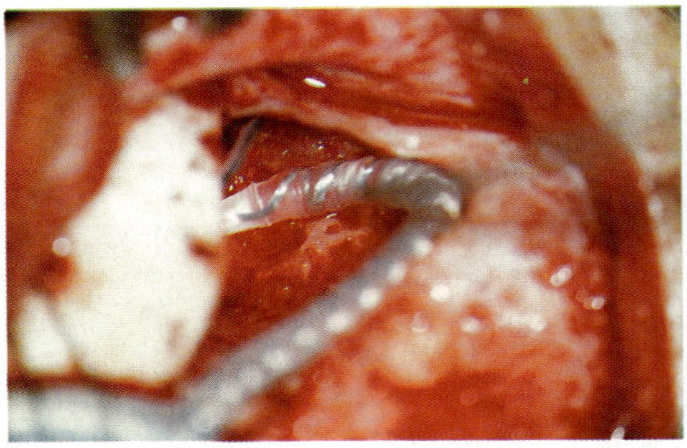

Fig. 8-39. The placement of the electrode is completed.

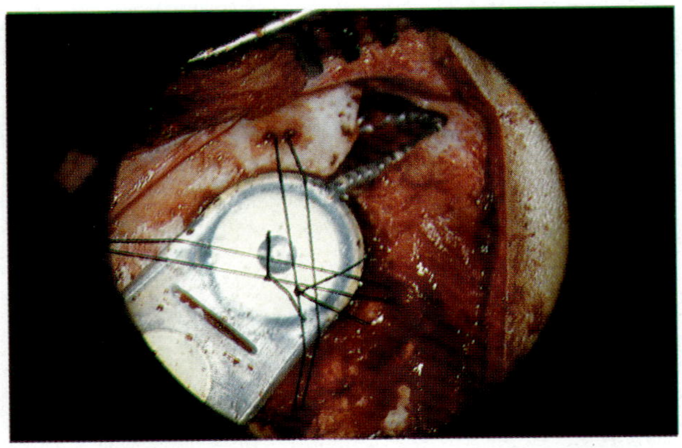

Fig. 8-40. The internal receiver is fixed in its seat with non absorbable sutures.

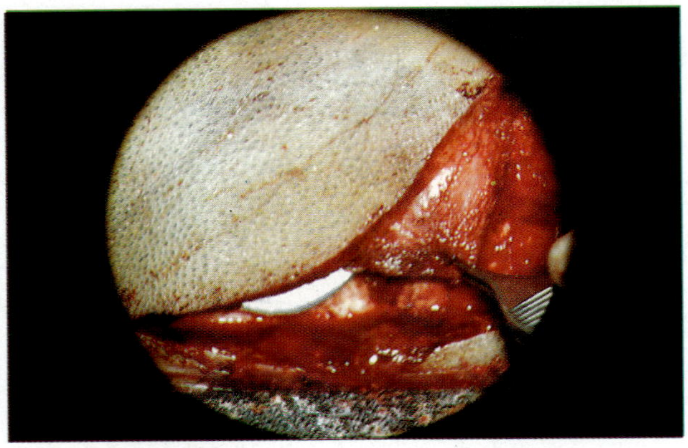

Fig. 8-41. The postauricular flap is closed in layers.

CHAPTER 14

Facial reinnervation techniques

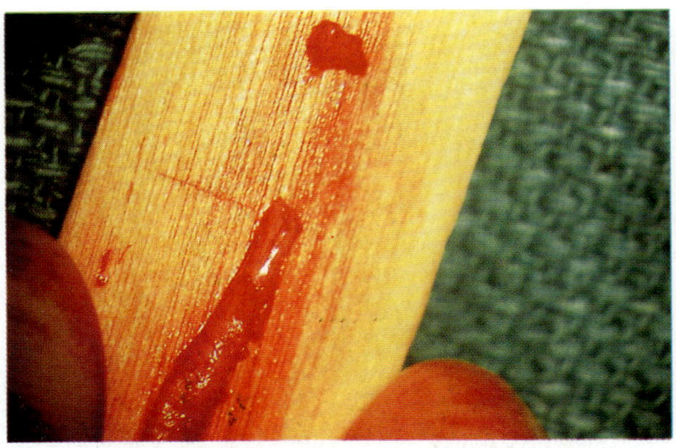

Fig. 14-12. The greater auricular n. graft is prepared on a moist tongue blade.

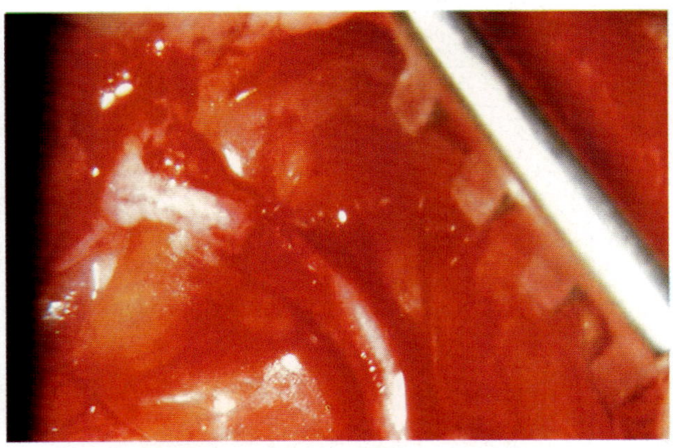

Fig. 14-13. Grafting of the facial nerve.

CHAPTER 18

Endolymphatic sac-mastoid shunt

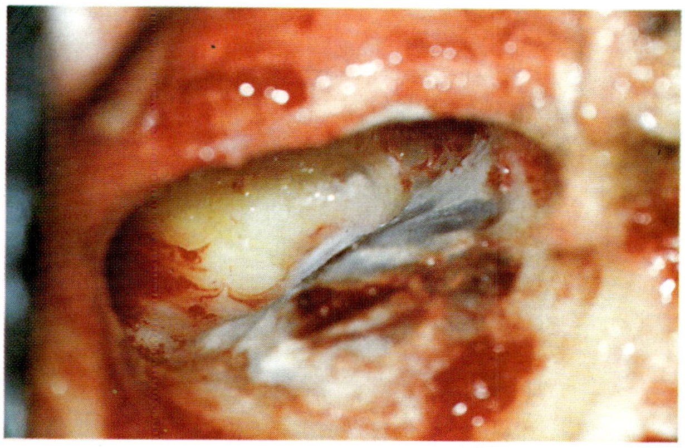

Fig. 18-21. Right endolymphatic mastoid shunt. The endolymphatic sac is found performing a simple mastoidectomy, skeletonizing the sigmoid sinus and exposing the posterior fossa dura medial to the sinus and posterior to the posterior semicircular canal.

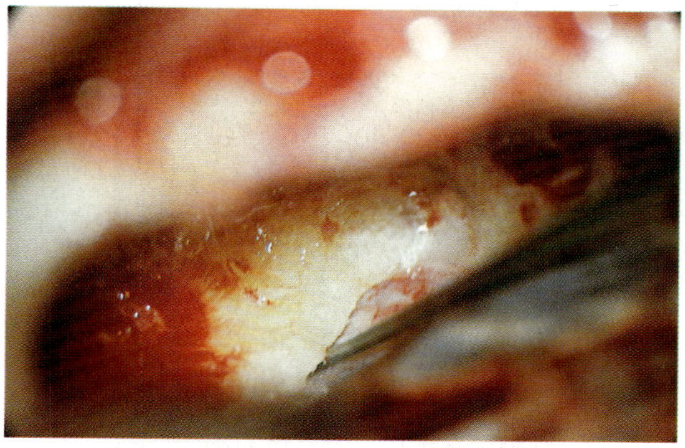

Fig. 18-22. The sac is identified as a thickened portion of posterior fossa dura. The ES is decompressed, below the posterior semicircular canal.

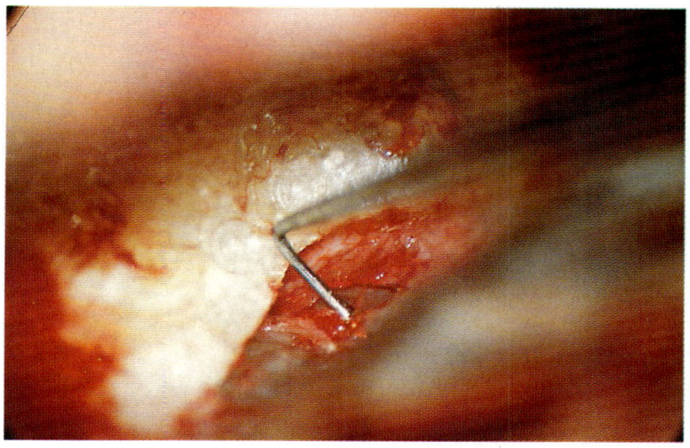

Fig. 18-23. The lateral wall of the sac is incised and the interior exposed.

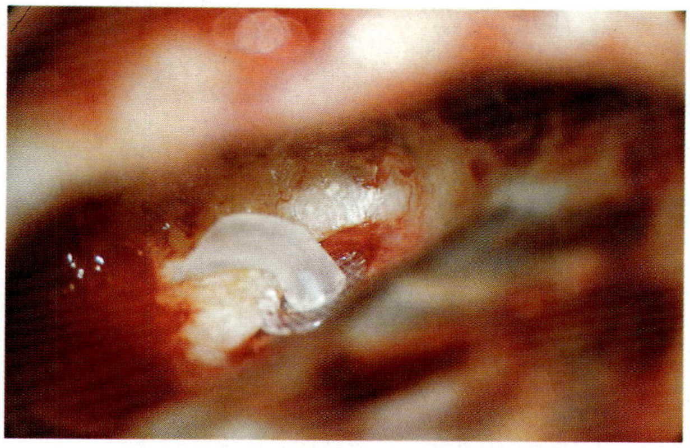

Fig. 18-24. A shunt tube or a silicone sheeting T-strut is placed within the sac.

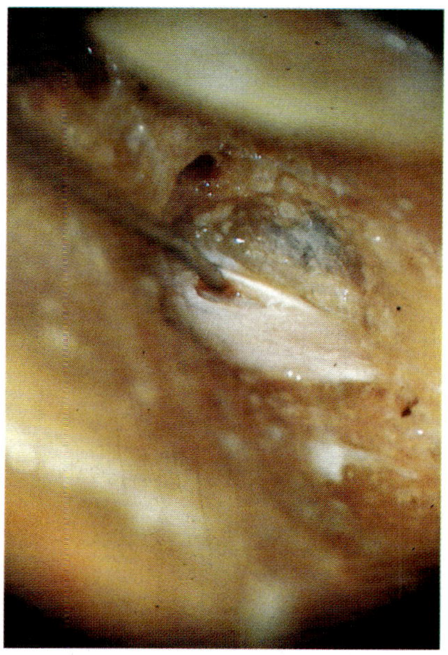

Fig. 18-25. The lumen of the sac is probed.

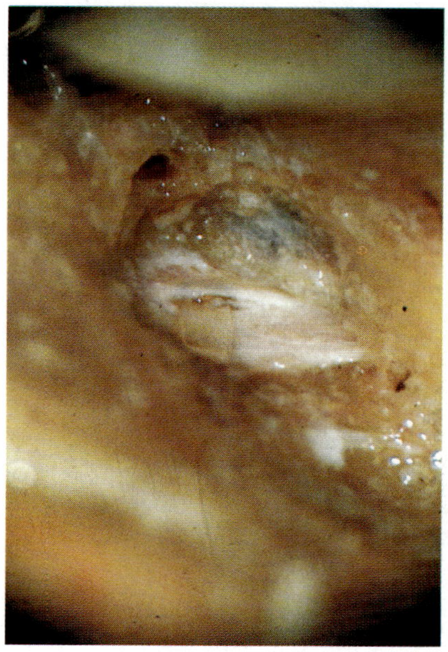

Fig. 18-26. A silicone sheeting T-strut is placed within the sac

CHAPTER 19

Vestibular nerve section. Retrolabyrinthine approach

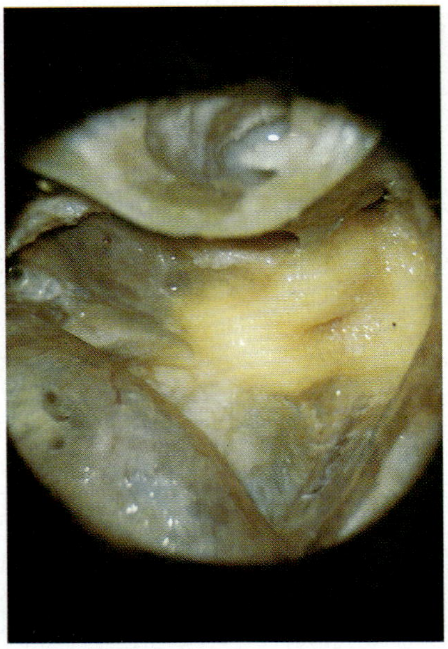

Fig. 19-25. Retrolabyrinthine vestibular nerve section. Left ear. A complete mastoidectomy is performed. The sigmoid sinus, the presigmoid dura, the semicircular canals and approximately 2 cm of dura posterior to the sigmoid sinus are exposed.

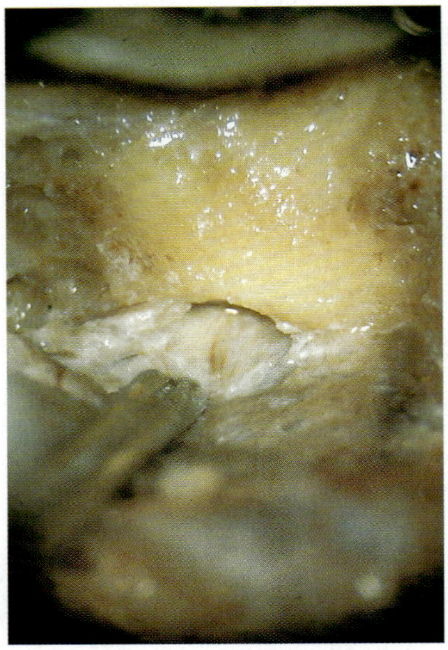

Fig. 19-26. The posterior fossa dura is exposed from the sinodural angle superiorly to the retrofacial air cells inferiorly. The posterior semicircular canal is skeletonized to gain the maximum anterior dural exposure.

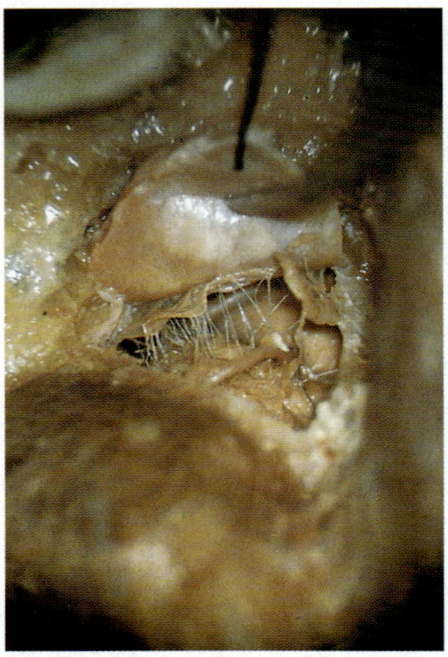

Fig. 19-27. The dura is incised in a U shape based on the posterior semicircular canal. The dural flap is elevated and suspended anteriorly with stay sutures.

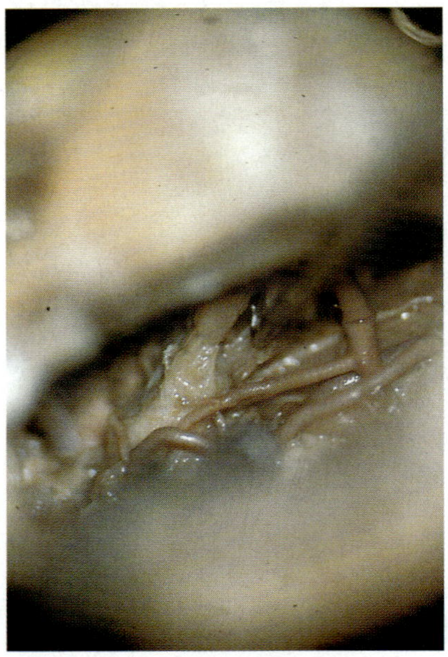

Fig. 19-28. The cleavage plane between the vestibular and the cochlear nerve is identified. The vestibular fibers are separated.

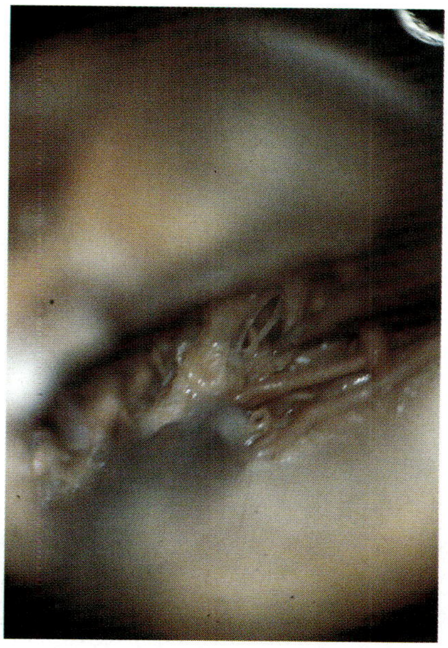

Fig. 19-29. The vestibular n. is transected. The labyrinthine artery is seen behind the cochleovestibular n. The IAA runs between the facial and cochlear nerves.

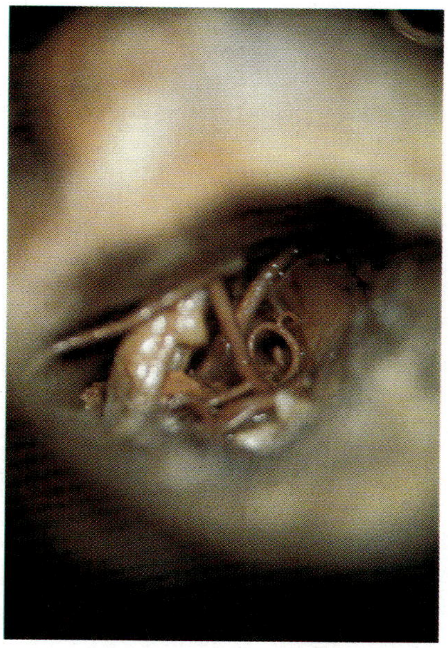

Fig. 19-30. The vestibular n. is cut, the cochlear n. is spared.

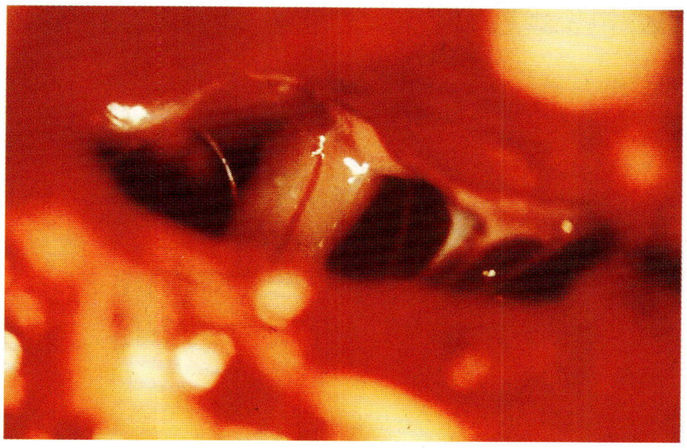

Fig. 19-31. Left cochleovestibular nerve.

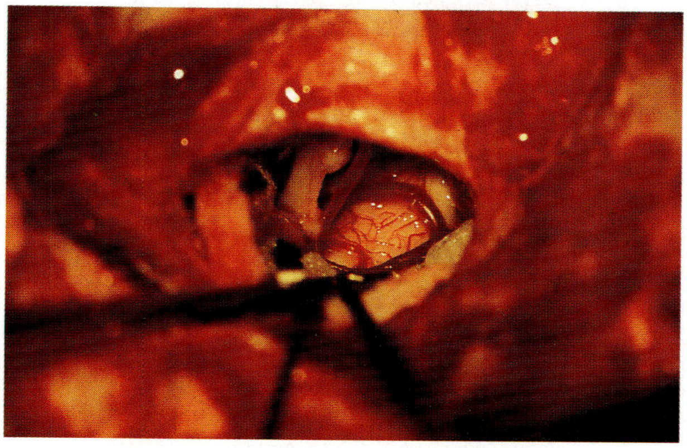

Fig. 19-32. The vestibular n. is cut, the cochlear n. is spared.

CHAPTER 19

Vestibular nerve section. Retrosigmoid approach

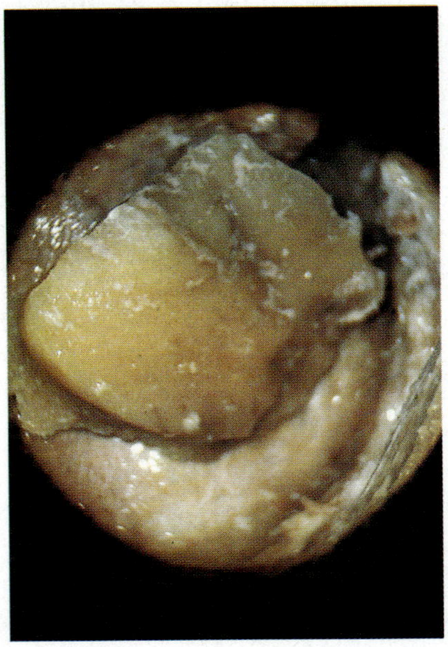

Fig. 19-33. Retrosigmoid approach. Right ear. A posterior fossa craniotomy window of approx. 3 x 3cm is made. The anterior limit is the sigmoid sinus, the superior limit is the transverse sinus.

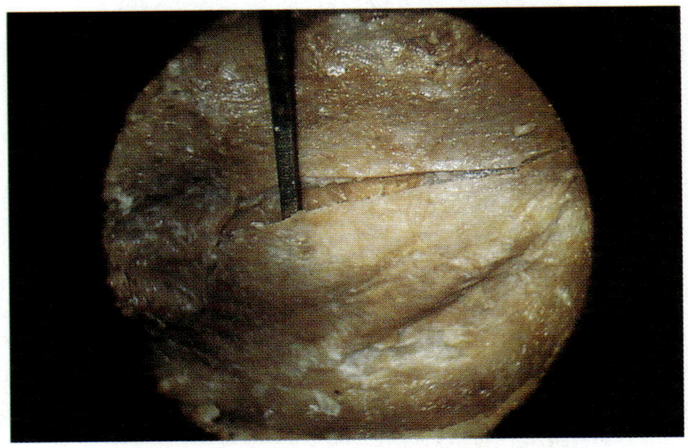

Fig. 19-34. The posterior fossa dura is incised. An anteriorly based dural flap is prepared, elevated and suspended anteriorly with stay sutures.

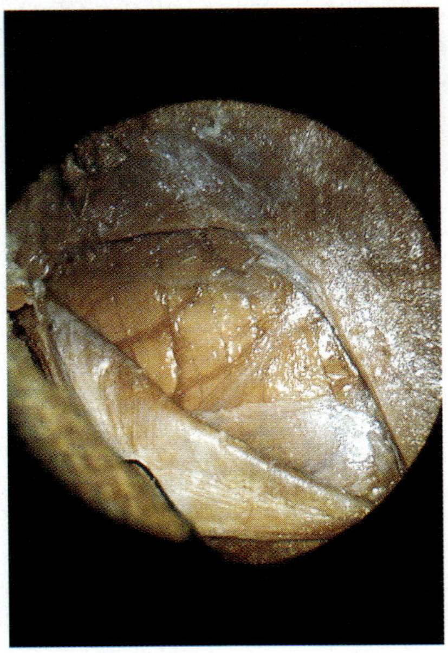

Fig. 19-35. The arachnoid of the cistern is lanced with a fenestrated suction-irrigator, CSF is aspirated and the cerebellum falls away medially.

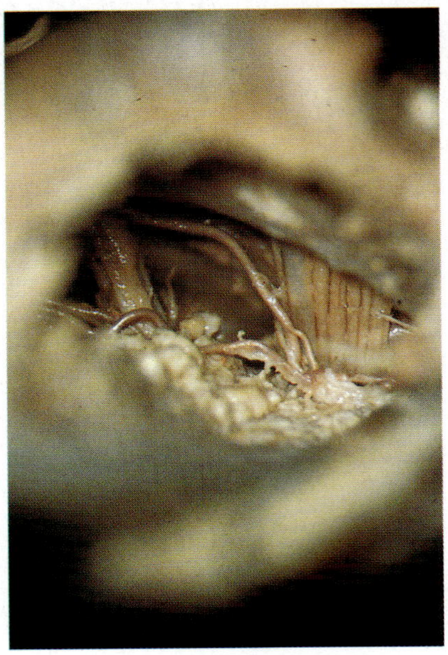

Fig. 19-36. The VIII CN and the IX-X-XI CNs are identified.

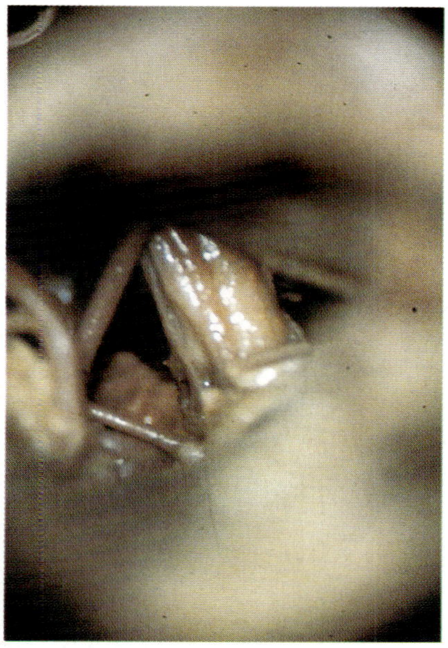

Fig. 19-37. Close up view of VIII CN.

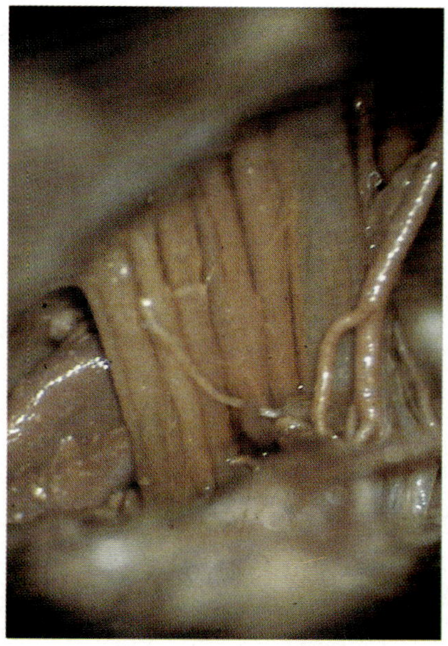

Fig. 19-38. Close up view of IX-X-XI CNs.

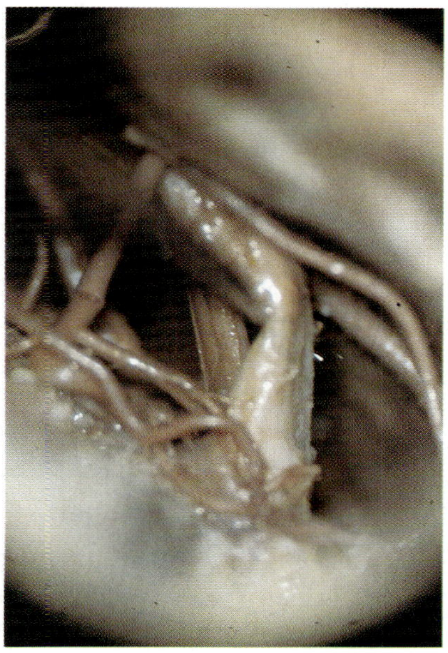

Fig. 19-39. The facial n. is identified by gentle retraction of the vestibulocochlear n.

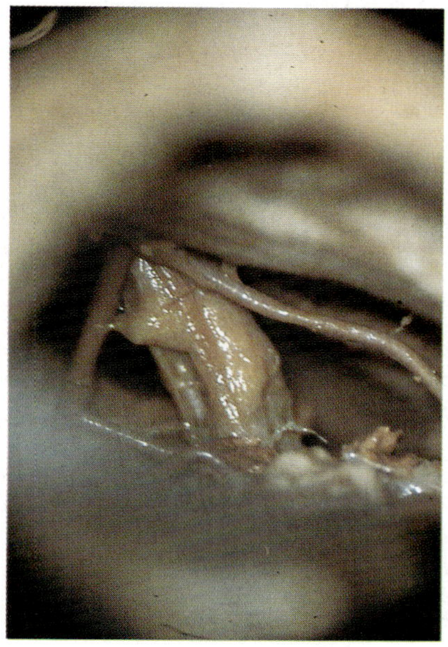

Fig. 19-40. Vestibular n. is cut. Internal auditory artery is seen behind the cochlear n.

CHAPTER 27

Surgical therapy of microvascular compression syndromes

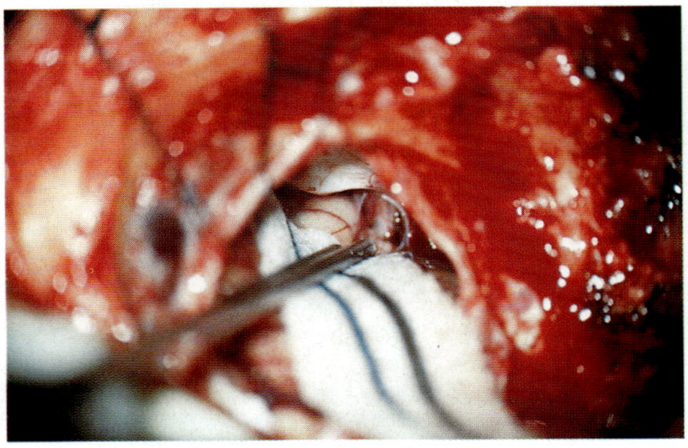

Fig. 27-4. Microvascular decompression of the VIII CN. Right ear. A partial mastoidectomy is performed and the sigmoid sinus is exposed. A retrosigmoid craniectomy, approx. 2.5 cm × 4 cm is performed. The dura is opened in a C shape. An anteriorly based dural flap is prepared, elevated and suspended anteriorly with stay sutures. To obtain a wide anterior exposure, it is important that the base of the dural flap be lateral enough to reach the edge of the sigmoid sinus.

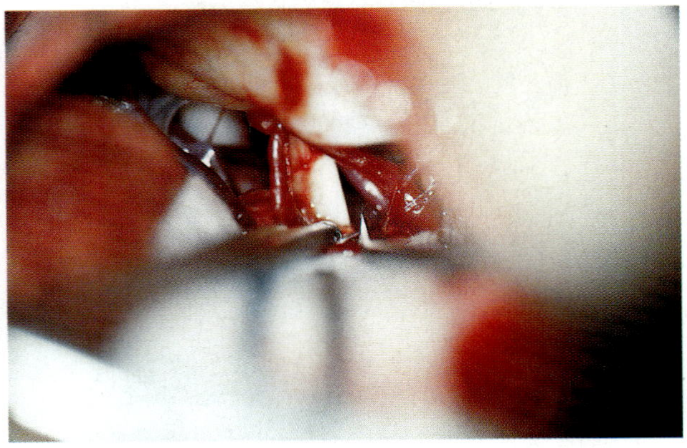

Fig. 27-5. The arachnoid is opened with sharp dissection, the cerebellum is gently depressed with the rod of a fenestrated suction-irrrigator, protected by a cottonoid. The vestibulocochlear nerve with the offending vessel is identified.

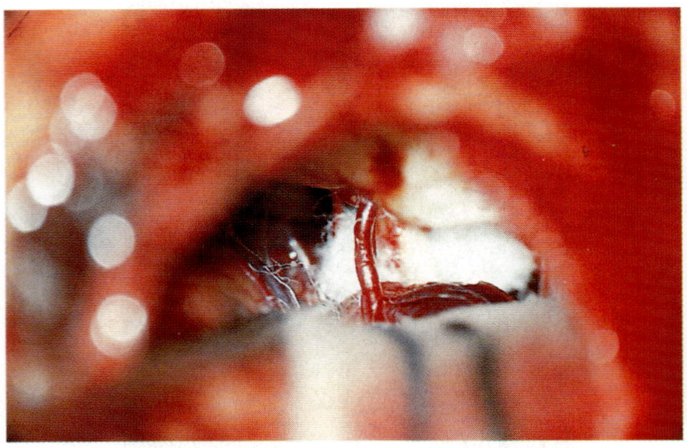

Fig. 27-6. The artery is mobilized and held away from the nerve with shredded Teflon felt.

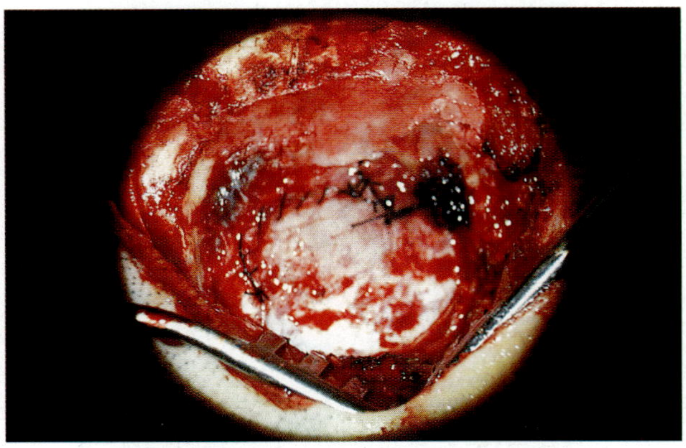

Fig. 27-7. The dural flap is sutured back into place with closely positioned, multiple 4.0 braided nylon sutures.

CHAPTER 28

Translabyrinthine approach to acoustic neuroma surgery

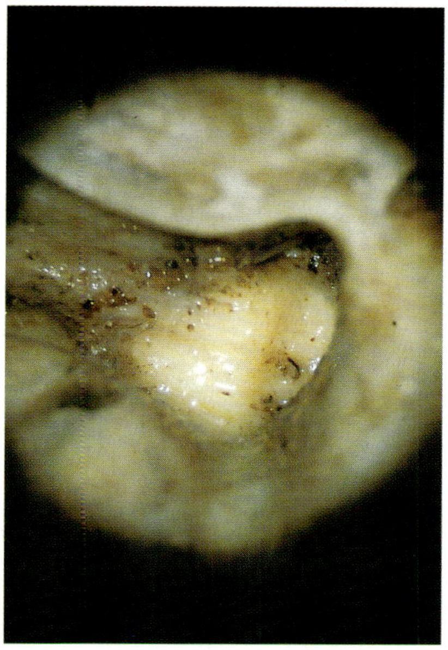

Fig. 28-39. Translabyrinthine approach. Left ear. Horizontal and posterior semicircular canals are exposed. The third part of the facial nerve is skeletonized: it is the anterior limit of the dissection.

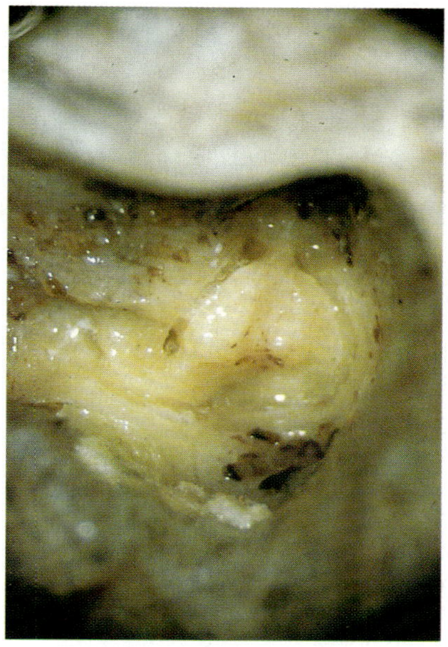

Fig. 28-40. Fenestration of the semicircular canals. The horizontal semicircular canal leads to the posterior canal which leads to the common crus and the superior canal. The anterior wall of the horizontal canal is kept intact, as a protection for the external genu and horizontal portions of the facial nerve.

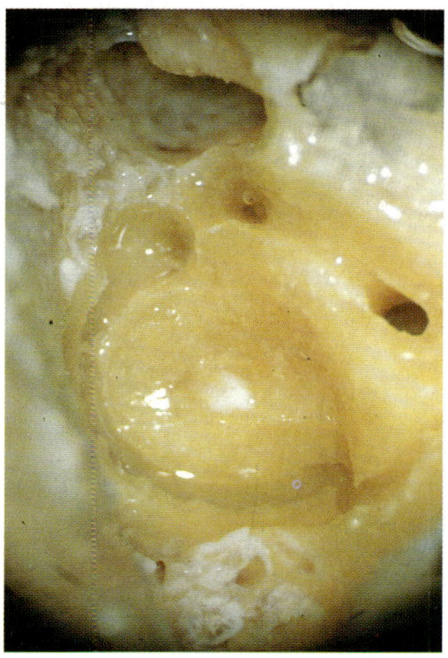

Fig. 28-41. The semicircular canals are completely opened. The subarcuate artery penetrates the labyrinthine bone in the center of the circle inscribed by the superior and horizontal semicircular canals.

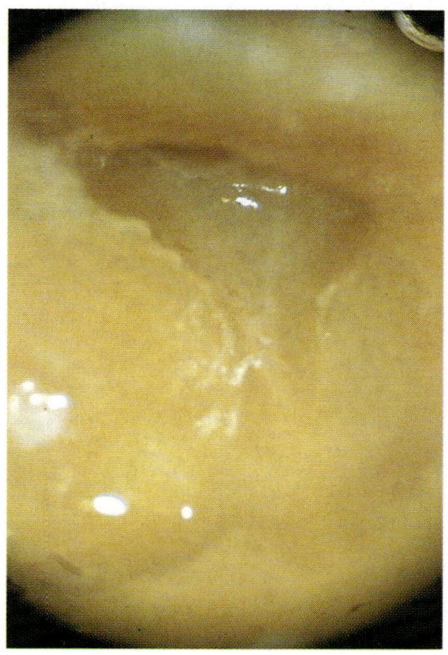

Fig. 28-42. The semicircular canals are completely connected, the bone over the facial nerve is thinned to provide good access to the vestibule, the vestibule is opened. The medial wall of the vestibule is the lateral wall of the IAC.

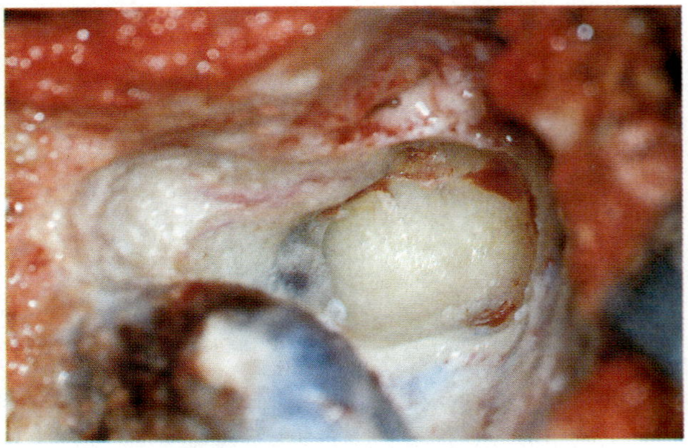

Fig. 28-43. Removal of the last dural plate over the IAC. The dura of the internal auditory canal is exposed for more then 180 degrees.

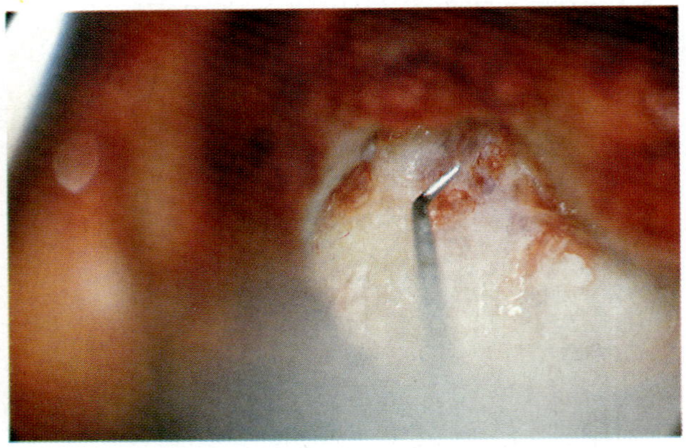

Fig. 28-44. The hook points out Bill's bar. The facial nerve is on the right, the superior vestibular nerve on the left.

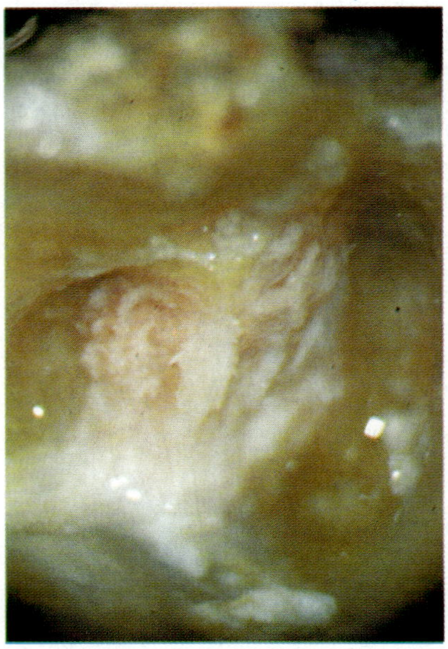

Fig. 28-45. IAC of a left temporal bone. Dura is still intact; transverse crest and Bill's bar can be seen.

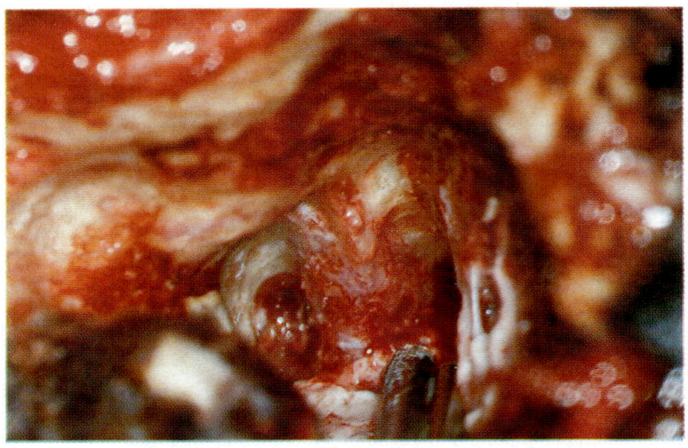

Fig. 28-46. The dura of the internal auditory canal is exposed for more then 180 degrees.

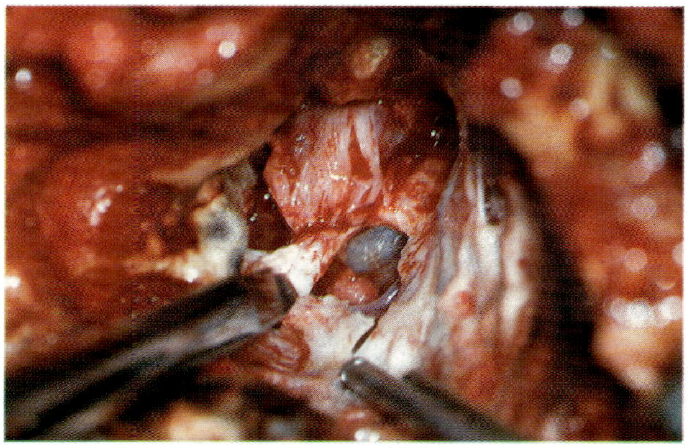

Fig. 28-47. The dura of the IAC is incised along the inferior border of the canal, far away from the facial nerve which is anterior inferior.

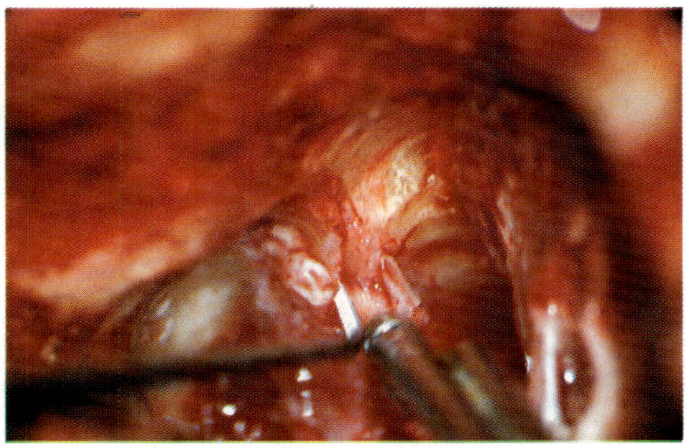

Fig. 28-48. Tumor is dissected away from the facial nerve rather then the facial nerve being retracted away from the tumor.

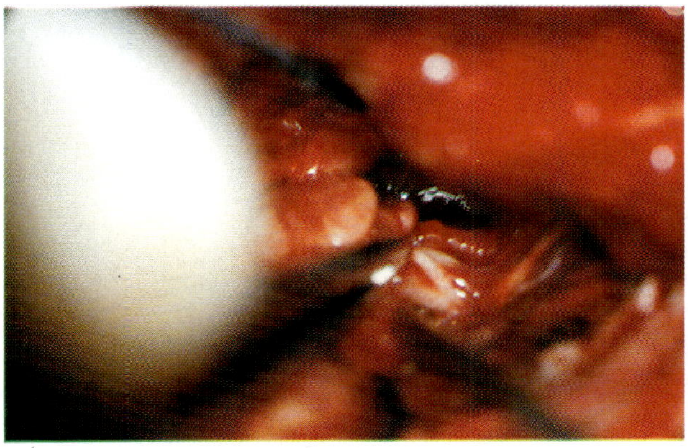

Fig. 28-49. The AICA is identified on the pons.

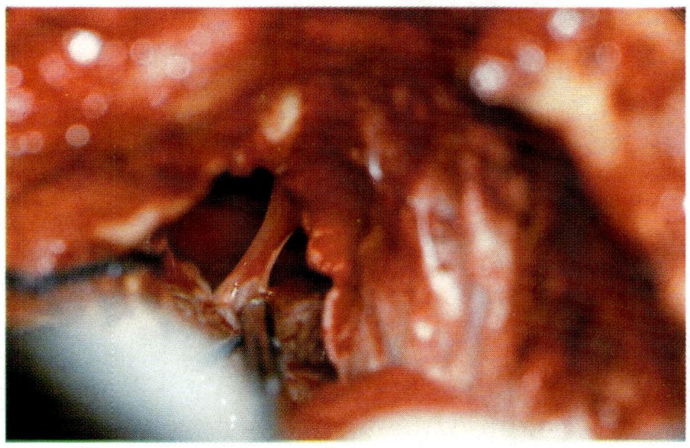

Fig. 28-50. Tumor has been completely removed. Facial nerve integrity is preserved.

CHAPTER 32

Middle cranial fossa approach

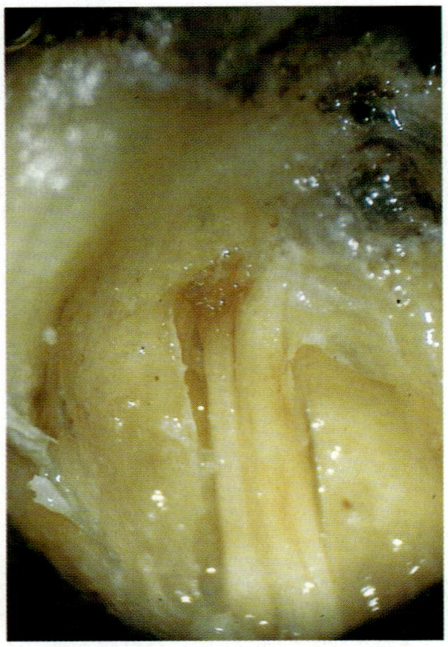

Fig. 32-27. Middle fossa approach. Left ear. The IAC is exposed, the dura is cut. Facial nerve, Bill's bar and superior vestibular nerve are exposed.

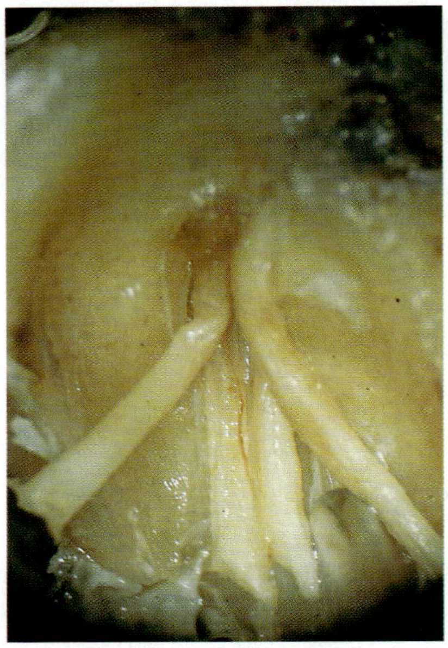

Fig. 32-28. Left ear. The facial nerve and the superior vestibular nerve are elevated to show the underlying inferior vestibular and cochlear nerves.

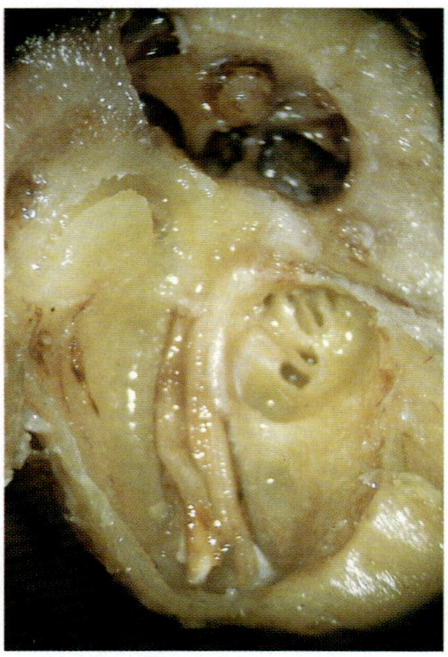

Fig. 32-29. The greater superficial petrosal n., the geniculate ganglion and the facial n. are exposed. The cochlea and the epitympanum are opened for demonstration.

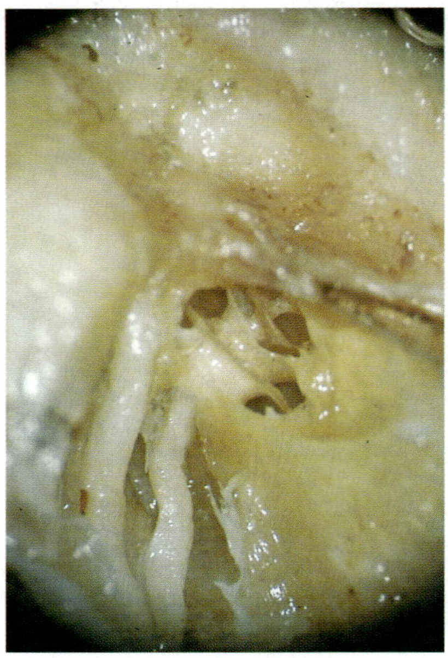

Fig. 32-30. The greater superficial petrosal n., the geniculate ganglion and the facial n. are exposed. The cochlea is opened to show the origin of the cochlear nerve.

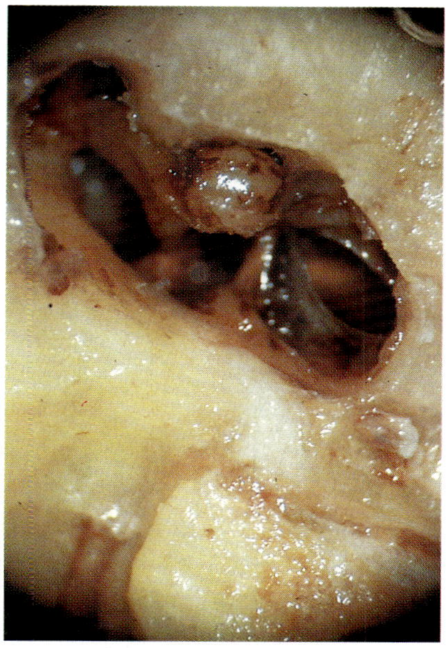

Fig. 32-31. Epitympanum is opened. The head of the malleus and the body of the incus are visible.

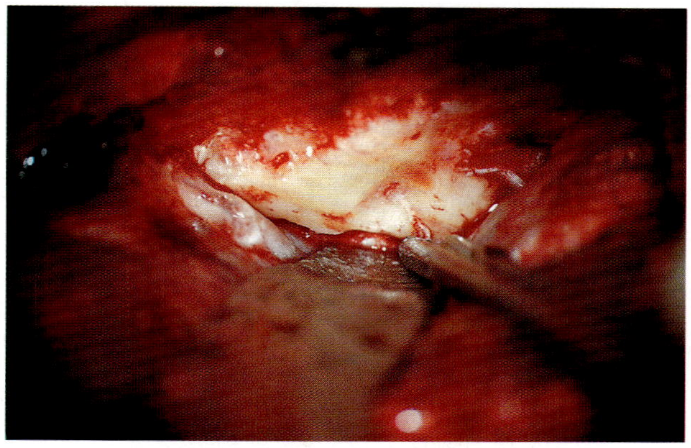

Fig. 32-32. The dura is elevated from the floor of the middle fossa with a blunt dural elevator and a suction irrigator. The House-Urban retractor is placed to gently support the temporal lobe.

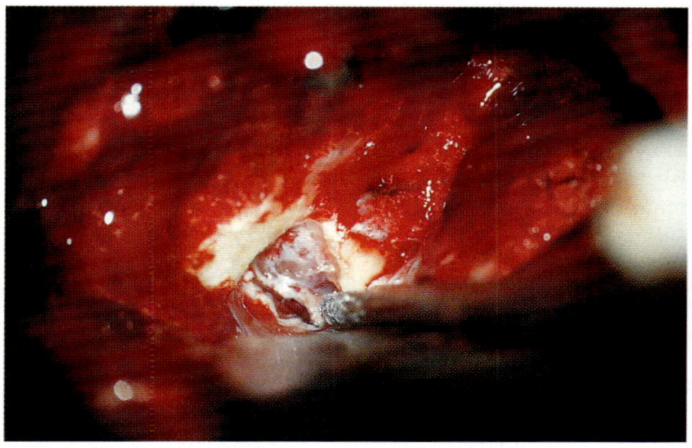

Fig. 32-33. The internal auditory canal is exposed. The dura of the IAC is incised along the posterior aspect, the CSF is aspirated and the temporal lobe is decompressed.

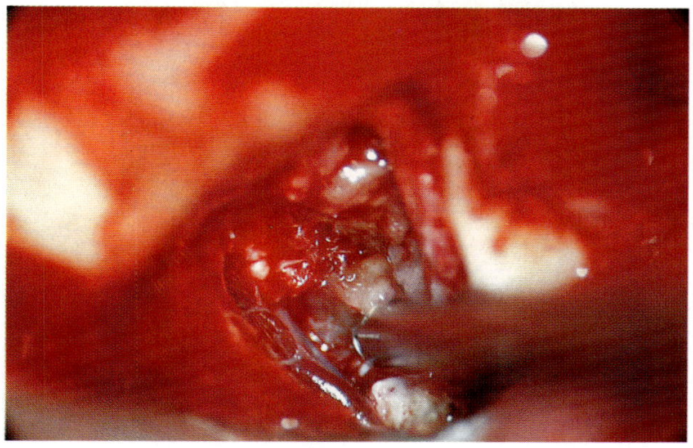

Fig. 32-34. Acoustic tumor. The facial n. is identified in the anterior superior portion of the IAC. The inferior vestibular nerve is divided and the tumor is freed from the fundus of the IAC.

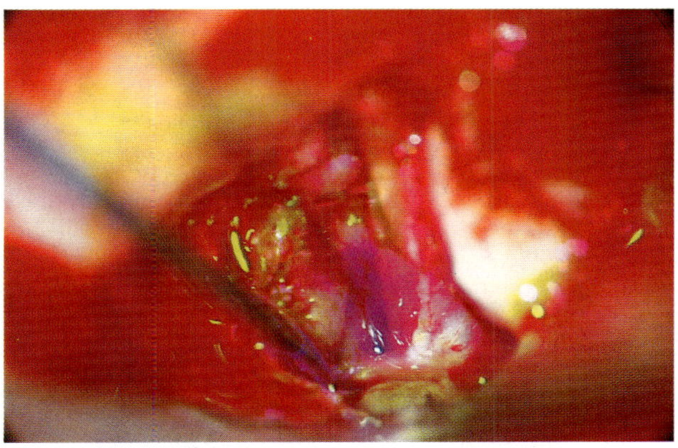

Fig. 32-35. Tumor is dissected away from the facial and cochlear nerves rather then the nerves being retracted away from the tumor. The dissection along the VIII n. is done in a medial to lateral direction, in order to avoid tearing the filaments of the nerve that pass through the holes of the lamina cribrosa, at the fundus of the IAC.

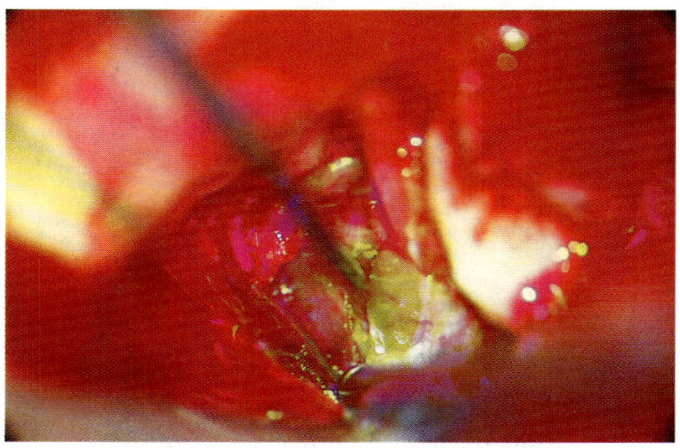

Fig. 32-36. Tumor is completely removed. Facial nerve, on the right, and cochlear nerve, on the left, are preserved.

CHAPTER 37

Transcochlear approach to cerebellopontine angle lesions

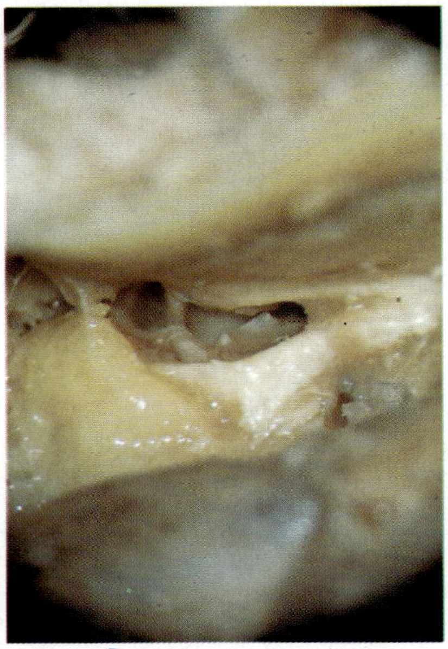

Fig. 37-27. Transcochlear approach. Right ear. Complete simple mastoidectomy. An extended facial recess opening is created.

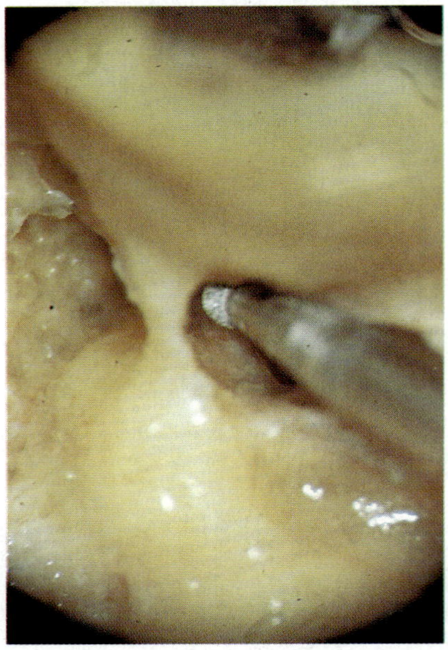

Fig. 37-28. The tympanic part and the mastoid part of the facial nerve are exposed, from the internal auditory canal to the stylomastoid foramen, including the geniculate ganglion.

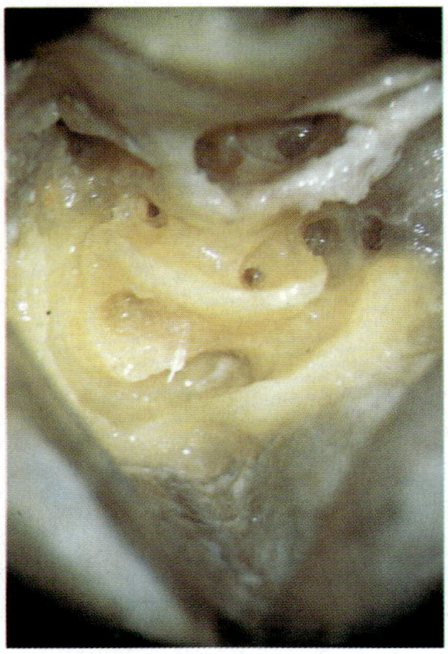

Fig. 37-29. Labyrinthectomy. The horizontal semicircular canal leads to the posterior canal that leads to the common crus and the superior canal. The semicircular canals are fenestrated and then removed.

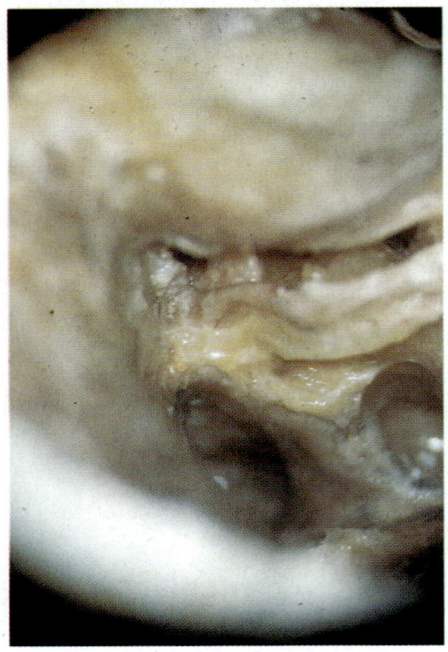

Fig. 37-30. The internal auditory canal is exposed. The facial nerve is exposed from the IAC to the stylomastoid foramen, including the geniculate ganglion.

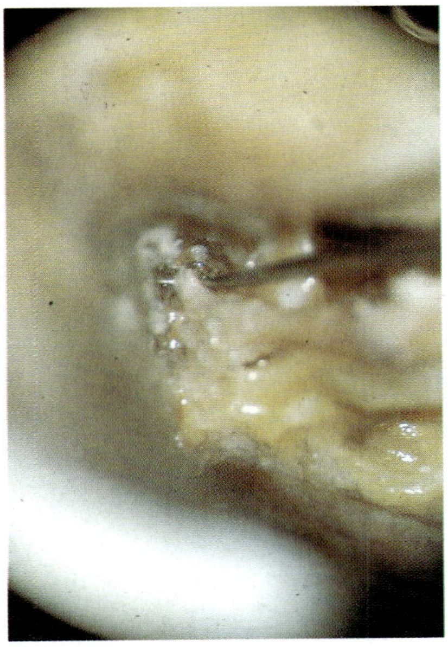

Fig. 37-31. The greater superficial petrosal nerve is cut at its origin from the geniculate ganglion with a sickle knife.

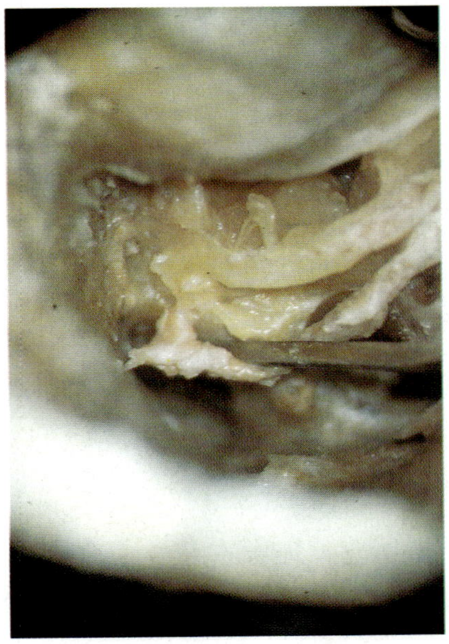

Fig. 37-32. The facial nerve is reflected posteriorly out of the bony fallopian canal, without exerting traction on it.

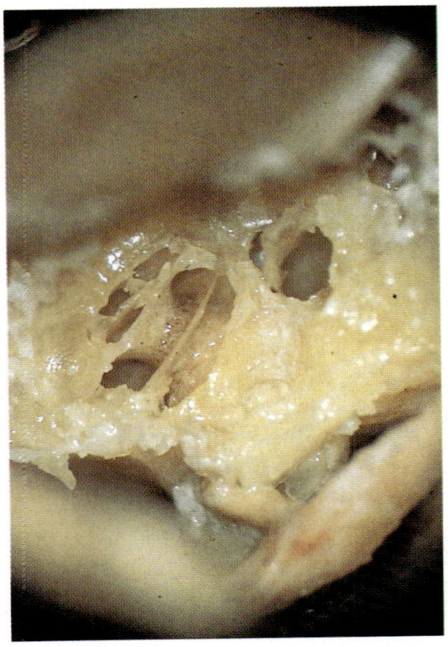

Fig. 37-33. Starting with the basal coil, the cochlea is completely drilled out. 1 mm. of bone approx. separates anteriorly the basal coil of the cochlea from the petrous carotid artery.

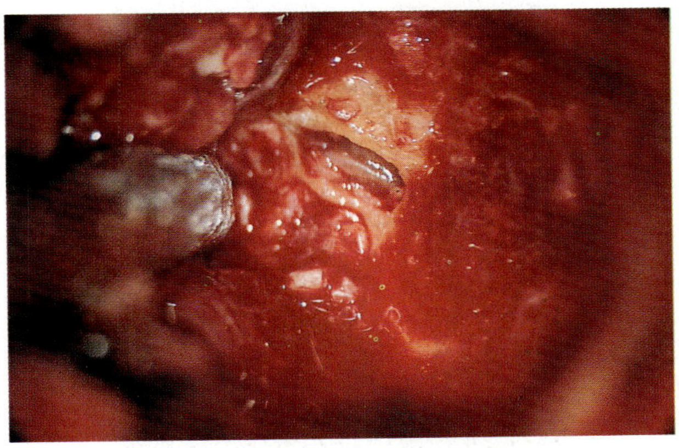

Fig. 37-34. The basal coil of the cochlea is opened.

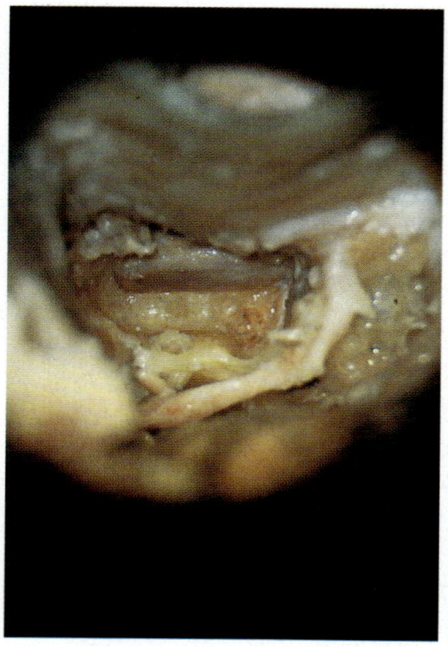

Fig. 37-35. Facial nerve is posteriorly rerouted.

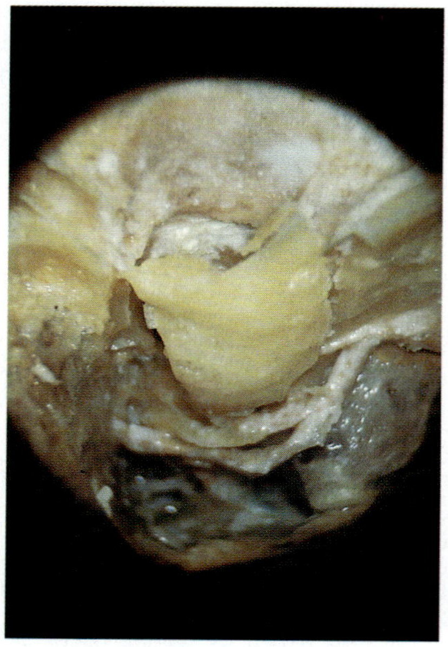

Fig. 37-36. When further anterior exposure is required, the external auditory canal is blind sac closed (chapter 16). The bony posterior EAC is drilled down.

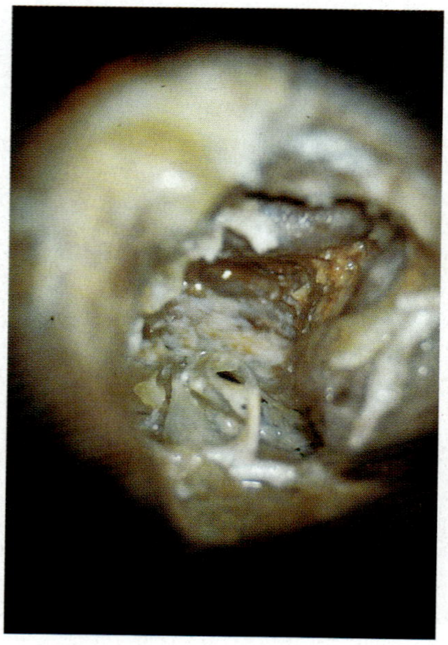

Fig. 37-37. The internal carotid artery and the jugular bone are exposed. The jugulocarotid bony spine (crotch) is drilled down.

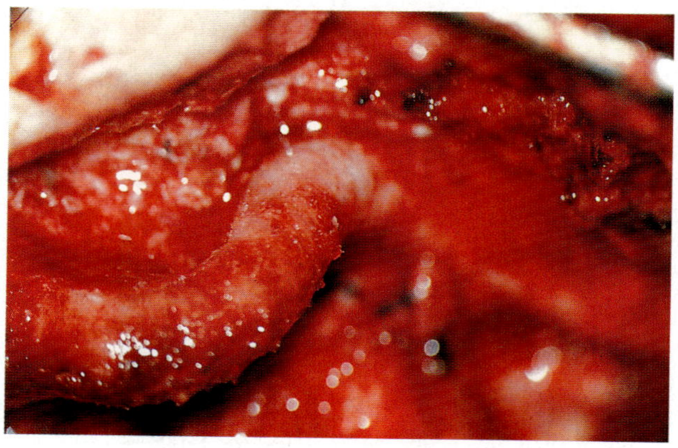

Fig. 37-38. Infratemporal fossa, transcochlear and intracranial approach for transdural right glomus jugularis tumor. The petrous carotid artery is exposed for 360 degrees. A transdural left glomus jugularis tumor of similar size is shown in figure 37-1.

CHAPTER 40

Petroclival tumors. Anterolateral approaches

Extended frontal approach

Pallini R., Patel S. (#), Salvinelli F. (*), De La Cruz A. (ç), Wright D.C. (@), Sekhar L. N. (@)
Institutes of Neurosurgery and (*) Otorhinolaryngology, Catholic University Medical School, Rome, Italy, (#) Neuro-Oncology Cranial Base Surgery, Department of Neurological Surgery, Medical University of South Carolina, Charleston, South Carolina, (ç) University of Southern California, St. Vincent Medical Center, LAC/USC Medical Center, USC University Hospital, Los Angeles, California, and (@) Department of Neurological Surgery, George Washington University Medical Center, Washington, D.C.

The extended frontal approach provides exposure of midline structures of the anterior, middle, and posterior skull base with minimal retraction of the frontal lobes. The operative field is limited laterally by the optic nerves, cavernous internal carotid arteries (ICAs), petrous apexes, cranial nerves (CNs) VI, and hypoglossal canals.

Indications for this approach are neoplasms of the orbito-fronto-ethmoidal region and of the middle and lower clivus that do not involve the cavernous sinus (CS). Tumors that involve the CS are first approached via a subtemporal-infratemporal trans-sylvian route, which allows proximal and distal control of the cavernous ICA, and then via the extended frontal approach.
Disadvantages include the sacrifice of the olfactory nerves, absence of proximal control of the cavernous ICA, poor exposure of the upper clivus (dorsum sellae), and risks for post-operative cerebro-spinal (CSF) fluid leaks.

The dissection will proceed as follows:
A: bifrontal craniotomy.
B: bilateral orbito-fronto-ethmoidal osteotomy;
C: exposure of the optic nerves, cavernous ICAs, and clival dura.

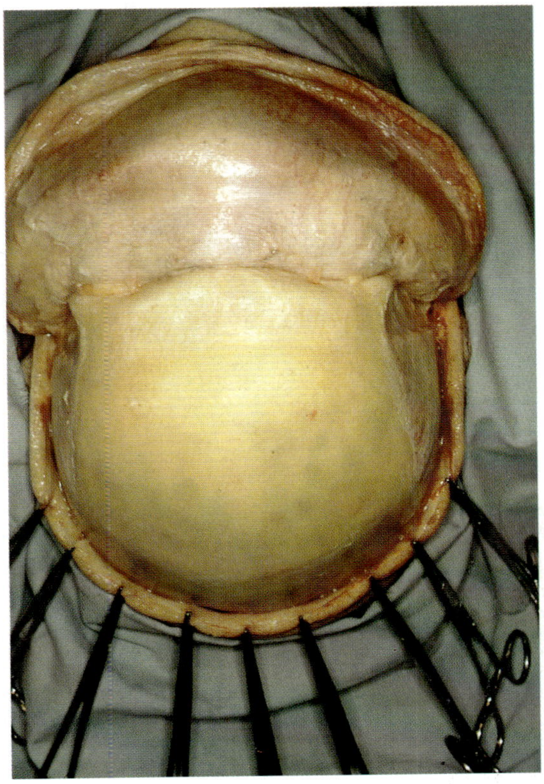

Fig. 40-14. A bicoronal skin incision is made 1 cm posteriorly to the coronal suture from one zygomatic arch to the other. The incision includes the skin and galea but spares the pericranium that is divided separately 3-4 cm posteriorly to the skin incision. This allows a longer vascularized pericranial flap for final reconstruction of the anterior skull base. The skin flap is elevated to the supraorbital rims. The superficial temporal fascia is incised and elevated along with the interfascial fat to preserve the frontal branches of the facial nerve.

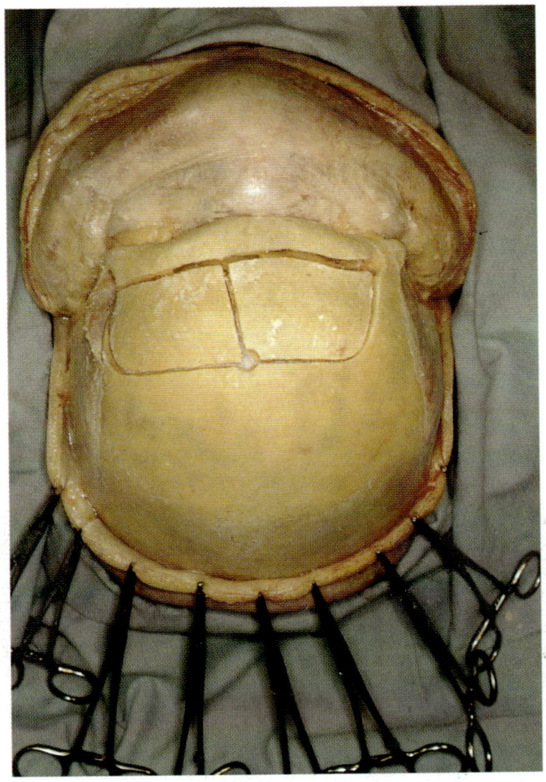

Fig. 40-15. A low bilateral frontal craniotomy is performed following these steps:
- Left frontal bone flap,
- Separation of superior sagittal sinus,
- Right frontal bone flap exposing the midline.

Such a bifrontal craniotomy is safe in preventing dural lacerations and injury to the right sinus. The craniotomy cuts must be performed after carefull dissection of the dura that in this area is usually thin and adherent to the bone.

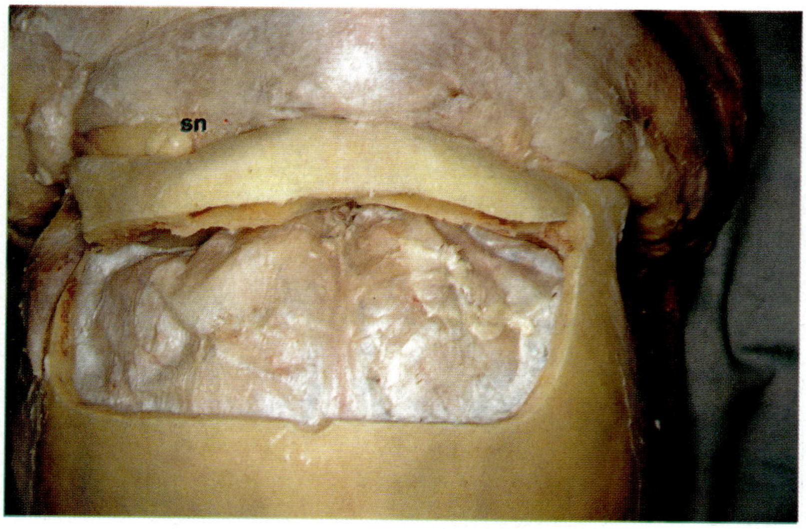

Fig. 40-16. The supraorbital nerves are released and the skin flap is further elevated down to the frontonasal suture. Care must be taken to avoid extensive lacerations of the periorbita. Dissection of the periorbita from the orbital roof starts from the supero-lateral corner and proceeds to the anterior ethmoidal artery medially. The periorbita is dissected from the roof of the orbit 2.5 cm posteriorly to the orbital rim.
sn: supraorbital nerve.

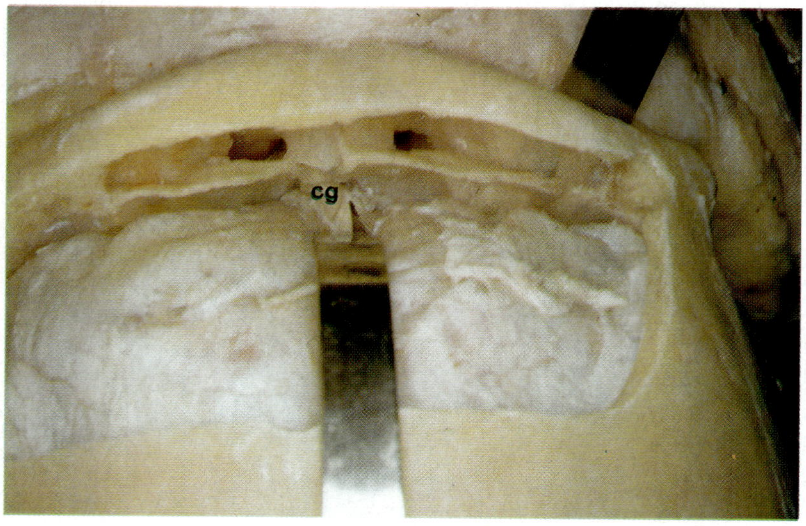

Fig. 40-17. The orbital content is protected with a malleable retractor and the subfrontal dura is dissected from the orbital roofs and planum ethmoidale. During surgery, this manouver is facilitated by CSF drainage. The crista galli (cg) is exposed.

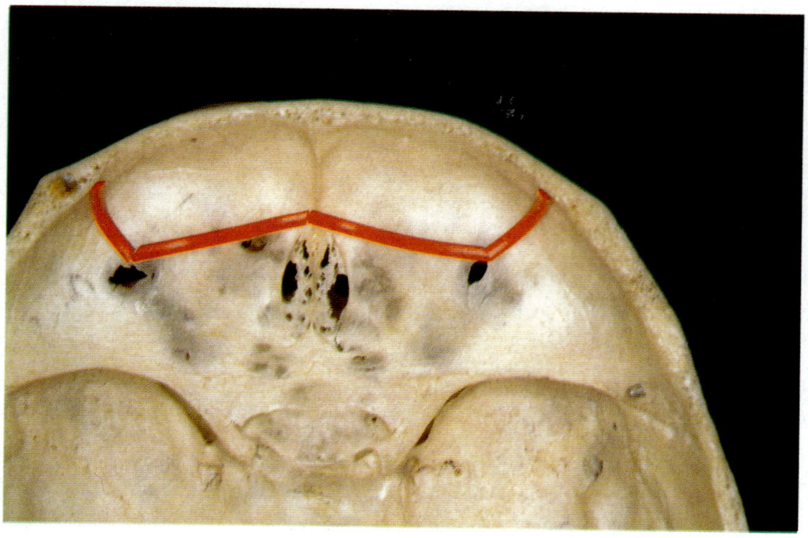

Fig. 40-18. Using a reciprocating saw, osteotomy cuts are made on each side through the orbital roofs from the supero-lateral corner of the orbit to the crista galli. It is important not to cut posteriorly to the crista galli to avoid injuries to the optic nerves. Incorporating approximately 2 cm of the orbital roof in the fronto-orbital osteotomy prevents post-operative en- or exophtalmos. A third bone cut is made over the frontonasal suture, from outside to inside, directed posteriorly and sligtly upward to enter the anterior cranial fossa in front of the crista galli. During sawing, both the orbital content and frontal dura have to be protected with malleable retractors.

Fig. 40-19. The orbito-fronto-ethmoidal osteotomy is mobilized with an osteotome and removed exposing the ethmoidal cells. At surgery, bleeding from the mucosa is easily controlled by packing the ethmoidal cells with muscle or fat.
or: orbital content.

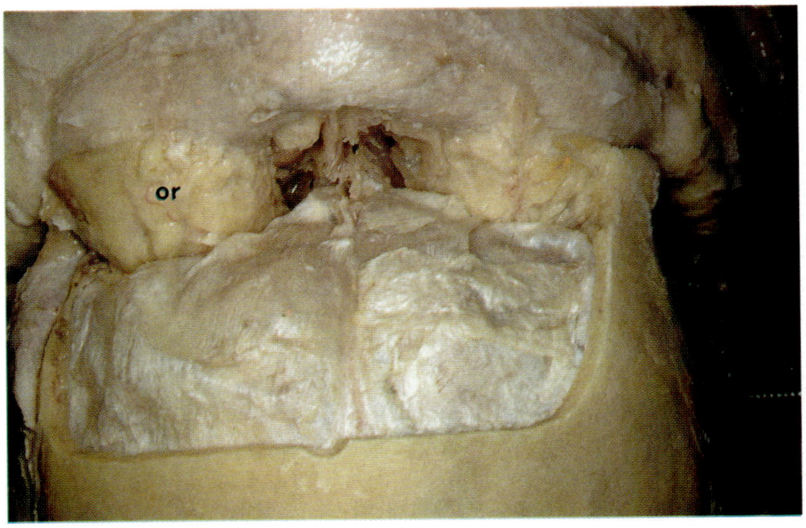

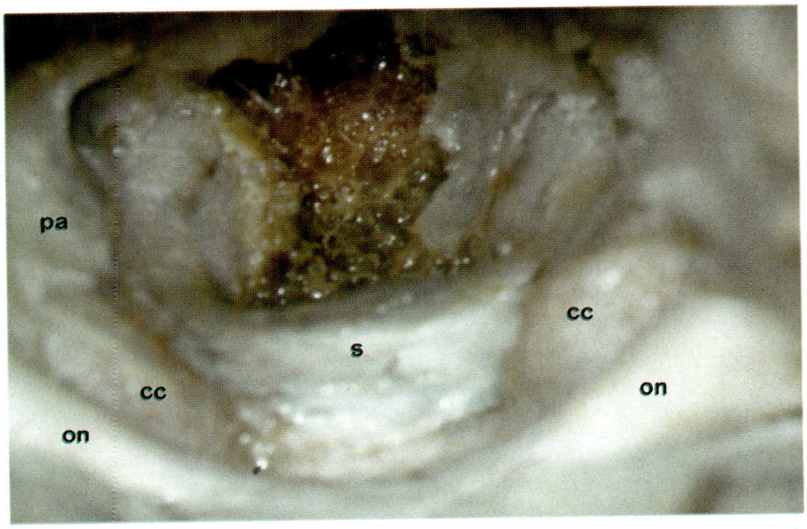

Fig. 40-20. Under the operating microscope, the dura is dissected along the planum ethmoidale. The branches of the olfactory nerves are progressively divided. Holes in the dura are closed with primary sutures. The posterior part of the planum ethmoidale that is not included in the orbito-ethmoidal osteotomy, is removed and the sphenoid sinus is opened.
The posterior orbital roof and the medial wall of the orbit are rongeured and the optic nerve canal is unroofed along its medial aspect. The bony walls of the sphenoid sinus are removed exposing the medial dura of the CS on both sides. The floor of the sella turcica is removed and the dura of the sella (s) is visualized.
The cavernous ICA (cc) is followed posteriorly resecting part of the petrous apex (pa). The clival bone is progressively drilled from superior to inferior working in between the clival dura and the submucosal nasopharyngeal plane that must be preserved.
on: optic nerve.

Fig. 40-21. The anterior rim of the foramen magnum (fm) is opened. The hypoglossal canals are unroofed to show the lower lateral limit of this approach. The hypoglossal canals are found 1.5 cm from the midline. At the end of dissection, the clival dura (cd) down to the foramen magnum can be seen without any brain retraction.

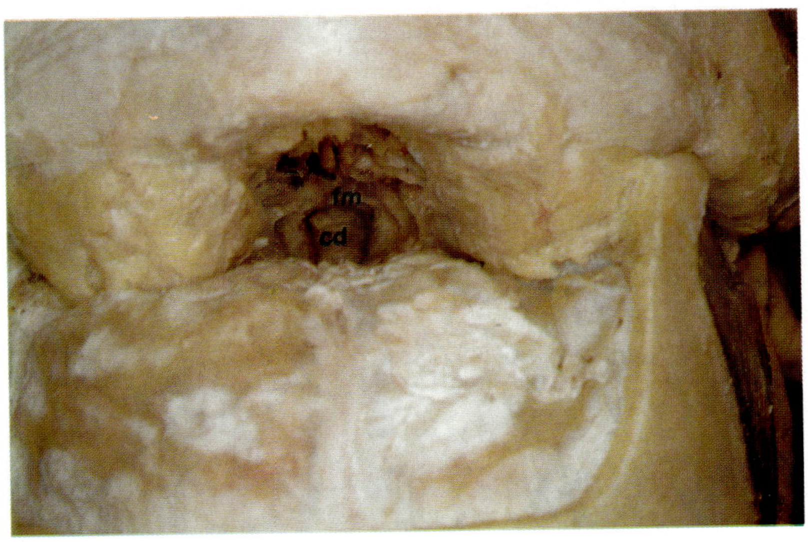

Sub temporal transcavernous and trans-petrous apex approach

Pallini R., Patel S. (*), Salvinelli F. (§), De La Cruz A. (ç), Wright D.C. (#), Sekhar L.N. (#)
Institutes of Neurosurgery and Otorhinolaryngology (§), Catholic University School of Medicine, Rome, Italy, (*) Neuro-Oncology Cranial Base Surgery, Department of Neurological Surgery, Medical University of South Carolina, Charleston, South Carolina, (ç) University of Southern California, St. Vincent Medical Center, LAC/USC Medical Center, USC University Hospital, Los Angeles, California, and (#) Department of Neurosurgery, George Washington University Medical Center, Washington D.C.

This approach provides exposure of the petrous apex and superior half of the clivus.
Indications for this approach are petro-clival and petro-spheno-clival meningiomas with cavernous sinus (CS) involvement and extension into the temporal fossa.

The dissection will proceed as follows:
A: extra-labyrinthine petrosectomy;

B: fronto-temporal craniotomy and orbito-zygomatic osteotomy;

C: removal of the petrous apex and exposure of the trigeminal root;

D: section of the tentorium, opening of the posterior CS, and exposure of CNs IV, III, VI, cavernous carotid, superior cerebellar, posterior cerebral, and basilar arteries.

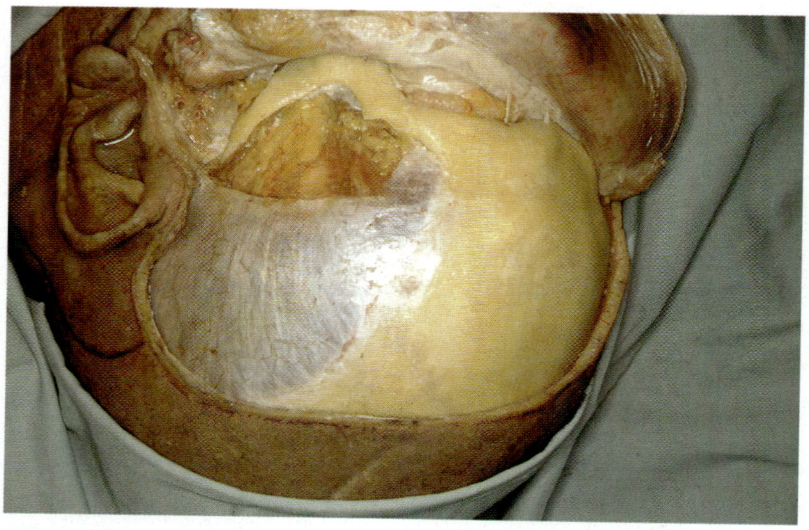

Fig. 40-22. A fronto-temporal preauricular skin flap is elevated exposing the orbital rim and zygoma. A second skin incision is made from the posterior temporal region to the mastoid tip.

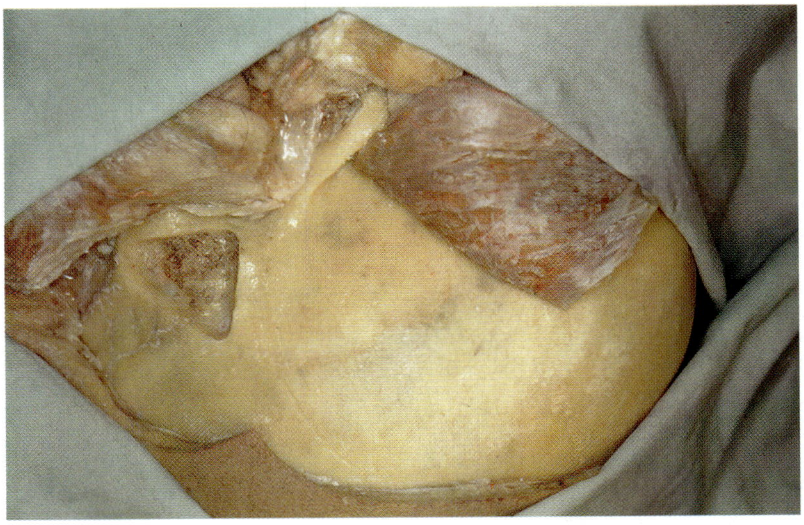

Fig. 40-23. The temporalis muscle is reflected, the lateral surface of the mastoid bone is exposed, and a simple mastoidectomy is performed. The semicircular canals are skeletonized.

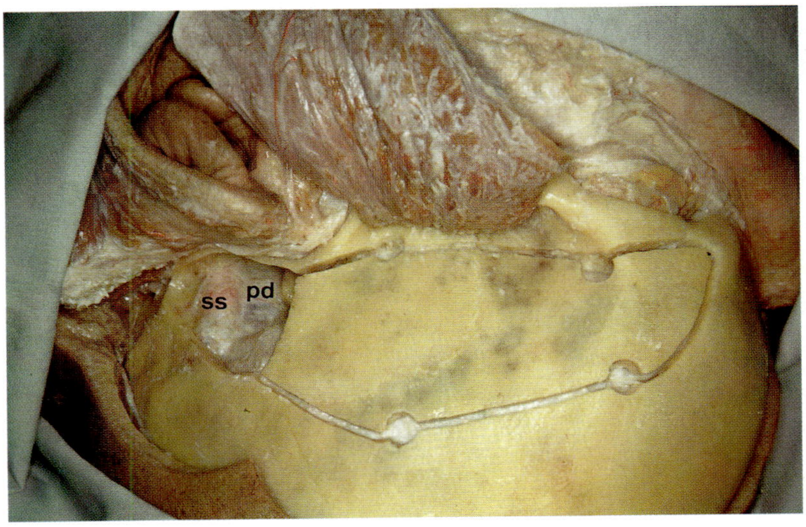

Fig. 40-24. After exposure of the presigmoid and temporal dura and removal of the petrous ridge, a fronto-temporal craniotomy is done.
ss: sigmoid sinus; ps: presigmoid dura.

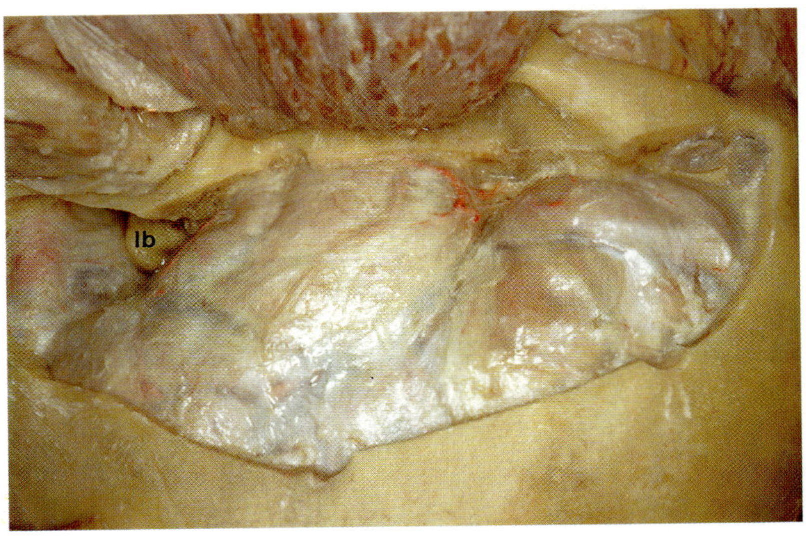

Fig. 40-25. A fronto-temporal bone flap is elevated.
lb: labyrinthine block.

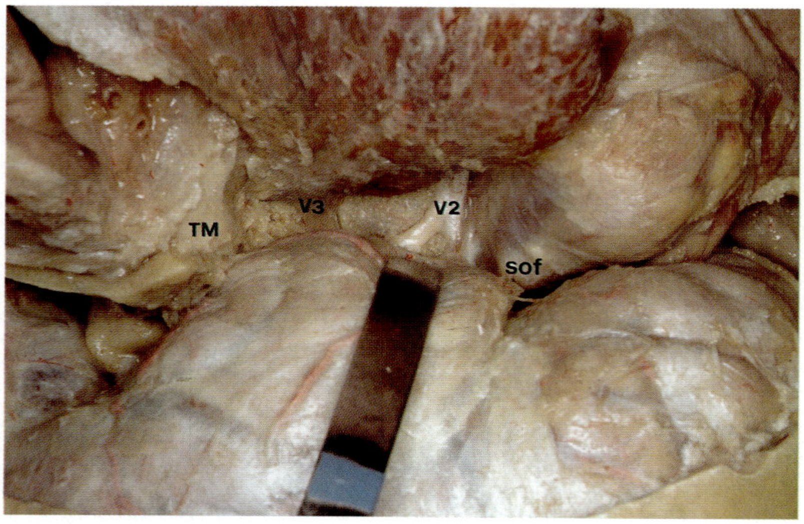

Fig. 40-26. An orbito-zygomatic osteotomy is performed and the floor of the middle fossa is removed unroofing the superior orbital fissure (sof), V2 (that in this specimem has two branches), and V3. By drilling bone between V2 and V3, the sphenoid sinus can be entered.
TM: temporo-mandibular joint.

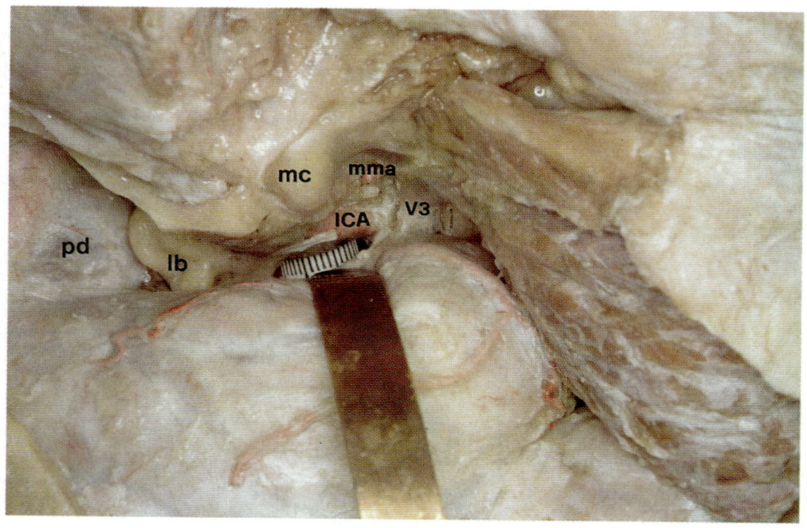

Fig. 40-27. The middle meningeal artery (mma) is ligated, the greater superfical petrosal nerve is cut, and the petrous ICA is exposed. The petrous apex, that lies medial to the horizontal segment of the petrous carotid, is drilled. About 15 mm of petrous apex can be safely removed without injuring the cochlea (see millimetric scale). The cancellous bone of the petrous apex ends posterolaterally with the compact bone of the otic capsule that surrounds the membranous cochlea.
lb: labyrinthine block; mc: mandibular condyle; pd: presigmoid dura.

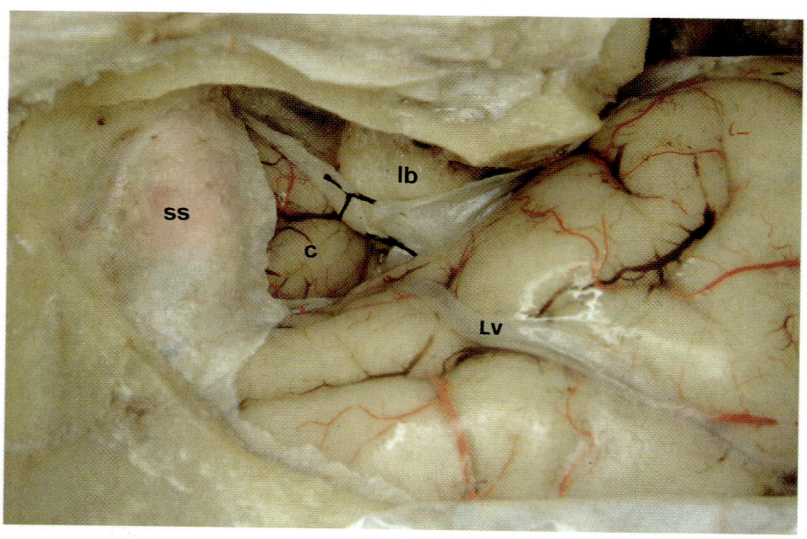

Fig. 40-28. The presigmoid dura and temporal dura are incised separately. The superior petrosal sinus is ligated and divided, and the tentorium is cut from lateral to medial up to the tentorial hiatus posterior to the CN IV. The CN IV must be recognized with gentle cerebellar retraction before completing the tentorial incision.
c: cerebellum; lb: labyrinthine block; Lv: Labbè vein; ss: sigmoid sinus.

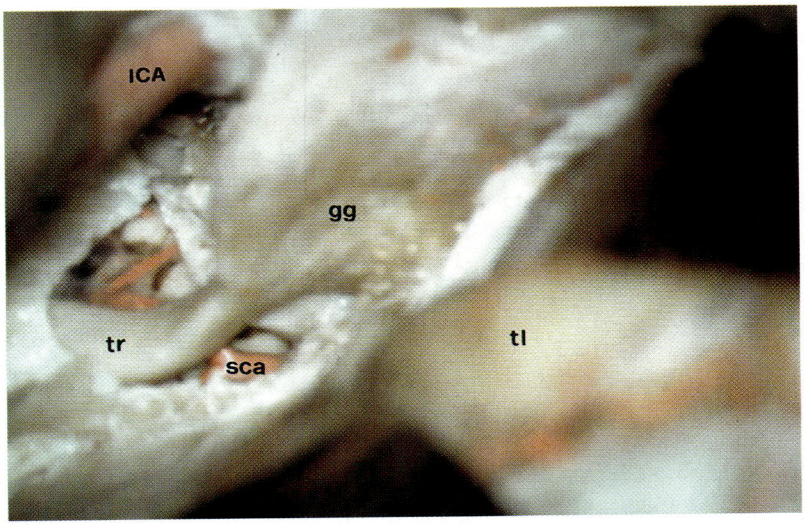

Fig. 40-29. The dura of the petrous apex is incised and the trigeminal root (tr) is dissected. At this stage, care must be taken to avoid injury to the superior cerebellar artery (sca).
gg: gasserian ganglion; tl: temporal lobe.

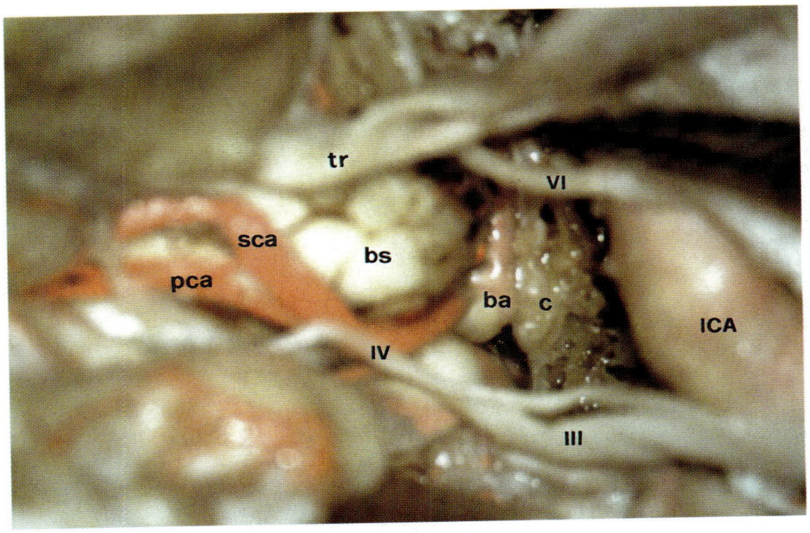

Fig. 40-30. The CN IV is dissected from the tentorial edge and the tentorium is stripped from posterior to anterior portion following the trigeminal root up to the petrous apex. The CNs IV and III are followed in the lateral wall of the CS. The dura of the Dorello's canal is also opened and the CN VI is followed in the posterior CS laterally to the cavernous ICA. The dura of the posterior clinoid is also removed and bone is drilled to expose the basilar artery (ba) with the origin of the superior cerebellar (sca) and posterior cerebral arteries (pca). The anatomical region being exposed is limited anteriorly by the cavernous ICA, posteriorly by the basilar artery, laterally by the trigeminal root (tr), medially and caudally by CN VI, and cranially by CNs III and IV.
bs: brain stem; c: clivus.

Sub-temporal infra-temporal approach

Patel S., Pallini R. (*), Salvinelli F. (#), De La Cruz A. (ç), Wright D.C. (@), Sekhar L.N.(@)
Neuro-Oncology Cranial Base Surgery, Department of Neurological Surgery, Medical University of South Carolina, Charleston, South Carolina, Institutes of (*) Neurosurgery and (#) Otorhinolaryngology, Catholic University Medical School, Rome, Italy, (ç) University of Southern California, St. Vincent Medical Center, LAC/USC University Hospital, Los Angeles, California, and (@) Department of Neurological Surgery, George Washington University Medical Center, Washington, D.C.

The sub-temporal infra-temporal approach provides exposure of the medial temporal fossa, cavernous sinus (CS), and superior orbital fissure with minimal retraction of the temporal lobe. It gives proximal and distal control of the internal carotid artery (ICA) for CS dissection and a lateral access to the clivus.

Indications for this approach are neoplasms of the temporal fossa and infratemporal area with extension to the CS, orbital apex, sphenoid sinus, and petroclival junction. Vascular lesions of the CS possibly requiring vein grafting procedures can also be treated with this approach.

The dissection will be as follows:

A: fronto-temporal craniotomy.

B: orbito-zygomatic osteotomy.

C: removal of the bony floor of the middle cranial fossa and decompression of superior orbital fissure, maxillary nerve (V2), and mandibular nerve (V3).

D: exposure of petrous ICA.

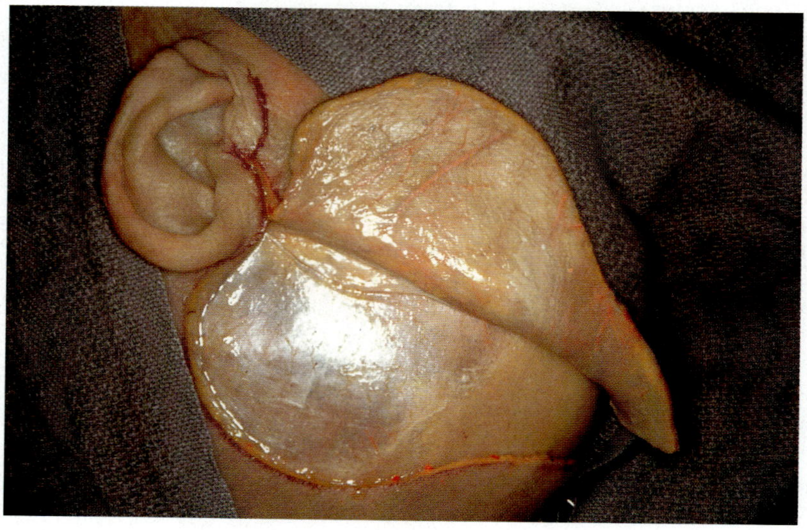

Fig. 40-31. The skin incision is marked in a curvilinear fashion extending from the forehead down to the preauricular area in front of the tragus just below the external auditory canal.

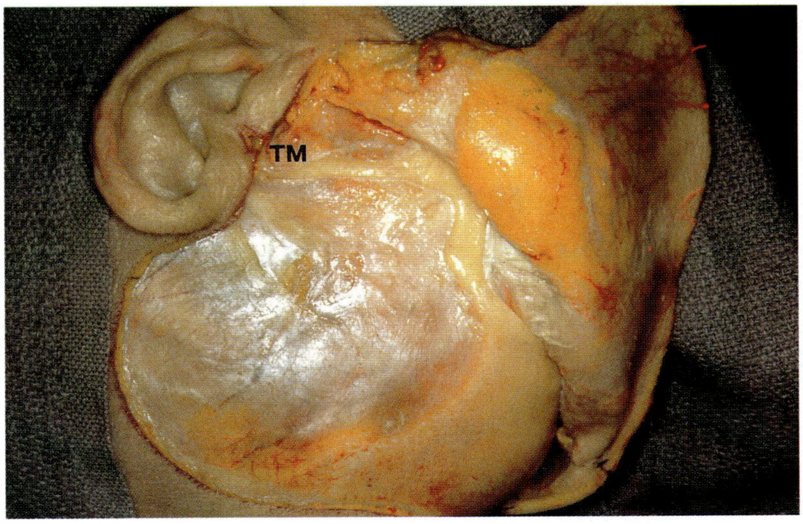

Fig. 40-32. The skin flap is elevated with the pericranium. To avoid damage to the frontal branches of the facial nerve, the superficial temporal fascia is incised down to the fat overlying the deep temporal fascia. The plane between the fat and the deep temporal fascia is dissected to reach the inner aspect of the zygomatic arc. The entire zygoma is then exposed by subperiosteal dissection from the inner aspect of the arc to the roots.
The skin flap is further turned forward along a line joining the supraorbital rim (medial to the supraorbital foramen) and the temporomandibular (TM) joint.

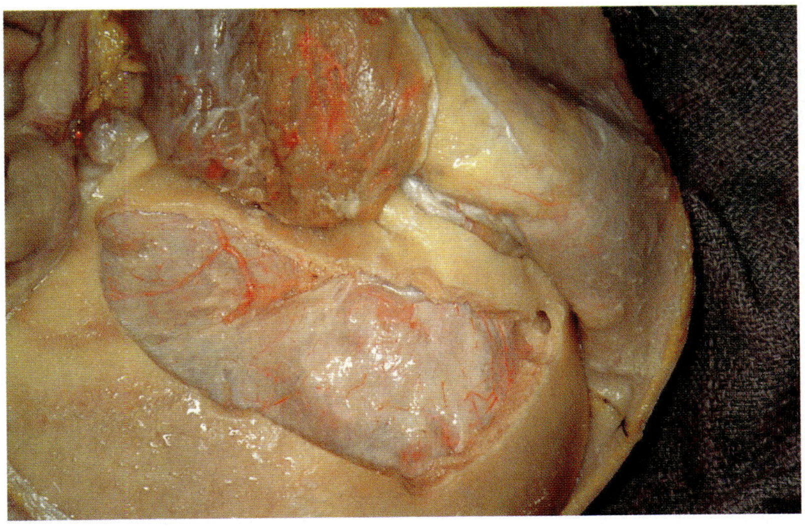

Fig. 40-33. The temporalis muscle with the deep fascia are elevated from the temporal fossa. A standard fronto-temporal craniotomy is then performed.

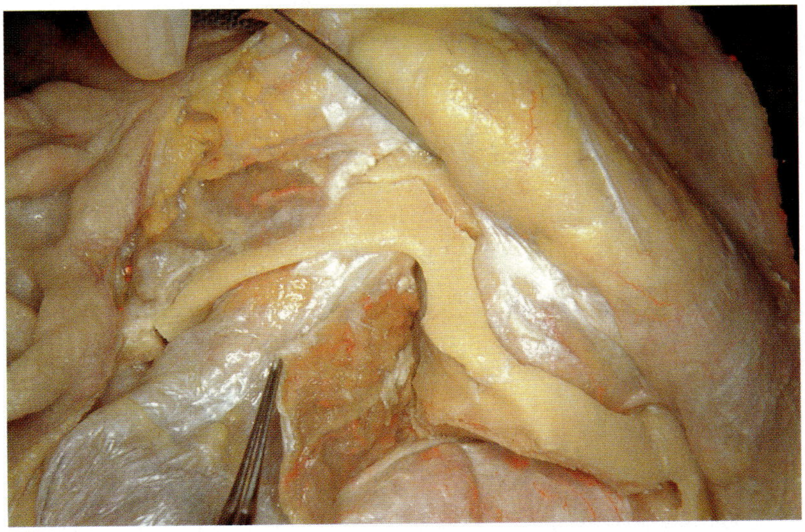

Fig. 40-34. The periosteum is incised and elevated over the lateral orbital wall down to expose the inferior orbital fissure.
The subfrontal dura is elevated from the orbital roof with gentle retraction of the frontal lobe. The periorbita is dissected from the lateral and superior wall of the orbit. To avoid lacerations of the periorbita and escape of orbital fat, it is convenient to start dissection from the lateral wall of the orbit, which is directed straight backwards, and then proceed superomedially.
Osteotomy incisions are made in the frontal bone just laterally to the supraorbital foramen, along the orbital roof 2.5 cm posteriorly to the orbital rim, and along the lateral orbital wall down to the inferior orbital fissure. The zygomatic bone is sawed anteroinferiorly from the inferior orbital fissure upwards without entering the maxillary sinus. The posterior root of the zygoma is cut at the level of the TM joint with two incisions medial and posterior to the glenoid fossa. Before sawing, the capsule of the TM joint is opened and the meniscus is dissected from the condylar fossa and is retracted downwards.

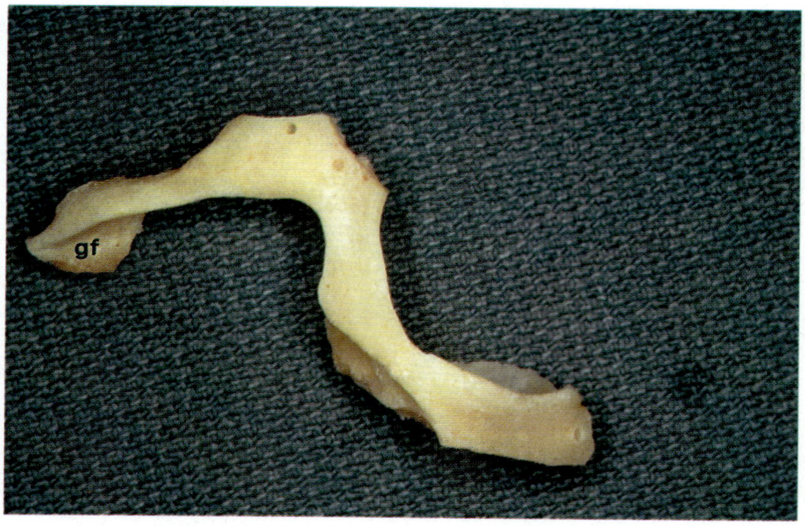

Fig. 40-35. The orbito-zygomatic osteotomy includes the orbital roof, the lateral orbital wall, the zygomatic arch, and the posterior zygomatic root with the glenoid fossa (gf).

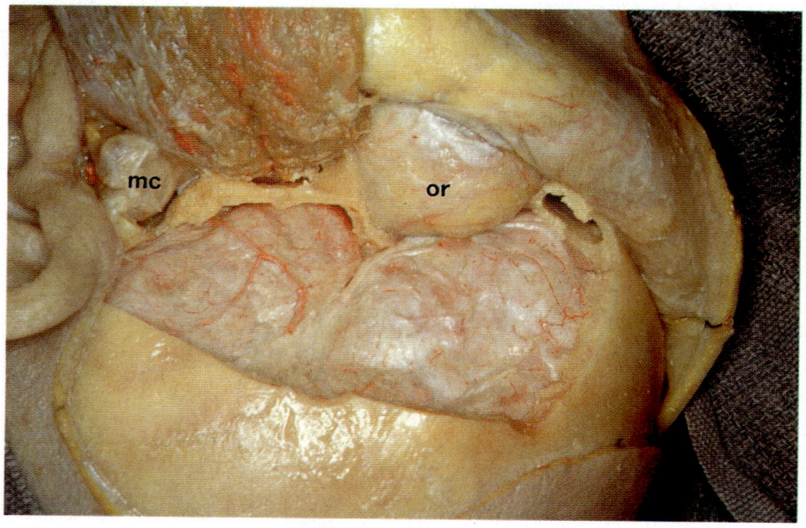

Fig. 40-36. After removal of the orbito-zygomatic osteotomy, the orbital content (or) and the mandibular condyle (mc) are exposed.

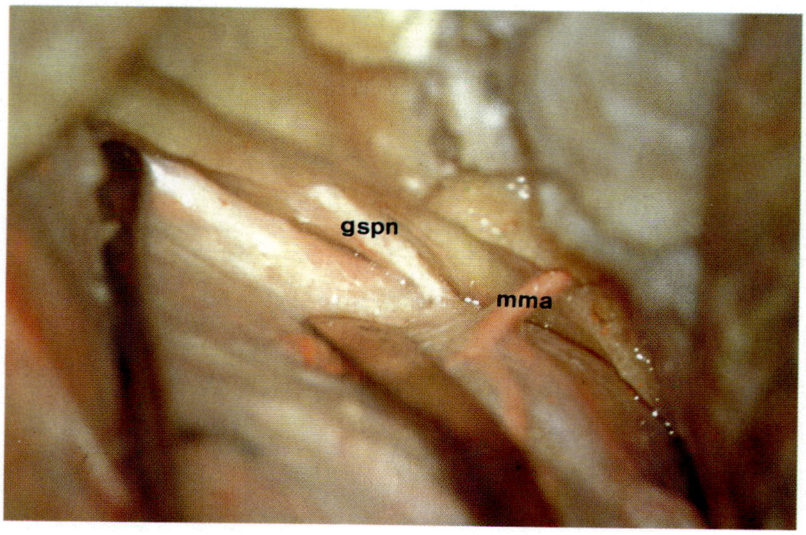

Fig. 40-37. Under the operating microscope, the floor of the middle fossa is rongeured to unroof the superior orbital fissure, the foramen rotundum, and the foramen ovale. The temporal dura is elevated posterior to foramen ovale (V3) exposing the middle meningeal artery (mma), the greater superficial petrosal nerve (gspn), and the arcuate eminence (tip of dissector).

Fig. 40-38. The mma is ligated and cut. The gspn is divided to avoid traction injury to the facial nerve. Bone is drilled medial to the glenoid fossa, anterior to the hiatus fallopi (exit site of GSPN), and the bony eustachian tube (*black thread inside*) and the tensor tympani muscle (*ttm: hold in the hook*) are exposed.

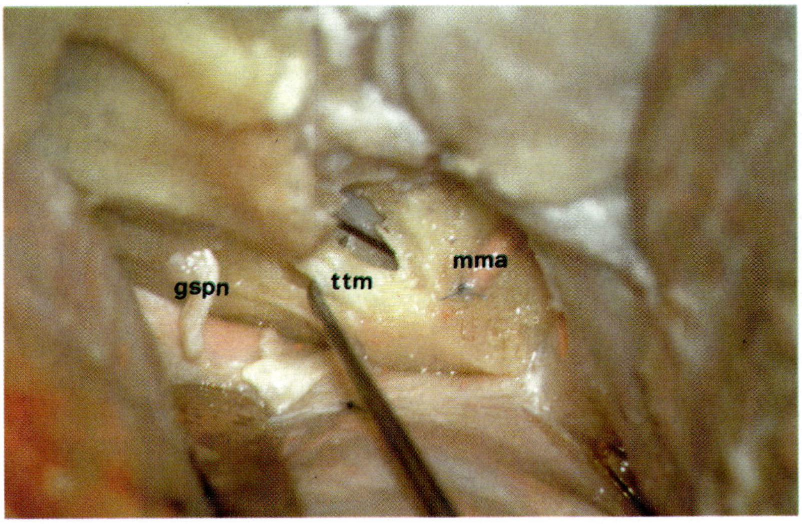

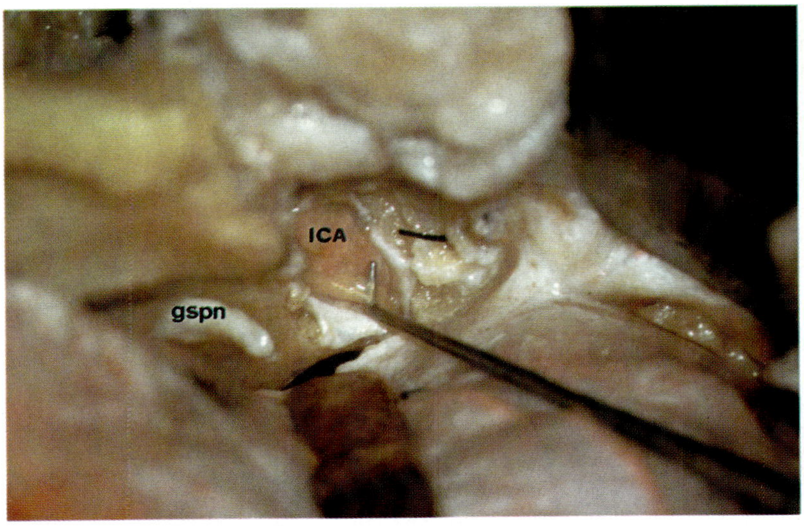

Fig. 40-39. The bony eustachian tube is packed, the cartilagineous segment of the tube is ligated tight, and the tensor tympani muscle is excised. The thin layer of bone medial to the eustachian tube is unroofed to expose the genu of the petrous ICA. The periosteal sheath of the carotid canal is opened showing a sympathetic nerve (held in the hook) from the internal carotid plexus.
gspn: greater superficial petrosal nerve.

Fig. 40-40. The horizontal segment of the petrous ICA is unroofed forward as are the posterior bend and vertical segments. Care must be taken not to drill bone posterior to the genu of the petrous ICA, in order to avoid injury to the cochlea and geniculate ganglion; the hiatus fallopi is a good landmark for this. To expose the entire vertical petrous ICA, the mandibular condyle has to be resected. After dividing the fibrocartilagineous ring at the cervical entrance of the carotid canal, the petrous ICA can be mobilized anteriorly exposing the petrous bone medial to the carotid canal. This can be removed to reach the lateral aspect of the clival bone. The horizontal segment of the petrous ICA can be followed forward to the CS working behind V3.

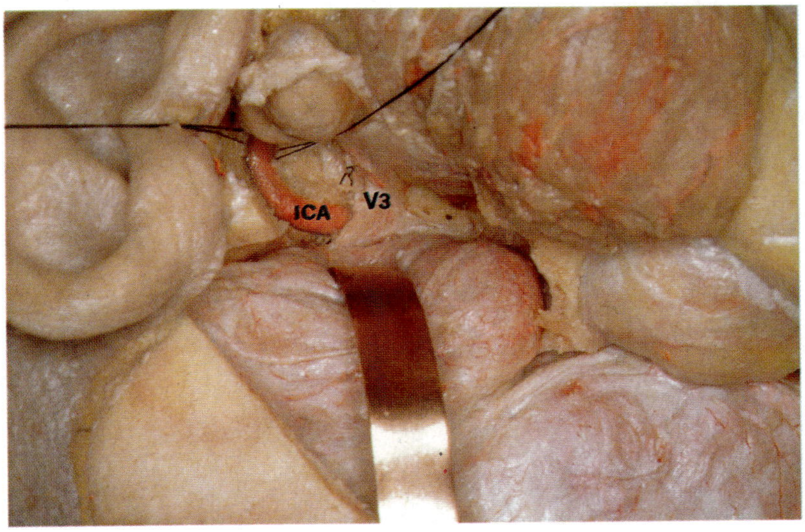

Extreme lateral transcondyle and transjugular approach

Patel S., Pallini R. (*), Salvinelli F. (§), De La Cruz A. (ç), Wright D.C. (#), Sekhar L.N. (#)
Neuro-Oncology Cranial Base Surgery, Department of Neurological Surgery, Medical University of South Carolina, Charleston, South Carolina, (*) Institutes of Neurosurgery and (§) Otorhinolaryngology Catholic University School of Medicine, Rome, Italy, University of Southern California, St. Vincent Medical Center, LAC/USC Medical Center, USC University Hospital, Los Angeles, California, and (#) Department of Neurosurgery, George Washington University Medical Center, Washington, D.C.

The Extreme Lateral Trans-Condylar Approach (ELTC) allows exposure of the ventral aspect of the foramen magnum, lower clivus, and upper cervical spine. Compared with standard approaches, the ELTC approach greatly reduces the need for cerebellar and medullary retraction. Elective *indications* for this approach are chordomas and meningiomas of the lower clivus that lie medial to the vertebral artery (VA) and displace the brainstem dorsally. Paragangliomas, basilar invagination, and vascular lesions of the VA, vertebro-basilar junction, and posterior inferior cerebellar artery (PICA) can also be treated with this approach. For tumors extending in the lower and mid clivus, the ELTC approach can be combined with the presigmoid petrosal approach. Resection of the dorsal third to half of the occipital condyle and lateral mass of C1 does not functionally compromise the atlanto-occipital joint.

The dissection will proceed as follows:

A: muscle dissection and exposure of the VA;

B: suboccipital craniectomy and C1 laminectomy;

C: partial resection of the occipital condyle and mobilization of the VA;

D: dural opening and exposure of the cranial nerves (CNs) XI, XII, X, IX, and PICA.

Fig. 40-41. An inverted J-skin incision is made following the superior occipital line and anterior border of the sternocleidomastoid (scm) muscle down to the transverse process of C2. The greater auricular nerve is dissected and kept for a possible interposition nerve graft repair.

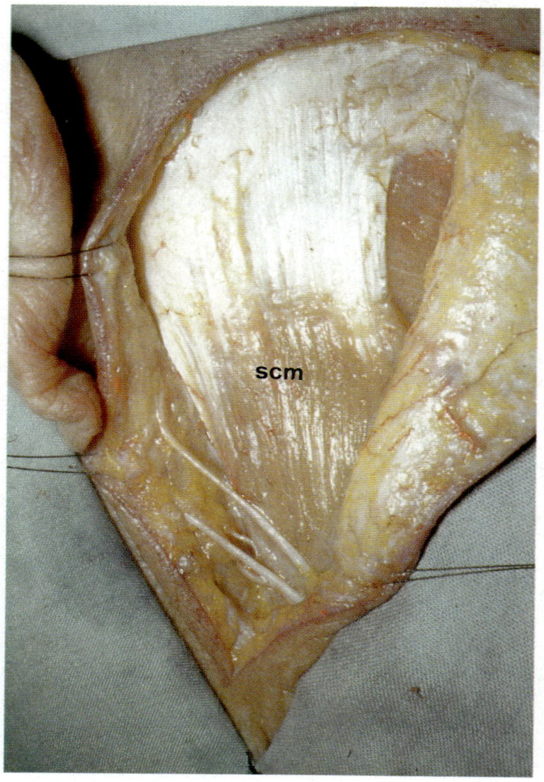

Fig. 40-42. The scm muscle is detached from the mastoid bone and reflected downwards. The splenius capitis (sc) muscle is reflected medially exposing the occipital artery that is prepared for a possible extra-intracranial arterial by-pass. Then, the semispinalis (ss) and longissimus capitis (lc) muscles are detached from the mastoid bone and elevated medially; the digastric (d) muscle is reflected downwards.

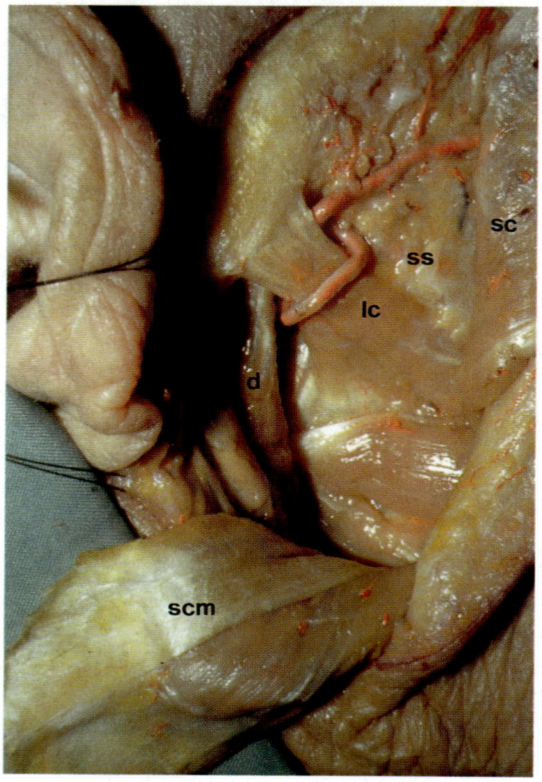

Fig. 40-43. The superior oblique, inferior oblique, and laevator scapulae muscles are detached from the transverse process (tp) of C1 and elevated medially, thus exposing the VA. The VA is prepared in the foramen transversarium of C1 with subperiosteal dissection (a dissector is placed in the foramen). The posterior condylar foramen (pcf) and the C2 root (C2r) are also exposed. Occasionally, muscle branches of the VA have to be ligated.

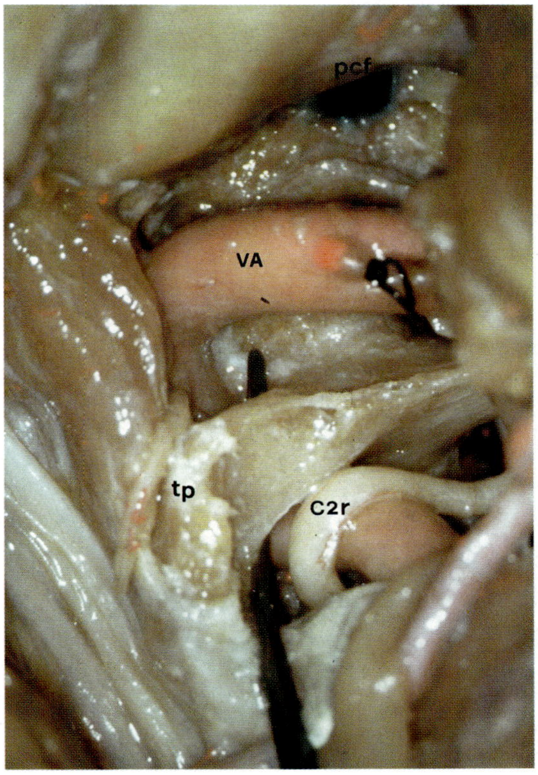

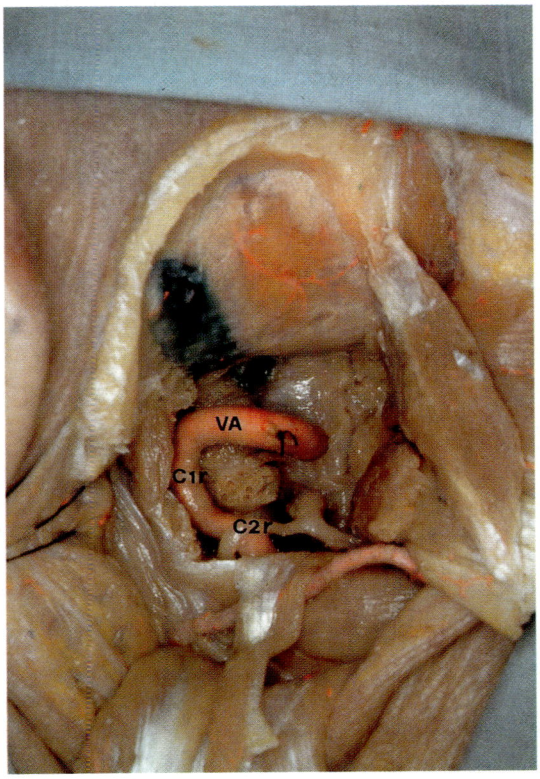

Fig. 40-44. A mastoidectomy unroofing the sigmoid sinus, a retrosigmoid craniectomy extending to the foramen magnum, and a C1 hemilaminectomy are performed. The foramen transversarium of C1 is opened dorsally. C1 root (C1r) is cut to mobilize the VA. Mobilization of the VA caudally to the C2 foramen implies division of the C2 root (C2r).

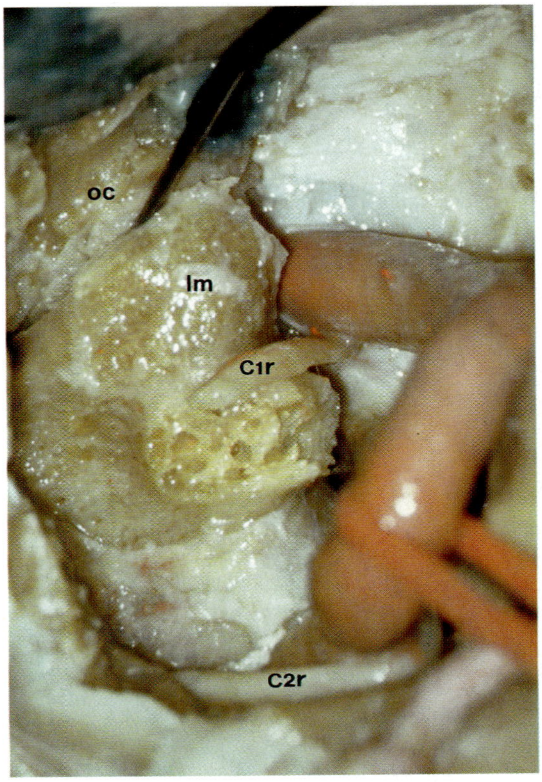

Fig. 40-45. A vessel loop is passed around the VA and the artery is mobilized medially and dorsally. The dorsal aspect of the occipital condyle (oc) and lateral mass (lm) of C1 are exposed. A dissector is placed in the atlo-occipital joint. Note that C1 root (C1r) pierces the dura just caudal to the VA.

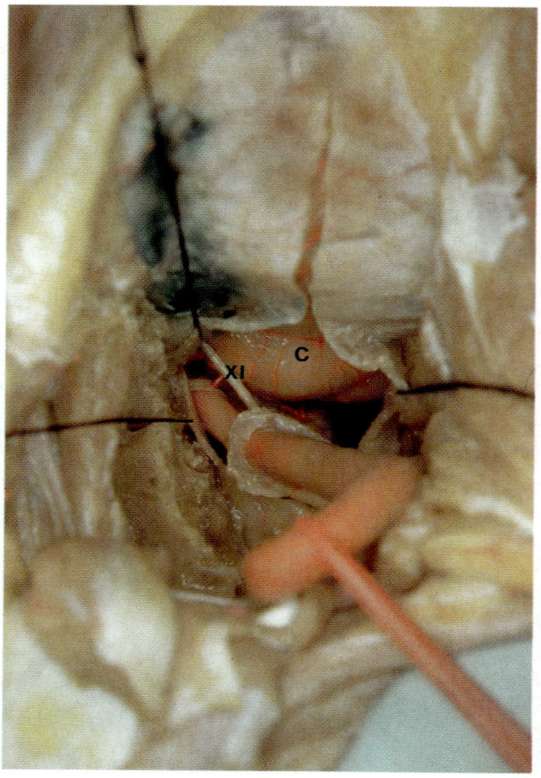

Fig. 40-46. The dorsal third to half of the occipital condyle and lateral mass of C1 are drilled to expose at least 1 cm of dura laterally to the point where the VA pierces the dura. The dura is opened parallel to the sigmoid sinus and all around the VA, leaving a ring of dura for watertight closure. *c: cerebellum; XI: cranial nerve XI.*

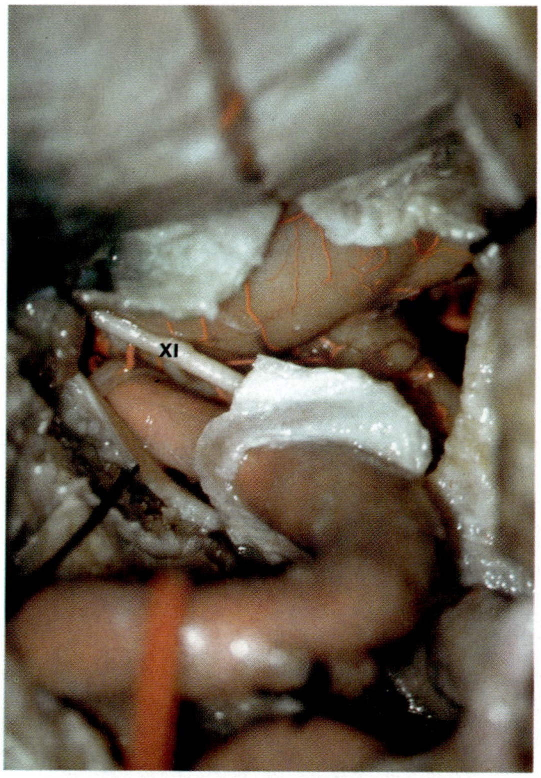

Fig. 40-47. Detail of the dural opening around the VA. Due to the oblique course of the VA, particular care must be taken when cutting the dura laterally to the vessel. The cranial nerve (CN) XI is the first one to come into view.

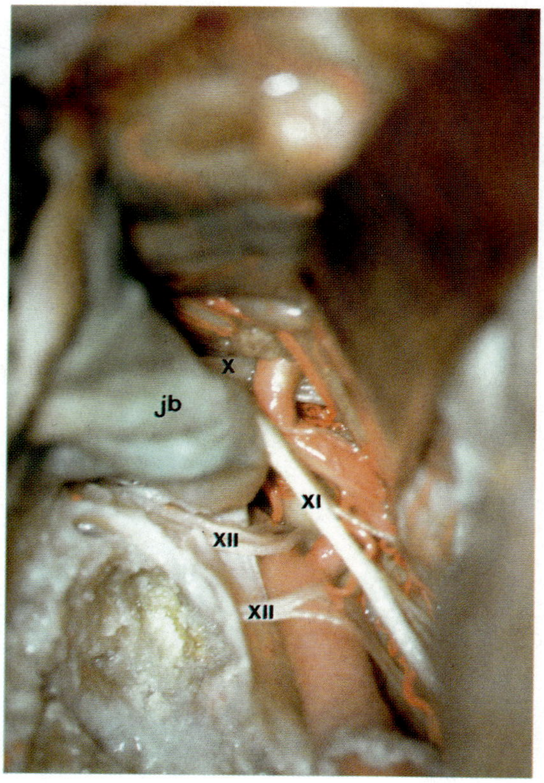

Fig. 40-48. After removal of the dentate ligament and gentle retraction of the cerebellum, the following structures are visualized: the full length of the subdural VA with the origin of the PICA, the CN XI that runs dorsally to the VA, the superior and inferior rootlets of the XII nerve that enter the hypoglossal canal through separate dural leaves, the dura of the jugular bulb (jb), and the CN X entering the jugular foramen.

REFERENCES

EXTENDED FRONTAL APPROACH

Derome PJ: The transbasal approach to tumors invading the base of the skull, in Scmidek HH and Sweet WH (eds): Current techniques in operative neurosurgery. New York: Grune and Stratton, 1977, pp 223-245.

Derome PJ, Guiot G: Surgical approaches to the sphenoidal and clival areas, in Krayenbuhl H (ed): Advances and technical standards in neurosurgery. Wien: Springer-Verlag, Vol 6, 1979, pp 101-136.

Jane JA, Park TS, Pobereskin L, et al: The supraorbital approach: technical note. Neurosurgery 11:537-542, 1982.

Persing JA, Jane JA, Levine PA, et al: The versatile frontal sinus approach to the floor of the anterior cranial fossa. Technical note. J Neurosurg 72:513-516, 1990.

Schramm VL Jr, Myers EN, Maroon JC: Anterior skull base surgery for benign and malignant disease. Laringoscope 89:1077-1091, 1979.

Sekhar LN, Nanda A, Sen CN, Snyderman CN, Janecka IP: The extended frontal approach to tumors of the anterior, middle, and posterior skull base. J Neurosurg 76:198-206, 1992

Smith RR, Klopp CT, Williams JM: Surgical treatment of cancer of the frontal sinus and adjacent areas. Cancer 7:91-994, 1954.

Snyderman CH, Janecka IP, Sekhar LN, et al: Anterior cranial base reconstruction: role of galea and pericranial flaps. Laryngoscope 100:607-614, 1990.

Tessier P, Guiot G, Derome PJ: Orbital hypertelorism. II: Definite treatment of orbital hypertelorism by craniofacial or by extracranial osteotomies. Scand Plast Reconstr Surg 7:39-58, 1973.

Wright DC, Sekhar LN: Cranial base meningiomas, in Salcman M (ed): Current Techniques in Neurosurgery. Philadelphia: Current Medicine, 1993, pp 2.1-2.13.

SUB-TEMPORAL TRANSCAVERNOUS AND TRANS-PETROUS APEX APPROACH

Al-Mefty O, Fox JL, Smith RR: Petrosal approach for petroclival meningiomas. Neurosurgery 22:510-517, 1988.

Bochenek Z, Kukwa A: An extended approach thriugh the middle cranial fossa to the internal auditory meatus and the cerebello-pontine angle. Acta Otolaryngol 80:410-414, 1975.

Fisch U, Mattox D: Microsurgery of the Skull Base. New York, Thieme Medical Publishers, Inc, 1988, pp 22-542.

Hakuba A, Nishimura S, Jang BJ: A combined retroauricular and preauricular transpetrosal-transtentorial approach to clivus meningiomas. Surg Neurol 30:108-116, 1988.

Hitselberger WE, House WF: A combined approach to the cerebello pontine angle. Arch Otolaryngol 84:267-285, 1966.

Javed T, Sekhar LN: Surgical management of clival meningiomas. Acta Neurochir (Suppl) 53:171-182, 1991.

Kawase T, Toaya S, Shiobara R: Transpetrosal approach for aneurysms of the lower basilar artery. J Neurosurg 63:857-861, 1985.

Malis LI: Surgical resection of tumors of the skull base, in Wilkins RH, Rengachary SS (eds): Neurosurgery. New York, McGraw Hill, 1985, vol 1, pp 1011-1021.

Mayberg MR, Symon LD: Meningiomas of the clivus and apical petrous bone. Report of 35 cases. J Neurosurg 65:160-167, 1986.

Miller CG, van Loveren HR, Keller JT, et al: Transpetrosal approach: surgical anatomy and technique. Neurosurgery 33:461-469, 1993.

Nelson R: Temporal Bone Surgical Dissection Manual. Los Angeles, House Ear Institute, 1984, pp 7-73.

Sakakai S, Takeda S, Jang BJ, et al: An extended middle fossa approach combined with a suboccipital craniectomy to the base of the skull in the posterior fossa. Surg Neurol 28:245-252, 1987.

Samii M, Ammirati M: The combined supra-infratentorial presigmoid sinus avenue to the petro-clival region. Surgical technique and clinical applications. Acta Neurochir 95:6-12, 1988.

Samii M, Ammirati M, Mahran A, Bini W, Sepehrnia A: Surgery of petroclival meningiomas: report of 24 cases. Neurosurgery 24:12-17, 1989.

Sekhar LN, Estonillo R: Transtemporal approach to the skull base: An anatomical study. Neurosurgery 19:799-808, 1986.

Sekhar LN, Schramm VL, Jones NF: Subtemporal-preauricular infratemporal fossa approach to large lateral and posterior cranial base neoplasms. J Neurosurg 66:488-499, 1987.

Spetzler RF, Daspit P, Pappas CTE: The combined supra- and infratentorial approach for lesions of the petrous and clival regions: experience with 46 cases. J Neurosurg 76:588-599, 1992.

SUB-TEMPORAL INFRA-TEMPORAL APPROACH

Al-Mefty O, Fox JL: Superolateral orbital exposure and reconstruction. Surg Neurol 23:609-613, 1985.

Al-Mefty O: Supratentorial-pterional approach to skull base lesions. Neurosurgery 21:474-477, 1987.

Al-Mefty O, Smith RR: Surgery of tumors invading the cavernous sinus. Surg Neurol 30:370-381, 1988.

Dolenc VV: A combined epi- and subdural direct approach to carotid-ophthalmic artery aneurisms. J Neurosurg 62:667-672, 1985.

Fujitsu K, Kubawara T: Zygomatic approachfor lesions in the interpeduncular cistern. J Neurosurg 61:340-343, 1985.

Hakuba A, Shu-Shan L, Nishimura S: The orbito-zygomatic infratemporal approach: a new surgical technique. Surg Neurol 26:271-276, 1986.

Hakuba A, Tanaka K, Suzuki T, Nishimura S: A combined orbitozygomatic infratemporal epidural and subdural approach for lesions involving the entire cavernous sinus. J Neurosurg 71:699-704, 1989.

House WF: Middle cranial fossa approach to the petrous pyramid. Report of 50 cases. Arch Otolaryngol 78:460-469, 1963.

House WF, Hitselberger WE, Horn KL: The middle fossa transpetrous approach to the antero-superior cerebello-pontine angle. Am J Otol 7:1-4, 1986.

Jane TA, Park TS, Pobereskin LH, Winn HR, Butler AB: The supraorbital approach: technical note. Neurosurgery 11:537-542, 1982.

Lesoin F, Thomas CE III, Pellerin P, Villette L, Autricque A, Jomin M: An orbital-zygomatic-malar bone flap approach: a technical note. Acta Neurochir 843:154-156, 1986.

Neil-Dwyer G, Shah M, Haskell R, Currie D, Hosseini M: Zygomatic-temporal approach to the basis cranii and basilar artery. Neurosurgery 23:20-22, 1988.

Pellerin P, Lesoin F, Dhellemmes P, Donazzan M, Jomin M: Usefulness of the orbito-frontomalar approach associated with bone reconstruction for fronto-temporo sphenoid meningiomas. Neurosurgery 15: 715-718, 1984.

Pitelli SD, Almeida GGM, Nakagawa EJ, Marchese AJT, Cabral ND: Basilar aneurysm surgery: the sub-temporal approach with section of the zygomatic arch. Neurosurgery 18: 125-128, 1986.

Sekhar LN, Schramm VL, Jones NF, Yonas H, Horton J Latchaw RF, Curtin H: Operative exposure and surgical management of the petrous and upper cervical internal carotid artery. Neurosurgery 19: 967-982, 1986.

Sekhar LN, Schramm VL, Jones NF: Subtemporal-preauricolar infratemporal fossa approach to large lateral and posterior cranial base neoplasm. J Neurosurg 67: 488-499, 1987.

Sekhar LN, Burgess J, Akin O: An anatomical study of the cavernous sinus emphasizing operative approaches and the related vascular and neural reconstruction. Neurosurgery 21:806-816, 1987.

Sekhar LN, Sen CN, Jho HD, Janecka IP: Surgical treatment of intracavernous neoplasms: a four-year experience. Neurosurgery 24:18-30, 1989.

Shiokawa Y, Saito I, Aoki N, Mizutani H: Zygomatic temporo polar approach for basilar artery aneurisms. Neurosurgery 25:793-797, 1989.

Smith RR, Al-Mefty O, Middleton TH: An orbitocranial approach to complex aneurisms of the anterior circulation. Neurosurgery 24:385-391, 1989.

Suzuki T, Tokuno H, Hakuba A: The orbito-zygomatic infratemporal approach (a new surgical technique), in Proceedings of International Symposium on Cavernous Sinus, Ljubljana, Yugoslavia, University Medical Centre, 1986, pp 390-398.

Uttley D, Archer DJ, Marsh HT, Bell BA: Improved access to lesions of the central skull base by mobilization of the zygoma: experience with 54 cases. Neurosurgery 28: 99-104, 1991.

EXTREME LATERAL TRANS-CONDYLE AND TRANSJUGULAR APPROACH

Babu RP, Sekhar LN, Wright DC: Extreme lateral transcondylar approach: technical improvements and lessons learned. J Neurosurg 81:49-59, 1994.

Bertalanffy H, Seeger W: The dorsolateral, suboccipital, transcondylar approach to the lower clivus and anterior portion of the craniocervical junction. Neurosurgery 29:815-821, 1991.

De Oliveira E, Rhoton AL Jr, Peace D: Microsurgical anatomy of the region of the foramen magnum. Surg Neurol 24:293-352, 1985.

George B, Dematons C, Cophignon J: Lateral approach to the anterior portion of the foramen magnum. Application to surgical removal of 14 benign tumors: technical note. Surg Neurol 29:484-490, 1988.

Heros RC: Lateral suboccipital approach for vertebral and vertebrobasilar artery lesions. J Neurosurg 64:559-562, 1986.

Perneczky A: The posterolateral approach to the foramen magnum, in Samii M (ed): Surgery In and Around the Brain Stem and the Third Ventricle. Berlin: Springer-Verlag, 1986, pp 460-466.

Sen CN, Sekhar LN: An extreme lateral approach to intradural lesion of the cervical spine and foramen megnum. Neurosurgery 27:197-204, 1990.

Sen CN, Sekhar LN: Surgical management of anteriorly placed lesions at the craniocervical junction, an alternative approach. Acta Neurochir 108:70-77, 1991.

Spetzler RF, Grahm TW: The far-lateral approach to the inferior clivus and upper cervical region: technical note. Barrow Neurol Inst Q 6(4):35-38, 1990.

Index

N

O

P

U

V

W

Y

Z